D0828469

Health Statistics

Shaping Policy and Practice to Improve the Population's Health

EDITED BY

Daniel J. Friedman

Edward L. Hunter

R. Gibson Parrish II

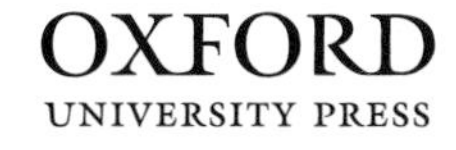

UNIVERSITY PRESS

2005

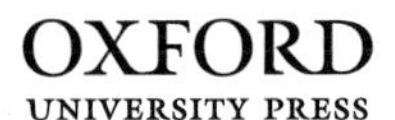

Oxford University Press, Inc., publishes works that further
Oxford University's objective of excellence
In research, scholarship, and education.

Oxford New York
Auckland Cape Town Dar es Salaam Hong Kong Karachi
Kuala Lumpur Madrid Melbourne Mexico City Nairobi
New Delhi Shanghai Taipei Toronto

With offices in
Argentina Austria Brazil Chile Czech Republic France Greece
Guatemala Hungary Italy Japan Poland Portugal Singapore
South Korea Switzerland Thailand Turkey Ukraine Vietnam

Published by Oxford University Press, Inc.
198 Madison Avenue, New York, New York 10016

www.oup.com

Library of Congress Cataloging-in-Publication Data
Health statistics : shaping policy and practice to improve the population's health / edited by
Daniel J. Friedman, Edward L. Hunter, R. Gibson Parrish II.
p. ; cm.
Includes bibliographical references and index.
ISBN-13 978-0-19-514928-9
ISBN 0-19-514928-9
1. Medical statistics. I. Friedman, Daniel J. II. Hunter, Edward L. III. Parrish, R. Gibson II.
[DNLM: 1. Statistics. 2. Data Collection—methods. 3. Health Surveys. WA 950 H43451 2005]
RA407.H443 2005
614.4'2—dc22 2004058315

1 3 5 7 9 8 6 4 2

Printed in the United States of America
on acid-free paper

FOREWORD

In 1998, several leaders in federal statistics met informally at the National Academy of Sciences to discuss the state of health statistics, one of the critical components of the federal statistical portfolio. Two main question were addressed: Are the federal health statistics enterprise and the scientific field of health statistics evolving in a direction to ensure that they will meet tomorrow's challenging health policy and research needs? Is the field of health statistics meeting current needs?

In 1998, our efforts to collect and apply health statistics were falling behind advances in informatics. The concept of the Internet as an *information highway* was already well established—but not in the health field. The National Center for Health Statistics (NCHS), part of the Centers for Disease Control and Prevention (CDC), other parts of CDC, and other components of the health information infrastructure were beginning to consider major changes in the collection and distribution of health information. The concept of a National Health Information Infrastructure, intended to bring the benefits of widespread access to the broad spectrum of health information, was also in its infancy. A few years earlier, during the debate on President Bill Clinton's health-care reform proposal, many recognized that the United States did not have all the data it needed to analyze new organizational forms or to predict the effect of new prevention policies. It was also recognized in many quarters that achieving healthy gains for different population groups (different by race, sex, geographic location, education, income, disability, and other factors) required more information specific to those populations and to a variety of local factors. A more detailed base of information was needed: in particular, the linkages among local, state, and national information needed to be effective.

Out of that 1998 meeting, CDC's NCHS, the National Committee on Vital and Health Statistics (the public advisory body on health information policy to the U.S. Secretary of Health and Human Services), and the U.S. Department of Health and Human Services' (USDHHS) committee on data issues (the USDHHS Data Council) developed an initiative to formulate a shared vision of a future health statistics enterprise. The goal was to formulate not only a vision espoused by these three groups, but one shared by those involved in the development, analysis, and dissemination of information vital to health policy and health research. The vision formulation initiative was, in fact, a series of opportunities for the many different stakeholders interested in health statistics, from users to researchers to policy analysts to data collectors, to voice their opinions and provide guidance on how health statistics could meet the needs of health policy and research and public and private health programs. The initiatives included a series of workshops, hearings, and public processes held across the country.

The initiative's first product was *Shaping a Health Statistics Vision for the 21st Century*, a report that presents the key elements of a shared vision—from a definition of health statistics to a vision of how the health statistics enterprise can operate and link with needs at the national, state, and local levels in both the public and private spheres, as well as development of a conceptual model of the factors that influence health. One of the most insightful, important, and telling conclusions—telling, that is, on the state of our efforts in health statistics—is that while there is formal literature on the constituent fields involved in collecting, compiling, and using health statistics, there is essentially no such literature focused on the health statistics enterprise. With this book that literature gap has been substantially filled. This volume formalizes the enterprise and, by discussing the approaches, data sources, uses, and issues in health statistics, helps give definition to the field and its importance. The hope of the editors (Dan Friedman, Ed Hunter, and Gib Parrish) and authors and, if I can take some license, the hope of those of us present at that meeting in 1998, is that this volume can serve both as a benchmark for participants in the health statistics enterprise and as a tool for attracting and teaching new entrants to the field about its intellectual underpinnings.

A field has come of age when it has a textbook. It is surprising that the field of health statistics, which (to stretch the point a bit) has been around since the biblical book of Numbers or, more to the point, since the early quantitative and epidemiologic work reported herein by Eyler, has not had a textbook of its own. Indeed, the gap is even more surprising given the exponential increase in health literature and the attendant growth of biostatistics, as well as the many issues now in front of us regarding the organization of health care, medical errors, health promotion, and disease prevention.

It is my belief that the careful crafting by the editors and this group of outstanding authors will enhance the academic base of the health statistics enterprise, giving it a formalism that has been lacking. The chapter headings, for example, form an outline for a curriculum in health statistics that focuses not only on epidemiology, but also on the many sources of health information, including administrative records and surveys, the principles underlying what the editors call the *health statistics enterprise*, preservation of confidentiality, dissemination and use of health statistics, and the potential for new mathematical methods.

Moreover, with this volume we are able to identify still more areas that need research and development. For example, an entire course could be devoted to assuring and reporting on data quality. The new opportunities and challenges of the Internet, discussed here in several chapters, is a topic on the cusp of developments that could radically change how we collect administrative information and conduct surveys. It has already radically transformed how we disseminate health statistics.

The delineation of 10 guiding principles for the health statistics enterprise in the joint report on *Shaping a Health Statistics Vision for the 21st Century* is one of the vision initiative's main accomplishments. This volume builds on these principles by calling on a distinguished group of scholars and health-related practitioners to flesh out the principles and offer new ideas to the field.

Enlarging our view of the breadth of health statistics from the collection of data with a more narrow focus on health status to encompass a broader group of factors that affect health and well-being, including functioning, is a major step forward in providing the information that will allow researchers and policymakers to understand more fully the evolution of health and how best to use resources to improve it.

My hope is that with an expanded concept of health statistics we can develop a clearer picture of the forces that cause transitions between health states and, with this knowledge, build models to inform health policy decisions about health well into the future.

Another important contribution of this volume is that it builds on and extends *Shaping a Health Statistics Vision for the 21st Century*'s conceptual model of *influences on the population's health* and suggests areas for future evolution and exploration to help us find ways to meet health's evolving needs. The conceptual model, however, is a static view of influences on health. Among our most challenging needs is to bring to the fore more information on the dynamics of health in the policy and program fields. I am convinced that the models included in *Shaping a Health Statistics Vision for the 21st Century* and in this text can be a significant step forward in helping us to develop this critical information on how health has evolved and will evolve (health state *transition probabilities*) as a function of the multiple influences.

We are indebted to this distinguished group of authors who have drawn on their special expertise in the context of field of health statistics. The authors range from present and former federal officials engaged in the operation and use of health information programs (Cohen, Deering, Fanning, Greenberg, Hunter, Koo, Madans, Parrish, Rothwell, Wingo), to academics (Ash, Detmer, Eyler, Feder, Iezzoni, Shwartz, Starfield, Steen), to state and local officials (Bailey, Corley, Friedman, Hargreaves, Lumpkin, Martin, Oswald), to private sector practitioners (Ketchel, Levitt, Moiduddin, Stoto), to international researchers (Black, Roos, Roos, Virani, Walker, Wolfson, Zelmer). Their broad range of disciplinary backgrounds demonstrates the interdisciplinary, collaborative aspect of the health statistics enterprise. I am particularly gratified to see the rigor they are bringing to this volume.

The health statistics enterprise is one of those elements of the infrastructure to which most of us pay little attention—but it supports a vast weight of policy, practice, and our health. With this volume we are taking a step toward making this important element of the foundation even stronger.

Edward J. Sondik

PREFACE

Health Statistics: Shaping Policy and Practice to Improve the Population's Health is the first book to provide an overview of health statistics and the health statistics enterprise for practitioners and students. It focuses on the development of health statistics and the health statistics enterprise, and explores the current status and future of this enterprise. The volume places health statistics within the conceptual and practical contexts of public and population health.

Although the editors live in the United States, we have strived to provide an international perspective on health statistics. Chapters have been contributed by experts who have worked in Australia, Canada, and the United Kingdom, as well as the United States. Examples from many countries of the uses of health statistics for public health practice, policy, and knowledge creation are incorporated.

The volume begins with three chapters devoted to Defining Health Statistics: Context, History, and Organization. In the first chapter, authored by the editors, we define health statistics and set forth an overarching conceptual framework based on a broad view of population health. In the second chapter, Eyler reveals the rich history of health statistics. Finally, we explain the health statistics enterprise and its components in the third chapter.

The second part focuses on Collecting and Compiling Health Statistics. Overviews are provided of the three data sources that form the core for most health statistics: Koo, Wingo, and Rothwell discuss notifications, registration systems, and registries; Madans and Cohen explain health surveys; and Iezzoni, Shwartz, and Ash address administrative health data. The chapters on those traditional health statistics data sources are complemented by additional chapters on other sources and approaches of increasing importance: health statistics from nonhealth sources by Bailey, Brock, Martin, Corley, Friedman, and Parrish; standards and their uses in health statistics by Greenberg and Parrish; and linking, combining, and disseminating data for understanding the population's health by Black and Roos.

The third part explicates Using Health Statistics. In the initial chapter, Friedman, Parrish, Moiduddin, and Ketchel explore knowledge creation and health statistics. The next chapter, by Feder and Levitt, focuses on health policy and health statistics. In the final chapter, Oswald, Friedman, and Hargreaves explain the multiple uses of health statistics in public health practice.

The chapters in the fourth part deal with Identifying Current and Forthcoming Issues in Health Statistics. Stoto discusses population health monitoring and the use of statistics in tracking community indicators and in summarizing health. Fanning then addresses privacy and confidentiality issues in health statistics. Detmer and Steen delve into the implications of new technologies and the Internet for health statistics. Wolfson reveals the potential for the use of modeling—especially microsimulation modeling—to maximum advantage in health statistics.

The chapters in the last part address Transforming Health Statistics through New Conceptual Frameworks. Zelmer, Virani, and Walker introduce readers to recent international developments in health information. Black, Roos, and Roos emphasize the need for population health-based, integrative approaches to health information and draw on the population-based research registry in Manitoba, Canada, as a central illustration of how this need can be met. Starfield argues for person-oriented rather than disease-oriented data systems, new characterizations of health services reflecting multiple providers and levels of care, and data collection approaches that yield data on systematic disparities in health across populations. Lumpkin and Deering discuss the concepts and development of a National Health Information Infrastructure in the United States, a framework that can facilitate significant advances in statistics for monitoring population health.

As Edward J. Sondik points out in his Foreword, this volume grew out of a national health statistics vision process conducted jointly by the U.S. National Committee on Vital and Health Statistics (NCVHS), the National Center for Health Statistics (NCHS) within the Centers for Disease Control and Prevention (CDC), and the Data Council of the U.S. Department of Health and Human Services (USDHHS). In developing this book, we have drawn on the substantial body of reports and articles developed through the vision process: the final report (Friedman et al. 2002); the commissioned papers (Black et al. 1999; Klerman 1999; Kronick 1999; Zelmer et al. 1999); the summary of the Committee on National Statistics workshop conducted as part of the vision process (Perrin et al. 2001); and testimony provided during vision process public hearings (NCVHS [hp] 21st Century Vision for Health Statistics Vision Documents). Some of the material initially developed through the vision process has been adapted, updated, and expanded upon as chapters in this book (Black et al. 1999; Friedman et al. 2002; Zelmer et al. 1999).

Even more important to us than the written materials produced through the health statistics vision process were the guidance, intellectual support, and encouragement provided by our colleagues: Edward H. Sondik, Director of NCHS; Don E. Detmer and John Lumpkin, NCVHS chairs; Paul Newacheck and Barbara Starfield, original members of the NCVHS workgroup on developing a twenty-first-century vision for health statistics; James Scanlon (USDHHS Office of the Assistant Secretary for Planning and Evaluation); and Marjorie Greenberg, Debbie Jackson, Rob Weinzimer, and Althelia Harris, all of NCHS; and Susan Kanaan, consultant to NCVHS. Bruce B. Cohen, Judy Kaplan, Denise Koo, and

Michael Shwartz provided collegial and extremely helpful reviews at various steps in the development of some of the chapters for this book. Beyond these individuals, the editors are also grateful for the institutional support provided by the Massachusetts Department of Public Health and two components of the CDC (the National Center for Health Statistics and the Epidemiology Program Office).

The contributing chapter authors have been uniformly gracious and generous in sharing their time, expertise, and intellectual energy. Jeffrey W. House, former vice president of Oxford University Press, provided friendship, sage advice, patience, and consistent and always appreciated good humor.

Brookline, Massachusetts D. J. F.
danieljfriedman@verizon.net

National Center for Health Statistics E. L. H.
Centers for Disease Control and Prevention
ehunter@cdc.gov

Peacham, Vermont R. G. P.
gib.parrish@earthlink.net

REFERENCES

Black C, Roos N, Roos L. From health statistics to health information systems: a new path for the 21st century [paper commissioned by the National Committee on Vital and Health Statistics]. Presented at Workshop on Toward a Health Statistics System for the 21st Century; 1999 Nov 4–5; Washington, DC. Washington, DC: National Research Council, Committee on National Statistics [cited 2004 May 25]. Available from: http://www.ncvhs.hhs.gov/hsvision/CP—Black.pdf.

Friedman DJ, Hunter EL, Parrish RG, eds. Shaping a Health Statistics Vision for the 21st Century. Final Report, November 2002. Hyattsville, MD: Centers for Disease Control and Prevention, National Center for Health Statistics; Washington, DC: U.S. Department of Health and Human Services Data Council; National Committee on Vital and Health Statistics; 2002 [cited 2004 Mar 17]. Available from: http://www.ncvhs.hhs.gov/reptrecs.htm.

Klerman LV. The State Children's Health Insurance Program: a case study, with additional material on data needs in the area of child health [paper commissioned by the National Committee on Vital and Health Statistics]. Presented at Workshop on Toward a Health Statistics System for the 21st Century; 1999 Nov 4–5; Washington, DC. Washington, DC: National Research Council, Committee on National Statistics [cited 2004 May 25]. Available from: http://www.ncvhs.hhs.gov/hsvision/CP-klerman.pdf.

Kronick, R. Numbers we need: health statistics and health policy [paper commissioned by the National Committee on Vital and Health Statistics]. Presented at Workshop on Toward a Health Statistics System for the 21st Century; 1999 Nov 4–5; Washington, DC. Washington, DC: National Research Council, Committee on National Statistics [cited 2004 May 25]. Available from: http://www.ncvhs.hhs.gov/hsvision/CP-kronick.pdf.

National Committee on Vital and Health Statistics [homepage on the Internet]. Washington, DC: U.S. Department of Health and Human Services; [updated 2003 Mar 23; cited

2004 May 25]. 21st century vision for health statistics, vision documents. Available from: http://www.ncvhs.hhs.gov/hsvision/visiondocuments.html.

Perrin EB, Kalsbeek WD, Scanlan TM, eds. Toward a health statistics system for the 21st century: summary of a workshop. Washington, DC: National Academy Press; 2001 [cited 2004 Jun 7]. Available from: http://books.nap.edu/catalog/10171.html.

Zelmer J, Virani S, Alvarez R. Recent developments in health information: an international perspective [paper commissioned by the National Committee on Vital and Health Statistics]. Presented at Workshop on Toward a Health Statistics System for the 21st Century; 1999 Nov 4–5; Washington, DC. Washington, DC: National Research Council, Committee on National Statistics [cited 2004 May 25]. Available from: http://www.ncvhs.hhs.gov/hsvision/CP-zelmer.pdf.

CONTENTS

PART V

Transforming Health Statistics Through New Conceptual Frameworks

CONTRIBUTORS

EDITORS

Daniel J. Friedman, Ph.D., is Principal, Population and Public Health Information Services, providing consulting and advisory services in the United States and Canada. He formerly served as Assistant Commissioner of the Bureau of Health Statistics, Research and Evaluation of the Massachusetts Department of Public Health, and chaired the Workgroup to Develop a 21st Century Vision of Health Statistics of the National Committee on Vital and Health Statistics. His work focuses on improving the population and public health information infrastructure, increasing access to population and public health information through e-public health, and models of population health.

Edward L. Hunter, M.A., is Associate Director for Planning, Budget, and Legislation at the National Center for Health Statistics (NCHS). In this capacity, Mr. Hunter is the senior policy and strategy official for the principal national health statistics agency in the United States, and has had leadership roles in data strategy for the U.S. Department of Health and Human Services (USDHHS). Since 2003, Mr. Hunter has also served as Acting Deputy Director of the Centers for Disease Control and Prevention's (CDC) Washington, DC, office, which serves as a liaison between the CDC and the Washington policy community.

R. Gibson Parrish II, M.D., retired in August 2001 from the CDC, where he had worked for 20 years, most recently as a Senior Public Health Scientist with the Epidemiology Program Office. Most of his career at the CDC was spent at the National Center for Environmental Health, where he devoted his time to various environmental problems, public health surveillance, and improving mortality data, often in collaboration with the NCHS. He now focuses on public health projects of interest and enjoying his family and the northeastern Vermont woodlands, where he lives.

CONTRIBUTORS

Arlene S. Ash, Ph.D., is a Research Professor at Boston University's Schools of Medicine (Division of General Internal Medicine) and Public Health (Department of Biostatistics) and a cofounder and Senior Scientist at DxCG, Inc., a company that licenses risk adjustment software. She is an expert in the development and use of risk adjustment methodologies and an experienced user of national research databases, especially for Medicare, where her Diagnostic Cost Group models have been adapted for use in health management organization (HMO) payment. Dr. Ash is a Fellow of AcademyHealth and of the American Statistical Association (ASA) and a recent Past Chair of ASA's Health Policy Statistics Section.

Walter Phillip (Pete) Bailey, M.P.H., is Chief of the Health and Demographics Section, Office of Research and Statistics, South Carolina Budget and Control Board. This office maintains an extensive array of health and human services data systems that are used both as stand-alone systems and as a fully integrated patient/client level warehouse.

Charlyn Black, M.D., Sc.D., is Director of the Centre for Health Services and Policy Research and Professor in the Department of Health Care and Epidemiology at the University of British Columbia (UBC). She came to UBC in 2002 from the University of Manitoba, where she was a founding member and ultimately, Co-Director, of the Manitoba Centre for Health Policy. In her work with the Manitoba Centre, she played a key role in working at the interface between research and policy and in ensuring policy relevance of the Centre's work. Her research interests focus on applications of population-based information systems, uses of administrative data to assess and monitor quality, effectiveness and outcomes of medical care, and the development of data-driven information tools to inform and improve health care delivery. Dr. Black obtained her M.D. from the University of Manitoba and her doctorate in health services research from the Johns Hopkins University.

Steven B. Cohen, Ph.D., is Director, Center for Financing, Access, and Cost Trends at the Agency for Healthcare Research and Quality. He has served as an Associate Professor in the Department of Health Policy and Management at Johns Hopkins University and the Department of Health Services Administration at George Washington University. He is also a Fellow of the ASA.

Elizabeth (Beth) H. Corley, M.A., has devoted her career to the development of health-care use and resources information systems and to the use of these systems for planning, evaluation and research. She has worked extensively in access to care and disparities, profiling treatment process and outcomes of care, creating a fully integrated health and human services statistical data warehouse for South Carolina, estimating supply and demand for the health-care workforce, and analyzing hospital planning for services and for physician recruitment. Retired as Assistant Chief of Health and Demographic Statistics, South Carolina Budget and Control Board, Office of Research and Statistics, she currently serves as a consultant for special projects.

Mary Jo Deering, Ph.D., is Special Expert for Informatics Dissemination and Coordination at the National Cancer Institute (NCI), National Institutes of Health, USDHHS. She works jointly out of the NCI Center for BioInformatics and the NCI Center for Strategic Dissemination. Previously, Dr. Deering was Deputy

Director for eHealth and Management in the USDHHS Office of Disease Prevention and Health Promotion. She is the lead staff for the National Committee on Vital and Health Statistics' National Health Information Infrastructure Work Group. She created the Science Panel on Interactive Communication and Health and developed and managed healthfinder.gov, the federal consumer health information gateway on the Internet that won the prestigious Hammer Award.

Don E. Detmer, M.D., M.A., is Professor Emeritus and Professor of Medical Education in the Department of Health Evaluation Sciences, University of Virginia. He is also Senior Associate of the Judge Institute of Management, University of Cambridge. His recent work focuses on national health information infrastructures, patient information policy, improving the performance of academic health centers, and health-care quality and safety. He is actively involved in a number of national and international health policy organizations. His past research contributions in addition to the above include vascular surgery, sports medicine, and the formal professional education of clinician-executives.

John M. Eyler, Ph.D., is Professor and Director of the Program in the History of Medicine at the University of Minnesota. His research has focused on the history of vital statistics, epidemiology, and public health, particularly in Great Britain. He has published books on William Farr, the Victorian statistician, and on Sir Arthur Newsholme, the epidemiologist and public health official, as well as articles and book chapters on related topics. He is currently studying the history of epidemiological research on influenza.

John P. Fanning, LL.B., recently retired as senior policy analyst in the Office of the Assistant Secretary for Planning and Evaluation of the USDHHS and serves as the Privacy Advocate of the Department. He has been involved in the development of policy for protection of personal information in health and research records since 1973.

Judith Feder, Ph.D., is Professor and Dean of the Georgetown Public Policy Institute. She has spent much of the past 20 years at Georgetown, conducting research on health and long-term care financing. Feder has also held senior government positions as staff director of the congressional Pepper Commission and as USDHHS Principal Deputy Assistant Secretary for Planning and Evaluation in the Clinton administration.

Marjorie S. Greenberg, M.A., is Chief of the Classifications and Public Health Data Standards Staff at the NCHS. She also serves as Executive Secretary to the National Committee on Vital and Health Statistics, which is the external advisory committee to USDHHS on health information policy, and as Head of the WHO Collaborating Center for the Family of International Classifications for North America. Her areas of interest and expertise include health data standardization, uniform health data sets, health classifications, data policy development, and evaluation policy. Ms. Greenberg is a founding member of the Public Health Data Standards Consortium, which represents the interests of public health and health services research in data standards setting processes, and serves as the Consortium's federal representative to the National Uniform Billing Committee.

Margaret B. Hargreaves is currently the Assessment Team Supervisor in the Health Protection Division of Hennepin County's Human Services Department. In this role, she is responsible for the County's population health assessment activities, including population health surveys and other public health planning, research and evaluation activities. Prior to this position, she worked as an evaluator and researcher for Abt Associates, in Cambridge, MA. She is currently a doctoral candidate in Multicultural Health Policy and Evaluation at the Union Institute and University.

Lisa I. Iezzoni, M.D., M.Sc., is Professor of Medicine at Harvard Medical School and Co-Director of Research in the Division of General Medicine and Primary Care, Department of Medicine, at Beth Israel Deaconess Medical Center in Boston. She has published and spoken widely on risk adjustment and disability policy. Dr. Iezzoni is a member of the Institute of Medicine in the National Academy of Sciences and served on the National Committee on Vital and Health Statistics from 1994 to 2001.

Alana E. Ketchel is a research assistant in the Health Survey, Program and Policy Research Department at the National Opinion Research Center (NORC).

Denise Koo, M.D., M.P.H., is currently Director of the Division of Applied Public Health Training in the Epidemiology Program Office at the CDC. Previously at the CDC, she served as Chief of the branch that runs the National Notifiable Diseases Surveillance System, as Director of the Division of Public Health Surveillance and Informatics, and as the Associate Director for Science in the Epidemiology Program Office. Dr. Koo initiated the CDC's public health informatics program and was responsible for CDC-wide implementation of the Health Insurance Portability and Accountability Act Privacy Rule.

Larry Levitt, M.A., is Vice President of the Kaiser Family Foundation, and Editor-in-Chief of kaisernetwork.org, the Foundation's online health policy information service. Before joining the Foundation, Mr. Levitt was a senior manager with The Lewin Group, where he advised public and private sector clients on health policy and financing issues. He previously served as a Senior Health Policy Advisor to the White House and the USDHHS, working on the development of President Clinton's Health Security Act and other health policy initiatives. Prior to that, he served as the Special Assistant for Health Policy with California Insurance Commissioner John Garamendi.

John R. Lumpkin, M.D., M.P.H., is the Senior Vice President and Director of the Health Care Group of the Robert Wood Johnson Foundation. He is responsible for the overall planning, budgeting, staffing, management, and evaluation of all activities of the Health Care Group. He has seen the health and health care system in operation first practicing emergency medicine and teaching medical students and residents at the University of Chciago and Northwestern University. After earning his M.P.H. in 1985, he began caring for the more than 12 million people of Illinois as director from 1991 to 2003 of the Illinois Department of Public Health, an agency with more than 1300 employees in seven regional offices, three laboratories, and locations in Springfield and Chicago. There he oversaw improvements in programs dealing with women's and men's health, information and technology, emergency and bioterrorism preparedness, infectious disease prevention and control, immunization, local health department coverage, and the state's laboratory services.

Jennifer H. Madans, Ph.D., is the Associate Director for Science, NCHS, where she is responsible for the overall planning and development of data collection and analysis programs. Since Dr. Madans joined the Center, she has concentrated her research efforts on data collection methodology, health services research, and chronic disease epidemiology. She has directed two national longitudinal studies (NHANES I Epidemiologic Followup Study and the National Nursing Home Followup Study) as well as the redesign of the National Health Interview Survey questionnaire. She has served as a lecturer in the Departments of Community and Family Medicine and Demography at Georgetown University. She is a Fellow of the ASA.

Amy Brock Martin, Dr.P.H., M.S.P.H., works with the South Carolina Office of Research and Statistics as a project manager to facilitate the use of integrated data systems by public and private entities to evaluate health programs. Previously, she served as Director of Education for a small rural hospital and as the Associate Director of the South Carolina Office of Rural Health, where she managed a cadre of programs aimed at improving the health-care infrastructure of rural communities. Ms. Martin consults as an evaluator on several federally funded projects that address the special health-care needs of mothers, infants, and children.

Adil Moiduddin, M.P.P., is a policy analyst and researcher at the National Opinion Research Center (NORC) at the University of Chicago, where he directs a range of projects relating to public health and health-care delivery and financing. Prior to joining NORC, Mr. Moiduddin served as a research assistant and consultant at The Lewin Group and as a health policy analyst for the Office of the Assistant Secretary for Planning and Evaluation of the USDHHS.

John W. Oswald, Ph.D., is currently the Director of the Center for Health Statistics at the Minnesota Department of Health. In this role, he is responsible for vital statistics, behavioral health surveys, and population health assessment activities in Minnesota. Prior to coming to this position, he worked for 9 years at Health Partners, a large managed care organization in the Twin Cities. He had management responsibilities for strategic planning and public policy and established a newly created research foundation.

Leslie L. Roos, Ph.D., is a Professor in the Department of Community Health Sciences, Faculty of Medicine, University of Manitoba. He was Director of the Population Health Research Repository at the Manitoba Centre for Health Policy from 1990 to 2004. Dr. Roos was a National Health Research Scholar and Scientist for over 20 years. He has been a Fellow of Academy Health and Associate of the Canadian Institute of Advanced Research. Dr. Roos has been named a Highly Cited Investigator by the Institute of Scientific Information. He is particularly interested in building on existing administrative data to create and maintain information-rich environments.

Noralou Roos, Ph.D., is a Professor in the Department of Community Health Sciences, Faculty of Medicine, University of Manitoba. She was founding Director of the Manitoba Centre for Health Policy. Dr. Roos has been an Associate of the Canadian Institute for Advanced Research and holds a Canada Research Chair in Population Health. For 24 years, she was a National Health Scientist supported by the National Health Research and Development Program. She was a member of the Prime Minister's Health Forum, the Medical Research Council, and the Interim Governing Council of the Canadian Institutes for Health Research. Her research interests include the use of administrative data for managing the health-care system and the relationship between health-care use and population health.

Charles J. Rothwell, M.S., M.B.A., is Director of the Division of Vital Statistics (DVS) within the NCHS, which is responsible for the National Vital Statistics System and the National Survey of Family Growth. Before becoming the Director of the DVS, he was an Associate Director of the NCHS, responsible for its information technology and data dissemination activities. Prior to coming to the NCHS, Mr. Rothwell formed and was the Director of the State Center for Health Statistics in North Carolina.

Michael Shwartz, Ph.D., is a Professor of Health Care and Operations Management at the Boston University School of Management. He was the founding director of the Institute for Health Care Policy and Research within the Boston Department of Health and Hospitals. He has done work in disease screening, risk adjustment, health-care costs and outcomes, quality of care, small area variations, substance abuse, and observational studies from large health-care databases.

Barbara Starfield, M.D., M.P.H., is University Distinguished Professor with appointments in the Departments of Health Policy and Management and Pediatrics at the Johns Hopkins University Schools of Public Health and Medicine, and is also Director of the Johns Hopkins University Primary Care Policy Center. Her overriding concerns are the impact of health services on health, especially the contributions of primary care and specialty care on reducing inequities in health. She focuses both on clinical care and on services to populations and the interrelationships between the two. Her major interests are health services research and its translation into health policy. Of particular note are her contributions in the areas of primary care, quality of care, health status assessment (particularly for children), and case-mix assessment and adjustment.

Elaine B. Steen, M.A., is a health policy analyst affiliated with the University of Virginia. Her recent work focuses on organizational performance of academic health centers, the national health information infrastructure, and improving health-care safety and quality. Previously Ms. Steen analyzed health-care use data for employer business coalitions, worked in administration and strategic planning at the University of Virginia Health Sciences Center, and served as a program officer at the Institute of Medicine.

Michael A. Stoto, Ph.D., is currently the Associate Director for Public Health in the RAND Center for Domestic and International Health Security and an Adjunct Professor of Biostatistics at the Harvard School of Public Health. As a professional staff member at the Institute of Medicine, Dr. Stoto edited numerous public health reports. He was also Professor of Epidemiology and Biostatistics at the George Washington University School of Public Health and Health Services, and was the founding director of the Metropolitan Washington Public Health Assessment Center. His research interests include meta-analysis, epidemiologic surveillance, community health assessment, performance measurement, infectious disease and immunization policy, bioterrorism, and public health preparedness.

Shazeen Virani has an undergraduate degree in health information science from the University of Victoria and a master's degree in health administration from the University of Toronto. She has worked for a variety of organizations, including the Canadian Institute for Health Information.

Jennifer Walker is a Ph.D. student in the Department of Community Health Sciences, University of Calgary, Canada. Ms. Walker is supported by a Health Research Studentship from the Alberta Heritage Foundation for Medical Research.

Phyllis A. Wingo, Ph.D., is Chief of the Cancer Surveillance Branch in the Cancer Division at the CDC. Previously, Dr. Wingo was the Director of Surveillance Research at the American Cancer Society and an epidemiologist at the CDC in the Division of Reproductive Health. She was the Principal Investigator for the data coordinating center in the Women's Contraceptive and Reproductive Experiences Study and the Project Director for the Cancer and Steroid Hormone Study. Dr. Wingo has appointments as Adjunct Professor in Epidemiology and in International Health in the Rollins School of Public Health at Emory University.

Michael C. Wolfson, Ph.D., is Assistant Chief Statistician, Analysis and Development, at Statistics Canada. Previously, he held a variety of positions in central agencies including the Treasury Board Secretariat, Department of Finance, Privy Council Office, House of Commons, and Deputy Prime Minister's Office with responsibilities in the areas of program review and evaluation, tax policy, and pension policy. In addition to his federal public service responsibilities, Dr. Wolfson was a Fellow of the Canadian Institute for Advanced Research Program in Population Health from 1988 to 2003. His recent research interests include income distribution, tax/transfer and pension policy analysis, microsimulation approaches to socioeconomic accounting and to evolutionary economic theory, design of health information systems, and analysis of the determinants of health.

Jennifer Zelmer, M.A., is Vice-President, Research and Analysis, at the Canadian Institute for Health Information. Ms. Zelmer is also an adjunct lecturer at the University of Toronto, a research associate at McMaster University, and a member of several health-related advisory committees and boards.

PART I

Defining Health Statistics: Context, History, and Organization

Chapters 1 through 3 lay the foundation for the rest of this book by introducing health statistics and the health statistics enterprise and by providing a thoughtful overview of the history of health statistics. In Chapter 1, Parrish, Friedman, and Hunter start by defining health statistics and delineating their scope. Health statistics are then compared and contrasted with health data, health information, health surveillance, and health informatics. This is followed by a description of the basic uses of health statistics. Next, the authors delineate the scope of health statistics through the presentation of a model of the influences on population health, which includes the environment; genetic and other biological characteristics; health services; community attributes; and the political and cultural contexts. Each of these influences is then described in detail together with one or more examples. The chapter concludes with examples of the use of the model in other chapters in this book.

In Chapter 2, Eyler provides a comprehensive overview of the history of health statistics, starting with the pioneering work of Graunt in London in the seventeenth century on the Bills of Mortality. Eyler then discusses the role of the census of population in various countries in the development of population-based statistics, followed by a description of early mortality statistics in the United States. It was not until the nineteenth century and the work of William Farr, however, that the intellectual basis of modern health statistics was laid. Eyler details Farr's contributions to the systematic collection, analysis, and interpretation of mortality and other data by the General Registrar Office in England, and his contributions to pubic health–based reforms through the application of health statistics to pressing social and health problems of his day. He continues with a discussion of the reporting of illness and the establishment of local health institutions in England. Next, the growth in morbidity statistics in the United States, including a remarkable series of studies by insurance companies of rates of illness in communities, is described. These morbidity studies were followed by numerous studies in the 1930s of health disparities in the United States during the Great Depression and of the accessibility, use, and cost of medical services. These studies, in turn, raised questions about the fairness and adequacy of the American health-care system and impacted discussions of national health policy. Eyler concludes with an account of the creation of the U.S. National Health Survey in 1956 and its influence on contemporary health statistics.

In Chapter 3, Hunter, Friedman, and Parrish describe the current health statistics enterprise in the United States. First, they define it and briefly enumerate its basic activities and the organizations and institutions that it comprises. The authors then list six defining characteristics of the health statistics enterprise, which include focusing on population health, serving the public interest, and striving for scientific objectivity. They introduce the *health statistics cycle*, which describes the steps that must be performed by the health statistics enterprise to meet its goal of providing useful numeric data on the health of the population under its purview. After a detailed description of each of the eight components of the cycle, Hunter, Friedman, and Parrish provide a more thorough account of the major public and private organizations and entities in the health statistics enterprise and their role in maintaining its day-to-day functioning. The authors conclude the chapter with an overview of the major issues and gaps currently confronting the U.S. health statistics enterprise, including such challenges as the lack of timeliness and geographic detail in many of our health statistics and the difficulty in locating, accessing, and using existing data.

CHAPTER 1

Defining Health Statistics and Their Scope

R. Gibson Parrish II, Daniel J. Friedman, and Edward L. Hunter

The collection, interpretation, and use of health statistics have been hampered by a lack of clarity about what is included in *health statistics* and what national health statistics priorities should be now and in the future. This is particularly the case in the United States, where only recently have efforts been made to define these concepts and provide a framework for the setting of priorities (Friedman et al. 2002). Few academic definitions exist, limited mainly to that by John Last in *A Dictionary of Epidemiology* (Last 2001). Providing a definition of health statistics and enumerating the scope of related efforts is important to ongoing discussion of frameworks and priorities, to promoting training and professional development, and to establishing greater cohesion in the national health statistics enterprise (see Chapter 3).

DEFINING HEALTH STATISTICS AND THEIR PURPOSE AND USE

We define health statistics as "numerical data that characterize the health of a population and the influences that affect its health." These influences include the environment; genetic and other biological characteristics; health services; community attributes; and the political and cultural contexts. Health statistics support the study of the interaction of these influences as well as the study of the way specific elements in each of these areas (such as the health services system or environmental exposures) influence the health of populations. Health statistics are used to design, implement, monitor, and evaluate specific health policies and programs. Properly organized and communicated, health statistics enable citizens, policymakers, public health workers, and health-care providers to assess local or national health, mobilize to improve it, and evaluate the success of their efforts.

Defining health statistics is difficult because there are other terms that are sometimes used interchangeably but have other meanings or connotations. For example, the term *health data* is often used to refer both to a single factual observation (such as the age of an individual) *and* to the aggregation of such observations (such as the age distribution of a population). Health statistics, which focuses on populations, is used to refer only to the latter.

Similarly, *health information* is very inclusive and may refer to either raw or analyzed, quantitative or qualitative, observations, records, or other facts on individuals, groups of individuals, or populations. For example, health information refers not only to the age of an individual or to the age distribution of a population, but also to knowledge derived from research on the health effects of aging and to patient-oriented information on how to treat illnesses associated with aging. Although health information includes health statistics, its broad and multiple uses render it overly general.

Another term in common use is *health surveillance.* As applied to health, "surveillance is a continuous and systematic process of collection, analysis, interpretation, and dissemination of descriptive information for monitoring health problems" (Buehler 1998, 435). Surveillance, unlike statistics, can refer to monitoring individuals, as well as groups and populations. Deciding whether an individual, a group, or a population is under surveillance depends on the situation (i.e., the health problem under surveillance) and what would be most useful for the control of the health problem: surveillance should be directed at individuals if individuals are the most appropriate group from which to gather information for monitoring and controlling a health problem; surveillance should be directed at a population if the population is the most appropriate group from which to gather information for monitoring and controlling a health problem. Surveillance can also focus on identification of cases (numerators), where health statistics focuses on placing cases, diseases, and other health events in a population context (numerators and denominators). Surveillance also relies on descriptive information that may not be quantitative in order to provide early signals of emerging health issues, where health statistics rely on quantitative methods.

Public health informatics is another term in increasingly frequent use. It can be defined as "the systematic application of information and computer science and technology to public health practice, research, and learning. Public health informatics is primarily an engineering discipline" (O'Carroll 2002, 5). Public health informatics, then, can be viewed as a set of tools, applications, and skills that are applied to health information, health surveillance, and health statistics (see Fig. 1.1).

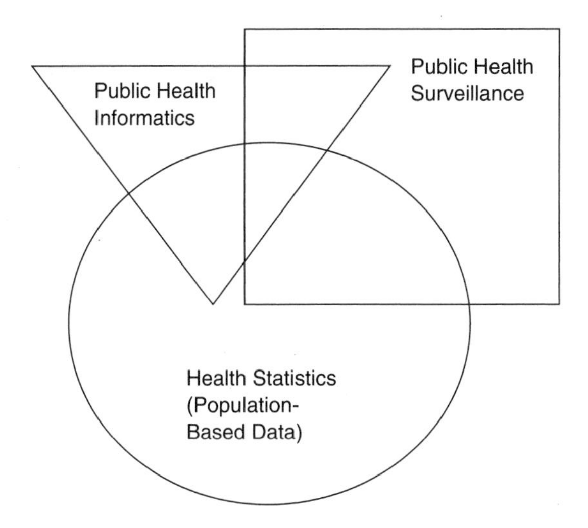

FIGURE 1.1
Relationship of health statistics to health data, health information, and health surveillance.

Health statistics, then, are distinguished by their focus on (*1*) quantification; (*2*) aggregation of data from observations on individuals, their communities, and the context of their communities; and (*3*) population health and the influences on it.

Health statistics provide information about aggregations of people, institutions, organizations, or health events rather than information about an individual person or event. Nevertheless, health statistics are typically created from raw data collected on or from individuals (or from the context in which they live and work). These data may, in turn, be linked with other data at either an individual or aggregate level using geographic, demographic, or other identifiers to construct data on a group of individuals (i.e., a population) and their context. Regardless of whether linkage occurs at the individual or aggregate level, health statistics provide information about populations and subpopulations but never about individuals.

Health statistics are based upon data sets derived from numerous data sources and collected through several different modes of data collection (see Tables 1.1 and 1.2 and Fig. 1.2). Health statistics are drawn from population-based health surveys (such as the Behavioral Risk Factor Surveillance System); surveys of health service institutions and individual health-care providers (such as the National Health Care Survey); administrative data generated through ongoing health service operations (such as Medicaid claims data or statewide hospital discharge data); reportable disease registries (such as state participants in the National Program of Cancer Registries); vital registrations; and other data collection systems not directly focusing on health. Health statistics may be based upon data originally intended to characterize the health of a population and the factors that influence it (such as those collected in the National Health Interview Survey), or they may be based upon data originally intended for other purposes (such as information collected through the Census of Population or

TABLE 1.1
Major Parameters of Health Statistics

Sources of Data	*Methods of Collecting Data*	*Geopolitical Level*	*Time Frame for Collecting Data*
Individual response	Record or transaction review	State or provincial	Continuous
Individual examination	Registration	Regional	Fixed time period (e.g., cohort followed over a 10-year period)
Environmental observations	Notification	National	Periodic
Laboratory measurements	Local		Point-in-time
Clinical observations			
Health-care financial transactions and administrative records			
Survey			

the Environmental Protection Agency's Aerometric Information Retrieval System). The data sets upon which health statistics are based may be collected on a periodic or an ongoing basis.

Some data sets that are sources of health statistics contain information that can be generalized to the entire population, or to a designated population subgroup. These gold standard data sets can also be evaluated for completeness of ascertainment. In practice, because gold standard data sets are not always available or affordable, specific data needs must be evaluated to determine the extent to which needs can be met with levels of completeness and quality less than this gold standard.

Identifying the Purposes of Health Statistics

Health statistics fulfill essential functions for public health, the health services system, and our society. Most basically, health statistics enable understanding of where we stand in terms of health. Health statistics allow individuals to place themselves in a broader context, and allow comparisons of subgroups and a better understanding of society. Through health statistics, we gain a collective understanding of our health, our collective experience with the health services system, and our public health problems and challenges. Health statistics establish a basis for comparisons among population subgroups or geographic areas. Health statistics enable us to look at the distribution of health in the United States, revealing, for example, the existence of health disparities among racial, ethnic, and socioeconomic groups; between Americans with and without substantial functional disabilities; and across rural, suburban, and central city areas. Health statistics document our current and

TABLE 1.2

Influences on the Health of Population, Typical Approaches for Gathering Information on these Influences, and Systems That Gather this Information in the United States at the National, State, and Local Levels

Influence on Health	*Typical Approaches*	*Examples of Systems: National Level*	*Examples of Systems: State Level*	*Examples of Systems: Local Level*
Context				
Natural environment				
Climate and weather (atmosphere)	Weather monitoring stations; satellite data	National Oceanographic and Atmospheric Administration and National Weather Service data files; private companies	National Oceanographic and Atmospheric Administration and National Weather Service data files; private companies	National Oceanographic and Atmospheric Administration and National Weather Service data files; private companies; local television and radio stations
Air quality; water quality; environmental contaminants	Environmental monitoring systems; sentinel surveys and special studies of vectors	Enviornmental Protection Agency: Aerometric Information Retrieval System; STORET	State environmental protection departments; state air quality control boards; state health departments	Local water districts; local sewer districts; local sanitation departments; local air quality monitoring programs; local health departments
Geology; topography; vegetative cover; and water resources	Land surveys; satellite images; aerial photographs	U.S. Geological Survey; U.S. Department of Agriculture; U.S. Environmental Protection Agency	State geology departments; state agriculture departments; state environmental protection departments	Local water districts; local land use planning programs
Animal vectors (biosphere)	Field surveys		State health departments; state agriculture departments	Local health departments; local animal control programs

(*continued*)

TABLE 1.2
Continued

Influence on Health	*Typical Approaches*	*Examples of Systems: National Level*	*Examples of Systems: State Level*	*Examples of Systems: Local Level*
Cultural context				
Norms and values		General Social Survey		
Racism		General Social Survey		
Political context				
Public policies and laws (social, economic, health, environmental)	Compilations and indexes	Thomas—U.S. Congress on the Internet	National Conference of State Legislatures	
Political culture		General Social Survey		
Community Resources				
Biological characteristics				
Population (number, geographic distribution)	Census and periodic population surveys	Decennial census; Current Population Survey	Decennial census; state vital statistics system;	Decennial census
Population (age and sex distribution)	Census and periodic population surveys	Decennial census; Current Population Survey	Decennial census; state vital statistics system;	Decennial census
Biological composition (e.g., genetic endowment, immune status)	Health care records; health examination surveys (e.g., hypertension, immune status)	Human Genome Project; research studies; outbreak investigations; National Health and Nutrition Examination Survey		

Fertility and natality (rate, geographic and demographic distribution, and temporal trends)	Vital registration; health-care records; periodic population or health-care provider surveys; periodic surveys of abortion providers	National Vital Statistics System; Centers for Disease Control and Prevention (CDC) Abortion Surveillance System; National Survey of Family Growth; Alan Guttmacher Institute	State vital statistics system; National Vital Statistics System; CDC Abortion Surveillance System	State vital statistics systems; National Vital Statistics System
Built environment				
Land use (deforestation, farming)	Land surveys; satellite images; aerial photographs; population surveys	U.S. Department of Agriculture; Decennial Census	State agriculture departments	
Urbanization (type, location, and extent) and housing		Department of Housing and Urban Development	Decennial census	Local land use planning programs
Workplaces	Surveys of the U.S. population; business and employer surveys; workplace regulatory inspections	Bureau of Labor Statistics; Occupational Safety and Health Administration; Mine Saftey and Health Administration; Census Bureau	Current Population Survey; County Business Patterns; Census of Industrial Sectors; Census of Agriculture; state labor departments	
Transportation infrastructure	Land surveys; satellite images; aerial photographs	U.S. Department of Transportation	State transportation departments	Local road and highway departments
Communication infrastructure (access to health information)	Surveys of population; government regulatory activities; mandated reporting by private organizations	Federal Communications Commission; Census Bureau; private telecommunication companies	Private telecommunication companies	Private telecommunication companies

(continued)

TABLE 1.2
Continued

Influence on Health	*Typical Approaches*	*Examples of Systems: National Level*	*Examples of Systems: State Level*	*Examples of Systems: Local Level*
Economic factors				
Economic development and equity (e.g., income distribution, employment, access to material resources)	Population surveys; national financial records; World Bank	Department of Commerce; Department of Labor, Bureau of Labor Statistics	State economic development departments	Local chambers of commerce
Work environment	Population surveys; business and employer surveys; workplace regulatory inspections	Bureau of Labor Statistics; Occupational Safety and Health Administration; Census Bureau; National Council on Compensation; National Agricultural Workers Survey	Current Population Survey; County Business Patterns; Census of Industrial Sectors; Census of Agriculture; state labor departments	
Population health programs				
Air quality; water supply and quality; waste disposal	Environmental laws and regulations; specific data collection specific programs during environmental cleanup; mandated reporting of locations of major sources of pollution; research studies of pollutants and their effects; environmental monitoring systems; sentinel surveys and special studies of vectors	Environmental Protection Agency: Aerometric Information Retrieval System and STORET	State environmental protection departments; state air quality control board; state health departments	Local water district; local sewer district; local sanitation department; local air quality monitoring programs; local health departments

Personal health practices				
Prevalence; geographic and demographic distribution	Populations surveys (e.g., behaviors, activities) observations of behavior; health examination surveys (e.g., body fat, nutritional status); qualitative research; behavioral risk factor surveys; exit surveys; focus groups	National Health Interview Survey; Youth Risk Behavior Survey; National Household Survey on Drug Abuse; Monitoring the Future Study; 1999 National Worksite Health Promotion Survey; Mothers' Survey, Abbott Laboratories, Inc., Ross Products Division	State health departments; state education departments; state Behavioral Risk Factor Surveys; Youth Risk Behavior Survey; School Health Policies and Programs Study; State Tobacco Activities Tracking and Evaluation System	Youth Risk Behavior Survey
Health services				
Providing effective health care (number and types of individuals and facilities; geographic distribution; type of care given; number of persons who can be served; use of health-care services)	Government health reports; licensure of health professionals; health facility and health-care provider surveys; populations surveys; studies of health-care quality and access to care; accreditation and licensing of health-care providers and facilities; reporting systems from professional associations; census of local health departments; reporting systems for physicians who treat end-stage renal disease	National Health Care Survey; American Hospital Association nnual Survey of Hospitals; American Medical Association Physician Masterfile; Healthcare Cost and Utilization Project; National Medical Expenditure Survey; Joint Commission on the Accreditation of Health Care Organizations; Clinical Preventive Services Guidelines; National Immunization Survey; National Profile of Local Health Departments; U.S. Renal Data System; American Association of Colleges of Osteopathic Medicine reports on osteopathic medical	National Immunization Survey	National Profile of Local Health Departments; U.S. Renal Data System

(continued)

TABLE 1.2
Continued

Influence on Health	*Typical Approaches*	*Examples of Systems: National Level*	*Examples of Systems: State Level*	*Examples of Systems: Local Level*
		education; American Association of Colleges of Pharmacy enrollment report; American Association of Colleges of Podiatric Medicine reports of colleges of podiatric medicine; American Dental Association surveys of dental educational institutions; Annual Census of Hospitals; Association of American Medical Colleges reports on enrollment; Association of Schools and Colleges of Optometry data on enrollment; Association of Schools of Public Health data on schools of public health; National Health Maintenance Organization Census; National League of Nursing annual survey of schools of nursing		

Population Health				
Disease				
Mortality (number, geographic and demographic distribution, temporal trends, causes) and life expectancy	Vital registration; health-care records; periodic population or health-care provider surveys; verbal autopsy	National Vital Statistics System; Bureau of Labor Statistics; National Institute of Occupational Safety and Health	State vital statistics systems; state medical examiners and coroners; Census of Fatal Occupational Injuries	Local (county) medical examiners and coroners
Morbidity (number, nature and severity, geographic and demographic distribution, temporal trends, causes)	General: registers of visits to health care facilities [1]; electronic health-care records; administrative or financial data derived from health-care records (e.g., insurance claims, data collected by payers from health-care providers in order to process payment for providing health care, and reports required by government or regulatory agencies); population surveys Hospitalizations: hospital records; hospital discharge surveys Ambulatory: health-care provider surveys Specific diseases: disease notifications; reporting of	General: databases maintained by managed care organizations; MEDSTAT research databases and other commercial health-care data sets; national Medicaid data files; Medicare data files Hospitalizations: National Hospital Discharge Survey; national Medicaid data files; Healthcare Cost and Utilization Project; Medical Expenditure Panel Survey Ambulatory: National Ambulatory Medical Care Survey and National Hospital Ambulatory Medical Care Survey Specific diseases: National Notifiable Disease Surveillance System; Drug Abuse Warning Network; National Electronic Injury Surveillance; Annual	General: databases maintained by managed care organizations; MEDSTAT research databases and other commercial health-care data sets; state Medicaid data files; Medicare data files Hospitalizations: state hospital discharge surveys; state Medicaid data files; Healthcare Cost and Utilization Project; Medical Expenditure Panel Survey Specific diseases: National Notifiable Disease Surveillance System; state notifiable disease programs; state cancer registries; state birth defects registries; Drug Abuse Warning Network; National Electronic Injury	General: databases maintained by managed care organizations; MEDSTAT research databases and other commercial health-care data sets; state Medicaid data files; Medicare data files Hospitalizations: state hospital discharge surveys; state Medicaid data files; Healthcare Cost and Utilization Project; Medical Expenditure Panel Survey Specific diseases: state notifiable disease programs; state cancer registries; state birth defects registries; Drug Abuse Warning Network; National Electronic Injury Surveillance

(*continued*)

TABLE 1.2
Continued

Influence on Health	*Typical Approaches*	*Examples of Systems: National Level*	*Examples of Systems: State Level*	*Examples of Systems: Local Level*
	sentinel disease by health-care providers; registries of patients with specific diseases kept by health-care providers or facilities or health agencies; employer surveys (occupational injury and illness records; laboratory reporting)	Survey of Occupational Injuries and Illnesses; HIV/AIDS Surveillance System; National Agricultural Workers Survey	Surveillance	
Function				
	Population surveys (self-reported health status)	National Health Interview Survey; National Health and Nutrition Examination Survey; National Crime Victimization Survey	State behavioral risk factor surveys; State and Local Area Integrated Telephone Survey	State and Local Area Integrated Telephone Survey
Well-being				

1. Type of health-care facility visited is often used as a surrogate for severity.
Source: Adapted from Friedman et al. (2002), Table 1, pp. 72–79.

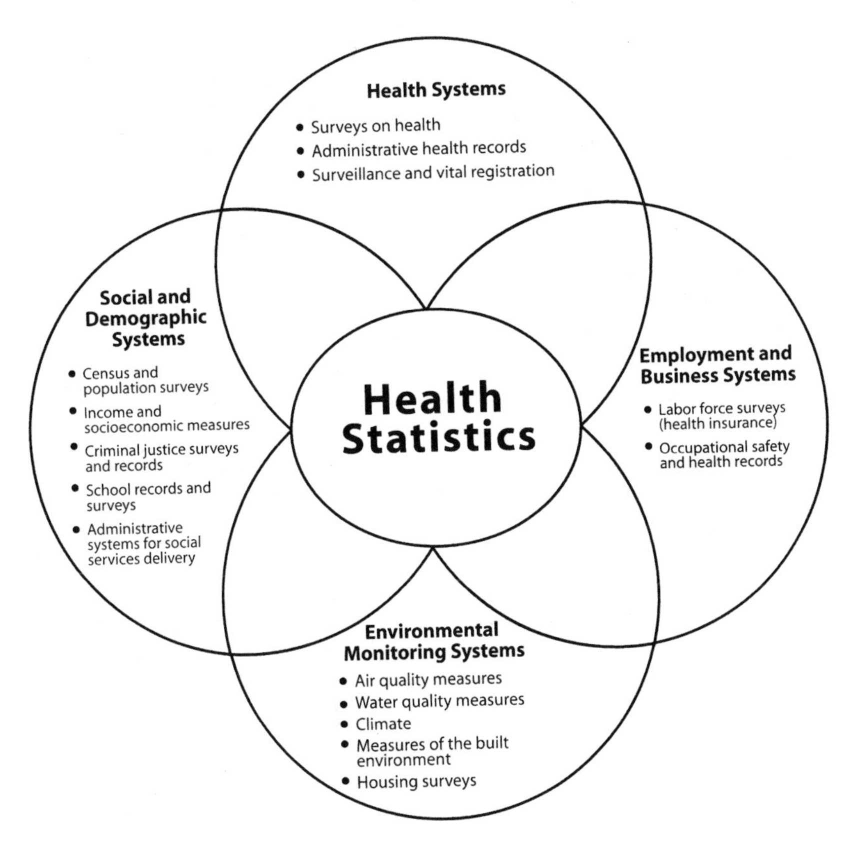

FIGURE 1.2
Health statistics: convergence of multiple systems.

past reality, and provide us with the ability to identify health trends so that we may anticipate future trends in health and health services.

Health statistics provide the information upon which we can base important public decisions at the local, state, and national levels. Once we have made those public decisions, health statistics make us accountable for the decisions that we have made. Health statistics thus enable us to evaluate the impact of health policies and health programs on the public's health. In short, health statistics give us the information we need to improve the population's health and to reduce health disparities.

Uses of Health Statistics

Health statistics have three major uses. The first use is *creating fundamental knowledge about the health of populations, influences on health, and interactions among those influences.* The fundamental knowledge created by health statistics is varied, and can contribute to increasing our understanding of the health-care system and the health of populations; of the influences on well-being, functional status, and disease; of relationships among community resources and health; and of changes in the health of a population and its health care, particularly as major changes are occurring in private markets and federal and state policies.

The second use of health statistics is *developing information to guide health policy development, assessment, and evaluation.* Health statistics help to establish health policy priorities based upon assessment of the health of a population and its health trends, disparities, and needs as well as the quality and efficiency of health services. Health statistics are used to project the impact of alternative policy choices on a population's health and to measure changes associated with policy implementation.

The third use of health statistics is *generating information to guide implementation, targeting, evaluation, and refinement of health programs and other interventions for populations and to guide personal health decisions.* Once policy directions have been established, health statistics are used to design public health programs that implement those policies. Health statistics enable identification and understanding of populations at risk of poor health and targeting of public health programs to those groups most in need of them. Once programs have been implemented, health statistics are used to evaluate them by determining their impact on target groups. Health statistics also enable information to be made available to inform personal decisions about health, helping individuals understand health promotion and disease prevention strategies, the consequences of health risk behaviors, and health-care outcomes associated with personal health-care decisions.

SCOPE OF HEALTH STATISTICS

Many factors influence the health of a population. In order to develop useful health statistics that accurately characterize the health of a population and the influences on its health, it is essential to have a comprehensive and coherent representation or model of these influences. To be comprehensive, this model must take a broad view of the health of populations and the factors that influence their health. Furthermore, it should guide the development, ongoing management, and evaluation of the health statistics enterprise so that the enterprise can provide data that are comprehensive and useful for characterizing health at all geopolitical levels. As Black, Roos, and Roos indicate in Chapter 18, when applied to a population of interest at any geopolitical level for a specific time period, this model can serve to identify gaps in data for the given population. In addition to being used to identify gaps, the model can be applied to a specific health issue (such as lung cancer, homicide, or depression) in order to identify the principal factors influencing it and potential approaches to preventing or ameliorating it.

Figure 1.3 presents a model of the factors that influence health that is based on the work of several authors (e.g., Berkman and Glass 2000; Evans and Stoddart 1994; Lalonde 1974; Starfield 1998; U.S. Department of Health and Human Services 2000) and an extensive consultative process (Friedman et al. 2002). Table 1.2 lists the influences on health from Figure 1.3 and provides examples of sources of data at the U.S. national, state, and local levels on many of these influences. The remainder of this chapter describes this model.

Overview of the Model

The model has three components: (*1*) the context or broad setting in which the population exists and acts, (*2*) factors acting at the community or individual level, and (*3*) measures of a population's health. The model positions a population's health as the central outcome variable (central oval in Figure 1.3). The health of a population is described by measures of disease, functional status, and well-being that reflect both the level and distribution of health in the population.

All variables in this model are either *aggregate* or *ecological.* Aggregate measures represent those community attributes that are derivable from the attributes of individual members of the community, such as the community age structure or the incidence rate for sexually transmitted diseases. Aggregate measures represent either averaged data on behaviors or attributes (such as the mean or median household income or the poverty rate) or a function of the distribution of behaviors or attributes (such as the ratio of the mean or median household income of the lowest fifth in the income distribution to the mean or median household income of the highest fifth). Ecological measures represent those community attributes that are not derivable from the attributes of individual members of the community. Levels of air or water pollutants, public policies, or the structure of health services are examples of ecological variables.

Social attributes, biological characteristics, the built environment, health services, economic factors, population-based health programs, and collective lifestyles and health practices (the major categories in the "community attributes" band immediately surrounding the population health oval in Figure 1.3) are factors that immediately affect the health of a population. Depending upon the specific health issue, these factors may interact in different ways and may influence the population's health in different ways. The built environment, health services, social attributes, and health programs for populations function predominantly as ecological variables in their influences on health. Biological characteristics, individual or family economic resources, and collective lifestyles and health practices function predominantly as aggregate variables.

The natural, cultural, and political contexts (the major categories within the outermost, "context" band in Figure 1.3) are ecological variables that affect both the population's health and the health of individuals.

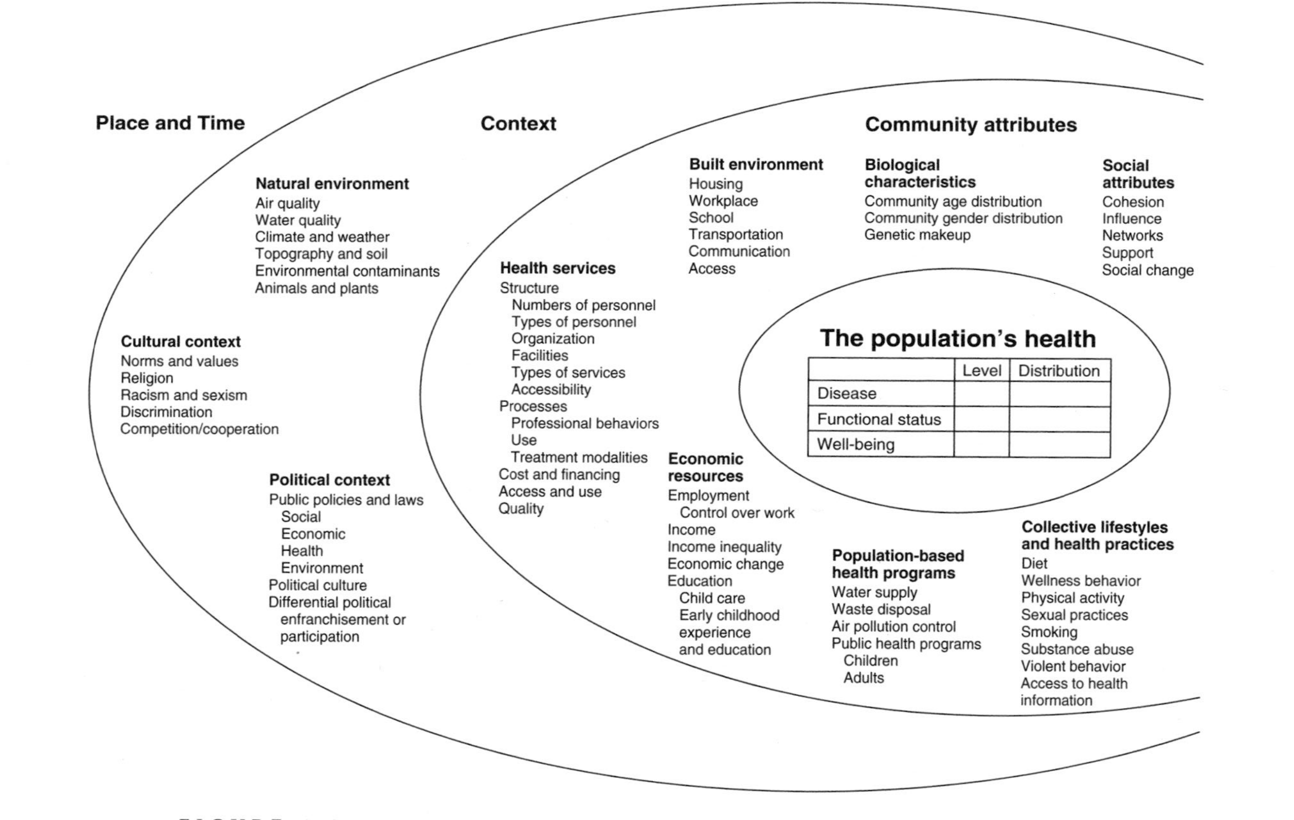

FIGURE 1.3
Influences on the population's health.

Finally, it is important to recognize that the influences portrayed in Figure 1.3 must be used to describe a particular place and time (Hayes 1994; Hayes and Dunn 1998). The configuration of the influences on the population's health will differ from place to place (in other words, from geopolitical area to geopolitical area) and will also differ by the particular time frame (in other words, the year or historic era). The location of a particular population in place and time will determine the specific constellation of contextual influences and community resource influences that most strongly affect the population's health.

The model does not presume causality, directionality, or interactions among its components. As indicated above, the purpose of Figure 1.3 is to provide a picture of the influences on a population's health for use in evaluating the availability of data and gaps in data at the national, state, or local level. A variety of research hypotheses can be developed to test the existence and direction of causality among elements in the model. Similarly, the model does not posit the relative weight or importance of different influences or combinations of influences. It leaves this work to analysts and researchers. The purpose of the health statistics enterprise is to ensure the availability of data to support such analysis and research.

The next three sections of this chapter provide a more detailed description of the elements within each of the three components of the model.

Model Overview—Context

Context consists of three major elements: the natural environment, the cultural context, and the political context. The natural environment has a strong overall influence on the population. Climate, topography, and water resources affect the animals and plants that can live in the area. These, in turn, affect food resources and the size and density of the populations that can be supported. Proximity to waterways, seas, and oceans and topography determine trade routes and the extent of interaction with other peoples (Diamond 1999). All of these influence health. The cultural context refers to the norms and values of a population; these, in turn, affect the level of competition and cooperation both within a population and between the population and other neighboring populations. The presence and extent of advantages held by or discrimination against particular population groups are manifestations of norms and values that can affect the health services use, health practices, and health of these groups.

The political context is the expression of norms and values in the overall political culture of a given population and geopolitical area. A society codifies its norms and values as the public policies and laws that guide the actions of its members. Thus, the political context can significantly shape the society's impact on the natural environment and how the society functions socially and economically. Policies and laws may also determine the availability and nature of health programs for the population and of health services. Finally, the extent to which individuals and groups within the population are enfranchised and participate in the political culture of a society has a strong influence on the responsiveness of the society to their health needs and other needs.

Model Overview—Community Attributes

Community attributes exist within and are determined by their environmental, cultural, and political contexts and the population that shares in these contexts. These attributes include the community's social attributes, biological characteristics of the population, the built environment, health services, economic resources, population-based health programs, and collective lifestyles and health practices of people in the community.

The social attributes of the community consist of the type and extent of social networks, the overall social cohesion of the community, and the support provided by the community or by subpopulations within the community to its members. Discrimination against particular groups within the community may adversely affect the health of these groups by excluding them from important social networks and support. The community's biological characteristics include its age and gender structures, the genetic makeup of its membership (such as the prevalence in the population of genes associated with hemoglobinopathy or hemochromatosis), and the immune status of its membership (such as the level of immunity to measles as a result of widespread childhood vaccination or infection). The community age structure affects the health outcomes of the population; for example, communities with relatively older populations are likely to have a higher prevalence of chronic diseases.

The built environment refers to modifications of the natural environment to support human habitation and activity, such as housing, roads and canals, telecommunications infrastructure, workplaces, and schools. These have a profound influence on the health of the community by determining the level of protection from weather and climate and the ability of the community to interact and trade with other communities. The quality of the physical structures available for schooling and work also influences the nature and quality of these activities. Some of these structures also provide the setting for important familial, community, and other social interactions (e.g., housing, schools, and workplaces).

The economic attributes of the community consist of the overall wealth of the community and its members, the distribution of this wealth, and the type, extent, and stability of employment of its members. As with social attributes, the extent of equity in the distribution of, and access to, economic attributes for individuals and groups is an important influence on community health. Furthermore, the control that members of the community can exercise over their work and economic status can profoundly affect health. Finally, educational opportunities for children and adults, and the level of education of members of the community, are both important influences on, and markers of, the economic and health status of the community. It has been suggested that child development be included as an influence on health (Hertzman 1998). The model in Figure 1.3 views child development as an outcome of influences on health and, therefore, as being a characteristic of the population's health (e.g., a subcategory of functional status). The model attempts to include all of the important influences on child development (e.g., nutrition, early childhood experience and education, and social support).

The cultural and political contexts and the social and economic attributes of a community exert a profound effect on the type, availability, and quality of health services and health programs for populations. The overall effectiveness or quality of health services depends on their structure and capacity (including factors such as the number, type, and training of personnel; the quality and availability of facilities; and the method and level of financing), their processes (organization of the delivery system, professional behaviors, and use), and accessibility. In addition to health services, which are usually delivered on an individual basis, population-based health programs and the provision of health-related information to the community exert important influences on health. Population-based health programs include systems for providing clean drinking water, waste disposal, or vector control and community health promotion and education programs, including those designed to influence personal health practices, such as smoking, sexual practices, and physical exercise.

Collective lifestyles and health practices include diet, wellness behaviors, physical activity, sexual practices and abstinence, smoking, violent behavior, and substance use (Frohlich and Potvin 1999; Frohlich et al. 2001). Collective lifestyles and health practices vary across communities as well as among individual members of those communities, and all of these attributes impact directly upon the population's health.

Model Overview—The Population's Health

The health of a population, the central focus of our model, is assessed using measures of disease, functional status, and well-being. These reflect both the level and distribution of health in a population. Measures of disease include rates of particular diseases within a population and how these rates vary over time, by place, and within subgroups of the population. The International Classification of Diseases provides a framework for undertaking and presenting these measurements (World Health Organization 1992). Functional status refers to the ability of people to engage in the activities of daily living and social life (Starfield 2001). The International Classification of Functioning, Disability and Health presents a framework for assessing function that takes into account the social aspects of functional status and provides a mechanism to document the impact of the social and physical environment on a person's functioning (World Health Organization 2001). The concept of well-being reflects the subjective aspects of health.

Unlike measures of disease and function, the measurement of well-being is less well defined and lacks an internationally agreed-upon framework.

Other chapters in this book illustrate the actual and potential uses of this and other similar models of population health. For example, in Chapter 3, the authors point out that the model is needed to focus the health statistics enterprise on appropriate data needs. In Chapter 7, the model is used to categorize the contents of health statistics derived from nonhealth sources. In Chapter 9, it is employed to demonstrate the importance of linking data sets to understand population health and the influences on it. In Chapter 19, another model of population health is presented and used to emphasize the interrelatedness of health risk factors and the importance of the social and political contexts in determining population health. Finally, Chapter 21 emphasizes the requirement for an overarching conceptual framework for health statistics, based upon a model of population health.

CONCLUSION

This chapter has provided a definition of health statistics, the purpose of health statistics, and an overview of their many uses. It has described the broad scope of health statistics and a model of population health to guide the health statistics enterprise in its goal of providing comprehensive, coherent, and useful data with which populations can create fundamental knowledge, guide their health policies, and implement and refine their health programs and other interventions to improve health. The remainder of this book elaborates upon these themes.

Acknowledgments

Much of the material in this chapter was originally published in Friedman et al. (2002, pp. 1–5, 8–13).

REFERENCES

Berkman L, Glass T. Social integration, social networks, social support, and health. In: Berkman L, Kawachi I, eds. Social Epidemiology. Oxford and New York: Oxford University Press; 2000, pp. 137–173.

Buehler J. Surveillance. In: Rothman K, Greenland S, eds. Modern Epidemiology, 2nd ed. Philadelphia: Lipincott Williams & Wilkins; 1998. pp. 435–457.

Diamond J. Guns, Germs, and Steel: The Fates of Human Societies. New York: W.W. Norton; 1999.

Evans R, Stoddart G. Producing health, consuming health care. In: Evans R, Barer ML, Marmor T, eds. Why Are Some People Healthy and Others Not? New York: Aldine de Gruyter; 1994, pp. 27–64.

Friedman DJ, Hunter EL, Parrish RG, eds. Shaping a Health Statistics Vision for the 21st Century. Final Report, November 2002. Hyattsville, MD: Centers for Disease Control and

Prevention, National Center for Health Statistics; Washington, DC: U.S. Department of Health and Human Services Data Council; National Committee on Vital and Health Statistics; 2002 [cited 2004 Mar 17]. Available from: http://www.ncvhs.hhs.gov/reptrecs.htm.

Frohlich K, Corin E, Potvin L. A theoretical proposal for the relationship between context and disease. Sociol Health Illn 2001:23(6):776–797.

Frohlich K, Potvin L. Collective lifestyles as the target for health promotion. Can J Public Health 1999:90 Suppl 1:S11–S14.

Hayes M. Evidence, determinants of health and population epidemiology: humming the tune, learning the lyrics. In: Hayes M, Foster L, Foster H, eds. The Determinants of Population Health: A Critical Assessment. Victoria, BC: Department of Geography, University of Victoria; 1994.

Hayes M, Dunn J. Population Health in Canada: A Systematic Review. Ottawa: Canadian Policy Research Networks, Inc.; 1998.

Hertzman C. The case for child development as a determinant of health. Can J Public Health 1998:89 (Suppl 1):S14–S19.

Lalonde M. A New Perspective on the Health of Canadians: A Working Document. Ottawa: Government of Canada; 1974.

Last J, ed. A Dictionary of Epidemiology, 4th ed. Oxford and New York: Oxford University Press; 2001.

O'Carroll PW. Introduction to public health informatics. In: O'Carroll PW, Yasnoff WA, Ward ME, Ripp LH, Martin EL, eds. Public Health Informatics and Information Systems. New York: Springer-Verlag; 2002, pp. 1–15.

Starfield B. Primary Care: Balancing Health Needs, Services, and Technology. Oxford and New York: Oxford University Press; 1998.

Starfield B. Basic concepts in population health and health care. J Epidemiol Community Health 2001;55(7):452–454.

U.S. Department of Health and Human Services. Healthy People 2010: Understanding and Improving Health. Washington, DC: U.S. Department of Health and Human Services; 2000.

World Health Organization. International Statistical Classification of Diseases and Related Health Problems, 1989 Revision. Geneva: World Health Organization; 1992.

World Health Organization. International Classification of Functioning, Disability, and Health. Geneva: World Health Organization; 2001.

CHAPTER 2

Health Statistics in Historical Perspective

John M. Eyler

The health statistics of the twentieth-first century are eminently evolutionary products. Knowing something of the evolutionary process helps us understand the nature of the data, the measures, and the expectations of health statistics in use today. In this context, the most simple-sounding questions can be the most meaningful. Should we collect information on the health of individuals at all? What information should we collect? And having amassed this information, what sense can we possibly make of it? These questions are as much political as technical. Realizing that fact is a key to understanding why the collection and use of health statistics are sometimes so controversial.

THE FIRST SYSTEMATIC POPULATION STATISTICS

Like most human activities, compiling health statistics has deep roots in our past. Ancient empires, including the Roman Empire, occasionally conducted censuses of their populations, and several nation-states of the sixteenth and seventeenth centuries tried to do the same. At certain times and places, both Catholic and Protestant clergy were required to keep records of marriages, baptisms, and burials in their parishes. These parish records were occasionally mined in the eighteenth century for information about population (Glass 1973, 11–77). Finally, beginning in the sixteenth century, there existed in certain cities, most famously London, a primitive system of disease surveillance. These Bills of Mortality consisted of published weekly lists of deaths and causes of death prepared by the Company of Parish Clerks, and they were sold to subscribers who wished to have early warning of outbreaks of disease, especially plague. By 1662 the Bills of Mortality and the parish records had been subjected to numerical analysis by the London haberdasher John Graunt, who demonstrated the remarkable fact that these seemingly individual vital events revealed in the aggregate consistent patterns (Graunt 1662).

Given these early data and the example of Graunt's research, we might be tempted to date the beginning of modern health statistics from the 1660s. Nothing could be further from the truth. In the first place, the data were not nearly as adequate as the description I have just given might suggest, and there was little prospect of improving their quality without fundamental institutional change. The causes of death listed in the Bills of Mortality were known to be inaccurate, even fanciful or deliberately falsified. Although a nation with a small, stable, and religiously homogeneous population like Sweden might compile complete and relatively accurate parish records, in England the parish records, which recorded only events in the Church of England, became increasingly inadequate as religious dissent grew in the eighteenth century. Furthermore, these records remained in isolated parishes, with all the problems of access and preservation that this condition suggests. Finally, census enumerations were rare, inaccurate, and unpublished. These problems of inaccuracy, incompleteness, and nonavailability might have been surmounted two centuries earlier had there been sufficient intellectual interest in problems of population and public health, and had there been a political consensus on the desirability for doing so. But before the nineteenth century, both were lacking (Glass 1973, 12–16).

Consider the example of the census, the most basic source of information on population and the source for the denominator for mortality and morbidity statistics. A nation unable or unwilling to conduct an accurate census is unlikely to produce any meaningful health statistics. A recent historical study yielded an estimate that at the end of the seventeenth century there were probably fewer than 100 men in England who can be said to have thought in numerical or quantitative terms and, even among these few, interest in the size of the population was slight; in fact, there was as yet no word in English for population (Cohen 1982, 39). The taking of a census was traditionally a means kings and emperors used to assess taxes and to raise armies. Being numbered in these circumstances carried distinct disadvantages to individuals. In addition, a census might be used as a way to encourage religious conformity or particular behavior, as when ecclesiastical authorities conducted local enumerations and gathered information on religious observance or illegitimacy (Arosenius 1918, 537–538; Cohen 1982, 36–37). The words *census* and *censor* have a common root and a shared history. Not surprisingly, although several nations succeeded in taking an occasional census during the eighteenth century, doing so frequently encountered resistance, sometimes outright rebellion (Buck 1982, 32–35; Cohen 1982, 35; Faure 1918, 257–258; Glass 1973, 12–13; Starr 1986, 10–13). Furthermore, the results of these early censuses were usually treated as state secrets and went unpublished. When bills to take a regular census were introduced in the English Parliament in 1753 and

1758, they were successfully opposed by defenders of liberty and property, one of whom promised "the discipline of the horse pond" for any official who came inquiring about the "number or the circumstances" of his family (Glass 1973, 20). These opponents saw a census as an unwelcome extension of royal authority. This political climate also contributed to the decline of political arithmetic. Political arithmeticians such as John Graunt, William Petty, and Samuel Gregory conceived of their research as a way to assist the monarch in managing his kingdom, a project with little appeal in eighteenth-century England, where the Whig establishment and dissenting merchant and manufacturing classes opposed the expansion of Crown authority. Clearly, major political change was necessary before accurate and complete data on the health of the population or even on its size could be collected and before the study of this information was deemed to be a project worthy of public support (Buck 1982, 35–45).

POLITICAL LEGITIMACY OF PUBLIC STATISTICS

History demonstrates that political legitimacy is a prerequisite for the collection of accurate and complete public statistics. The absolute monarchies of the seventeenth and eighteenth centuries and the totalitarian states of the twentieth century both failed to win the necessary cooperation of their populations. This need for political legitimacy helps to explain why reasonably full, complete, and accurate statistics of the health of populations were first collected in the young liberal democracies of the late eighteenth and early nineteenth centuries. Here for the first time, the needs of the state did not conflict with the individual interests of the people.

The Census in the United States

In 1790 the United States became the first modern nation to initiate and publish regular, periodic censuses of its entire population. The census was essential to the legitimacy of the new government and was required by the Constitution to reapportion the lower chamber of Congress. Its requirement was part of a delicate process the framers of the Constitution used to balance the interests in civil society. There was thus every incentive to be counted, because it increased one's political clout. James Madison hoped that this provision would encourage accurate returns and serve as a counterweight to the second purpose of the census: to apportion taxes among the states (Starr 1986, 16). This political purpose helps to explain the early appearance of the U.S. census, but it also accounts for the limited nature of the early U.S. censuses (Anderson 1988, 1991). The first four censuses were ad hoc enterprises, loosely supervised by the Secretary of State and consisting of only six questions narrowly conceived for the purpose of reapportionment. Census information was not collected on an individual level until the

Census of 1850, which was also the first to be planned by statistical advisors, and to employ a central processing office in Washington, DC. It was a long time before the census-taking apparatus was considered important enough to be made permanent. The Census Bureau was not made a permanent federal agency until 1902.

Early Mortality Statistics in the United States

While the United States collected and published basic information on its population before other modern nations, it was slow to collect information on deaths and causes of death. Given the federal nature of American government and the fact that information on births and deaths was not a constitutional necessity, information on deaths, if it was to be collected at all, would be collected by the states. In 1842 Massachusetts, which had passed, although seldom enforced, registration statutes in the colonial period, became the first state to require the registration of births and deaths (Blake 1955, 46, 57; Gutman 1958, 374–381). Expansion at the state level eventually was encouraged by the federal government, which created a registration area for death in 1880. At the time of its creation only two states, the District of Columbia, and several cities had records considered accurate and complete enough to be included. By 1900 the Census Bureau proposed standardized birth and death certificates, and in 1902 it was given authority to develop the registration area and to publish reports on the vital statistics for that area. The first of its annual reports on mortality appeared in 1906 and covered the period 1900–1904 (U.S. Department of Commerce and Labor 1906). It was not until 1933, however, that the entire nation was in the registration area (Cassedy 1965; 1984, 194–204; Krieger and Fee 1996, 393–394). In the United States, the Census Bureau continued to be responsible for the nation's mortality statistics until 1946, when responsibility was transferred to the Public Health Service.

NINETEENTH-CENTURY FRANCE: STATISTICAL EXPERTISE WITHOUT A SOCIETAL MANDATE OR SUPPORT

While European nations were slower to begin collecting information on their populations, they developed health statistics faster and more fully than the United States. The crucial changes occurred in the 1820s and 1830s in response to the troubling social problems produced by the Industrial Revolution. Developments in Britain and France took different paths and provide instructive contrasts. France was the world leader in mathematical statistics, numbering among its savants Laplace and Fourrier, and it had in Phillippe Pinel and Pierre Louis early and influential proponents of the numerical method in medicine (Matthews 1995, 8–38; Rosen 1955, 34–39, 42–44). It also had a tradition of strong central government committed to directing the development of the French economy and institutions. But despite an early start in the collection of statistics, France failed to provide the stable and continuous institutional framework that would have enabled the proponents of the statistical study of health and welfare to build a robust system like the one that developed in England. In 1800 as part of Napoleon's wartime mobilization of the national economy, France created a central statistical office in Paris, Statistique Générale de la France (SGF), which produced the first published census of France in 1801 (Coleman 1982, 139–141; Desrosières 1991, 517–518). The SGF did not survive Napoleon's fall, however, and the collection of national social statistics, including the census, stopped under the Restoration government. The SGF was not revived until 1833, and this time it was modeled on the English Board of Trade. Under the revived SGF the census was taken again, this time every 5 years beginning in 1836. A similar pattern of an early beginning with a long hiatus before a national system of data gathering appeared occurred with the registration of causes of death. As early as 1802, doctors in Paris were asked to state the cause of death on printed forms, but this practice was not extended to the rest of France until 1885, and then only to towns of 5000 or more people. The inability to collect adequate data was not the only problem with French health statistics in the nineteenth century. More important were the priorities of its central statistical agency. Throughout the nineteenth century the SGF was in the Ministry of Commerce, and it placed a much lower priority on the study of health than did the statistical agencies of other European nations (Desrosières 1991, 529, 530). Clearly, in France the strong intellectual interest in statistics was insufficient to ensure the development of a strong national system of health statistics in the absence of a favorable political and administrative environment.

On the local level, however, committed investigators with the support of sympathetic civil servants produced some of the earliest analytical studies of mortality and morbidity. During the 1820s and 1830s, Louis René Villermé and fellow contributors to the *Annales d'hygiène publique et de medicine légale* produced a series of remarkable studies of the health and social condition of French workers and their families. These early investigators were able to use statistics, including several censuses taken by direct enumeration, for the city of Paris, collected by the Department of the Seine (Coleman 1982, 141–148). They supplemented these local statistics with personal investigations of prisons, workshops, and factories. These studies were clearly inspired by growing anxieties about the effects of industrialization on the French working class. Villermé and his colleagues documented the poverty, misery, and poor health of working-class families and generated series of differential mortality rates by locality, occupation, and income. These early investigators struggled to reconcile their faith in the market and the new industrial order with the evidence they found of the misery and early death among industrial workers. They never succeeded, and their commitment to political economy kept them from recommending any regulation of the free market or of working conditions (Coleman 1982, 271–276). Their efforts also were not extended to the nation, nor were they sustained. It was in Britain, not France, that the most effective and sustained work in health statistics was undertaken in the nineteenth century. Methods and conventions developed there would become world standards by the end of the century.

VICTORIAN ENGLAND AND THE BUILDING OF MORTALITY STATISTICS

"It was the business of the thirties to transfer the treatment of affairs from a polemical to a statistical basis, from Humbug to Humdrum" (Young 1963, 32). In the 1830s, major political and administrative reform in England, following the enfranchisement of the middle classes, coincided with a momentary popular enthusiasm for statistics, which drew most of its adherents from the same commercial, manufacturing, and professional classes that were making their influence felt in the reform of government. The activists were appalled by the ignorance, inefficiency, and incompetence of the government that had heretofore excluded them, and they longed to bring to its management the skills and techniques they believed were succeeding in the marketplace, where success and advancement depended on merit, and where businesslike mastery of facts and record keeping were essential. They found, for example, that the English census, which had begun decennial enumerations in 1801, was both poorly conceived and riddled with errors (Census of the population 1829). The census report for 1831, for example, gave two different acreages for England, with the discrepancy between the two figures the size of Berkshire; meanwhile, the government continued to calculate the value of imports using the prices of 1690 (Young 1963, 32). According to these middle-class critics, the government needed better information and better advice. Statistics, they were coming to believe, would serve both purposes. In the 1830s, the more representative government had a legitimacy it had lacked in the 1750s, and public-spirited men now demanded rather than opposed official fact-gathering.

Building Institutions for Statistical Investigation

In the 1830s, statistical investigation was institutionalized both outside government and then inside. A statistical section, Section F, was added to the British Association for the Advancement of Science in 1833, and within a few years statistical societies were established in London, Manchester, and several other provincial cities. The societies had their origin in concern about public affairs, especially the social problems of early industrial societies: urban poverty, civil unrest, crime, epidemic disease, and education. Statistics were seen as a tool to address these problems (Cullen 1975). The leaders of the statistical movement might claim to be following the example of the Belgian statistician Adolph

Quetelet, who visited England in 1833 and appeared as a star witness at the meeting of the British Association, when the formation of a statistical section was under discussion, but they made no attempt to employ the statistical concepts, such as the law of normal distribution, that Quetelet had pioneered. Statistics for these statistical society members denoted less a set of numerical methods or mathematical concepts than the objective study of problems of government by the collection of facts. These early statistical activists asserted that they could remove the treatment of public affairs from the partisan bickering and the competing interests that characterized legislation and administration and produce an objective science of government that could guide the legislator and the administrator in dealing with even the most practical and specific problems (Introduction 1838; Sixth annual report of the Council 1840).

From our vantage point in the early twenty-first century, these claims seem both naive and self-serving—little more than transparent demands to be listened to in the name of expertise. This initial wave of statistical enthusiasm did not last. It proved to be more difficult to collect reliable and objective data on complex social problems than many of these first British statisticians had anticipated, and the provincial statistical societies quickly disbanded. But the statisticians' demands that government do a better job of minding its business had lasting effects. In the 1830s, the Civil Service began more systematically to collect and publish statistics, to establish bureaus and offices, and to fill these with officials to collate and analyze the growing mountains of data. These government statisticians, along with a group of London actuaries, were the sustaining members of the Statistical Society of London, which survived the demise of the provincial societies and transformed the fantasies of the 1830s into the hard working realities of official statistics at midcentury.

It was in the midst of this reforming legislation and in the heyday of popular statistical enthusiasm that the foundations were laid for the English system of health statistics. The initial political force came from an unexpected quarter: the demands of dissenters, that is, non-Anglicans, to have a legally recognized means to prove family relationships and establish inheritances (Cullen 1974). Members of the Church of England could rely on the parish records of marriage, baptism, and burials, but this option was not attractive to dissenters, who lobbied for a public system independent of the Church. Their demand was seconded by some professional men who saw other legal or statistical benefits from a national system of civil registration. The Registration Acts of 1836 established a national system of civil registration for England and Wales (Act for marriages in England 1836; Act for registering births 1836). It permitted the registration of marriages and births and required the registration of deaths with local registrars who served in registration districts, which were themselves based on the newly established Poor Law Unions. But as often happens during legislation, the registration bills were endowed with additional purposes as they moved through Parliament. The Registration Acts provided not only for registering the fact of death but also its cause. Edwin Chadwick, one the of the chief architects of the

New Poor Law of 1834 and the future author of the famous *Report on the Sanitary Condition of the Labouring Population of Gt. Britain* of 1842 (Chadwick 1842), recognized that records of causes of death, along with the name, address, age, and occupation of the deceased, would be an invaluable resource for social investigation, and he claimed to have suggested the inclusion of cause of death in the legislation.

The law called for the registration data to flow to a new bureau in London, the General Register Office (GRO), whose job was to compile summaries and an annual report for Parliament. Registration began in July 1837, but the Registrar-General, a political appointee, soon discovered that he needed someone with statistical experience to bring order to the rapidly accumulating data. The person hired was a young doctor and medical journalist, William Farr, who had recently published a string of articles on vital statistics. Farr quickly became the intellectual leader in the GRO, and before his retirement in 1880 he established basic practices in health statistics and produced some of the finest studies of mortality patterns and disease outbreaks to be published in the nineteenth century (Eyler 1979).

Making Statistical Use of Registration Systems

The registration system had not been created for research, so Farr had to exercise much creative energy and administrative persistence to turn it to such uses. First of all, the inaccuracy of the reported causes of death was a perennial problem. The Registration Acts permitted laymen to determine and report the cause of death to the Registrar. Under Farr's leadership, the GRO sought the cooperation of the medical profession in certifying the causes of death, and in 1845 it began to distribute to all legally qualified practitioners printed forms for that purpose. This voluntary system worked very well. By 1870, 92% of all English deaths and 95% of deaths in London were medically certified using these forms (Farr 1872, 408). Then there was the major problem of classifying deaths by cause. In 1839, his first year at his post, Farr devised a statistical nosology to classify deaths by their cause (Farr 1839, 92–99). He revised the nosology in 1842 and again in 1853 (Farr 1842, 1856). These nosologies have cast a long shadow on health statistics. They were adopted by other English-speaking nations in the nineteenth century and, along with the nosology of Marc D'Espine of Geneva, formed the basis of the first edition of the International List of Causes of Death that Jacques Bertillon drew up in 1893 and that, after several revisions, is still in use today (Eyler 1979, 53–60). Finally through the weekly, quarterly, annual, and decennial supplements the GRO published, Farr helped to establish many of the standard conventions for recording and comparing mortality rates.

Farr was not only a dedicated and creative statistician; he was also a passionate public health reformer. Under his leadership, the GRO effectively used its reports as propaganda to strengthen the hands of public health activists and to shame local government into action (Szreter 1991). This was done most often by publishing in rank order the crude death rates of towns, rankings that newspapers began to reprint, much as they did the weather reports. Farr found an especially effective way to publicize the preventable loss of human life in the use of an arbitrary standard of health, a crude mortality rate of 17 per 1000. By 1850, 10% of the districts of England and Wales, the so-called Healthy Districts, had rates at or below this level, so such rates were undeniably possible. Farr used the Healthy District Rate to dramatize the poor health of other districts by calculating their degree of insalubrity, one degree for each death per 1000 above 17 per 1000, and by computing the number of deaths in excess of the number that would have occurred if the town had met the Healthy District standard (Table 2.1). Used in such ways, local death rates became political weapons, and the GRO's use of mortality rates in this way provoked predictable controversy (Eyler 1976).

Farr was aware, of course, that comparisons of crude mortality rates, however effective as political propaganda, were not strictly accurate, because the populations in different districts were not comparable, especially in their age composition. Especially problematic was the concentration in industrial towns of infants and young children, groups with the highest mortality. In many of his

TABLE 2.1
Deaths in 30 Large Town Districts in the Years 1851–60; and Also the Deaths Which Would Have Occurred in the 10 Years if the Mortality Had Been at the Same Rate as Prevailed in the 63 Healthy Districts (1849–53)

Ages	*Deaths in 10 Years 1851–60*	*Deaths Which Would Have Occurred in the 10 Years at Healthy District Rates*	*Excess of Actual Deaths in 10 Years over Deaths at Healthy District Rates*
All Ages	711,944	384,590	327,354
0–	388,950	135,470	203,520
5–	31,319	19,290	12,029
10–	14,240	11,020	3,220
15–	43,807	37,550	6,237
25–	48,623	36,150	12,475
35–	50,071	30,320	19,751
45–	49,638	26,680	22,958
55–	49,763	27,020	22,743
65–	47,445	31,510	15,935
75–	30,583	22,920	7,663
85 & upwards	7,463	6,660	803

Source: Farr (1864).

comparative studies, especially those in the annual reports, Farr attempted to overcome this problem by using age- or cause-specific mortality rates to compare the health of different places and to identify the causes of disease and premature death. But it is in his massive supplements to the 25th and 35th annual reports for the years 1851–1860 and 1861–1870 that we see Farr's statistical methods in their fully developed form (Farr 1864, 1875). In preparing these supplements, the GRO had at its disposal unprecedented sources of data—not only the vast and ever-growing data from registration but also the results of the census, whose supervision the GRO took over in 1841. To analyze these rich data, Farr adapted the life table techniques of British actuaries. In the 1830s, Farr had learned from the publications of the actuary Thomas Rowe Edmunds that human mortality changed with age in three geometric series (Eyler 2002). Edmunds had shown how this law of mortality could be used to construct model life tables and suggested that life tables for the general population could be used to assess the health and vitality of population groups. Farr used Edmunds's suggestions in constructing his own life tables from the census and registration returns: two for the entire nation, one for the Healthy Districts, several for places with notably high mortality such as Liverpool and the London metropolis, and several for specialized groups such as the one he composed from British miners for the Royal Commission on Mines (Eyler 1979, 77–80, 81–83, 133–135). He adopted the life table as the best measure of the health and vitality of a population (Fig. 2.1). A life table not only gave him figures for life expectancy and age-specific mortality rates, it also allowed him to produce standardized mortality rates, typically using the nation or the Healthy Districts as standards, which allowed him to compare the mortality of places and to avoid the disturbances caused by great differences in age structure. It was the use of such standardized rates that distinguished the GRO's decennial supplements and typified the best work in nineteenth-century health statistics.

Farr understood the life table to be a statistical tool of wide application, and he put it to some very novel uses: to study human fertility, to describe patterns of promotions in the army and in the civil service, and to describe the duration of English governments (Eyler 1979, 80–81). Perhaps most important, life tables and the law of mortality he used to construct them were the strongest proof of something that Farr fervently believed. The phenomena of life, disease, and death were regular, law-abiding, and predictable, and statistics had the power to unlock their secrets. This conviction lay behind some of the results he prized most: formulae to describe and to predict the waning of epidemics of smallpox and rinderpest, another numerical expression that showed how human mortality varied with population density, with mean proximity between persons to be more precise (Fig. 2.2), and yet another that described with great precision how mortality from Asiatic cholera varied with soil elevation (Eyler 1979, 111–117). From our perspective, there seems to be no biological reason why cholera mortality should depend on elevation of soil or why mortality from all causes should be related to mean proximity of people. But in the decades when the modern public

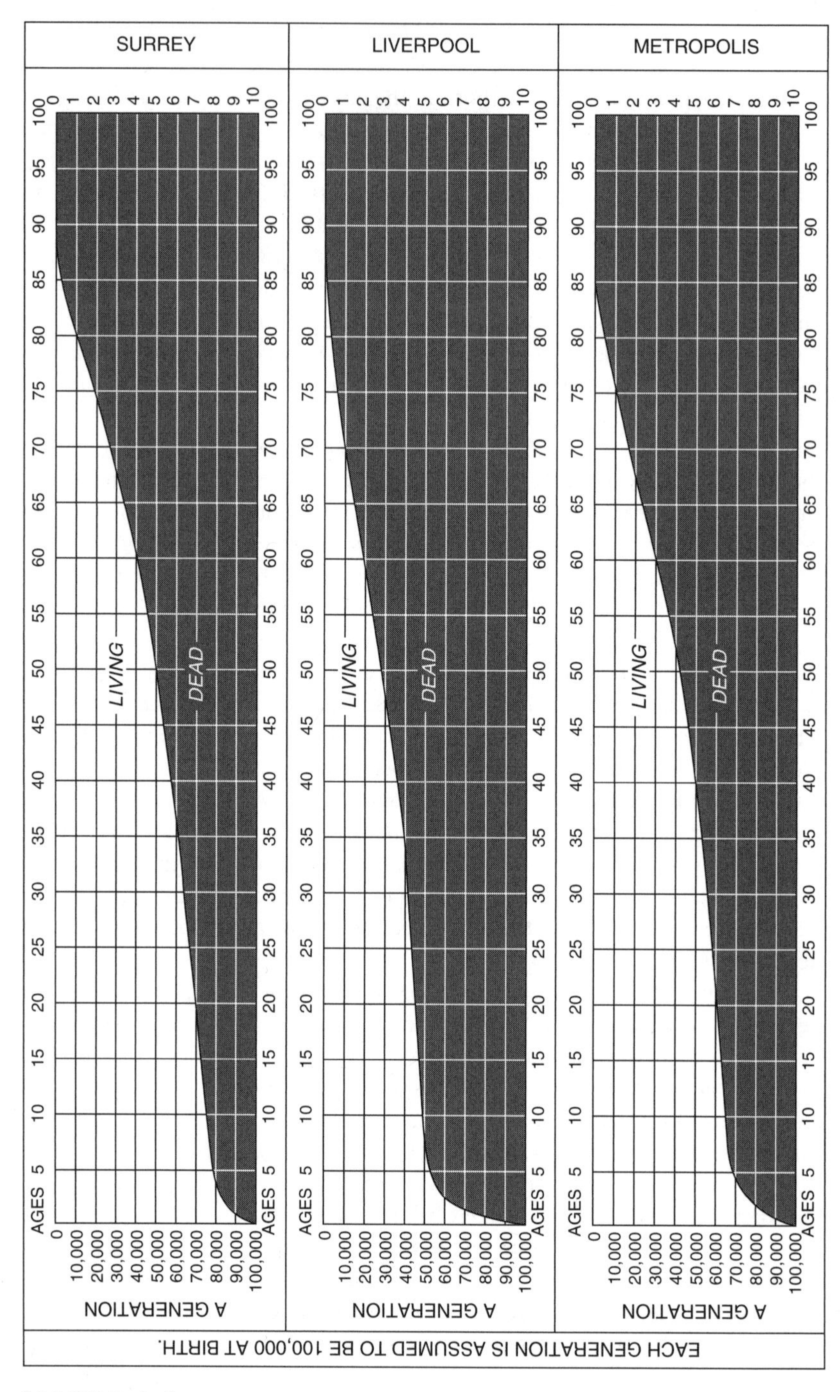

FIGURE 2.1
Farr's diagram for local life tables. (Source: Registrar-General of Births, Deaths, and Marriages in England 1843, pp. 50–51 [Parliamentary Papers 1843, xxi].)

health movement was getting underway, that is, just before the bacteriological revolution and the general acceptance of the germ theory of infection, these were entirely plausible relationships. Farr, like the majority of the medical profession, believed that diseases of public health concern were caused by miasmata—nonliving organic material produced by the decomposition of organic waste and suspended in the air. Farr named these epidemic, endemic, and contagious diseases *zymotic*, because of their assumed relationship to fermentation, and he made them the first class in his nosologies and the primary focus of his studies of disease.

Farr began his career as a committed miasmatist, anticontagionist, and sanitary reformer, but unlike many other sanitary reformers, he was open-minded and capable of changing his position in the face of convincing evidence. Perhaps the best example is found in his studies of the three epidemics of Asiatic cholera that occurred during his career. During the first, in 1848–1849, he formulated his elevation law for cholera mortality and took this law as confirmation of a miasmatic model for cholera causation. However, over the next two outbreaks, in 1853–1854 and 1866, he not only provided John Snow, an English physician, with data that enabled Snow to provide statistical evidence that cholera was water-borne, but in the 1866 epidemic, after Snow's death, Farr produced further evidence that helped to convince many of the truth of Snow's theory. Along the way, Farr gradually moved to a microbial model for the causation of the zymotic diseases (Eyler 1973, 2001).

Applying Statistics to Emerging Public Health Efforts

Victorian interest in mortality data was seldom just theoretical. It was almost always related to surveillance and to public health intervention. As the public health enterprise grew during the nineteenth century, that connection became more conspicuous. At the most fundamental level, crude mortality rates served to justify the intervention of the central government in the affairs of local government. Most public health legislation in the nineteenth century was permissive, leaving to the local authorities the option of doing what the law authorized. But Section 8 of the Public Health Act of 1848, the general legislation permitting towns to establish health departments and to undertake sanitary improvements, permitted the central government to step in and to put the other provisions of the act into effect if a town's crude annual mortality rate exceed 23 per 1000, then the national average (An act for promoting the public health 1847–1848). That provision was seldom enforced, but the central health authority soon began to exert its influence by monitoring local mortality rates and pressuring local authorities to act. Under the leadership of Sir John Simon, Medical Officer of the Privy Council, and his successors at the Local Government Board, the central health authority reviewed weekly, quarterly, and annual morality rates published by the GRO (Lambert 1963, 350–355, 424–437). If either a town's crude mortality or mortality from a specific cause, diarrheal diseases for example,

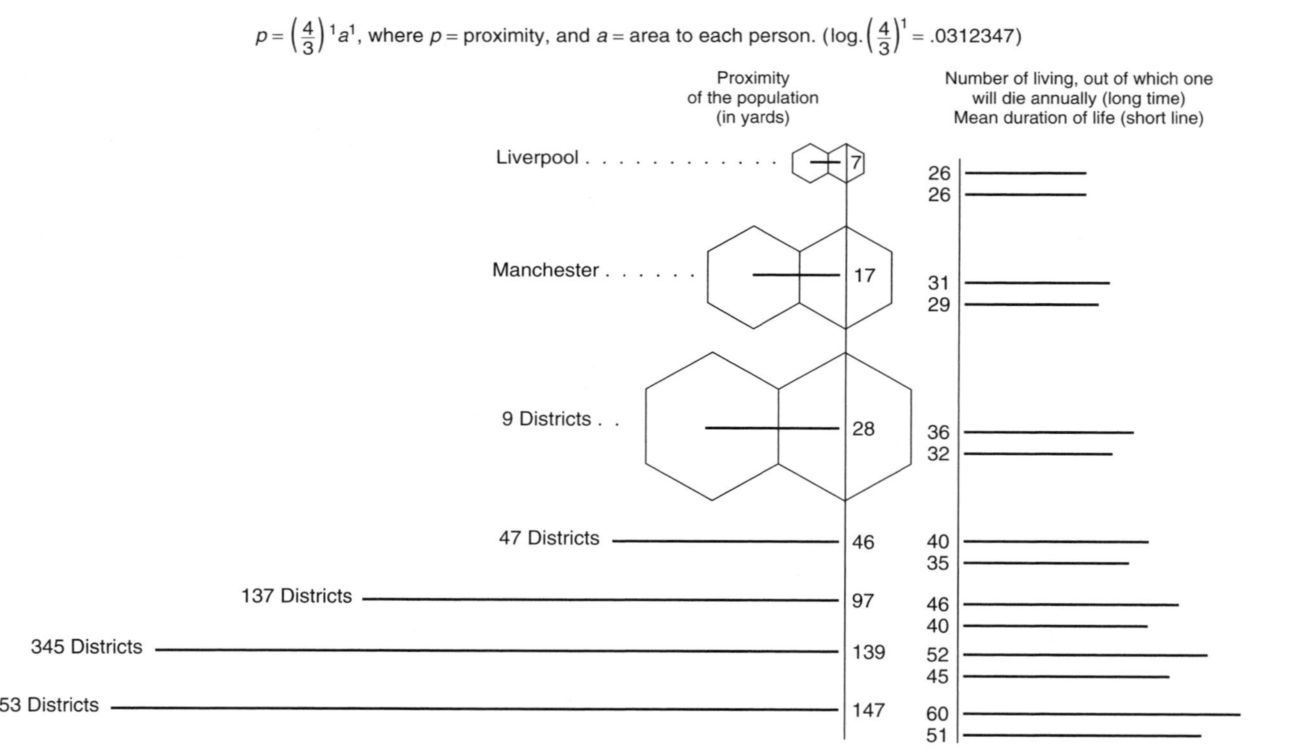

FIGURE 2.2
Farr's diagram for relation of proximity to mortality.(Source: Registrar-General of Births, Deaths, and Marriages in England. Fortieth Annual Report of the Registrar-General of Births, Deaths, and Marriages in England. London, HMSO; 1879, p. 237. [Parliamentary Papers 1878–1879, xix].)

suddenly increased or seemed abnormally high, the central authority might send medical inspectors to conduct a local investigation. The fact that an investigation was called for, and the weight of the inspector's report, were often enough to convince a budget-cautious town to build a sewer system, to protect its drinking water, or to improve its housing stock. Under this constant pressure from the center, the public health infrastructure and services improved incrementally during the second half of the century. Systems of surveillance also appeared at the local level, and these were often very responsive. Consider, for example, the system of surveillance Arthur Newsholme developed in Brighton in the opening years of the twentieth century to prevent milk-borne outbreaks of scarlet fever (Eyler 1986, 577–578). Scarlet fever was by then a notifiable or reportable disease, and Newsholme immediately visited every house in which a case had been notified, that is, reported, to inquire, among other things, about the source of the family's milk. He also bullied the town's dairies into keeping the milk from different farms separate and recording which milk was used on each milk route. Using this simple system in 1905, the health department detected the source of a milk-borne outbreak after only six cases had been registered. By immediately banning milk from one farm, it was able to limit the outbreak to a total of 20 cases.

Reporting of Illness

As the above examples suggest, during the nineteenth century health statistics, even the most comprehensive and rigorous, like these from the GRO, were based entirely on mortality and census data. The GRO knew almost nothing about the incidence of sickness. By the 1860s, reformers in the medical profession were calling for a system of reporting human illness for purposes of both prevention and research (Rumsey 1875, 47–55, 99–107). But the collection of information on individual cases of illness by a public authority was much more problematic in a democratic society that prided itself on its respect for privacy and local self-government than even the registration of births and deaths had been. When the reporting of illnesses finally began at the end of the century, it applied only to a small number of illnesses deemed dangerous to the community, and the data were put in the hands not of a central authority, but the local health authority. Furthermore, the initial legislation of 1889 was adoptive, that is, permissive (Infectious Disease Notification Act 1889). It permitted, but did not require, outside the London metropolis, local authorities to require medical practitioners to notify cases of a small list of infectious diseases to the local Medical Officer of Health (MOH). It was a full decade before the legislation was made mandatory over the entire nation (Infectious Disease [Notification] Extension Act 1899). Thus, well into the twentieth century, morbidity statistics were collected and used separately from mortality statistics, making impossible the sorts of studies of morbidity that the GRO had produced for mortality.

This division of data reflects major changes in the professional landscape. When the GRO was established and for several decades thereafter, there were no local health departments, and the GRO's role as a research facility on mortality was one it had created for itself out of the vagueness of the original legislation. By the 1880s, health departments existed in all towns, and public health was a rapidly professionalizing field with widening responsibilities. In their role as protectors of the public's health, local MOHs had a special claim on registration data and received weekly reports from the registrars of deaths from dangerous diseases in their areas. Once their town had adopted the Notification Act, they also collected reports of nonfatal infectious cases. The Local Government Board (LGB), the central public health agency, began a voluntary system of sharing information on reported illnesses among local authorities, but not all towns cooperated and no central data on reported illness existed.

As the public health profession grew in the last quarter of the nineteenth century, some of the most creative uses of health statistics were undertaken by public health officials working both at the local level and at the LGB. The best example may be the work of Sir Arthur Newsholme. While Newsholme was MOH of the town of Brighton in 1888–1908, he published a series of remarkably insightful studies of infectious disease by combining mortality and morbidity data with intense fieldwork. By these means he was able to demonstrate that scarlet fever spread through the town's unpasteurized milk supply, how typhoid fever was transmitted by raw oysters from beds at the outlets of a neighboring town's sewers, and how tuberculosis spread within households (Eyler 1997, 119–191). After Newsholme moved to the LGB to head the English public health system, he continued his intense statistical investigations. Perhaps the most important are the five comprehensive and timely monographs he produced between 1910 and 1916 on infant, childhood, and maternal mortality (Eyler 1997, 295–316).

Newsholme freely acknowledged that he had developed his statistical skills by studying the publications of the GRO. It was through his efforts in part that the methods Farr developed at the GRO became standards in public health work. In 1889 Newsholme wrote a practical textbook of statistical methods for health officers. It was widely read throughout the English-speaking world, going through three editions in its first decade and having new English and American editions as late as 1923–1924 (Newsholme 1889, 1924).

THE GROWTH OF AMERICAN MORBIDITY STATISTICS, 1910–1935

Given the decentralization of American government, the tenuous existence of the Census Bureau before 1902, and the absence of a complete national system of registering births and deaths before the 1930s, America produced nothing in the nineteenth century like the systematic studies of mortality patterns for the entire population that emerged from the General Register Office of England. In the early twentieth century, some of the best American studies of mortality were in fact undertaken outside government by actuaries such as Louis I. Dublin of the Metropolitan Life Insurance Company.

Private Initiatives in Collecting Morbidity Statistics

Beginning about 1910, Dublin prepared a series of studies of the mortality experience of Metropolitan Life Insurance policy holders, distinguishing causes of mortality and a variety of risk factors such as occupation (Dublin 1917; Dublin and Lotka 1937; Dublin et al. 1919). Although the studies were based on the experience of a subset of the nation's population, that subset was very large and arguably quite representative. Met Life industrial policies, after all, were sold throughout the nation to families of very modest means and were issued without a medical examination. Dublin's studies of mortality were well designed and carefully analyzed, and they constituted important and influential contributions to American health statistics. More remarkably, Dublin and his colleagues at Met Life were among the first Americans to investigate rates of sickness in communities. Their strategy for collecting this information was simple. Company agents visited the homes of industrial policy holders every week to collect a small premium payment. Between 1915 and 1917, agents in seven communities, five large cities, and two composite study groups of smaller villages were asked to fill out a simple form for each family they visited on current illness among family members. The surveys gathered information on 637,000 individuals who represented between 2.5% and 25% of their communities. Unlike many of the surveys undertaken in the following 20 years, these surveys included both black and white families and attempted to disaggregate the data by race from the composite study group of Pennsylvania and West Virginia. Although illness was self-reported, the surveys included length of illness to date, whether the sick person was able to work, and whether a physician had been consulted (Frankel and Dublin 1914, 1916a, 1916b; 1916c; 1917a, 1917b; Stecker 1917).

Early Public Sector Morbidity Statistics

Public health officials soon followed suit in collecting morbidity statistics. The great influenza pandemic of 1918–1919 gave an impetus to these studies, since it was known that during the outbreak, vital records of all types were incomplete and inaccurate, and since it seemed to be impossible to answer some fundamental epidemiologic questions about the epidemic from mortality data alone. After the first wave of the pandemic, the U.S. Public Health Service (USPHS) undertook a sickness survey in 18 locations. The first results to be published were for Baltimore and four smaller towns and two rural areas of Maryland (Frost and Sydenstricker 1919). Information was collected by survey from households containing some 48,000 people during November and December 1918. The diagnosis, of course, had to be made retrospectively on the basis of symptoms and sick time reported by the family. The authors of the report, W.H. Frost and Edgar Sydenstricker, concentrated on providing basic mortality, morbidity, and case fatality rates, distinguishing locality, age, and gender. A much more intensive study was undertaken 2 years later, during a recurrent epidemic of influenza, by Warren T. Vaughan of Harvard's Department of Preventive Medicine with financial support from the Metropolitan Life Insurance Company (Vaughan 1921). Vaughan and his assistants did surveys of households containing 10,800 persons in six neighborhoods of Boston. Family spokespersons were asked not only to report on cases of illness during the present epidemic but also to recall illness during the great epidemic a year and a half earlier. Using this survey's data and employing strict case definitions, Vaughan produced what is probably the best epidemiologic analysis of a local influenza outbreak before the virus was isolated in the 1930s. His studies clearly suggested that lack of herd immunity was paramount in determining the explosive nature of the great flu pandemic.

Both of these sickness surveys of influenza outbreaks were based on sampling procedures. But it is typical of the state of health statistics in the 1910s and 1920s that neither report explains very much about how the selections were made. Characteristic of the age, these choices seemed to have been made rather intuitively. Frost and Sydenstricker explain nothing about how neighborhoods in the Maryland towns were selected for inclusion. Vaughan is much more explicit. He chose six neighborhoods based on their reputation for ethnic composition and level of prosperity: one Italian neighborhood, one Irish neighborhood, one poor Jewish neighborhood, one ethnically mixed middle-class neighborhood, one moderately well-to-do Jewish neighborhood, and one prosperous white Protestant neighborhood. Neither study discusses the significance of the size of its sample or its bearing on the reliability of its results. Formal discussions of sampling theory were at least a decade off.

Initiation of Formal Morbidity Studies in the United States

By the 1920s, the Statistical Division of the USPHS was becoming very interested in charting the burden of ordinary, nonfatal illness on a community's health. In beginning a report in February 1925, USPHS statistician Edgar Sydenstricker decried the dependency of epidemiology on mortality statistics. "The effect has been to foster a fallacious premise for public health work, namely, that a low death rate indicates the presence of health. Obviously it does not" (Sydenstricker 1925, 279). To support his claim, he pointed to areas of the South with ordinary death rates but where the population was chronically incapacitated by hookworm, malaria, or pellagra. Unlike their European counterparts, who could rely on the administrative records of national health insurance schemes, which had been created between 1880 and 1920, American researchers had to rely on social survey methods to collect data on rates of illness. One of the first ventures of the USPHS into this new field was a sickness survey it undertook in what it deemed to be a typical small American city in a period of ordinary health conditions. The Statistical Division followed 7200 white individuals in 1600 families in Hagerstown, Maryland, from December 1921 through March 1924. Following an initial survey in which demographic and socioeconomic information was gathered and a health history taken of each subject, each household was visited every 6 to 8 weeks for a total of 16 times to collect information on illnesses that had taken place since the last visit (Sydenstricker 1926). The reliance on self-reporting of complaints was typical. What set the study apart was its prospective nature and its duration. The results fully justified the agency's expectations. A disease's importance as a cause of death proved to be a poor indicator of its importance as a cause of illness. The most striking example was the class of respiratory diseases, which during the study period accounted for only 20% of deaths but about 60% of illnesses lasting 3 days or longer. Such results suggested to Sydenstricker that change was needed in research priorities and public health efforts.

Identifying and Documenting Health Disparities in the United States in the 1930s

While such morbidity statistics as these were important precedents, it was only during the Great Depression of the 1930s that morbidity statistics of the American population began to be energetically collected. The apparent failure of industrial capitalism and its institutions and massive unemployment forced statisticians and other students of society in the 1930s to ask some of the same questions about the relationship between economic condition and human health and welfare that had prompted the pioneering European studies of mortality in the 1820s, 1830s, and 1840s. In the economic crisis of the 1930s, the crude mortality rate for the American people continued to fall. That fact proved to some observers that human health was not suffering. The statisticians at the USPHS cautioned, however, that the decline in mortality for the whole population might mask an increase for a segment living in the worst conditions or, more likely, that rates of illness might have increased even though the death rate continued on its downward trajectory (Perrott and Collins 1935, 595–596; Sydenstricker 1933, 273–274). Concern over the effects of the Depression on public health prompted two joint research projects between the Office of Statistical Investigations of the USPHS and private research groups: the Committee of the Costs of Medical Care (CCMC), the Milbank Memorial Fund, and International Health Organization of the League of Nations.

The CCMC had begun its deliberations before the Depression began, and its primary purpose was to assess the adequacy and cost of the health care

Americans received. It was, in fact, the first, and for a long time the only, attempt to study the American health-care system as a whole. Inevitably its work was swept up in the debates over economic and welfare policy that the Depression fostered. This joint study of the prevalence of sickness proved to be the longest and most costly of all the CCMC research projects. It was a prospective study of sickness of nearly 9000 families living in 130 communities in 17 states plus the District of Columbia, and it formed the basis of the CCMC's Monograph No. 26 and an article in *Public Health Reports* by the USPHS statistician Selwyn Collins (Collins 1933; Falk et al. 1933). Between 1928 and 1931, families in the study areas recorded information on schedules provided to them for a full year. An enumerator, usually a public health nurse, visited at 2-month intervals to interview an adult family member and to fill out the permanent record. In keeping with the CCMC's original purpose, this sickness survey gathered information not only on the occurrence and duration of sickness but also on the use and cost of medical services and their accessibility to the families studied. While the CCMC's analysis of data was hastily undertaken to meet the general Committee schedule, the analysis was still among the most sophisticated of the period. The researchers contacted attending physicians to confirm the diagnosis of 64% of illnesses seen by a physician or 51% of all illnesses reported. They also carefully assessed the difference between the sample population and the general American population, using demographic and economic measures, and adjusted their results to more accurately reflect the experience of the general population (Collins 1933, 289–292; Falk et al. 1933, 29–39). They also recognized that the numerical results might be influenced by the fact that the survey was not taken simultaneously in all communities. This survey revealed an incidence of illness significantly lower than what resulted from the Hagerstown survey of 1921–1924. The chief reason was a higher rate of respiratory illness in Hagerstown, which Collins attributed to the period and methods of observation there and to two local outbreaks of respiratory disease during the study (Collins 1933, 298–299).

In its collaboration with the Milbank Memorial Fund and the International Health Organization of the League of Nations, the Statistical Division of the USPHS addressed directly the question of how the Depression was affecting the health of the American people. For this study it selected poor but not slum neighborhoods in 10 communities: 8 cities and 2 collections of small industrial settlements, a group of mining villages near Morgantown, West Virginia, and a set of mill villages near Greenville, South Carolina. Enumerators made a single visit to the homes of nearly 12,000 families to collect a 3-month history of illness for each family member and a 4-year income and employment history of each adult. Altogether, data for 49,136 individuals were coded and transferred to punch cards and formed the basis for an important string of publications (Perrott and Collins 1933, 1934a, 1934b, 1935; Perrott et al. 1933). The study grouped families into a small number of broad income classes and into groups according to rate of full or part-time employment. The investigation provided ample evidence that sickness increased with economic hardship. Not only were families in the "poor" class sick more often than those in the "moderate" or "comfortable" classes, but families whose incomes had fallen the most had the highest rates of illness. Families who between 1929 and 1932 had fallen from the comfortable class into the poor class had rates of disabling illness 45% higher than the rates of those who remained in the comfortable class, while the formerly comfortable whose incomes had fallen still further, so far that they qualified for relief by 1932, had rates 73% higher than those who remained in the comfortable class (Perrott, Collins 1935, 612, 616). The formerly comfortable who had become poor or had gone on relief suffered even more illness than the chronically poor, those who remained in the lowest economic class throughout the whole period.

The Political Context for Emerging Health Statistics Efforts

These studies raised troubling questions about the justice of American society and the adequacy of the American health-care system. They cannot be understood today without reference to the social and political context in which they were conducted. Best known is the stormy reception of the CCMC's report. The CCMC was an independent research group supported by several foundations. Its membership was chosen to be broadly representative of academic, professional, and public interests in health care: economists and other social scientists with expertise in health care, representatives of organized medicine, practicing physicians and dentists, public health experts, hospital administrators, and a few representatives of the public. Predictably, serious fault lines developed early in the CCMC's deliberations over medical politics and economics (Starr 1982, 261–266; Walker 1979;). Questions about how much of the nation's budget should go to treating disease and whether Americans were receiving the care they needed are controversial at any time. They were especially controversial in the 1930s, when Americans' inability to pay deprived them of care and physicians and hospitals of the revenues they counted on. Furthermore, by the time the CCMC concluded its work, it was known that President Franklin D. Roosevelt was considering adding medical care to his social security proposal, an idea that was anathema to the American Medical Association's leadership, which was struggling to protect private practice, even to waging war with local medical societies, whose financially pinched members were considering initiating voluntary health insurance schemes on their own.

Despite its extensive empirical research, the CCMC could arrive at no consensus, and ended its work by issuing a majority report and two minority reports (Committee on the Cost of Medical Care 1932). The majority report signed by the social scientists, the public health officials, and the hospital representatives, concluded that America needed to spend much more on disease prevention; it needed more general practitioners and fewer specialists; it needed to organize its health care into groups; and it needed to provide for care through some scheme of prepayment. The minority reports rejected both the principles of prepayment and health insurance and the proposal to organize medical services into groups. Organized medicine's hostility can be gauged by the editorials of Morris Fishbein, the editor of the *Journal of the American Medical Association*, who viewed the majority report as a radical document that threatened the physician's right to practice and attempted to replace the basic freedoms of Americans with "Sovietism" (Report of the Committee on the Cost of Medical Care [editorial] 1932).

Given this environment, the CCMC proceeded cautiously. The study of the incidence of sickness was the first field investigation it initiated, and it decided to use communities in West Virginia as a trial of its methods. The secretary of the American Medical Association, who was a member of the CCMC, contacted county medical societies throughout the state society, asking for the cooperation of their members. Following this procedure in other states, the CCMC first obtained the approval of the state medical society and the state public health department before approaching local health departments, whose nurses it relied on to do most of the canvassing. But even these precautions did not ensure the cooperation of medical practitioners. Some physicians refused to confirm the diagnoses their patients reported to the canvassers, while in a few areas health officials asked that nurses not attempt to contact any local physicians. Faced with general opposition, the CCMC soon abandoned its plans to confirm the costs of care that families reported (Falk et al. 1933, 12–13).

These studies of morbidity undertaken during the Great Depression reflect not only the highly charged issue of health-care policy, they also reflect basis social assumptions of the statistical investigators themselves. Consider, for example, the issue of race. None of the studies we have discussed thus far, other than the sickness surveys by the Metropolitan Life Insurance Company, included African Americans. Americans of African descent were nearly as invisible in America's mortality statistics as they were in American public life. All the studies in which the USPHS participated explained why they did not include African Americans. The report on the Hagerstown survey stated that blacks formed too small a minority in Hagerstown to be included (Sydenstricker 1926, 2071). The joint study with the Milbank Fund explained that it excluded black families, because it wanted to keep the influence of race separate from the influence of family income (Perrott and Collins 1935, 597). The joint study with the CCMC suggested that it was not their number in society but their nature or the nature of their families that kept African Americans from being fit subjects. "It was considered that the procedure adopted could not procure satisfactory information from negro families" (Falk et al. 1933, 5). The report did not elaborate, but it seems that the researchers did not believe that black families could be relied upon to supply accurate or complete information.

These studies also reflect deep-seated hereditarian attitudes toward human misfortune that were characteristic of the age. In spite of the firm connection between a fall in the standard of living and high rates of sickness that their data established, the authors of the Sickness and the Depression study were reluctant to conclude that economic privation increased the risk of sickness. In part, their reluctance sprang from the problems inherent in inferring causation from correlation. High rates of sickness among the poor might simply reflect that illness caused poverty. In this case, the authors believed that their data did not support the conclusion that illness had caused most families to plunge into poverty. But they also entertained the nagging suspicion that the Depression had simply exposed the inherent weakness of the unfit. Despite acknowledged exceptions, the authors considered that those who kept their jobs were "on the average, the more vigorous, capable, and intelligent ones" and those who lost their jobs the "less efficient" (Perrott and Collins 1935, 620). They maintained this view while acknowledging that, if one considered the "new poor" in 1929, families that would fall into poverty by 1932, one found that their household heads had lower educational levels and less skilled employment, and that they lived in more crowded quarters in 1929 than other members of the comfortable classes. But even this evidence was perceived through the filter of eugenic attitudes. "Some of these findings appear to indicate that families of certain *types* were least successful in weathering the depression. However, it seems highly improbable that a theory of selection contains the sole explanation of the results of the present survey" (Perrott and Collins 1935, 620). In the post–World War II period, after eugenics had been thoroughly discredited, statisticians in America faced with the evidence this study gathered would not have paid a hereditarian theory of economic hardship so much attention.

The publications springing from the Sickness and the Depression study were still appearing when the USPHS initiated its most important study of sickness to date, the National Health Survey of 1935–1936, which was part of its new National Health Inventory (Perrott et al. 1951, 1–24). The initiation of the National Health Survey was made possible not only by the Roosevelt administration's growing interest in health, but also by its activist policy of using federal employment to support the unemployed. The National Health Survey used unemployed white-collar workers as canvassers and paid them with money from the Works Project Administration. This great expansion in the labor force for fieldwork made it possible to work on a much larger scale. This survey dwarfed all previous sickness studies. Whereas the largest completed sickness survey, the Sickness and the Depression study, had collected data on 49,000 individuals at 10 study sites, the National Health Survey included 2.5 million individuals in 83 cities. This portion of the study population represented 3.6% of the urban population in the United States according to the census of 1930. The survey was not as complete for the rural population, but it still collected information on 140,418 persons in 23 rural counties. The conduct of the survey can be regarded as the culmination of the research interests and methods developed by the Statistical Department of the USPHS and its collaborators during the past half-dozen years. Like the Sickness and the Depression study, it used trained enumerators who collected their information retrospectively, in this instance for a full year, during a single visit to households. Also, like the joint study with the CCMC, it included information on the receipt of health care as well as on the incidence of illness, and it attempted to confirm a portion of the reported diagnoses by contacting hospitals, clinics, and physicians. The canvassing took place between October 1, 1934, and March 3, 1936. In small towns, every household was canvassed. In towns with a population of over 100,000, the survey canvassed only households in randomly selected districts used in the 1930 census enumeration.

THE CREATION OF THE U.S. NATIONAL HEALTH SURVEY, 1956: A MAJOR INFLUENCE ON CONTEMPORARY HEALTH STATISTICS

The National Health Survey of 1935–1936 provided an unprecedented fund of data, and it proved to be of great importance to public health and medical services researchers for two decades. Appearing before the Subcommittee on Health of the Senate Committee on Labor and Public Welfare in August 1951, the Surgeon General estimated that the National Health Survey of 1935–1936 had provided the data for some 200 papers, reports, and book chapters (Perrott et al. 1951, 25–65; U.S. Public Health Service 1963, 26). In fact, it was the last major study of morbidity until after the Second World War and remained a major source of data well into the 1950s. However, by the time the Surgeon General made this observation, public health statisticians were growing acutely aware that the data this survey had collected were out of date and, furthermore, that the methods that had been used to collect them, especially the sampling techniques, could be improved upon. Through the U.S. National Committee on Vital and Health Statistics, which had been established in 1949, they began to study the problem with an eye toward proposing a major expansion and a restructuring of the nation's health statistics. The National Committee's Subcommittee on National Morbidity Survey issued a report in October 1953 that served as the blueprint for this important change (U.S. Public Health Service 1963, 19–38). After acknowledging the importance of the National Health Survey of 1935–1936, the report discussed the advances in research methods that had taken place since 1935, and several recent local projects aimed at either updating the data or improving the techniques used in the mid-1930s. The Subcommittee recommended that the collection of national morbidity statistics be made an ongoing function of the USPHS and that both a set of ongoing surveys of illness and disability and special studies of health problems and methodological issues be initiated. Probability sampling and other modern statistical techniques were to be employed.

This was a bold proposal that would require congressional authorization and funding, but it was an auspicious time to be lobbying for such changes. The immediate postwar years witnessed a rapid expansion of federal activity in health that mirrored the growth of the American economy and Americans' newly demonstrated faith in modern science and medicine. In this political environment and with the orchestrated pressure from lobbyists like the Laskers and the Mahoneys of the American Cancer Society, Congress expanded its appropriations for medical research at a dizzying pace. In the first 6 full postwar years, 1947–1953, the budget of the National Institutes of Health increased by a factor of 10, from $7 to $70 million, and by 1961 it had multiplied by a factor of 10 again to more than $700 million (Bordley and Harvey 1976, 425; Strickland 1972, 75, 97). The epidemiologic and preventive arm of the federal health enterprise also grew in significant ways. The Centers for Disease Control and Prevention, for example, had its origins during the war in the very limited mission of controlling malaria around defense installations in the South. After the war, not only was the project retained, but its mission was redefined and its staff was expanded significantly by absorbing in 1947 USPHS's Plague Laboratory with its Epidemiological Division, by instituting the Epidemic Intelligence Service during the Korean War as a defense against germ warfare, and by a policy of answering all calls from the states for help in investigating disease outbreaks (Etheridge 1992, 1–48). Such expansion of federal initiatives and expenditures would have been unthinkable in the prewar years.

The Eisenhower administration responded favorably to the recommendations of the Subcommittee on National Morbidity Survey. It included the broad outline of the Subcommittee's report in the President's legislative package to Congress in 1956, and with the unanimous endorsement of Lister Hill's Senate Committee on Labor and Public Welfare, the bill authorizing the these changes passed without opposition in July 1956 (Haywood 1981, 196; U.S. Senate Committee on Labor and Public Welfare 1956). The National Health Survey Act authorized the Surgeon General to undertake, on a noncompulsory basis, continuing surveys and special statistical investigations of the occurrence of sickness and disability and to make special studies of the survey methods and techniques that would refine the statistical methods in use (National Health Survey Act 1956). With this broad authorization, the USPHS was soon able to implement the recommendations of the Subcommittee on National Morbidity Survey.

What emerged was a family of surveys that both built on the pioneering work undertaken in the 1920s and 1930s and broke much new ground. By 1961 three continuous surveys were functioning: the Health Interview Survey, the Health Examination Survey, and the Health Records Survey (U.S. Public Health Service 1963, 8–14). The Health Interview Survey most closely resembled the prewar work. It was based on household interviews in selected survey districts, but its research methods were refined. The questionnaires used, for example, had been improved, but, most significantly, the methods of sampling used in this and in the other surveys reflected the growth since the 1930s of sampling theory and the growing use of probability sampling in government statistics (Duncan and Shelton 1978, 35–73). The Health Records Survey, like the CCMC and the National Health Survey of 1935–1936, gathered information on how Americans used the nation's health-care facilities, but its capacity to gather data was more robust with the compilation and maintenance of a master and complementary lists of American health-care facilities whose records it monitored. Also, in the changed political climate of the 1960s, it was much less controversial than it had been in the 1930s. The Health Examination Survey gathered information on Americans' health, especially on chronic and nonmanifest illness, through screening and physical examinations using mobile screening units. The goal in undertaking these continuous surveys was to be able to provide quarterly reports on the health of the nation and biannual reports on the health of regional survey areas. There were, in addition, special studies of specific health problems and methodological studies aimed at improving the collection, analysis, and distribution of survey data.

The National Health Survey was run by a small, highly qualified staff in the USPHS, and it undertook much of its fieldwork by contract with other governmental agencies, particularly the Census Bureau, and with nongovernmental entities as well (U.S. Public Health Service 1963, 7–8). The National Health Survey found its permanent administrative home in 1960, when it was combined with the National Office of Vital Statistics, a product of the transfer of the census to the USPHS in 1946, to form the National Center for Health Statistics (NCHS) (U.S. Department of Health and Human Services 2000, v). The NCHS and its program of health surveys were further detailed in federal law in 1973. Today, the NCHS is part of the Centers for Disease Control and Prevention, and its surveys are more commonly known as the National Health Interview Survey, the National Health and Nutrition Examination Survey, and the National Health Care Survey.

The move to establish an ongoing, nationally sponsored program of broad, multipurpose health surveys has been augmented over time by a series of more specialized surveys addressing more narrowly defined health topics or population groups, paralleling the growth and specialization of federal health programs. Similarly, state and local governments have established ongoing survey programs to meet data needs for program and policy purposes, and foundations and other private organizations have often filled gaps in publicly sponsored health surveys in order to support research and advocacy. These surveys are described in Chapter 5; the organizations and entities that carry forward the long evolution in health statistics are described in Chapter 3.

The surveys currently conducted by the NCHS and others involved in the health statistics enterprise provide the basic intelligence system for American medical research and public health activity, and this work forms the basis for health statistics in the twenty-first century. In this work we can detect both the long tradition of statistical thinking and research leading back to the early nineteenth century and the rapid development of statistical methods and federal initiatives in health care that has taken place since the Second World War.

REFERENCES

Act for marriages in England. Great Britain. Statutes at large. 6 & 7 Wm IV, c. 85. 1836.
Act for registering births, deaths, and marriages in England. Great Britain. Statutes at large. 6 & 7 Wm IV, c. 86. 1836.
An act for promoting the public health. Great Britain. Statutes at large. 11 & 12 Vict, c. 63. 1847–1848.
Anderson MJ. The American Census: A Social History. New Haven, CT: Yale University Press; 1988.
Anderson MJ. The U.S. Bureau of the Census in the nineteenth century. Soc Hist Med 1991;4(3):497–513.
Arosenius E. The history and organization of Swedish official statistics. In: Koren J, ed. The History of Statistics: Their Development and Progress in Many Countries. New York: Macmillian; 1918, pp. 535–569.
Blake JB. The early history of vital statistics in Massachusetts. Bull Hist Med 1955;29(1):46–68.
Bordley J, Harvey AM. Two Centuries of American Medicine, 1776–1976. Philadelphia: W.B. Saunders; 1976.
Buck P. People who counted: political arithmetic in the eighteenth century. Isis 1982;73:28–45.
Cassedy JH. The registration area and American vital statistics: development of a health research resource, 1885–1915. Bull Hist Med 1965;39:221–231.
Cassedy JH. American Medicine and Statistical Thinking, 1800–1860. Cambridge, MA: Harvard University Press; 1984.
Census of the population—law of mortality. Edinb Rev 1829;49:1–34.
Chadwick E. Report on the Sanitary Condition of the Labouring Population of Gt. Britain. London: HMSO; 1842.
Cohen PC. A Calculating People: The Spread of Numeracy in Early America. Chicago: University of Chicago Press; 1982.
Coleman W. Death Is a Social Disease: Public Health and Political Economy in Early Industrial France. Madison: University of Wisconsin Press; 1982.
Collins SD. Causes of illness in 9,000 families, based on nationwide periodic canvasses, 1828–1931. Public Health Rep 1933;48:283–308.
Committee on the Cost of Medical Care. Health Care for the American People: The Final Report of the Committee on the Cost of Medical Care. Chicago: University of Chicago Press; 1932.
Cullen MJ. The making of the Civil Registration Act of 1836. J Ecclestiast Hist 1974;25:39–59.
Cullen MJ. The Statistical Movement in Early Victorian Britain: The Foundations of Empirical Social Research. New York: Barnes and Noble; 1975.
Desrosières A. Official statistics and medicine in nineteenth-century France: the SGF as a case study. Soc Hist Med 1991;4:515–537.
Dublin LI. Causes of Death, by Occupation: Occupational Morality Experience of the Metropolitan Life Insurance Company, Industrial Department, 1911–1913. Washington, DC: GPO; 1917.
Dublin LI, Kopf EW, Van Buren GH. Mortality Statistics of Insured Wage-Earners and Their Families. New York: Metropolitan Life Insurance Co; 1919.
Dublin LI, Lotka AJ. Twenty-Five Years of Health Progress: A Study of the Mortality Experience Among the Industrial Policyholders of the Metropolitan Life Insurance Company 1911 to 1935. New York: Metropolitan Life Insurance Co; 1937.
Duncan JW, Shelton WC. Revolution in United States Government Statistics 1926–1976. Washington, DC: GPO; 1978.

Etheridge EW. Sentinel for Health: A History of the Centers for Disease Control. Berkeley: University of California Press; 1992.
Eyler JM. William Farr on the cholera: the sanitarian's disease theory and the statistician's method. J Hist Med 1973;28:79–100.
Eyler JM. Mortality statistics and Victorian health policy: program and criticism. Bull Hist Med 1976;50:335–355.
Eyler JM. Victorian Social Medicine: The Ideas and Methods of William Farr. Baltimore: Johns Hopkins University Press; 1979.
Eyler JM. The epidemiology of milk-borne scarlet fever: the case of Edwardian Brighton. Am J Public Health 1986;76:573–584.
Eyler JM. Sir Arthur Newsholme and State Medicine, 1885–1935. Cambridge: Cambridge University Press; 1997.
Eyler JM. The changing assessments of John Snow's and William Farr's cholera studies. Soc Prev Med 2001;46:225–232.
Eyler JM. Constructing vital statistics: Thomas Rowe Edmonds and William Farr 1835–1845. Soc Prev Med 2002; 47:6–13.
Falk IS, Klem MC, Sinai N. The Incidence of Illness and the Receipt and Costs of Medical Care Among Representative Families: Experiences of Twelve Consecutive Months during 1828–1931. Publications of the Committee on the Costs of Medical Care, No. 26. Chicago: University of Chicago Press; 1933.
Farr W. Letter to the Registrar-General. Annual report of the Registrar-General of Births, Deaths, and Marriages in England 1839;1:86–118 [63–81 in House of Commons Sessional Papers].
[Farr W.] Statistical nosology. Annual report of the Registrar-General of Births, Deaths, and Marriages in England 1842;4:147–166 [93–105 in House of Commons Sessional Papers].
Farr W. Project de classification. Compte rendu de la deuxième session du Congrès International de Statistique. Paris: Congrès International de Statistique; 1856, pp. 147–165.
Farr W. Letter to the Registrar-General on the mortality in the registration districts of England during the 10 years 1851–61. In: Supplement to the Twenty-Fifth Annual Report of the Registrar-General of Births, Deaths, and Marriages in England. London: HMSO; 1864, pp. iii–xxxvi.
Farr W. Letter to the Registrar-General. Annual report of the Registrar-General of Births, Deaths, and Marriages in England 1872:403–413.
Farr W. Letter to the Registrar-General on the mortality in the registration districts of England during the years 1861–70. In: Supplement to the Thirty-Fifth Annual Report of the Registrar-General of Births, Deaths, and Marriages in England. London: HMSO; 1875, pp. iii–lxxxii.
Farr W. Proximity of population. Annual report of the Registrar-General of Births, Deaths, and Marriages in England 1878–1879;40:231–246.
Faure F. The development and progress of statistics in France. In: Koren J, ed. The History of Statistics: Their Development and Progress in Many Countries. New York: Macmillian; 1918, pp. 215–329.
Frankel LK, Dublin LI. Sickness Survey of West Virginia Cities. New York: Metropolitan Life Insurance Co; 1914.
Frankel LK, Dublin LI. Community sickness survey. Rochester, N.Y., September, 1915. Public Health Rep 1916a;31:423–438.
Frankel LK, Dublin LI. A Sickness Survey of Boston, Mass. New York: Metropolitan Life Insurance Co; 1916b.
Frankel LK, Dublin LI. A sickness survey of North Carolina. Public Health Rep 1916c;31: 2820–2844.
Frankel LK, Dublin LI. Sickness Survey of Pittsburgh, Pennsylvania. New York: Metropolitan Life Insurance Co; 1917a.

Frankel LK, Dublin LI. Sickness Survey of Principal Cities in Pennsylvania and West Virginia. New York: Metropolitan Life Insurance Co; 1917b.
Frost WH, Sydenstricker E. Influenza in Maryland: preliminary statistics of certain localities. Public Health Rep 1919;34:491–504.
Glass DV. Numbering the People: The Eighteenth-Century Population Controversy and the Development of Census and Vital Statistics in Britain. Farnborough (Hants, UK): Saxon House; 1973.
Graunt J. Natural and Political Observations Mentioned in a Following Index, and Made upon the Bills of Mortality. London: John Martin; 1662.
Gutman R. Birth and death registration in Massachusetts. II. The inauguration of a modern system, 1800–1849. Milbank Mem Fund Q 1958;36:373–402.
Haywood A. The National Health Survey—in the beginning. Public Health Rep 1981; 96(3):195–209.
Infectious Disease Notification Act. Great Britain. Statutes at large, 52 & 53 Vict, c 72. 1889.
Infectious Disease (Notification) Extension Act. Great Britain. Statutes at large, 62 & 63 Vict, c 8. 1899.
Introduction. J Statist Soc Lond 1838;1:1–5.
Krieger N, Fee E. Measuring social inequalities in health in the United States: a historical review, 1900–1950. Int J Health Serv 1996;26:391–418.
Lambert R. Sir John Simon 1816–1904 and English Social Administration. London: MacGibbon & Kee; 1963.
Matthews JR. Quantification and the Quest for Medical Certainty. Princeton, NJ: Princeton University Press; 1995.
National Health Survey Act, Pub. L. No. 652. Stat. 3076. 3 July 1956.
Newsholme A. Elements of Vital Statistics. London: Sonnenchein; 1889.
Newsholme A. Elements of Vital Statistics in their Bearing on Social and Public Health Problems. Revised edition. London: George Allen and Unwin; 1923 and New York: D. Appleton; 1924.
Perrott GSJ, Collins SD. Sickness and the depression. Milbank Mem Fund Q 1933;11:281–298.
Perrott GSJ, Collins SD. Sickness among the "depression poor." Am J Public Health 1934a; 24:101–107.
Perrott GSJ, Collins SD. Sickness and the depression. Milbank Mem Fund Q 1934b;12:28–34, 99–114, 218–224.
Perrott GSJ, Collins SD. Relation of sickness to income and income change in 10 surveyed communities: health and depression studies no. 1: method of study and general results for each locality. Public Health Rep 1935;50:595–622.
Perrott GSJ, Collins SD, Sydenstricker E. Sickness and the economic depression: preliminary report on illness in families of wage earners in Birmingham, Detroit, and Pittsburgh. Public Health Rep 1933;48:1251–1264.
Perrott GSJ, Tibbitts C, Britten RH. The National Health Survey: scope and method of the nation-wide canvass of sickness in relation to its social and economic setting. In: U.S. Public Health Service, Division of Public Health Methods. The National Health Survey 1935–36. Washington, DC: GPO; 1951.
Registrar-General of Births, Deaths, and Marriages in England. Fifth Annual Report of the Registrar-General of Births, Deaths, and Marriages in England. London, HMSO; 1843.
Report of the Committee on the Cost of Medical Care [editorial]. JAMA 1932;99:1950–1952, 2034–2035.
Rosen G. Problems in the application of statistical analysis to questions of health: 1700–1880. Bull Hist Med 1955;29:27–45.
Rumsey HW. Essays and Papers on Some Fallacies of Statistics Concerning Life and Death, Health and Disease with Suggestions Towards an Improved System of Registration. London: Smith, Elder; 1875.

Sixth annual report of the Council of the Statistical Society of London. J Statist Soc Lond 1840;3:1–13.
Starr P. Social Transformation of American Medicine. New York: Basic Books; 1982.
Starr P. The sociology of official statistics. In: Alonso W, Starr P, eds. The Politics of Numbers. New York: Russell Sage Foundation; 1986, pp. 7–57.
Stecker ML. Some Recent Morbidity Data: A summary of Seven Community Sickness Surveys Made Among Policy Holders of the Metropolitan Life Insurance Company, 1915 to 1917. New York: Metropolitan Life Insurance Co; 1917.
Strickland SP. Politics, Science, and Dread Disease: A Short History of United States Medical Research Policy. Cambridge, MA: Harvard University Press; 1972.
Sydenstricker E. The incidence of illness in a general population group: general results of a morbidity study from December 1, 1921 through March 31, 1924 in Hagerstown, Md. Public Health Rep 1925;40:279–291.
Sydenstricker E. A study of illness in a general population group: Hagerstown morbidity studies No. 1: the method of study and general results. Public Health Rep 1926;41:2069–2088.
Sydenstricker E. Health and the depression. Milbank Mem Fund Q 1933;11:273–280.
Szreter S. The GRO and the public health movement in Britain, 1837–1914. Soc Hist Med 1991;4:435–463.
U.S. Department of Commerce and Labor, Bureau of the Census. Mortality statistics 1900 to 1904. Washington, DC: GPO; 1906.
U.S. Department of Health and Human Services, Centers for Disease Control and Prevention, National Center for Health Statistics. Current Legislative Authorities of the National Center for Health Statistics Enacted as of November 1999. Hyattsville, MD: National Center for Health Statistics; 2000.
U.S. Public Health Service, National Center for Health Statistics. Origin, Program, and Operation of the U.S. National Health Survey. National Center for Health Statistics Series 1, Number 1. Washington, DC: GPO; 1963.
U.S. Senate Committee on Labor and Public Welfare. Continuing Survey and Special Studies of Sickness and Disability in the United States. Report of the Senate Committee on Labor and Public Welfare, 84th Congress, 2nd Session, 26 March 1956.
Vaugan WT. Influenza: An Epidemiologic Study. Baltimore: American Journal of Hygiene Monograph No. 1; 1921.
Walker FA. Americanism versus sovietism: a study of the reaction to the Committee on the Costs of Medical Care. Bull Hist Med 1979;53:489–504.
Young GM. Victorian People: Portrait of an Age. 2nd ed. London: Oxford University Press; 1963.

CHAPTER 3

The Health Statistics Enterprise

Edward L. Hunter, Daniel J. Friedman, and R. Gibson Parrish II

The health statistics needed to understand the dynamics of and influences on the U.S. population's health involve the efforts of a diverse and decentralized enterprise. Individually, the organizations and people involved in producing health statistics are responsible for specific data systems and focused efforts to use and disseminate data, with the measure of success often defined as meeting a specific need or use. Collectively, these organizations and individuals constitute the health statistics enterprise. The measure of success of this enterprise is the extent to which these individual components work in concert to meet the broader mission of understanding the population's health and influences on it.

DEFINING THE HEALTH STATISTICS ENTERPRISE

The U.S. health statistics enterprise consists of the public and private organizations and individuals at all geopolitical levels that perform the processes (that is, carry out the activities) of health statistics. The U.S. health statistics enterprise is highly decentralized and diverse, without the overall organization and direction that often characterize corporate enterprises. The health statistics enterprise includes the many organizations that collect, analyze, and disseminate data on the health of populations and on the factors that influence health: (*1*) federal agencies, such as the National Center for Health Statistics (NCHS) of the Centers for Disease Control and Prevention (CDC), for which the generation of statistics and research is a central focus of their mission; (*2*) other federal activities that generate statistics as by-products of the agency mission, such as the Center for Cost and Financing Studies of the Agency for Healthcare Research and Quality and the Office of Applied Studies of the Substance Abuse and Mental Health Services Administration; (*3*) national private organizations, such as the American Hospital Association; (*4*) state and local public agencies, such as state centers for health statistics within state health departments, and county public health departments; (*5*) private third-party payers, such as health maintenance organizations and other health plans; and (*6*) private foundations and their grantees.

National health statistics enterprises generally reflect governmental organization in each country. An especially important influence on the nature of the health statistics enterprise in each country is the organization of health insurance and the health-care delivery system. Countries such as the United States, characterized by less centralized organization of health services and larger private roles in the provision of health insurance and health services, can be expected to have more decentralized health statistics enterprises. Countries such as Australia, Canada, and the United Kingdom, with greater governmental roles in the provision of health insurance and consequently of health services, can be expected to have health statistics enterprises characterized by more national planning and greater sustained national coordination of health statistics processes.

The activities of the health statistics enterprise include the collection of data from institutions, organizations, and individuals; aggregation and compilation of those data into health statistics; analysis and translation of health statistics in order to make them comprehensible to varied users; and evaluation of health statistics and the health statistics enterprise in order to improve them.

CHARACTERISTICS OF NATIONAL HEALTH STATISTICS ENTERPRISES

National health statistics enterprises can be described by the following major characteristics.

1. *Focus on the health of the population and the influences and actions that affect it.* While different organizations, individuals, and processes within the health statistics enterprise may focus on different influences and actions, ultimately all parts of the enterprise contribute to better understanding and characterizing the population's and subpopulations' health.
2. *Serve the public interest and generate products that are public goods.* The health statistics enterprise may include both public and private sector entities, all of which can contribute to the collection, aggregation, analysis, and translation of data. Government agencies, private sector health-care providers, insurers, and purchasers develop health statistics. Each of the organizations and individuals comprising the health statistics enterprise ultimately contributes to better understanding and characterizing the population's health. Data made available in the public domain by these entities become public

BOX 3.1

The National Health Statistics Enterprise

1. Focuses on the health of the population and subpopulations
2. Serves the public interest and generates products that are public goods
3. Engages in systematic and organized inquiry
4. Strives for scientific objectivity
5. Involves multiple disciplines
6. Links national health statistics activities to those of international partners in health and health statistics

goods in the economic sense, in that once they are made available, multiple users can use them for multiple purposes.

3. *Engage in systematic and organized inquiry.* The health statistics enterprise relies upon systematic data collection, aggregation, analysis, and translation. Health statistics entail organized inquiry, not unsystematic collection of anecdotes and personal impressions.
4. *Strive for scientific objectivity.* The health statistics enterprise strives for scientific objectivity in data collection, aggregation, analysis, and translation and attempts to minimize or eliminate any explicit political biases in its activities. The choice of priorities within the health statistics enterprise is necessarily based upon a series of choices about what constitutes and how to measure the health of a population, and what influences on health merit study and how to assess their influences (Krieger 1992). These choices of priorities within the health statistics enterprise may be made at the societal level, at the health agency level, or occasionally by health statistics practitioners themselves. Such choices are inherently based upon values and judgments; however, once the choices of priorities are made, health statistics practitioners make scientific objectivity a preeminent concern.
5. *Involve multiple disciplines.* The practice of health statistics involves multiple disciplines, including statistics, epidemiology, health services research, demography, public health informatics, information technology, and economics.
6. *Link national efforts to those of international partners in health and health statistics.* The national health statistics enterprise is guided by international health statistics standards and policies, such as periodic revisions to the International Classification of Diseases codes. The national health statistics enterprise also contributes to international discussions of health statistics methods and provides health statistics to international agencies for comparative purposes.

BOX 3.2
Health Statistics Cycle Hub—Integrating the Health Statistics Enterprise

Elements:

- Defining data needs
- Specifying necessary data attributes
- Identifying appropriate data sources and strategies
- Collecting, aggregating, and compiling data
- Analyzing statistics
- Translating statistics for users
- Evaluating extent to which user needs are met

THE HEALTH STATISTICS ENTERPRISE AND THE HEALTH STATISTICS CYCLE

The performance of the health statistics enterprise, as well as of many individual programs that collect data and manage statistics, involves a number of key elements that are described in the health statistics cycle (Fig. 3.1). This model can be used to describe the steps required to define and meet data needs, to evaluate the strengths and weaknesses of current programs, and to suggest ways in which different components of the health statistics enterprise can be tied together into a more cohesive whole (Friedman et al. 2002).

Elements in the Health Statistics Cycle

Figure 3.1 depicts seven elements in the health statistics cycle, arrayed in a circle, with each element leading to the next. Importantly, there is no first or last step; the model recognizes that the health statistics enterprise needs to be in a constant state of evolution, evaluation, and regeneration. The model is applicable both to the development of new statistical efforts and to efforts to make existing data systems that produce health statistics more effective. The model is also equally applicable to looking at the overall health statistics enterprise and to focusing on individual data systems or data needs.

Defining Data Needs

In the aggregate, the data needs to be met by the health statistics enterprise are determined by an ongoing and iterative process. The overall data

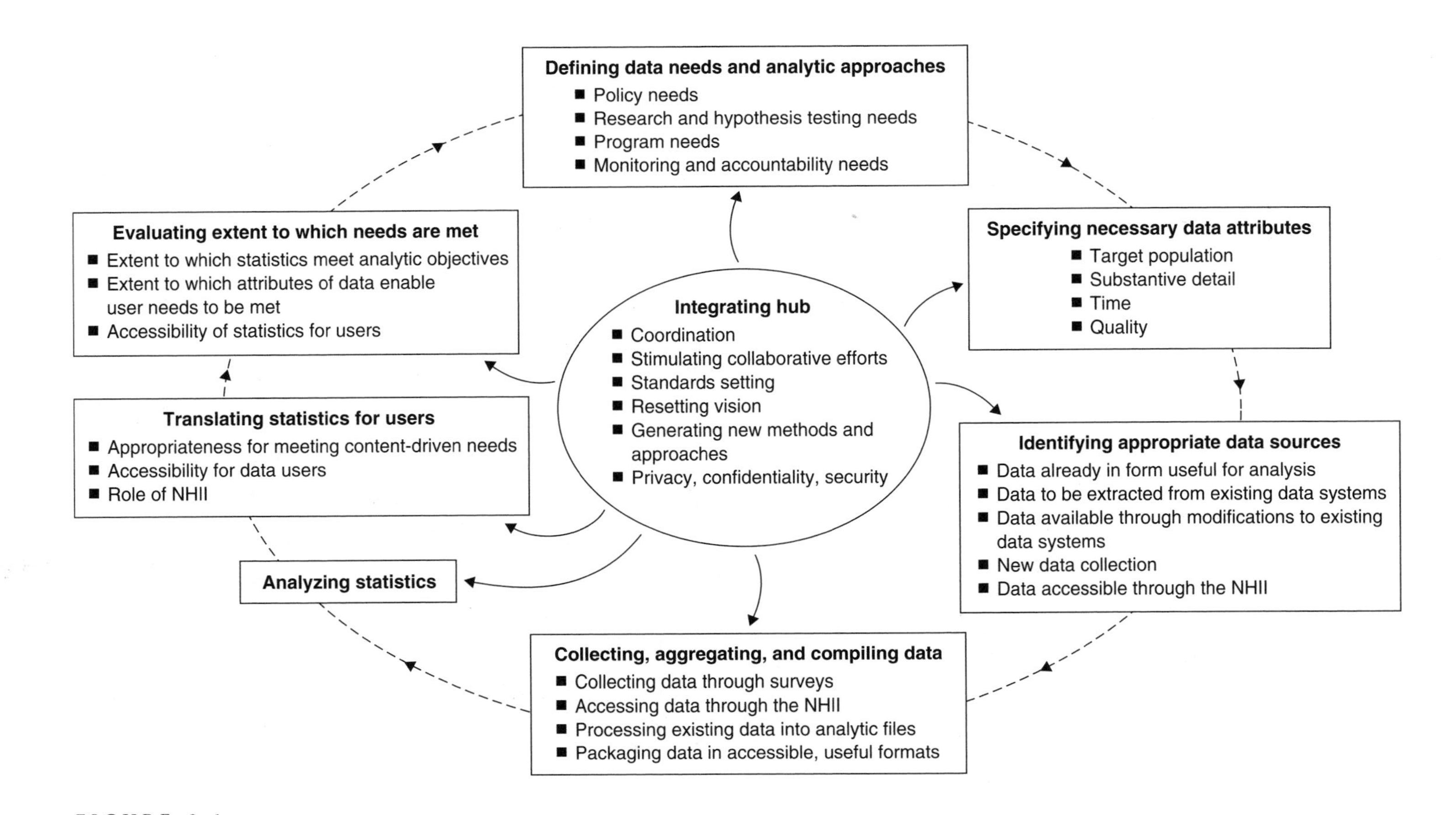

FIGURE 3.1
Health statistics cycle. NHII = National Health Information Infrastructure. (Source: Friedman et al. 2002, p. 21.)

needed to promote understanding of the population's health and the influences on the population's health are reflected by the scope of Figure 1.3. In working to address more specific needs, organizations that collect and compile statistics help add specificity to often generally stated needs of data users, and work with data providers (such as respondents to surveys and managers of healthcare records) to help translate these needs into detailed definitions and specifications. Each of these needs is grounded in specific data uses: knowledge development (see Chapter 10); health policy, such as data to document the lack of health insurance or the relationship between the lack of health insurance and access to care, and to evaluate alternative programs to address lack of coverage (see Chapter 11); and public health practices such as monitoring community health status and outcomes, assessing community health, designing public health programs and targeting interventions, evaluating public health programs and policies, and informing the public (see Chapter 12).

Specifying Necessary Data Attributes

Data needed to support these uses can be further specified in terms of the attributes resulting statistics must have to fulfill the required use. This greater specificity is needed so that systematic efforts can be made to identify appropriate data sources. Data attributes include:

- Characteristics of the populations under study, such as racial/ethnic and socioeconomic subgroups, and age/sex breakdowns.
- Degree of geographic detail, such as national, regional, community, or even more granular levels.
- Depth and complexity of information required to meet the need, such as the number of questions to be asked regarding a particular topic in a telephone survey or the level to which data are coded in a classification system.
- Length of time to be observed, ranging from a single point in time to a full calendar year to a range of years.
- Data quality, such as timeliness of reporting of results, both in terms of the turnaround time for data processing and in terms of the currency of the time period for which data are collected; degree of sensitivity and specificity needed to meet user needs; and extent to which observations need to be validated, verified, tested for reliability, or subjected to other methods of ensuring data quality.
- Type of data source, such as an individual or a family member, health records, or other administrative records.
- Mode of data collection, such as a survey of individuals; notifications, registries, or registration systems; administrative health records systems; or other mechanisms.

Identifying Appropriate Data Sources and Strategies

With detailed specifications, various data sources or strategies can be evaluated in order to rapidly and efficiently meet user needs. Strategies, in increasing order of cost and complexity, may include:

- Identifying existing data that are already in formats meeting user specifications and accessible for analysis.
- Extracting data from existing data sets.
- Identifying opportunities to use data initially collected for nonstatistical purposes (such as administration or patient care).
- Adapting existing data collection systems to meet new needs.
- Designing and implementing new data collection systems.

These sources and strategies are further detailed in the chapters in Part 2.

Collecting, Aggregating, and Compiling Data

Depending on the strategy selected, this element in the health statistics cycle includes steps ranging from simple data acquisition to the management of complex, ongoing data systems:

- Establishing data use agreements with (or purchasing data from) organizations that manage existing data systems. In Canada, for example, the Canadian Institute for Health Information works to facilitate data sharing and aggregation.
- Creating user-accessible analytic files from existing data sets. An example would be processing administrative health records into formats useful for data analysis.
- Aggregating statistics from multiple sources and creating new statistical products that, because of the synergy created by combining data sets, have analytic usefulness beyond that of any one component data set. An example is the linkage of data about local air or water quality to surveys of human health.
- Managing ongoing surveys and other data collection systems to meet the needs of multiple users.
- Launching surveys or other data collection approaches to meet specific user needs, such as targeted surveys to measure immunization status in communities.

Analyzing Statistics

Once data are in usable form, analysts must carefully define and apply analytic approaches. Individual components of the health statistics enterprise devote considerable resources to developing analytic packages and tools that can be directly applied to specific data sets or data that are derived from individual data systems, such as those established for analysis of the National Household Survey on Drug Abuse (Substance Abuse and Mental Health Services Administration [hp]). Fewer efforts have been devoted to development of more widely applicable analytic tools and approaches that minimize the learning curve for individual users; efforts like the Federal Electronic Research and Review Extraction Tool (FERRET) of the U.S. Bureau of the Census achieved success but failed to gain broad acceptance or adoption by other producers of data (U.S. Bureau of the Census [hp] Welcome to DataFERRETT!).

Translating Statistics for Use

Organizations that collect and compile health statistics bear responsibility for ensuring that the data collected are translated into forms that maximize their appropriate and successful use. Professional statisticians and data processing specialists typically staff organizations that collect and compile data, while many users are untrained in statistics and techniques for accessing them. The translation function seeks to bridge this gulf. For systems geared to meeting narrowly defined needs of specific users (e.g., when a specific set of questions is added to a multipurpose survey to meet address a programmatic use), this element of the health statistics cycle involves a direct relationship between producer and user. More generally, the health statistics enterprise is responsible for steps including:

- Making data available in forms appropriate to the level of sophistication of potential users. These forms range from raw micro-level data, such as detailed individual-level files from the National Medical Expenditure Survey that could be downloaded from the Internet for analysis and used in microsimulation modeling, to tabular or graphic presentations of the same data, such as a table depicting health expenditures by source of payment (Agency for Heathcare Research and Quality [hp]).
- Providing easy access for potential users, for example through interactive World Wide Web systems designed to provide community users with access to health statistics data, such as Massachusetts' MassCHIP system, Missouri's MICA system, and Washington State's Vista/PH (Friedman, et al. 2001).
- Making it easier for users to locate available data, for example through World Wide Web portals that provide users with topical listings of data sources, such as a U.S. federal government effort to direct users to statistical resources and the Illinois Project for Local Assessment of Needs Web site highlighting indicators available at the state and local levels in Illinois (FedStats [hp]; Illinois Department of Public Health [hp] IPLAN). Such efforts simplify the task of "identifying appropriate data sources" described earlier in the cycle.

- Providing technical assistance, training, and coaching to users, for example through distance training techniques such as World Wide Web–based interactive courses, through video-based training resources such as CDC's "Public Health Data: Our Silent Partner," through in-person training in conducting community health assessments, or through providing adequate explanations of statistical concepts such as confidence intervals in written reports (Centers for Disease Control and Prevention 1999).

In the United States, many of these steps will be facilitated by further development of an overall National Health Information Infrastructure (NHII), which will provide greater interconnectivity between health providers and establish a framework for data access and exchange (see Chapter 20).

Evaluating the Extent to Which Needs Are Met

An integral component in the health statistics cycle is the continuing evaluation of the extent to which needs are met and the identification of improvements that can be made. Without this explicit step, systems for collecting or compiling health statistics risk stagnation and irrelevance. This element involves multiple strategies and approaches, relying on direct feedback from users and extensive links outside the health statistics enterprise. Questions to be addressed in such an evaluation include:

- Are individual data collection systems meeting defined analytic objectives? In other words, are the data collection systems actually addressing the data questions that have been asked?
- Are the specific data attributes necessary or sufficient for addressing analytic objectives? In other words, are we collecting too much detail or not enough?
- Have analytic objectives changed, requiring change in or elimination of data collection systems? (If other systems have evolved since the initial selection of a data strategy, can they meet these needs?)
- Are data accessible enough for users, and are the tools available to support a level of analysis that meets user needs?
- Is the health statistics enterprise as a whole meeting its mission and addressing broadly defined data needs required for understanding influences on health?
- Is the health statistics enterprise as a whole operating in an efficient manner?

Hub—Integrating the Health Statistics Enterprise

At the core of the health statistics enterprise is a set of activities and functions that collectively represent an integrating *hub*. These efforts must ensure that the diverse and decentralized set of organizations and individuals in the health statistics enterprise work in concert to meet a broader agenda. An effective hub, which may involve multiple organizations, approaches, and influences, can serve as a center of gravity for diverse elements, holding the health statistics enterprise together and ensuring that the cycle of development and improvement continues to move in constructive ways. If the movement from element to element in Figure 3.1 can be viewed as driven by the winds of a hurricane, the integrating hub is the "eye" around which these elements move.

Critical functions of the integrating hub include:

- Fostering information sharing among diverse players spanning different levels of government, public and private entities, and related functions.
- Stimulating collaborative statistical efforts.
- Facilitating the process of locating and accessing data from diverse sources.
- Developing and maintaining common definitions, technical standards, classifications, methodological benchmarks, and so forth, that facilitate data sharing, systems integration, and comparability of data.
- Renewing and revisiting the overall vision for the health statistics enterprise at defined intervals and evaluating whether the overall enterprise is meeting its mission.
- Stimulating research and development directed toward new methods and approaches.
- Providing guidance and policy on privacy, confidentiality, and security as they apply to health statistics and the organizations that collect, compile, and disseminate them.
- Ensuring user and wider public input into decisions that affect the overall performance of the health statistics enterprise and of its individual component systems.

MAJOR ORGANIZATIONS AND ENTITIES IN THE HEALTH STATISTICS ENTERPRISE

In the United States, the diversity and number of organizations and entities that are involved in the health statistics enterprise make a simple categorization difficult. A large number of organizations are involved in defining data needs, analyzing data, and using health statistics. A comparatively smaller number are involved in the direct operation of data collection systems, while still fewer are involved in the process of defining and integrating health statistics from an enterprisewide perspective. In this section, these organizations are described in order to aid in identifying functional gaps in the overall health statistics enterprise.

It is worth noting that some other countries have engaged in more concerted and ongoing data set integration and national health information priority-setting than the United States. Canada, for example, is now in its second round of national consultations to identify health services and policy issues requiring research (Canadian Health Services Research Foundation 2003). Australia, for example, has developed a National Health Information Agreement and a National Health Information Development Plan that are used to develop work plans and benchmarks for health information at national, state, and territorial levels (Australian Institute for Health and Welfare [hp] Development Priorities; Australian Institute for Health and Welfare [hp] Work Plan).Chapter 17 provides many more examples of such national health information planning and coordination activities in various countries.

Table 3.1 reflects the major functional elements in the health statistics cycle, and provides U.S. examples of the organizations and entities carrying out these functions at the national, state, and local levels. At the national level, data needs are often expressed in broad terms by Congress and the executive branch; by advocacy groups; by the business community; by the research community; and by managers of federal health programs. These broadly stated needs are translated into specifications for individual data collection systems by a large number of public and private entities that are engaged in data collection and dissemination. Federal statistical agencies are charged with the continuing operation of large-scale national data system that are geared to meeting multiple (as opposed to specific, categorical) data needs, but these agencies are augmented by many other research and programmatic entities. The NCHS within the CDC is the only federal agency with a singular mission of providing health statistics, but the NCHS is actually responsible for only about one-tenth of the spending on health statistics by its parent department, the U.S. Department of Health and Human Services (DHHS) (Office of Management and Budget 2001). Other centers, institutes, and offices within the CDC also maintain major ongoing surveys and data collection systems. Ongoing national health-related data systems are managed by virtually every other agency within the DHHS, and administrative data from the Medicare program and other federally administered programs are often made available for research and statistical purposes. Data from nonhealth agencies, such as the Census Bureau (e.g., data on population demographics and health insurance coverage) and the Bureau of Labor Statistics (e.g., data on work-related injury and employee health benefits) are important for the study of health, and private data sources, often funded by foundations, provide data frequently used by policy analysts and researchers. Professional associations, such as the American Medical Association and the American Hospital Association, provide widely used information from surveys of their members. Similarly, private organizations, often supported by foundations, frequently conduct significant studies and surveys, such as the Center for Studying Health Systems Change's Community Tracking Study and the Urban Institute's National Survey of America's Families (Center for Studying Health Systems Change [hp]; Urban Institute [hp]).

At the state level in the United States, the complexity of interaction within the health statistics enterprise is similar. All states have a vital statistics function and conduct population surveys of behavioral risk factors, maintain ongoing

TABLE 3.1

Programs and Activities that Contribute to the Health Statistics Cycle in the United States at the National, State, and Local Levels

Step in Cycle	*Examples of Programs and Activities: National Level*	*Examples of Programs and Activities: State Level*	*Examples of Programs and Activities: Local Level*
Define data needs	Legislation and congressional support organizations (e.g., Congressional Research Service, General Accounting Office, Congressional Budget Office); administration policy priorities; federal agency policy and regulatory agendas; operational and research needs of program managers of federal program operations; advisory bodies (e.g., the National Committee on Vital and Health Statistics [NCVHS]); findings of review and study panels (e.g., the National Academy of Sciences and Institute of Medicine); reports of commissions; scientific literature	State legislatures; executive agency policies; managers of State program operations; advisory bodies operational and research needs of program managers	County and city councils; local executive agency policies; managers of local program operations; Turning Point grantees
Specify necessary data attributes	Centers and programs within the Centers for Disease Control and Prevention (CDC), including the National Center for Health Statistics; Agency for Healthcare Quality and Research; other federal statistical agencies; other Department of Health and Human Services (DHHS) components	State Centers for Health Statistics; state epidemiologists; state chronic disease epidemiologists; Robert Wood Johnson Foundation–funded State Health Access Data Assistance Center; Urban Institute-Assessing New Federalism	

TABLE 3.1
Continued

Step in Cycle	*Examples of Programs and Activities: National Level*	*Examples of Programs and Activities: State Level*	*Examples of Programs and Activities: Local Level*
Identify appropriate data sources	FedStats, a gateway to statistics from federal agencies	State Centers for Health Statistics; state epidemiologists; state chronic disease epidemiologists	
Collect, aggregate, and compile data	Multiple centers and programs within the CDC, including the National Center for Health Statistics; Agency for Healthcare Quality and Research; other federal statistical agencies; other DHHS components; foundation-supported entities and organizations such as the Center for Studying Health Systems Change	State Centers for Health Statistics; state epidemiologists; state chronic disease epidemiologists	
Analyze and interpret data	Centers and programs within the CDC, including the National Center for Health Statistics; Agency for Healthcare Quality and Research; other federal statistical agencies; other DHHS components; foundation-supported organizations such as the Center for Studying Health Systems Change	State Centers for Health Statistics; state epidemiologists; state chronic disease epidemiologists	
Communicate and translate findings (statistics)	FedStats, a gateway to statistics from federal agencies	State Centers for Health Statistics; state epidemiologists; state chronic disease epidemiologists; state health department	County and other local health department Web sites

(*continued*)

TABLE 3.1
Continued

Step in Cycle	*Examples of Programs and Activities: National Level*	*Examples of Programs and Activities: State Level*	*Examples of Programs and Activities: Local Level*
		Web sites (e.g., Missouri's Missouri Information for Community Assessment [MICA], Massachusetts' MassCHIP, VistaPH, Illinois Project for Local Assessment of Needs)	
Evaluate extent to which needs are met	DHHS Data Council; Committee on National Statistics, National Academy of Sciences; NCVHS		
Integrating statistics	DHHS Data Council; NCVHS; standards development organizations; CDC's National Electronic Disease Surveillance System (NEDSS) program; Public Health Standards Data Consortium		

surveillance systems for communicable diseases, and collect data on newly diagnosed cases of cancer. Many state health departments have well-developed health data centers that produce or integrate data from multiple sources. As providers or financers of care, states maintain systems from which statistical information can be derived, collecting data as by-products of the Medicaid program and the State Children's Health Insurance Program (SCHIP) and patient-level data from the provision of clinical care. As protectors of the public's health and as regulators of health-care providers, state agencies also maintain systems that gather public health surveillance reports as well as data collected through the oversight and enforcement arms of state government (such as licensing, certification, insurance oversight, worker compensation enforcement, and overseeing nursing home quality). Nonpublic sources also play an important role; for example, in many states, hospital associations aggregate data on hospital discharges and make them available for statistical analysis. At the local and community levels, statistical efforts are more episodic and sporadic. Health departments in larger cities and counties—such as New York City, Boston, Seattle/King County, and Los Angeles County—have well-developed health statistics offices.

Finally, a number of organizations are involved in efforts to integrate and coordinate efforts across the U.S. health statistics enterprise. At the national level, the National Committee on Vital and Health Statistics (NCVHS) provides advice to the Secretary of the DHHS and serves as a bridge to the private sector on health information policy issues, while the internal DHHS Data Council brings together the DHHS agencies to coordinate statistical efforts. Individual agencies have funded data planning and integration efforts, such as CDC's Public Health Information Network and its component, the National Electronic Disease Surveillance System (Centers for Disease Control and Prevention [hp] NEDSS; Centers for Disease Control and Prevention [hp] PHIN). National standards development organizations, such as the American National Standards Institute and its subject matter–oriented subgroups, facilitate processes for arriving at data standards that transcend public and private organizations and functions (see Chapter 8), and professional associations such as the National Association for Public Health Statistics and Information Systems, the Association for Maternal and Child Health Programs, the Council of State and Territorial Epidemiologists, and the Association of State and Territorial Health Officers undertake data planning initiatives that have impact in all states. The Public Health Data Standards Consortium is a coalition of more than 30 national and state organizations committed to promoting and developing common data standards for pubic health and human services research (Public Health Data Standards Consortium [hp]). Both nationally and in many states, some health statistics agencies influence the coordination and integration of data collection efforts, including the NCHS and some state centers for health statistics. Finally, foundations often provide leadership in data planning and coordination; for example, the Robert Wood Johnson Foundation has funded the Information for State Health Policy program and the recently established State Health Access Data Assistance Center, and the Robert Wood Johnson Foundation and the Pew Charitable Trusts fund the Trust for America's Health, which has stimulated efforts to better coordinate data related to the environment and health (Trust for America's Health [hp]; University of Minnesota [hp]).

MAJOR ISSUES AND GAPS IN THE U.S. HEALTH STATISTICS ENTERPRISE

A U.S. nationwide process began in 1999 to inform the development of *Shaping a Health Statistics Vision for the 21st Century*, a joint report of the NCVHS, the NCHS, and the DHHS Data Council (Friedman et al. 2002). The process relied on input from a wide range of experts in health statistics and their uses, and documented significant gaps and issues in the health statistics enterprise.

Participants in the national process generally agreed that the U.S. health statistics enterprise possesses many positive features. Many participants noted the completeness and usefulness of data systems in the United States, and some felt that sufficient data were already available for a large number of specific policy and programmatic purposes. Other participants noted improvements in the availability and usability of data sets, gains made in making data more widely available through the Internet and other electronic media, and the burgeoning efforts to develop data standards through the Health Insurance Portability and Accountability Act (HIPAA) and other mechanisms.

Despite the perceived strengths of the U.S. health statistics enterprise and the masses of data collected by various systems, experts in health statistics and their uses noted gaps in the availability of data and in the ability of the current components of the health statistics enterprise to fully address needs expressed by data users. In a sense, these gaps indicate that the health statistics enterprise may be rich in data but poor in information. Major criticism of the current health statistics enterprise focuses on the difficulty in identifying appropriate data resources and in translating raw data into information useful for action at appropriate geographic levels. The major issues, and resulting gaps in the health statistics cycle, as identified in the national process to develop the NCVHS report *Shaping a Health Statistics Vision for the 21st Century*, are described here (Friedman et al. 2002).

Insufficient Connections Between Data Sources (the Suppliers of Data, Such as Individual Respondents to Surveys, Hospitals Holding Patient Records, and So Forth), Organizations That Collect or Aggregate Data (Such as Organizations That Conduct Surveys or Compile Data from Administrative Systems), and Data Users

The traditional view of health statistics has been limited to the collection, compilation, analysis, and processing of data—a static view that lacks explicit connections to users on both the front end (defining data needs and specifying necessary attributes) and the back end (translating statistics and evaluating the extent to which needs are met). In recent years, there has been a constructive trend toward more formal reviews of data needs associated with important health issues. More often than not, however, these data reviews focus on a single subject (such as a U.S. General Accounting Office study on environmental health statistics) or on specific statistical issues. Furthermore, the data reviews are generally but one of many topics addressed in the context of a more broadly focused study of a health issue (e.g., a discussion of issues in racial and ethnic data was included in the recent Institute of Medicine report on disparities in health care (Smedley et al. 2002; U.S. General Accounting Office 2000). While these efforts are valuable, they are not useful in evaluating priorities across different health data needs or in integrating the efforts of data collection mechanisms that address multiple topics. Few are formally established as ongoing mechanisms that address enterprisewide issues more broadly.

Lack of Geographic Detail and Other Specificity

Some data are available on many influences on the population's health and on many aspects of the working of the health services system. While such data may exist at the national level for many research purposes, it is clear that these data are not sufficiently detailed to meet most research, policy, or programmatic purposes. The relative lack of data on major health issues and trends at the state and community levels is a clear concern, and participants maintained that this lack of data has hampered the effective pursuit of public health goals.

Similarly, participants noted the lack of sufficient detail on race/ethnicity, income, and other sociodemographic factors in existing health statistics even in large national efforts to collect health-related data; an expert panel convened by the National Research Council's Committee on National Statistics is currently examining these gaps (National Research Council [hp] Panel on DHHS). The lack of such detail has hampered research into the underlying causes of differentials in health; limited efforts to target interventions to groups at greatest risk for poor health; and made more difficult the task of monitoring and evaluating the effectiveness of public programs to improve health.

Lack of Timeliness in Making Data Available

Data users express frustration with the chronic inability of existing systems at all levels of geography and detail to produce results that can be used to rapidly identify and address current health problems. While progress has been made in improving the timeliness of many data systems (e.g., the NCHS has reduced the time required to produce results from the National Health and Nutrition Examination Survey from 3 years to 1 year after a completed survey year for many findings), many systems lag decades behind in implementing technology that is in widespread use in other sectors. For example, though efforts are underway to make improvements, many state vital statistics systems still rely on outmoded electronic systems to process some of the most widely used health statistics.

Existing Data Are Unnecessarily Difficult to Locate, Access, and Use

For the health statistics enterprise to be efficient and to avoid unnecessary duplication of effort, it is important to make maximum use of all relevant data that are collected. Three major impediments exist. First, knowledge of data resources is limited, and there are few comprehensive and readily available guides to finding existing data. While some data collection agencies make data available in searchable formats on the Internet, others do not; even when data are available, it is not readily apparent to many users how to search the Internet to find them. Data collected for specific analytic purposes—or for proprietary purposes—are often not widely publicized or referenced in searchable form. Second, once found, data are often not available in a user-friendly format, placing burdens on the user that can discourage use or make it more likely that a new data collection mechanism will be developed to meet the user's need. Making data widely and easily available can be expensive for data collection organizations, limiting access even to data collected for public purposes and for the public good. Third, barriers due to legal, administrative, and proprietary concerns as well as to organizational practices inhibit the use of existing data resources.

Resource Constraints Have Placed the Performance and Usefulness of Major Data Collection Systems at Risk (Rice 2001)

Data systems that have multiple purposes and address multiple health topics, such as the National Health Interview Survey, can be efficient mechanisms for meeting data needs. By sharing a basic infrastructure, these systems address multiple issues and can often be used to meet specialized needs for more detailed data. For example, many DHHS major surveys include a core of content designed to meet general needs, along with supplements or specialized components developed to meet a defined research or programmatic need. Yet these shared systems face chronic resource limitations, and have in some cases deteriorated to the point where they are at risk. Losing these workhorse data systems would cause an interruption in the data needed to monitor trends, lead to a lack of comparability across years, reduce opportunities for integration of diverse data activities, and spawn multiple, less efficient efforts more narrowly focused on specific needs or uses. Efforts to support funding for core data systems of the NCHS, for example, often note the multiple purposes served by single survey mechanisms (U.S. Department of Health and Human Services 2004).

Existing health statistics enterprisewide coordinating and integrating efforts in the United States have been of limited utility, hampering potential collective efforts of the diverse elements in the health statistics enterprise to move toward needed improvements in health statistics. A great deal of effort has been devoted to such mechanisms in recent years, and organizations at the national and state levels have made progress in bringing about greater cohesion in the health statistics enterprise. Nonetheless, there is wide agreement on several issues.

First, despite recent CDC efforts to better coordinate the health statistics enterprise, there is still insufficient attention to developing consensus approaches and standards that would simplify collecting, protecting, and accessing data and make more efficient the process of developing methods, software, and specifications for individual data systems. Important topics to be addressed or continue to be addressed include, for example, standards for systems architecture, comparable questionnaires, common classification and coding systems, standards for the way in which data will be exchanged over the Internet, and conventions for presenting and formatting data that reduce the learning curve for users of multiple data sets.

Second, the health statistics enterprise, because it is decentralized as well as underfunded, has insufficiently invested in new methods (such as more efficient sampling approaches), technologies (such as Web-enabled, meta-data repositories, electronic data access initiatives), and integrated approaches (such as combining survey field operations, unifying data entry systems for clients served by multiple state programs) that could reduce costs, improve data quality and availability, and provide added confidentiality protection.

Third, insufficient attention has been given within the health statistics enterprise specifically and within public health more generally to developing and implementing training in health statistics. For example, testifiers at the NCVHS public hearings could cite no U.S. school of public health that currently offers even an introductory course devoted to health statistics. Graduate-level training is needed to introduce health statistics to masters and doctorate students. Additionally, expanded in-service training is needed for professionals already engaged in any elements of the health statistics cycle beyond the valuable training already offered to state department of health employees by the NCHS. In order to be most useful, such in-service training should rely upon a range of training modalities, including short courses at regular professional meetings and Web-based courses.

Fourth, participants in the health statistics enterprise have not been effective in working with decision makers who influence the processes that ultimately determine the availability of much of the data needed for studying health-related issues. Data sources for health statistics are often by-products of decisions made primarily for nonhealth or nonstatistical reasons, such as the structure or content of a medical claim; the laws and regulations governing access to medical records for research and statistical purposes; the standards for legal or administrative records; or the data elements included in data systems focused on the labor force or population demographics. Given the wide scope of influences on health, the ability to use nonhealth data sources constitutes a strength of the health statistics enterprise; however, this often requires the major task of piecing together a patchwork of data resources. The current health statistics enterprise largely lacks the capacity to develop and articulate effective statements about the need for data, to engage with the producers of nonhealth sources of data, and to effectively pursue opportunities to use data that flow from these other producers.

Fifth, the health statistics enterprise lacks a consistent, effective confidentiality and data-sharing framework that would facilitate the integration and linkage of information while protecting the privacy of individual data (see Chapter 14). Current systems for public health data, as well as underlying health records, are covered by a patchwork of state and federal laws and regulations. These protections rarely address issues associated with the creation and use of large databases with both the potential for important public purposes and the risk of individual disclosure.

Sixth, insufficient support, training, and assistance are available to users of health statistics. Most data are released in a form that requires users to have a high level of statistical sophistication as well as direct experience with the individual data set. Comparatively few resources are devoted to *help desks*, to the development of materials accompanying a data file that give users a clear description of how the data were collected and their limitations, to the development of meta-data Web sites to enable identification of data sources, or to training of users. Many system managers invest resources in meeting the specialized needs of their own users, but few address more general issues of building a competent user community that can effectively use data resources to inform policy and program management. There are constructive, though limited, examples. The NCHS offers the University Visitation Program and the biennial NCHS Data Users Conference, though these conferences are directed to a relatively small group of technically sophisticated users (National Center for Health Statistics [hp]). The Manitoba Centre for Health Policy has created an on-line *concepts dictionary* to aid programmers, helping to create an institutional memory to facilitate analysis (Manitoba Centre for Health Policy [hp]).

Seventh, a suboptimal allocation of resources—or an undue burden on providers of data—results from the lack of coordination among elements of the health statistics enterprise. If users are unable to identify and use existing data or work with organizations to modify existing data systems, there is a tendency to initiate new, single-purpose data collection systems. This can lead to duplication of effort, lost opportunities for efficient shared systems, and the failure to gain maximum value from data that are collected.

Eighth, the health statistics enterprise lacks flexibility and adaptability. For a number of reasons, it is difficult for organizations that operate systems that produce health statistics to adapt quickly to meet new needs. The funding for health statistics is distributed throughout the decentralized health statistics enterprise, and many key data sources are not principally designed to address health issues. As a result, it is often difficult to reallocate funding to emerging health needs. Managers of data systems must balance the need for stable trend data against the need to address new issues. Further, in the absence of new resources, data system managers may choose to tinker with existing systems rather than to introduce fundamental changes.

Finally, these issues—and the persistent presence of data gaps—provide evidence of a fundamental lack of a health statistics enterprisewide planning forum in the United States. Some entities have gained a measure of success in planning for specific elements of health statistics. For example, public/private standards development organizations are effective forums for developing consensus standards in specific areas, such as uniform billing records and standards for electronic transactions. The role of the NCVHS has expanded in providing advice to the DHHS on the implementation of the data standards aspects of recent congressionally mandated administrative simplification initiatives, and the DHHS Data Council provides a forum for coordinating activities within the Department, playing a role in reviewing agency budget initiatives. However, there is no single place in the United States where these efforts are all tied together. While the existence of these and other separate planning and coordination efforts can be taken as an indication of the widespread view that such functions are needed, these multiple initiatives and forums themselves add to the perception of fragmentation and disorganization in the overall health statistics enterprise.

An effective planning and decision-making effort can improve integration and coordination, help set systemwide goals and expectations, establish common frameworks and standards, and find ways to develop funding sources to ensure that the enterprise meets the needs of users in an effective and efficient manner. The NCVHS has made a number of recommendations in this regard (NCVHS 2002).

CONCLUSION

The health statistics enterprise is best viewed as an assemblage of diverse organizations and individuals that, though often operating in an independent and decentralized manner, share common characteristics, goals, and functions. This chapter attempts to define the characteristics of a national health statistics enterprise and develops a framework (the health statistics cycle) to describe the relationship of the various functions carried out within this enterprise. At the core of this enterprise is an integrating hub that provides for coordination of diverse organizations, standards, and integration of separate statistical efforts. This integrating hub is stronger in countries with more central direction of health services. In the United States, a wide range of entities shares the functions of this hub, and the creation of a strong central focus for planning and coordination of national health statistics efforts is an ongoing challenge.

NOTE

Much of the material in this chapter was originally published in Friedman et al. (2002), pp. 13–34. The "vision" process reflected input from a lengthy consultative process documented at http://www.ncvhs.hhs.gov/hsvision/visiondevelopment.html.

REFERENCES

Agency for Healthcare Research and Quality [homepage on the Internet]. Rockville, MD: Agency for Healthcare Quality and Research [cited 2004 Feb 15]. Medical Expenditure Panel Survey. Available from: http://www.meps.ahrq.gov.

Australian Institute for Health and Welfare [monograph on the Internet]. National Health Information Development Priorities Canberra: Australian Institute for Health and Welfare; 2002 [cited 2004 Mar 5]. Available from: http://www.aihw.gov.au/publications/hwi/nhidp/index.html.

Australian Institute for Health and Welfare [homepage on the Internet]. Canberra: Australian Institute for Health and Welfare [cited 2004 Mar 5]. National health information agreement work program 1995–96. Available from: http://www.aihw.gov.au/publications/index.cfm?type=detail&id=168.

Canadian Health Services Research Foundation [monograph on the Internet]. Listening for Direction II: A National Consultation on Health Services and Policy Issues. Ottawa: Canadian Health Services Research Foundation; 2003 [cited 2004 Mar 5]. Available from: http://www.chsrf.ca/other_documents/listening/pdf/LfD_II_Summary_e.pdf.

Center for Studying Health System Change [homepage on the Internet]. Washington, DC: Center for Studying Health System Change [cited 2004 Mar 5]. Design and methods for the Community Tracking Study. Available from: http://www.hschange.org/index.cgi?data=01.

Centers for Disease Control and Prevention. Public Health Data: Our Silent Partner. Atlanta: Centers for Disease Control and Prevention; 1999.

Centers for Disease Control and Prevention [homepage on the Internet]. Atlanta: Centers for Disease Control and Prevention [cited 2004 Mar 5]. National Electronic Disease Surveillance System. Available from: http://www.cdc.gov/programs/research12.htm.

Centers for Disease Control and Prevention [homepage on the Internet]. Atlanta: Centers for Disease Control and Prevention; [cited 2004 Mar 5]. Public Health Information Network. Available from: http://www.cdc.gov/phin.

FedStats homepage on the Internet; [cited 2004 Mar 5]. Available from: http://www.fedstats.gov.

Friedman DJ, Anderka M, Krieger J, Land G, Solet D. Accessing population health information through interactive systems: lessons learned and future directions. Public Health Rep 2001;116(2):132–141.

Friedman DJ, Hunter EL, Parrish RG, eds. Shaping a Health Statistics Vision for the 21st Century. Final Report, November 2002. Hyattsville, MD: Centers for Disease Control and Prevention, National Center for Health Statistics; Washington, DC: U.S. Department of Health and Human Services Data Council; National Committee on Vital and Health Statistics; 2002.

Illinois Department of Public Health [homepage on the Internet]. Springfield: Illinois Department of Public Health [updated 2004 Feb 24; cited 2004 Mar 5]. Illinois project for local assessment of needs. Available from: http://app.idph.state.il.us.

Krieger N. The making of public health data: paradigms, politics, and policy. J Public Health Policy 1992;13(4):412–427.

Manitoba Centre for Health Policy [homepage on the Internet]. Winnipeg: Manitoba Centre for Health Policy [cited 2004 Mar 5]. Concept dictionary. Available from: http://www.umanitoba.ca/centres/mchp/concept.

National Center for Health Statistics [homepage on the Internet]. Hyattsville, MD: National Center for Health Statistics [cited 2004 Mar 5]. Catalog of university presentations. Available from: http://www.cdc.gov/nchs/products/catalogs/unipres.htm.

National Committee on Vital and Health Statistics. NCVHS recommendations for achieving the health statistics vision for the 21st century. In: Friedman DJ, Hunter EL, Parrish

RG, eds. Shaping a Vision for Health Statistics for the 21st Century: Final Report. Washington, DC: Department of Health and Human Services; 2002, pp. 49–68.

National Research Council, Council on National Statistics [homepage on the Internet]. Washington, DC: The National Academies [cited 2004 Mar 5]. Panel on DHHS Collection of Race and Ethnicity Data. Available from: http://www7.nationalacademies.org/cnstat/DHHS_Panel.html.

Office of Management and Budget. Statistical Programs of the United States Government, Fiscal Year 2002. Washington, DC: Office of Management and Budget; 2001.

Public Health Data Standards Consortium [homepage on the Internet]. Hyattsville, MD: National Center for Health Statistics [cited 2004 Mar 5]. Public Health Data Standards Consortium. Available from: http://phdatastandards.info.

Rice D. Health statistics: past, present, and future. In: Perrin EB, Kalsbeek WD, Scanlon TM, eds. Toward a Health Statistics System for the 21st Century: Summary of a Workshop. Washington, DC: National Academy Press; 2001, pp. 7–30.

Smedley BD, Stith AY, Nelson AR, eds. Unequal Treatment: Confronting Racial and Ethnic Disparities In Health Care. Washington, DC: National Academy Press; 2002.

Substance Abuse and Mental Health Services Administration, Office of Applied Studies [homepage on the Internet]. Rockville, MD: Substance Abuse and Mental Health Services Administration [cited 2004 Mar 5]. Substance Abuse and Mental Health Data Archive. Available from: http://www.samhsa.gov/oas/SAMHDA.htm.

Trust for America's Health [homepage on the Internet]. Washington, DC: Trust for America's Health [cited 2004 Mar 5]. Available from: http://healthyamericans.org.

U.S. Bureau of the Census [homepage on the Internet]. Washington, DC: U.S. Bureau of the Census [cited 2004 Mar 5]; Welcome to DataFERRETT!. Available from: http://ferret.bls.census.gov.

U.S. Department of Health and Human Services [monograph on the Internet]. Justification of Estimates for Appropriations Committees, Fiscal Year 2005, Centers for Disease Control and Prevention; February 2004 Washington: U.S. Department of Health and Human Services; 2004. [cited 2004 Feb 9]. Available from: http://www.cdc.gov/nchs/data/budget/nchs2005bdgtreq.pdf.

U.S. General Accounting Office. Toxic Chemicals: Long-Term Coordinated Strategy Needed to Measure Exposures in Humans. Report #GAO/HEHS-00-80. Washington, DC: General Accounting Office; 2000.

University of Minnesota [homepage on the Internet]. Minneapolis: University of Minnesota [cited 2004 Mar 5]. State Health Access Data Assistance Center. Available from: http://www.shadac.umn.edu.

Urban Institute [homepage on the Internet]. Washington, DC: Urban Institute [cited 2004 Mar 5]. Assessing the new federalism. Available from: http://www.urban.org/Content/Research/NewFederalism/NSAF/Overview/NSAFOverview.htm.

PART II

Collecting and Compiling Health Statistics

The approaches commonly used for gathering health-related information fall into four categories: (*1*) systems for notification or registration, (*2*) surveys, (*3*) administrative data systems, and (*4*) data systems outside the health sector (Table II.1). Notifications are reports of one or more health-related events, usually specified by law or regulation with reporting required by a specific group (e.g., health-care providers are required to report any patients with cholera whom they see), to an official—usually governmental—agency responsible for their prevention and control. *Notifiable* or *reportable* events usually require close monitoring by the health or other agency to ensure that they are controlled and do not spread to, or adversely affect, others. Certain communicable diseases (e.g., plague, cholera) are most commonly the object of notification systems, but other hazardous events or conditions (e.g., adverse reactions to a drug or another pharmaceutical agent, a hazardous roadway condition, or the downing of electrical power lines following a storm) may also be the subject of notifications. Registrations are similar to notifications in that specific events are the subject of registrations, but the registration of these events is not usually for the immediate control of a specific health problem or hazardous condition, but rather for the long-term tracking of events or persons for administrative, legal (e.g., registration of births and marriages), scientific (e.g., to facilitate the identification of a cohort exposed to a hazardous substance for future study), or statistical purposes. The registration of some events is required by law or regulation (e.g., births and deaths), but the registration of other events may not be. Chapter 4 by Koo, Wingo, and Rothwell addresses notifications and registrations through detailed examples of one notification system—the national notifiable disease system in the United States—and two registration systems: the U.S. national vital statistics system and the North American system of cancer registries.

Surveys constitute a particularly important source of health statistics because they can be tailored to meet a variety of health information needs. Chapter 5 by Madans and Cohen provides an overview and examples of the major kinds of surveys in current use: population-based surveys that obtain information directly from the subject; surveys that obtain information about entities such as health-care providers; and surveys that are based on administrative records. This is followed by a discussion of the objectives, content, and design of surveys that must be considered so that questions about populations or events can be answered accurately and appropriately. Finally, the authors highlight some current issues, including technological advances that are affecting methods of data collection and raising concerns about the public release of detailed survey data.

The two final approaches in Table II.1 range from health-care data systems that collect and compile administrative and health-data necessary for the financing and overall administration of hospitals, clinics, and other health-care delivery settings to systems that routinely collect detailed data about air and water quality through environmental sampling and testing. Two chapters are devoted to these approaches: Chapter 6 by Iezzoni, Shwartz, and Ash describes administrative health systems in the United States and the use of data derived from them

TABLE II.1
Approaches for Gathering Health Statistics

Approaches for Gathering Health Statistics
Notifications and registrations
Disease notifications
Sentinel notifications
Vital-event registration
Disease registries
Surveys
Population surveys
Health-care provider surveys
Population and household censuses
Administrative data systems for health care
Admissions
Health-care claims
Health-care encounters
Hospital discharges
Data systems outside the health sector
Environmental monitoring
Transportation related surveys and studies
Urbanization, land use, and housing surveys
Economic surveys

in formulating health policy; and Chapter 7 by Bailey et al. provides an overview of a host of data systems that are not traditionally maintained or used by public health agencies but that contain a wealth of information on many of the influences on health described in Chapter 1. Examples of the use of data from these systems in public health practice follow this overview.

Finally, chapters on standards by Greenberg and Parrish and linkage by Black and Roos round out this part. Standards and data linkage are critical to taking full advantage of the data collected through the approaches listed in Table 1. Standards can provide common language and definitions, guide the collection and processing of data to ensure their quality and usefulness, and facilitate the exchange and sharing of data among varied users. Linkage is a technique that makes possible more complete use of health and other data by bringing together data from many sources at the level of individual persons, populations, events, or places, which is often needed to fully understand a population's health.

CHAPTER 4

Health Statistics from Notifications, Registration Systems, and Registries

Denise Koo, Phyllis A. Wingo, and Charles J. Rothwell

This chapter describes two types of data collection that are critical for monitoring the population's health and generating health statistics: notifications and registrations. Notifications are reports of one or more health-related events that typically require close monitoring by health or other agencies to ensure that they are controlled and do not spread to, or adversely affect, others. The first part of this chapter provides a brief overview of notifications and a detailed description of one notification system, the U.S. National Notifiable Disease Surveillance System, to illustrate the history, practice, and uses of one important example of these systems.

Registrations are similar to notifications in that a specific event is the subject of a registration system, but the registration of events is not usually for the immediate control of a specific health problem or hazardous condition. Rather, it is for documenting and tracking events or persons for administrative, legal (e.g., registration of births and marriages), scientific (e.g., to facilitate the identification of a cohort exposed to a hazardous substance for future study), or statistical purposes. The second part of this chapter provides a brief overview of registration systems and then presents detailed descriptions of two registration systems, the U.S. national vital statistics system and the U.S. system of cancer registries, to illustrate the history, practice, and use of registration systems.

NOTIFICATIONS

Notifications cover a variety of health-related events. Table 4.1 provides a classification of notification systems by topic and examples of different health events within each topic. Which health-related events are subject to notification often differs by government jurisdiction, depending on its laws or regulations.[1] These notification systems, often referred to as *surveillance systems* by public health practitioners, may address occurrences of specific diseases or injuries, adverse effects of specific treatments, or the presence of specific hazards in the environment, which without intervention are likely to lead to disease or injury in exposed populations (Teutsch and Churchill 2000). They may also address members of the population who have already been exposed to a hazard and who, through screening or other measures, are found to be at risk for a particular disease or health condition. In all cases, the goal of these notifications is to identify situations in which immediate action may be required to treat those affected and to prevent others from exposure to the hazard, whether it is an infectious agent or a hazardous environmental condition.

Notification systems use different methods for gathering information, including direct reports by individuals or health-care providers, ongoing surveys composed of representative samples of health-care facilities, and sentinel report-

TABLE 4.1
Types of Notification Systems

1. Disease or hazard specific notifications
    a. Communicable diseases
        i. WHO: International Health Regulations require reporting of cholera, plague, and yellow fever (World Health Organization [hp] International health regulations)
        ii. National: United States: (Centers for Disease Control and Prevention [hp] Nationally notifiable infectious diseases); Canada: (Health Canada [hp] National notifiable diseases for 2000)
        Provincial, state, or subnational (e.g., coccidiodomycosis in California)
    b. Chemical and physical hazards in the environment
        i. Childhood lead poisoning (Meyer et al. 2003)
        ii. Occupational hazards (National Institute for Occupational Safety and Health [hp] Health hazard evaluations)
        iii. Firearm-related injury (Fox et al. 1998; Mercy et al. 1998)
        iv. Consumer product-related injury (U.S. Consumer Product Safety Commission [hp] Report unsafe products)
2. Treatment notifications
    a. Adverse effect of drugs or medical products (U.S. Food and Drug Administration [hp] Reporting adverse reactions and medical product problems to the FDA; Vaccine Adverse Event Reporting System [hp])
3. At-risk notifications
    a. Adult blood lead elevation (National Institute for Occupational Safety and Health [hp] ABLES)

ing sites. The rest of this part of the chapter presents a detailed example of the approach taken to monitor communicable diseases of public health importance in the United States.

Notifiable Diseases

Overview

Notifiable diseases generally are defined as those diseases or conditions for which regular, frequent, and timely information on individual cases is considered necessary for their prevention or control (Centers for Disease Control 1993b). Currently, most notifiable diseases in the United States are communicable diseases, and state laws usually require that health-care providers or laboratories report them to the state health department, often within 24 hours, so that public health officials can take appropriate, timely action to prevent further cases. Systems set up within individual state health departments systematically collect these reports of notifiable diseases; these systems are sometimes referred to as *notifiable* or *reportable* disease surveillance systems.

Some noninfectious conditions, such as elevated blood lead levels or pesticide poisoning, are reportable in many states. However, most of the National Notifiable Disease List consists of diseases or conditions that are infectious in etiology, including most vaccine-preventable diseases such as hepatitis A and measles; sexually transmitted diseases (STDs) such as syphilis and chlamydia; enteric diseases such as salmonellosis and botulism; tuberculosis (TB) and other respiratory diseases; and arthropod-borne or zoonotic diseases such as plague and the encephalitides. Some diseases that are of strong interest to public health, but that are very uncommon, are not specified on the national list, but there is clearly an expectation that any case of smallpox or viral hemorrhagic fever, for example, would be immediately reported to public health authorities (Broome et al. 2003).[2] Some state laws specify that these uncommon conditions are reportable to the state health agency; others specify that "any unusual condition or disease" is reportable.

Historical Development

As described below, the utility of vital records for public health practice was demonstrated by the mid-1800s in England. However, health authorities also recognized that registration of deaths was not sufficient for the early identification and control of disease outbreaks. Thus, in the 1870s, Massachusetts and Michigan required notification to their respective boards of health of several diseases "dangerous to the public health" (Trask 1914). In 1893 Congress gave the U.S. Marine Hospital Service (the precursor of today's U.S. Public Health Service) the authority for collecting and publishing weekly morbidity data from states and municipal authorities (Hampton 1923). However, the traditional tension between federal authority and the states' autonomy led to conflicts over the reporting of notifiable diseases and the use of the information (Smillie 1955). For example, when plague first appeared in the United States in San Francisco in 1900, the U.S. Marine Hospital Service's Dr. Joseph Kinyoun, who was based in San Francisco, was stymied in his efforts to control the disease by state officials who denied that there was plague in California (Mullan 1989, 39–40). Thus, in 1902 Congress enacted a law directing the U.S. Surgeon General to increase the uniformity of the reporting by providing forms for data collection and publishing national morbidity statistics, although the law also stipulated that the federal government must consult with state and territorial health authorities on these matters (U.S. Public Health and Marine Hospital Service 1903).

Gradually state health authorities realized that they needed to know not only what diseases were prevalent in their own state but also in other states, and they recognized that the federal government was indeed a useful common agent for the collection and dissemination of this information. By 1928 all states, the District of Columbia, Hawaii, and Puerto Rico were participating in national reporting of 29 specified diseases (Centers for Disease Control 2000). At their annual meeting in 1950, the state and territorial health officers authorized the Council of State and Territorial Epidemiologists (CSTE) to determine which diseases should be reported to the U.S. Public Health Service. In 1961, the U.S. Communicable Disease Center (CDC, which is currently named the Centers for Disease Control and Prevention) assumed responsibility for the collection and publication of data concerning nationally notifiable diseases.

Current Practices

AUTHORITY

Disease reporting is mandated by legislation, regulation, or health officer declaration at state and local levels, but reporting by states to the CDC is voluntary. Nevertheless, public health officials at state health departments and the CDC continue to collaborate in determining what diseases should be nationally notifiable. The CSTE, with input from the CDC, annually revises the list of nationally notifiable diseases, but the list of diseases considered notifiable varies slightly by state (Roush et al. 1999). All states generally report the diseases (i.e., cholera, plague, and yellow fever) whose notification to the World Health Organization (WHO) is required of WHO member states under the International Health Regulations.

FUNDING

National funding for reporting notifiable diseases has historically been disease-specific. Congress provides *categorical* funding for reporting, studying, and controlling specific diseases (e.g., TB, STDs, cancer, and acquired immunodeficiency syndrome [AIDS]), which has led to independently developed disease-specific computer applications for use at the state (and sometimes local) level for the collection, entry, and analysis of disease reports, and for transmission of data to the CDC. General notifiable (or *noncategorical*) disease reporting receives very little direct funding, and must be supported with general funds for communicable disease prevention and control. Because the quality and completeness of reporting on a given disease are often related to the funding level, the quality and completeness of notifiable disease data vary by disease.

POPULATION BASIS

Given the caveat of state-by-state variability, reporting of notifiable diseases that relies on health-care providers to initiate reports covers the population of the entire country. However, the completeness of this coverage must be interpreted in light of reporting practices. Certain diseases that cause severe clinical illness (e.g., plague and rabies) are more likely to be reported because patients with these diseases are more likely to be seen and diagnosed by clinicians. Diseases that are clinically mild and infrequently associated with serious consequences (e.g., salmonellosis) are less likely to be reported because patients with these diseases are less likely to seek clinical care. Finally, even if these less severe diseases are diagnosed, they are less likely to be reported because clinicians often perceive them as less of a public health threat.

CASE DEFINITION ISSUES

While the tradition of reporting communicable diseases dates back over a century, uniform criteria for defining and reporting occurrences of individual diseases (also known as *cases* of disease) was not provided until 1990, when the CDC collaborated with the CSTE to publish recommended "Case definitions for public health surveillance" (Centers for Disease Control and Prevention 1990). These case definitions generally include clinical, epidemiologic, and laboratory criteria for assigning status as a confirmed, probable, or suspected case. The availability of data to verify the classification of a reported case of disease often varies by funding levels for the disease. For example, data on diseases that receive specific funding for their control, such as AIDS, include information that allows public health officials to pinpoint the rationale by which a case is classified as a confirmed case (e.g., what laboratory test verified the diagnosis). For other diseases, such as salmonellosis, the only information available at the national level may be the final classification of the case. Case definitions do not remain static and can change, for example, when new diagnostic methods for, or etiologies of, a disease are discovered (Centers for Disease Control and Prevention 1997).[3]

SOURCES OF DATA AND TYPES OF DATA COLLECTED

Regardless of what diseases are considered reportable in a given state, notifiable disease reporting originates with health-care providers (clinicians and laboratories). Information requested generally includes disease name; patient name, address, date of birth, age, race, ethnicity, and sex; date of onset of illness; and the results of diagnostic laboratory tests. For diseases such as hepatitis A, information about whether the patient works as a food handler is often included. The state or local health department follows up with the provider, as appropriate, and collects additional information such as sexual or other contacts, vaccination status, and risk factors for disease. Health department officials must do their best to reconcile potentially duplicative reports originating separately from clinicians and laboratories. However, these two data sources are both critical for notifiable disease systems, because while laboratory-based reporting is usually more reliable than clinician-based reporting, the data reported from laboratories often lack demographic information, and the laboratory usually has no access to information about risk factors for contracting the disease.

SYSTEM OVERVIEW

Reports from providers and laboratories about individual cases of notifiable diseases are generally sent to the local health department (by telephone, facsimile, or morbidity report card), and the local health department passes the information on to the state health department. (Outbreaks or cases that require an urgent response [e.g., a suspected case of botulism, a case of meningococcal meningitis, or a multistate outbreak of food-borne disease] are immediately reported to the health department by telephone.) Each state health department reports electronically to the CDC on a weekly basis via a system that uses a standard record format, accepting records generated by the different software programs used in the states, whether for general communicable diseases or categorically funded diseases (e.g., for STDs and TB) (Koo and Wetterhall 1996). States do not transmit names or addresses of cases to the CDC.

For certain notifiable diseases, state or local health departments in conjunction with the CDC undertake supplemental activities to identify cases of disease—for example, contacting health-care providers in a specified geographic area. Data from these efforts are often collected separately from the notifiable disease reporting system, although they can be linked. The information collected through such activities is usually more extensive and may include information on potential risk factors of the patient and laboratory analyses of specimens taken from the patient, such as species type, antibiotic-resistance pattern, or DNA fingerprinting. Such efforts generally require additional disease-specific funding and involve partnerships between health departments and universities or laboratories.

Uses of Reports of Notifiable Diseases

Reporting of notifiable diseases plays a critical role in the early identification of outbreaks. For example, in early 1993 in Washington State, disease notifications and the subsequent investigation of an outbreak of *Escherichia coli* O157:H7 infections led within a week of the first report to the identification of hamburgers from a fast-food restaurant chain as the cause of the outbreak (Bell et al. 1994). This quick response resulted in removal of more than 250,000 potentially contaminated hamburgers and prevented an estimated 800 cases of infection. Subsequent testing showed that most regular hamburgers cooked according to the chain's policy did not attain the internal temperature (68.3°C) required by the state to kill infectious agents, which led to a change in restaurant policy nationwide.

Outbreak detection is only one—but perhaps the most publicized—use of reports of notifiable diseases. Reports of notifiable diseases also provide crucial information for estimating the burden of disease, following the natural history of a disease, and determining its geographic distribution. For example, in the late 1940s, improvements in the quality of the reporting of cases demonstrated that, despite beliefs to the contrary, malaria had disappeared as an endemic disease in the southern United States (Langmuir 1963). When an outbreak is detected, reports of disease can sometimes help pinpoint the cause. For example, a system for reporting cases of polio, quickly developed following initial reports from a few health-care providers, provided critical evidence that the vaccine-associated poliomyelitis found after initiation of a nationwide polio vaccination program was limited to a single brand, which had been contaminated with live virus. This finding was critical for rescuing the nascent vaccination program (Thacker and Berkelman 1988). Typically, programs that receive reports of notifiable diseases generally do not identify the etiology, but they can generate hypotheses for further investigation. For example, reporting of cases of measles facilitated the recognition, after further investigation, that a single dose of measles vaccine was insufficient for lifelong immunity in the late 1980s (American Academy of Pediatrics 1989; Centers for Disease Control and Prevention 1989).

Reports of notifiable diseases, because they are often collected for acute or communicable diseases, are quite useful for directing immediate or intermediate control and treatment measures. For example, as part of the response to detected cases of infection, health departments use reports to locate and treat persons who have been exposed to a disease (especially critical for STDs and infectious respiratory diseases such as TB and measles). Recognition of changes in the resistance to antibiotics of *Mycobacterium tuberculosis* and *Neisseria gonorrhoeae* resulted in important recommendations for changes in the initial drug treatment of TB and gonorrhea (American Thoracic Society, Centers for Disease Control and Prevention 1994; Centers for Disease Control and Prevention 1993a, 1998a). Regardless of the types of control measures, notifiable disease data provide additional information to monitor the effectiveness of interventions.

Current Issues in Notifiable Disease Reporting

DEFICIENCIES OF CURRENT SYSTEMS

Current systems that gather reports of notifiable diseases generally capture only a fraction of cases, in a delayed and labor-intensive fashion (Birkhead et al.

1991; Kimball et al. 1980; Rosenberg et al. 1977). Underreporting to public health agencies, particularly by physicians, has been well documented (Alter et al. 1987; Campos-Outcalt et al. 1991; Kirsch and Shesser 1991; Konowitz et al. 1984; Marier 1977; Simpson 1996). Many providers do not know how or to whom to report diseases or feel that it detracts from their clinical responsibilities. Few health-care providers understand the importance of reporting, the role of the provider as the principal source of reports, and the role of the health department in response. The degree of completeness of reporting is also influenced by the diagnostic facilities available; control measures in effect; public awareness of a specific disease; and the interests, resources, and priorities of state and local officials responsible for receiving reports and controlling disease. Finally, factors such as changes in the criteria for diagnosing and reporting a disease, the introduction of new diagnostic tests, or the discovery of new disease entities can cause changes in disease reporting that are independent of the true incidence of disease.

More importantly, this disease-based approach to prevention and control has made it more difficult for state and local health departments to efficiently and comprehensively assess the diseases and health problems in their communities. To evaluate the overall health of their jurisdictions, local and state health officials must use and access multiple sources of information. For example, maternal and child health programs cannot easily access data in the independent systems that receive reports of childhood lead poisoning, diarrheal diseases, and vaccine-preventable diseases. In addition, these disease notification systems are event-based, which is useful for monitoring incidence but not for measuring prevalence or conducting longitudinal follow-up. It was clear by the mid-1990s that a more efficient, nonduplicative change in the approach to obtaining and analyzing reports of disease was needed (Morris et al. 1996; Thacker and Stroup 1994).

INTEREST IN NEW DATA

Public health will benefit by collecting more timely and complete data not only from current sources, but also from new sources. Highly critical is the need for more information for public health—for example, for detecting bioterrorist events and emerging infectious diseases. In the past, public health designated specific conditions or syndromes as important for notification to public health. However, concerns about bioterrorism and the relative uncertainty about the exact biological or chemical agent that a terrorist might choose to use as a weapon give rise to an interest in capturing somewhat less specific data in a more timely fashion, such as collecting real-time data on the occurrence of suspicious respiratory syndromes (i.e., possible early anthrax, plague, smallpox, or tularemia) in order to generate a more rapid and effective public health response (Rotz et al. 2000). Early access to these data in electronic format, *as they are entered* into the computer systems of health-care providers, is desired, although the true public health usefulness of this approach is not yet proven (Reingold 2003; Sosin 2003).

PROLIFERATION OF INFORMATION SYSTEMS

The increasingly widespread use of computerized health information systems by state and local health departments, as well as health-care providers, is another motivator for a change in the approach to obtaining data for public health. Many state and local health departments have developed information systems to meet a range of internal data needs and wish to simplify reporting to CDC programs by using a single electronic approach, such as secure Internet transmission without re-entry of data into CDC systems. This problem is even more pressing for health-care providers and diagnostic laboratories. Technological advances provide the possibility of an integrated approach to gathering public health data from key primary data sources, one that facilitates capture and use of data that are already electronic. Of necessity, such an approach will also acknowledge the interdependence of the public health and health-care systems and should improve the efficiency of systems to support both.

INTEGRATION OF SURVEILLANCE SYSTEMS: THE NATIONAL ELECTRONIC DISEASE SURVEILLANCE SYSTEM

The CDC is spearheading a new initiative in integrated disease reporting and in other data collection. The National Electronic Disease Surveillance System (NEDSS) initiative promotes the use of data and information system standards to advance the development of efficient, integrated, and interoperable surveillance systems at federal, state, and local levels. A primary goal of NEDSS is the ongoing, automatic capture and analysis of data that are already available electronically (National Electronic Disease Surveillance System Working Group 2001).

This more comprehensive approach would support efficient data collection via access to multiple critical sources—such as computerized medical and laboratory records as well as sources of data outside the health arena (e.g., environmental monitoring systems, highway traffic crash data)—for multiple programmatic uses, but *not* through the building of myriad independent systems for single diseases or programs. It would involve a much closer and more integrated working relationship between the public health and health-care systems, which should lead to improved provision of health care as well as public health (for more detail, see Centers for Disease Control and Prevention [hp] NEDSS). This vision is consistent with that of the National Health Information Infrastructure (see Chapter 20).

CONCERNS ABOUT SECURITY AND CONFIDENTIALITY

Discussion of direct electronic access to clinical data and improved integration of public health with the health-care system may raise concerns among consumers about the security and confidentiality of their personal health data.

In reality, use of electronic information systems actually provides an opportunity to improve the security and confidentiality of health data (Barrows and Clayton 1996). In its new data systems, the CDC is building in security standards for the transmission of data that are consistent with security standards of the Health Insurance Portability and Accountability Act. It is hoped that these standards will facilitate secure electronic exchange of appropriate data between public health and the health-care system (see also Chapters 8 and 14).

REGISTRATION SYSTEMS AND REGISTRIES

Registrations are similar to notifications in that specific events are the subject of registrations, but the registration of these events is not usually for the immediate control of a specific health problem or hazardous condition, but rather for documenting and tracking events or persons for administrative, legal (e.g., registration of births and marriages), scientific (e.g., to facilitate the identification of a cohort exposed to a hazardous substance for future study), or statistical purposes.[4] The registration of some events is required by law or regulation (e.g., births and deaths), but the registration of other events may not be. In his review of registers and registries, Weddell (1973) described the broad scope of the types of registers—defined as books or other records of "details of any kind sufficiently important to be exactly recorded"—and the kinds of health conditions covered by these registers.[5] Table 4.2 summarizes his scheme with a few additions for completeness.

To illustrate the nature and usefulness of registration systems and registries, the remainder of this chapter provides detailed descriptions of two registration systems: the U.S. national vital statistics system and the U.S. system of cancer registries.

Vital Registration and Statistics in the United States

Overview

USES AND IMPORTANCE

Birth, marriage, divorce, and death are not only vital events on a personal level but also provide public health officials with critical data from which to ascertain information about the circumstances of these events and in the aggregate create what is known as the *vital statistics system.* Since the turn of the twentieth century, the United States has operated a decentralized vital statistics system as an essential component of public health. The system of vital registration was created for—and its primary function remains—the recording of vital events at the state and local levels for various administrative and legal purposes. Nevertheless, as Graunt did with the Bills of Mortality in London in the 1600s and Farr with the records of the General Register Office in England in the 1800s

TABLE 4.2
Types of Registration Systems and Registries with Examples of Selected Types

1. Vital event registration
    a. Birth registration
    b. Marriage and divorce registration
    c. Death registration
2. Registers used in preventive medicine
    a. Immunization registries
    b. Registers of persons at risk for certain conditions
    c. Registers of persons positive for genetic conditions
3. Disease specific registers and registries
    a. Blind registers
    b. Birth defects registries
    c. Cancer registries
    d. Psychiatric case registers
    e. Ischemic heart disease registers
4. Treatment registers
    a. Radiotherapy registers
    b. Follow-up registers for detection of iatrogenic thyroid disease
5. After care registers
    a. Handicapped child
    b. Disabled
6. At-risk or exposure registers
    a. Children at high risk of developing a health problem
    b. Occupational hazards registers
    c. Medical hazards registers
    d. Elderly or chronic sick registers
    e. Atomic bomb survivors (Japan)
7. Skills and resources registers
8. Prospective studies
9. Specific information registers

Source: Adapted from Weddell (1973).

(see Chapter 2 and below), the administrative system has been further used as the primary source of information to track the health status of the U.S. population; to plan, implement, and evaluate health and social services for children, families, and adults; and to set health policy at the national, state, and local levels. Data on access to prenatal care, maternal risk factors, infant mortality, disparities in health status, changes in the rankings of causes of death, life expectancy, years of potential life lost, and other pregnancy and mortality indicators have informed public policy and programmatic debates about improving health and health service delivery. Unlike any other public health data system, vital statistics provide almost complete, continuous, and comparable federal, state, and local data to public health officials and programs. The strength of the vital records and statistics system is that it provides a complete census of events allowing for population-based analysis and comparisons at the national, state, and local levels by age, race, ethnicity, and gender (NCHS 2001b; NCHS [hp] HIST290A; NCHS [hp] NVSS; Rothwell 2003).

HISTORICAL DEVELOPMENT

Vital registration was carried out in limited fashion in ancient Egypt, Greece, and Rome for revenue and military purposes. Historically, two types of vital registration have been undertaken: ecclesiastical and civil. Prior to the rise of the modern nation-state, ecclesiastical registers were kept by religious officials. With the evolution of the nation-state, there arose increased public concern about the legal and civil rights of individuals, which led to increased importance of, and documentation of proof of, birth and death. Civil registration, that is, registration administered by the government, became compulsory, continuous, and permanent. In the Massachusetts Bay Colony in 1639, civil registration was carried out by government clerks. It was not until the work of John Graunt in 1662 in England, however, that information from vital registration activities was used to collect statistical information to measure the demographic structure and health status of the population. In the American colonies, one of the earliest statistical users of burial records was Cotton Mather, who in 1721 demonstrated the protective effect of smallpox inoculation during a smallpox epidemic in Boston. In 1789 Edward Wigglesworth, using vital registration data, developed the first American life table, which showed a life expectancy of 28.15 years. Yet not until 1839 in England, when William Farr used vital statistics to initiate sanitary reform through measuring the impact of premature death, did vital registration become a systematic means for measuring the health of the population (Public Health Service 1954).

The Bureau of the Census created the first U.S. standard certificate of death, and recommended its adoption by states and cities by January 1, 1900 (Public Health Service 1954). No coordinated, nationwide vital registration system for births and deaths existed until 1902, when the Bureau of the Census was made a permanent agency of the federal government. Legislation authorized the director of the Bureau of the Census to obtain copies of records filed in states, cities, and towns with adequate death registration systems and to publish data from the records. By 1933, all states were registering live births and deaths with reasonable completeness and providing the data to the Bureau for reporting of national birth and death statistics (Hetzel 1997; Public Health Service 1954).

Collection and publication of vital statistics at the federal level was transferred to the National Office of Vital Statistics, in the U.S. Public Health Service, in 1946. The National Center for Health Statistics (NCHS) was created in 1960, and assumed responsibilities for the national vital statistics collection and its reporting functions. In 1987, the NCHS became part of the CDC, within the U.S. Department of Health and Human Services, and continues to carry out these responsibilities (NCHS 2000a).

Current Practices and Activities

AUTHORITY

The federal government has no express constitutional authority to enact vital statistics legislation of national scope and therefore is reliant on states to enact laws and regulations for the collection of vitals statistics, which are comparable among states. However, under Section 306 of the Public Health Service Act, the NCHS is charged with the "annual collection of data from births, deaths, marriages and divorces in registration areas" (NCHS 2000a). In addition, the federal government plays a significant role in coordinating and ensuring that comparable data of high quality are collected at the state level through the development of model state vital statistics acts, model U.S. standard vital certificates, reports, and data edit standards, and providing training and technical assistance (NCHS [hp] NVSS).

Each state creates its own laws regarding collection of and access to vital records and statistics. State laws must be put in place to specify the duties of physicians, funeral directors, hospitals, and other providers of information to the vital statistics system and to establish a state registrar's office and its functions. State legislation needs to specify the process of the recording of marriages, divorces, annulments, and amendments to vital records; the requirements for reporting of fetal deaths; the registration and certification process for births and deaths; and the procedures for disclosure of vital records. State legislation is also enacted to process adoptions and issues relating to paternity. Without concise and consistent legislation concerning all the processes surrounding the registration of vital events, the completeness and accuracy of statistics derived from the registration of vital events would suffer and there could be little consistency of reporting among states. For these reasons, the Model State Vital Statistics Act was developed by the NCHS in partnership with the states (NCHS 1995). In developing and implementing the act and other measures that encourage consistency of practice, the sharing of information between states, and the collective responses to national interests, states frequently work collectively through the professional association that represents vital statistics professionals, the National Association for Public Health Statistics and Information Systems (NAPHSIS), which has existed under various names since 1933. The NAPHSIS is one of the affiliates of the Association of State and Territorial Health Officials, which represents broader interests of state health departments (Hetzel 1997; NAPHSIS [hp] About NAPHSIS; NCHS 1995).

The Model State Vital Statistics Act serves as proposed legislation, which states can then use to enact vital statistics legislation specific to their singular situations. The first model act was developed by the Bureau of the Census in 1907 and covered births and deaths. Since then, model acts have been modified frequently and expanded to deal with emerging registration and statistical needs. In 1942, the Model Act was modified to include marriages and divorces; in 1977, it was modified to ensure that centralized state systems existed for collecting, processing, registering, and certifying vital records. The Model State Vital Statistics Regulations were first issued in 1977. The Model Act and Regulations were most recently updated in 1992 (NCHS 1995).

At its annual meeting in 2000, NAPHSIS adopted Model Act modifications supported by the NCHS, including the use of electronic signatures, standardized worksheets for data collection, and electronic submission of records from the data provider to the state registrar (NAPHSIS 2000). The major components of the current version of the Model Act reflect the major functions of a vital registration system: the authorization of a central vital statistics office and a statewide system; requirements for birth and death registration; marriage registration; divorce, marriage dissolution, and annulments; issues of enforcement; and the appropriate use of technology (Hetzel 1997; NAPHSIS 2000; NCHS 1995).

Funding

The primary support for vital statistics at the state level comes from state appropriations and receipts for providing certified copies of birth and death certificates (NCHS 2000a). Through contracts under the Vital Statistics Cooperative Program (VSCP), the NCHS reimburses states for the provision of standard data items that are transmitted to the NCHS in accordance with specified timeliness and quality requirements. This limited financial support helps states to maintain their vital statistics data collection systems (NCHS 2000a). Regardless of the source of funds, the providers of the information—whether physicians, hospitals, next of kin, mothers, or funeral directors—are not paid for providing the information.

Standards and Consensus Practices

U.S. STANDARD CERTIFICATES AND REPORTS

To ensure comparability across states, federal law provides for the issuance of model U.S. standard certificates that specify the data required by the VSCP. The standard certificates are periodically updated through a national consensus process convened by the NCHS involving data providers and public health experts. Since the issuance of the first standard certificates of birth and death in 1900, there have been 12 versions of the standard certificate of live birth, 11 of the standard certificate of death, 8 of the standard report of fetal death, 4 of the standard certificates of marriage and divorce, and 2 of the standard report of induced termination of pregnancy (Hetzel 1997; Public Health Service 1954). States are currently converting from the 1989 standard birth, death, and fetal death standard certificates to the 2003 versions (see NCHS [hp] 2003 revisions) (NCHS 2000b; NCHS [hp] NVSS). Because of the complexity and expense of changing certificates and processing systems, many states are linking the implementation of these new certificates to more a fundamental overhaul of their overall vital registration and statistics systems. This "re-engineering" effort is described in more detail later in this section. The 2003 revision emphasizes the submission of electronic data and improvements in data quality. Over the years, the standard certificates have become more complex, with the number of items increasing from just over 30 on the birth certificate and 40 on the death certificate in 1900 to more than 60 and 70 items, respectively, in the 2003 versions. For births, many of the additions relate to information concerning the mother's pregnancy and the condition of the infant. For deaths, more information is now collected concerning the circumstances of deaths due to injuries (NCHS 2000b).

To improve the quality of the data, the NCHS issues instruction manuals and handbooks that define the duties and responsibilities of those involved in the registration process and provide guidelines for accurate registration of the events (NCHS [hp] NVSS). In implementing the 2003 revisions of the birth certificate and the fetal death report, the NCHS, working with state colleagues, recommended standardized worksheets to help hospital personnel in the collection of information required on birth certificates, including separate worksheets for the mother or patient and the facility where the delivery occurred (NCHS 2000b). A guidebook has also been developed that provides information on the best sources for the data items (NCHS 2003a). Re-engineered vital statistics systems include detailed edit specifications for each data item with guidelines for editing and querying data at the source (NCHS 2000b, 2003a). Each state adapts these materials to meet its unique requirements.

INTERNATIONAL CLASSIFICATION OF DISEASES AND AUTOMATED MEDICAL CODING SYSTEMS

The cause-of-death information on death certificates is classified for statistical purposes by use of the World Health Organization's International Classification of Diseases, Injuries and Causes of Death (ICD). Since 1900, there have been 10 revisions to the ICD. The ICD provides definitions of terms and guidelines for coding and classifying the causes of death; rules for determining the underlying cause of death; and groupings for compilation and publishing of death statistics. The current ICD-10 revision provides a list of 113 selected causes for identifying, ranking, and publishing the leading causes of death. See Chapter 8 for a fuller discussion of the ICD and its role in health data standards.

In order to enhance the comparability, timeliness, and quality of cause-of-death data, the NCHS has developed a family of electronic medical classification systems, which are provided along with training to states and many foreign countries to automate the entry, classification, and retrieval of the medical information provided on the death certificate. These systems contain the decision tables used to automatically select the underlying cause of death; format and edit the multiple cause-of-death data in preparation for analysis; and enable entry of literal text and abbreviations for cause-of-death information (Chamblee and Evans 1986; Hetzel 1997).

Types of Data Collected

Over the years, the information contained in the vital registration certificates and reports has expanded greatly. For births, detailed data pertaining to the characteristics of the mother and the birth event are now collected, such as methods of delivery, obstetric procedures, complications of labor and delivery, behavioral (e.g., prenatal smoking) and medical risk factors (e.g., hypertension, diabetes), number of prenatal visits, month prenatal care began, birth weight, and plurality, as well as demographic characteristics of both the mother and the father. When states implement the 2003 standard certificate for live birth, new data will be collected on the principal source of payment for the delivery, participation in the Women, Infants and Children (WIC) nutrition program, breast-feeding, maternal morbidity, and fertility therapy, along with improved data on cigarette smoking, method of delivery, congenital anomalies, and maternal weight gain (NCHS 2000b; NCHS [hp] NVSS). (See NCHS [hp] 2003 revisions for the statistical items on the 2003 standard birth certificate.)

Significant additions have been made to the standard certificate of death since the issuance of the first standard certificate in 1900. Changes to the standard death certificate as a result of the last two revisions have, however, been slight. (See NCHS [hp] 2003 revisions for statistical items on the 2003 standard death certificate.) For the fetal death report, improved information on maternal morbidity, smoking, and cause of death will be collected under the latest revision (see NCHS [hp] 2003 revisions) (NCHS 2000b).

Records and Data Flow

The registration of vital events, the generation of statistics about these events, and the subsequent flow of information involve the cooperation of many governmental and private organizations and individuals. The process varies by state, depending on the presence of local or country registrars and the involvement of local or country health departments. Although differences exist among states, the registration of a birth is typically the responsibility of the professional attendants at birth (Hetzel 1997). With the advent of automated birth records in hospitals, local registrars and health departments may play less important roles in the process. Because most births occur in hospitals, all states have implemented automated hospital birth certificate systems to speed reporting and improve data quality and completeness through editing when the data are initially collected. However, automated hospital birth certificate systems are usually independent of other hospital information systems and often do not connect to or obtain data from these systems. Although automation has improved data processing speed, duplicate data entry by hospital staff still occurs. Once the records are received at the state level, hospitals are queried about any records with incomplete or inconsistent information. A permanent automated file is then created, which enables correcting and issuing certified copies of certificates and developing a statistical file for analysis of state and local data. The state registrar electronically sends birth records to the NCHS, which in turn creates the national data file of birth outcomes. It is anticipated that as states re-engineer their data collection systems, the editing and querying of data will be increasingly carried out at the source, namely, the hospital or birth facility.

The record and data flow for deaths differs considerably from that of births. The funeral director has primary responsibility for completing the demographic and administrative information on the death certificate, and a physician or medical examiner has responsibility for providing information on the cause of death. Because of this split responsibility and the many data providers involved, no state has been able to completely automate the collection of death information. As was the case at the beginning of the twentieth century, death certificates continue to be paper-based at the local level and are not automated until they reach the state registrar. There data from death certificates are entered into automated registration systems that can issue certified copies, create statistical files for state and local analysis, and electronically transmit nonidentifying death information to the NCHS for the creation of the national mortality database. Although there have been many technological advances at the state level for providing certified copies and for displaying and analyzing state vital statistics through the Internet, the conversion of paper vital records into an electronic format remains complex and labor intensive, with the all the delays and inflexibilities inherent in such systems (Rothwell 2003).

States have agreements with other states so that they can receive vital event data for state residents who have vital events in another state. The interstate exchange enables states to complete their statistical files for all events to their residents, regardless of the states in which those events occurred.

Uses and Applications of Vital Statistics

The strength of vital statistics is their coverage for all population groups and their geographic specificity. Unlike national surveys, both the researcher and the public health practitioner can employ vital statistics to examine disparities between population groups within subnational areas. An important use of vital statistics data is for monitoring and tracking progress in achieving Healthy People 2010 (HP2010) goals (USDHHS 2000). Forty-three of the 467 HP2010 objectives—or more than 9%—rely on vital statistics data for monitoring. Because vital statistics data are comparable among states, health outcomes can be examined for high-risk groups in different geographic settings. For mortality data, because of the specificity of the ICD and the large number of deaths nationally (nearly 2.5 million deaths in the United States per year), rare causes of death can be explored at the national level, or differentials in major causes of death can be examined for small racial and ethnic groups or within small geographic regions. Because substantial consistency has existed over time in the collection of mortality data and because comparability ratios have been developed to adjust for periodic revisions in the ICD, it is possible to analyze the trends in the major causes of death over time. With the advent of automated medical coding systems, data on both the underlying cause of death and the contributing or secondary causes of death have become available, enabling study of the impact of conditions such as hypertension, atherosclerosis, and diabetes on mortality.

With over 4 million live births each year in the United States, birth outcomes and prenatal care can be examined by demographic and behavioral characteristics of the mother. Infant deaths, of which there are approximately 28,000 per year, are linked to their corresponding birth records to examine differentials in infant mortality by the characteristics of the mother and the medical treatment provided. The annual linked file of births and infant deaths provides critical information on the relationship of birth weight to gestational age-specific mortality and on the impact of other high-risk conditions on infant mortality (Mathews et al. 2003). To study early infant loss, perinatal mortality files are created through combining into single data files late fetal deaths (>28 weeks), live births, and early neonatal deaths (<7 days) (NCHS 2004). As the proportion of multiple births has increased, files of multiple births have been created in order to examine birth outcomes, maternal characteristics, and prenatal care (NCHS 2003b).

With their universal coverage, substantial specificity, and flexibility for linkage to other data files, vital statistics are used to measure a broad spectrum of public health and societal issues, such as changes over time in teenage pregnancy rates, homicide rates, prematurity rates, motor vehicle fatality rates, and maternal smoking patterns; racial differentials in infant mortality; differentials in causes of death by age, race, and sex; and the increases in deaths due to emerging diseases, such as human immunodeficiency virus disease (HIV) in the 1980s and early 1990s. Vital statistics provide the basis for the most basic population health indicators, such as premature mortality rates and infant mortality rates.

New Directions—Re-engineering Vital Records Record and Data Flow

Vital statistics remain a critical element in the health statistics portfolio of data sources. The collection of detailed data on more than 6 million vital events annually in the United States, however, is accompanied by concerns about the quality of vital statistics data, their timeliness, and difficulties in immediately linking to other health data systems and screening programs. In order to resolve these issues, as with the other systems mentioned in this chapter, vital registration requires more complete automation at the level of the primary data providers and changes in the basic relationships among the providers of the source records, the state registration offices, and the NCHS.

Increasingly, vital records are being used in the administration of many benefit and entitlement programs and services. Examples include Social Security, child support enforcement, and welfare reform, among others. Vital records data have long been used to estimate the U.S. population between decennial censuses and to project school populations. Vital records data are also used to manage social welfare and pension programs, administer life insurance policies, and control access to passports. Recent terrorist events and criminal actions have heightened the need for this system to deal with identity theft and fraud.

Despite the expanding importance of the vital records and statistics system, it continues to be based on outmoded registration, records, and data flow processing systems and underlying business practices. For almost 20 years, electronic birth certificate (EBC) systems have been used by some states and are now used in all states, with over 95% of birth records electronically recorded at the hospital and transmitted to state offices. While a significant step forward, EBCs are electronic certificates rather than electronic registration systems. Even with EBCs, all states continue to operate dual paper and electronic systems, with the paper record being the official legal document. The collection of death information continues to be basically a paper-based process, unchanged at the local level for the past half century. To compound these problems, current electronic systems have been difficult to modify, causing many states to delay the implementation of the 2003 revisions to the U.S. standard certificates.

To address these problems, the NCHS, the NAPHSIS, and the Social Security Administration have established a partnership to examine the responsiveness of state vital registration systems to current and anticipated data needs (NAPHSIS [hp] About NAPHSIS; NCHS 2001a). The partners have concluded that states need to fundamentally re-engineer the process through which vital statistics are produced; simply modifying existing systems is no longer sufficient. The partners have agreed that collaboration is essential to success. The primary objective of the re-engineering initiative is to improve the timeliness, quality, and sustainability of the decentralized vital statistics system through adopting nationally developed, consensus standards and guidelines. The driving concept of the activity is that business practices within state vital records offices must be documented and then updated to be more efficient and effective in light of today's technology. These systems will be driven by national standards and guidelines. The resulting re-engineered state systems will use the 2003 version of the U.S. standard certificates of live birth, death, and fetal death. Re-engineered systems will include efficient methods for capturing data and standard data collection instruments; coding specifications; query guidelines; standardized definitions; and Health Level 7–based standardized messaging. Re-engineered systems will need to be integrated with other health information systems, such as those for immunizations, newborn screening, and hearing screening, and with electronic systems used by data providers themselves, including hospitals, physicians, and funeral homes.

The national partnership and its consensus process have already had some notable accomplishments, including the development of functional requirements for re-engineered birth and death registration. The consensus national requirements will serve as the foundation for the design, development, and implementation of re-engineered, Internet-based vital records and statistics systems for states. The most daunting problem still to be solved is the funding of the development and implementation of new systems, especially the automated reporting of deaths by funeral directors and physicians (Rothwell 2003).

Once these re-engineered systems are operational, the dissemination of vital statistics will no longer be tied to the production of annual files for analysis but will be available as soon as they are filed (i.e., in real time). Changes in availability of the data will require new methods of analysis, display, and dissemination in order to take advantage of the enhanced timeliness of vital statistics while protecting the confidentiality of individual subjects. In the more distant future, with the full implementation of electronic health records and the knitting together of the Public Health Information Network and the National Health Information Infrastructure (NHII), the national vital statistics system may evolve into primarily an administrative registration system with direct links to electronic health records to extract the necessary health information surrounding these fundamental societal events (Rothwell 2003). (For additional information on the PHIN see CDC [hp] PHIN; for additional information of the NHII see Chapter 20 and USDHHS [hp] NHII.)

Cancer Registries

Cancer registries collect information through passive and active approaches about the occurrence (incidence) of cancer, the types of cancers that occur and their locations within the body, the extent of cancer at the time of diagnosis (disease stage), and the kinds of treatment that patients receive. These data are reported to a central or statewide registry from various medical facilities, including hospitals, physician office practices, therapeutic radiation facilities, freestanding surgical centers, and pathology laboratories. Data from state cancer registries are used to monitor trends over time and determine cancer patterns in various populations for the nation, in states, and in local communities. Cancer registry data are also useful for guiding the planning and evaluation of cancer control programs, determining priorities for the allocation of health resources, and advancing clinical, epidemiologic, and health services research (Centers for Disease Control and Prevention 2003a).

Historical Development

Cancer registration in the United States began early in the twentieth century with the establishment of a bone sarcoma registry to track etiology, treatment, and survival among patients diagnosed with this rare condition (Clive and Miller 1997). Other specialized registries for cancers of the breast, mouth, tongue, colon, and thyroid soon followed. In the 1930s, the American College of Surgeons initiated clinical surveys and approvals programs for monitoring cancer patient care, although participating hospitals were not required to maintain a cancer registry. The Yale New Haven Hospital was the first hospital-based registry in the United States in 1942, and the Connecticut Tumor Registry, which has diagnoses dating to 1935, was the first population-based cancer registry. In 1971, Congress passed the National Cancer Act that mandated the collection, analysis, and dissemination of data useful for the prevention, diagnosis, and treatment of cancer (National Cancer Act of 1971). This mandate led to the establishment of the Surveillance, Epidemiology, and End Results (SEER) Program at the National Cancer Institute (NCI) (Hankey et al. 1999).

SURVEILLANCE EPIDEMIOLOGY AND END RESULTS PROGRAM

A continuing program of the NCI, SEER consists of population-based cancer registries that routinely collect data on all cancers that occur among residents of the participating geographic areas. Thirty-year trends in cancer incidence and patient survival in the United States are derived from this database.

Case ascertainment for SEER began on January 1, 1973, in Connecticut, Hawaii, Iowa, New Mexico, and Utah and in the metropolitan areas of Detroit and San Francisco-Oakland. Table 4.3 shows the current location of SEER registries in the United States and the first diagnosis year for which data were reported to the NCI for each SEER area. The SEER Program currently collects and publishes cancer incidence and survival data for 26% of the U.S. population, including 23% of African Americans, 40% of Hispanics, 42% of American Indians and Alaska Natives, 53% of Asians, and 70% of Native Hawaiians and Pacific Islanders (U.S. Cancer Statistics Working Group 2003). Information on more than 3 million in situ and invasive cancer cases is included in the SEER database, and approximately 170,000 new cases are accessioned each year within SEER catchment areas. The SEER registries routinely collect data on patient demographics, primary tumor site, morphology, stage at diagnosis, and first course of treatment. They also actively follow all patients for information on vital status (alive or dead) (Surveillance, Epidemiology, and End Results [hp]).

NATIONAL PROGRAM OF CANCER REGISTRIES

Recognizing the need for more complete local, state, regional, and national cancer incidence data, Congress established the National Program of Cancer Registries (NPCR) in 1992, which required the CDC to provide funds to states and territories to improve or enhance existing cancer registries; plan for and implement registries where they did not exist; develop model legislation and regulations for states and territories to enhance the viability of registry operations; set standards for data completeness, timeliness, and quality; provide training for registry personnel; and help establish a computerized reporting and

TABLE 4.3

First Diagnosis Year for Which Cancer Cases Were Reportable to the NPCR or SEER, Federal Funding Source for Cancer Registries in 2004, and the Quality of Data Contributed by Cancer Registries to *United States Cancer Statistics: 2000 Incidence* by State, Territory, and Selected Metropolitan Area, United States

State, Metropolitan Area, or Territory	*First Diagnosis Year for Which Cancer Cases Were Reportable to the NPCR or SEER*	*Federal Funding Source, 2004*	*Registry Met High Quality Data Criteria for Publication in* United States Cancer Statistics: 2000 Incidence
Alabama	1996	NPCR	Yes
Alaska	1996	NPCR	Yes
Arizona	1995	NPCR	Yes
Arkansas	1996	NPCR	No
California	1995/2000	NPCR/SEER	Yes
Los Angeles	1992	SEER	Yes
San Francisco-Oakland	1973	SEER	Yes
San Jose-Monterey	1992	SEER	Yes
Colorado	1995	NPCR	Yes
Connecticut	1973	SEER	Yes
Delaware	1997	NPCR	No
District of Columbia	1996	NPCR	Yes
Florida	1995	NPCR	Yes
Georgia	1995	NPCR	Yes
Atlanta	1975	SEER	Yes
Hawaii	1973	SEER	Yes
Idaho	1995	NPCR	Yes
Illinois	1995	NPCR	Yes
Indiana	1995	NPCR	Yes
Iowa	1973	SEER	Yes
Kansas	1995	NPCR	Yes
Kentucky	1995/2000	NPCR/SEER	Yes
Louisiana	1995/2000	NPCR/SEER	Yes
Maine	1995	NPCR	No
Maryland	1996	NPCR	Yes
Massachusetts	1995	NPCR	Yes
Michigan	1995	NPCR	Yes
Detroit	1973	SEER	Yes
Minnesota	1995	NPCR	Yes
Mississippi	1996	NPCR	No
Missouri	1996	NPCR	Yes
Montana	1995	NPCR	Yes
Nebraska	1995	NPCR	Yes
Nevada	1995	NPCR	Yes
New Hampshire	1995	NPCR	Yes

(*continued*)

TABLE 4.3
Continued

State, Metropolitan Area, or Territory	*First Diagnosis Year for Which Cancer Cases Were Reportable to the NPCR or SEER*	*Federal Funding Source, 2004*	*Registry Met High Quality Data Criteria for Publication in* United States Cancer Statistics: Incidence 2000
New Jersey	1995/2000	NPCR/SEER	Yes
New Mexico	1973	SEER	Yes
New York	1996	NPCR	Yes
North Carolina	1995	NPCR	Yes
North Dakota	1997	NPCR	Yes
Ohio	1996	NPCR	Yes
Oklahoma	1997	NPCR	No
Oregon	1996	NPCR	Yes
Palau	1999	NPCR	No
Pennsylvania	1995	NPCR	Yes
Puerto Rico	1998	NPCR	No
Rhode Island	1995	NPCR	Yes
South Carolina	1996	NPCR	Yes
South Dakota	2000	NPCR	No
Tennessee	1999	NPCR	No
Texas	1995	NPCR	No
Utah	1973	SEER	Yes
Vermont	1996	NPCR	Yes
Virgin Islands	1999	NPCR	No
Virginia	1996	NPCR	No
Washington	1995	NPCR	Yes
Seattle-Puget Sound	1974	SEER	Yes
West Virginia	1995	NPCR	Yes
Wisconsin	1995	NPCR	Yes
Wyoming	1996	NPCR	Yes

NPCR = National Program of Cancer Registries; SEER = Surveillance, Epidemiology, and End Results.
Source: U.S. Cancer Statistics Working Group (2003).

data-processing system (Cancer Registries Amendment Act, Public Law 102-515). Before the NPCR was established, 10 states had no cancer registry and many states with a cancer registry lacked the resources and legislative support to collect needed data (Centers for Disease Control and Prevention 1994). In 2004, the CDC funded a total of 45 states, the District of Columbia, and three U.S. territories; and NPCR registries covered 96% of the U.S. population, including 96% of whites, 99% of blacks, 91% of Asians/Pacific Islanders, 92% of American Indians/Alaska Natives, and 96% of Hispanics (Table 4.3).

The NPCR registries routinely collect data on patient demographics, primary site, morphology, stage at diagnosis, and first course of treatment. They also conduct passive follow-up for vital status (confirming deaths through linkage with state and national death records). In January 2001, NPCR registries began annually reporting incidence data to the CDC. In January 2004, the CDC received information on more than 7.6 million invasive cancer cases diagnosed during 1995–2001, including 1.2 million invasive cancer cases diagnosed in 2001 (Centers for Disease Control and Prevention [hp] National Program of Cancer Registries).

NORTH AMERICAN ASSOCIATION OF CENTRAL CANCER REGISTRIES

Established in 1987, the North American Association of Central Cancer Registries (NAACCR)is an umbrella organization for population-based cancer registries, governmental agencies, professional associations, and private groups in North America interested in improving the quality and use of cancer registry data. The mission of the NAACCR is to support and coordinate the development, enhancement, and application of cancer registration techniques in population-based groups in a consistent manner, so that quality data may be used for cancer control and epidemiologic research, public health programs, and patient care to reduce the burden of cancer in North America. All state and metropolitan area registries participating in the NPCR and SEER are members of the NAACCR (North American Association of Central Cancer Registries [hp]).

Current Practice and Activities

AUTHORITY

Cancer registration now occurs in all 50 states, the District of Columbia, and selected U.S. territories (Table 4.3). All states, except one—South Dakota—have a law authorizing the formation of a statewide central cancer registry, making cancer a reportable disease (Centers for Disease Control and Prevention 1994; Hutton et al. 2001).

FUNDING AND OTHER SOURCES OF SUPPORT

In addition to technical and financial resources from both the SEER Program and the NPCR, states provide partial financial support to cancer registries. Under the Federal Cancer Registries Amendment Act, the state, or the academic institution or private organization designated by the state to operate the cancer registry, contributes not less than 25% of the federal funds (Cancer Registries Amendment Act, Public Law 102-515). That is, this maintenance of effort requires that the state provide no less than $1 for every $3 of federal funds. In addition, cancer registries work closely with the NAACCR to promote standards for cancer surveillance in the United States and Canada.

SOURCES OF DATA AND TYPES OF DATA COLLECTED

Potential new diagnoses of cancer are identified through active and passive methods of case ascertainment (Potts et al. 1997). Active case finding occurs in hospital- and population-based registries and involves the thorough examination of various hospital and nonhospital sources (Menck and West 1997; Potts et al. 1997). Hospital sources include pathology reports (histology, pathology, cytology, hematology, and autopsy), health records (admission reports, discharge summaries, disease indices), radiation therapy reports (radiation therapy logs, treatment summaries), surgery schedules, outpatient reports, diagnostic radiology and nuclear medicine logs and reports; nonhospital sources include outpatient treatment facilities, independent pathology laboratories, radiation and surgery facilities, physician office practices (oncology and dermatology offices), out-of-state facilities, and various sources related to end-of-life care (hospices, nursing homes, Vital Statistics offices, coroners' offices) (Menck and West 1997; Potts et al. 1997). Data collection from nonhospital sources is challenging and requires extensive resources. The primary advantage of active case finding includes more complete and accurate information as coded by persons, usually certified tumor registrars, who have extensive knowledge of terminology that identifies potential cases. The primary disadvantage is the high financial and personnel costs.

Passive case ascertainment involves reports from other health care professionals who notify the registries of potential new cases of cancer (Potts et al. 1997). The primary advantage and disadvantage are the opposite of active case finding: possibly decreased financial and labor costs and potentially less complete information. Cancer registries in the United States typically use both active and passive case ascertainment procedures.

Data on newly identified potential cases from hospital and nonhospital sources are reported to regional or statewide population-based registries in the United States. Because information about a particular cancer case usually derives from multiple sources, registrars use hands-on approaches and computer software to consolidate these data and to resolve discrepancies among sources. Selected metropolitan areas and all states provide information about all cancer cases diagnosed in their geographic area to the NPCR or SEER.

DATA QUALITY

Published cancer incidence data for the United States must meet selected high quality data criteria (Hotes et al. 2003; U.S. Cancer Statistics Working Group 2003). More specifically, the data must be population-based and meet these minimum requirements:

- Case ascertainment is 90% or more complete.[6]
- No more than 5% of cases are ascertained solely on the basis of a death certificate.

- No more than 3% of cases are missing information on sex, 3% on age, and 5% on race. The completeness of basic demographic information (e.g., gender, age, and race) is essential for describing the cancer burden in all populations.
- At least 97% of the registry's records pass a set of single-field and interfield computerized edits. These edits test the validity and logic of data components, such as consistency in age, as reported by various sources.[7]

In 1997, the NAACCR began voluntary annual reviews of member registries to determine their ability to produce complete, accurate, and timely data. Registries report their data to the NAACCR in early December each year. The NAACCR evaluates the data using standard, objective measures and then recognizes through certification those registries that meet the highest standards for data quality (Tucker and Howe 2001; Tucker et al. 1999).[8]

CASE DEFINITION

The NPCR and SEER cancer registries consider as reportable all incident in situ or invasive cancers with the exception of in situ cancer of the cervix and basal and squamous cell carcinomas of the skin, with the exception of those on the skin of the genital organs (Hultstrom 2002).

Both NPCR and SEER data are collected and reported using uniform data items and codes as documented by the NAACCR, which provides for comparability of data items collected by the two federal programs (Hultstrom 2002; Surveillance, Epidemiology, and End Results Program 1998). All information on primary cancer sites is coded according to the ICD-O-2 (Percy et al. 1990). Cancers in patients of unknown sex or age are excluded. The classification of childhood cancer differs from that used for adult cancers.[9]

Use of Cancer Registry Data for Public Health Practice

In 2000, more than 1 million invasive cancer cases in adults and 10,456 cases in children less than 20 years old were diagnosed and reported by 42 state cancer registries (37 NPCR and 5 SEER), the District of Columbia (NPCR), and 6 SEER metropolitan areas (U.S. Cancer Statistics Working Group 2003). These data are reported in the *United States Cancer Statistics.* In total, the population-based cancer registries that met the high quality data criteria for inclusion in the report covered 84% of the U.S. population (Table 4.3) (84% of the U.S. white population, 81% of the U.S. black population, 91% of the U.S. Asian/Pacific Islander population, and 79% of the U.S. Hispanic population).

Data collected by state cancer registries enable local, state, and national public health professionals to better understand and address the cancer burden in their jurisdictions (Centers for Disease Control and Prevention 2003a). Registry data are critical for targeting programs focused on risk-related behaviors (e.g., tobacco use and exposure to the sun) or on environmental risk factors (e.g., radiation and chemical exposures). The Minnesota registry, for example, noted an excess of mesothelioma, a rare cancer with only one known cause—asbestos—in the northeastern part of the state (Centers for Disease Control and Prevention 2001). Registry data are also essential for identifying when and where cancer screening efforts should be enhanced and for monitoring the treatment provided to cancer patients. Some states, Arizona and New Jersey, for example, have used registry data to identify geographic areas with excess late-stage breast cancers for increased mammography screening (Centers for Disease Control and Prevention 2001; Roche et al. 2002). In addition, reliable registry data are fundamental to a variety of research efforts, including those aimed at evaluating the effectiveness of cancer prevention, control, or treatment programs.

Current Issues

DEFICIENCIES OF THE CURRENT SYSTEM

Although the cancer registration infrastructure in the United States is highly developed, there is a pressing need for more timely data—a common theme and need among health statistics systems. As medical records are the source of most of the data in cancer registries, meeting this need would be facilitated by more complete implementation of the electronic health record using accepted national electronic messaging and clinical coding standards (Williams 2002). Application of state-of-the-art technologies and national standards will yield more timely and efficient collection of higher-quality data for cancer registries. Other needs include support to states for increasing their use of data in more sophisticated ways, such as geo-coding, linkages with Medicare and other health claims systems to access additional patient information about treatment and a history of comorbid conditions, and increased use of registry data for cancer control planning and research.

NEW APPROACHES FOR REPORTING DATA

Increased application of information technology transfer, including electronic pathology reporting and data quality, are issues of current importance and interest to registries. Health Level 7 (HL7) is being used as a data messaging standard, and standardized vocabularies such as the Logical Observation Identifiers Names and Codes (LOINC) and the Systematized Nomenclature of Medicine (SNOMED) are already being used by some pathology laboratories (Health Level Seven [hp]; LOINC [hp]; SNOMED International [hp]). A cancer registries workgroup met to explore the development and application of an alternate reporting protocol to the NAACCR format that would use HL7 messages, LOINC identifier codes, standard demographics, and local value responses. The workgroup produced an implementation guide using the HL7 approach (Centers for Disease Control and Prevention 1998b), which promoted pilot projects to test the use of this alternative standardized approach for reporting data to cancer registries. Additional work has focused on the development and use of a comprehensive medical record vocabulary, including the educational, practical, and technical concerns of implementing a vocabulary that accommodates both ICD-O and SNOMED. While it is important for cancer registries to promote and use national standardized coding schemes and reporting structures, it is equally important for the standards organizations to integrate into their standards, as appropriate, the practical reporting needs of cancer registries. Thus, the development and use of messaging approaches and clinical coding sets for cancer registries that follow national standards will require a transitional approach. Finally, cancer registries need to be broadly educated about the use and benefits of controlled vocabularies, and national standards organizations educated about coding schemes for specific program data needs.

NATIONAL HEALTH INFORMATION INFRASTRUCTURE

Achieving the NHII vision (see Chapter 20) requires synergy and interplay among many organizations. Active coordination efforts are needed to strengthen the reporting of clinical data to cancer registries and build upon various components of the NHII. For example, the College of American Pathology (CAP) has developed and published standardized reporting protocols. These are designed to help the surgical pathologist achieve completeness, accuracy, and uniformity in collecting and reporting pathology-related tumor data. In 2001, the CDC funded two state registries to work with two pathology laboratories to evaluate the use of code sets and structured data entry for pathology reports submitted to cancer registries. As a collaborative effort in public health practice, this 3-year project is expected to result in improvements in the completeness, timeliness, and quality of cancer data from pathology laboratories (Centers for Disease Control and Prevention 2003b). Additional evaluation and educational efforts are needed to demonstrate the practical benefits of standards supporting the NHII.

IMPROVING DATA QUALITY

Applications of electronic pathology reporting and national standards for the transmission of medical data will contribute to more timely and higher-quality data. Two areas of data quality that are of current interest in cancer registries are the quality of data for specific racial and ethnic populations and stage of disease at diagnosis.

Providing accurate estimates of disease burden in specific racial and ethnic populations poses unique challenges, particularly with the 2000 census question allowing respondents to identify more than one race. Information on detailed race is coded at state cancer registries according to standard definitions, consistent with current federal agency standards (Hultstrom 2002; Office of Management and Budget 1997). Although standardized data items and codes for both race and Hispanic ethnicity are used in state registries across the country, the initial collection of information on a patient's race and ethnicity by reporting health-care facilities and practitioners is variable. Some institutions report only white, black, and other race; others, such as some pathology labs, do not report race at all (O'Malley et al. 2002). In addition, state registries do not follow identical procedures for assigning the standard codes for race and ethnicity: some registries use either surname lists or birthplace to improve the reporting of specific racial and ethnic populations, while others do not (O'Malley et al. 2002). Inconsistencies in the collection and coding of data on race and ethnicity and the subsequent impact on incidence and mortality statistics have been documented (Minino et al. 2002).

Stage at diagnosis is variously reported according to different systems meeting different needs (Hultstrom 1997). Three systems are consistently used by the cancer registry community: tumor, nodes, and metastasis stage from the American Joint Committee on Cancer by clinicians for assessing prognosis and making treatment decisions; extent of disease by the SEER Program; and SEER summary stage by the NPCR. Hospital registrars in some facilities are responsible for providing stage at diagnosis according to all three systems. To promote coordination, to reduce the burden on registrars, and to ensure better quality for staging data across the cancer registry community, the concept of *collaborative stage* was introduced in 1998.

Collaborative stage was designed to address differences in guidelines among the major staging systems used in the United States (Collaborative Staging Task Force of the American Joint Committee on Cancer 2004). The American Joint Committee on Cancer formed the Collaborative Staging Task Force to develop the crosswalk among TNM, SEER extent of disease, and SEER Summary Stage and determined that nine basic data elements (tumor size, extension, tumor size/extension evaluation, lymph nodes, regional nodes evaluation, regional notes positive, regional nodes examined, site of metastases at diagnosis, method of diagnosing metastases) plus six site-specific factors could be translated by a computer algorithm into any of these three systems. Collaborative stage was implemented in 2004.

INTEGRATION OF SYSTEMS

Hospital- and population-based cancer registries provide the infrastructure for identifying patterns and trends in cancer occurrence and treatment and for directing cancer control interventions in the United States, including broad geographic regions, individual states, and local communities. Support for this infrastructure derives from many sources: (*1*) hospitals that maintain tumor registries; (*2*) American College of Surgeons standardized data collection in hospital cancer registries through participation in the Approvals Program and the National Cancer Database (American College of Surgeons [hp] Commission on cancer information); (*3*) certification by the National Cancer Registrars Association and continuing education programs for cancer registrars (National Cancer Registrars Association [hp]); (*4*) state mandates for public health reporting for all residents with new diagnoses of cancer and partial financial support from states for cancer registries; (*5*) NAACCR consensus standards and measures of data quality for central registries (Hotes et al. 2003; Howe 2001; Tucker and Howe 2001; Tucker et al. 1999); and (*6*) funding and technical assistance to population-based registries from the NPCR and SEER. Collaboration among these entities is essential for maintaining high-quality, complete, and uniform cancer reporting. With the expanding adoption of the electronic health records, systems maintained by these entities must also be coordinated with data received from radiation therapy facilities, physician office practices, and other nonhospital sources of cancer diagnostic and treatment information. Complete integration can occur only with the adoption of national standards for electronic messaging and coding.

CONCERNS ABOUT SECURITY AND CONFIDENTIALITY

Security and confidentiality are key issues for cancer registries, the research community that uses registry data, and the public (Deapen 2004; North American Association of Central Cancer Registries 2002). Historically, cancer registries have done an excellent job of protecting patient privacy (Deapen 2004). They have given extensive consideration to physical security procedures for confidential data, physical data security, and electronic data security (North American Association of Central Cancer Registries 2002). The public is concerned that breaches of confidentiality may lead to financial losses, such as loss of employment or health insurance, or to embarrassment and psychological harm (Deapen 2004). The Cancer Registries Amendment Act that created the NPCR requires that confidentiality regulations and legislation be enacted in states before the states receive federal funds for a statewide cancer registry (Cancer Registries Amendment Act of 1992). States must provide assurances (Cancer Registries Amendment Act of 1992, Sec. 3 (c) (2) (D) (v–vi)):

> (v) for the protection of the confidentiality of all cancer case data reported to the statewide cancer registry, including a prohibition on disclosure to any persons of information reported to the statewide cancer registry that identifies, or could lead to the identification of, an individual cancer patient, except for disclosure to other State cancer registries and local and State health officers;
>
> (vi) for a means by which confidential case data may in accordance with State law be disclosed to cancer researchers for the purposes of cancer prevention, control, and research.

In addition, the cancer registry data provided to the CDC from states that participate in the NPCR are protected by a federal Assurance of Confidentiality that covers routine surveillance activities and that is provided to only a few data collection efforts. While it is a matter of principle for the CDC to guard sensitive information, and while federal statutes such as the Privacy Act provide a degree of protection, Section 308 (d) of the Public Health Service Act, which describes the federal Assurance of Confidentiality, enables the CDC to provide the highest level of confidentiality protection for sensitive and mission-significant research and surveillance data, such as the data collected by cancer registries.

CONCLUSION

The example notification system and these two registration systems illustrate common themes among health statistics systems today that are also emphasized in other chapters in this book. There is an increasing expectation of timely electronic sharing of data to maximize efficiency of the systems and effective, comprehensive use of data to improve the health of the public. Efforts directed at these goals in the United States fall under the rubric of the NHII, a critical framework for successful implementation of fully electronic, interoperable, and useful systems.

NOTES

1. Notifications of some events may be voluntary, rather than required, and may be received from any member of the population. In this situation, a government agency is often responsible for follow-up investigation and intervention.
2. For the most up-to-date list of nationally notifiable diseases, see http://www.cdc.gov/epo/dphsi/phs/infdis.htm.
3. The CDC maintains up-to-date case definitions at http://www.cdc.gov/epo/dphsi/casedef.
4. See also Bellows (1948). Ms. Bellows, in her article on case registers, considered their distinguishing feature to be the recording of changes in status over a period of time. Thus, she did not consider reports of births, deaths, or other single events in the life of a person as fitting her definition of a case register. Nevertheless, these events are fitting for a register and registration if they are intended to be used for long-term tracking of the event or person.
5. See also Stroup et al. (1994) for further discussion and examples of different kinds of registries.
6. Case ascertainment assessed by methods developed by the NAACCR (Hotes et al. 2003; Howe 2001; Tucker and Howe 2001; Tucker et al. 1999).
7. The SEER Program originally developed these edits; they were expanded in the 1990s and incorporated into NAACCR standards (North American Association of Central Cancer Registries [hp] Data standards and data dictionary).
8. In 2003, after the NAACCR evaluated the 2000 incidence data, 36 NPCR registries and all 10 SEER registries were certified. For more information on the certification program, see North American Association of Central Cancer Registries [hp] Registry certification.

9. Childhood cancers are presented in 12 groups that are classified by morphology, while adult cancers are categorized mainly by primary site. Most cases (94%) are confirmed by positive microscopic findings (histology, cytology, or unspecified microscopy method) indicative of cancer (Hultstrom 2002).

REFERENCES

Alter MJ, Mares A, Hadler SC, et al. The effect of underreporting on the apparent incidence and epidemiology of acute viral hepatitis. Am J Epidemiol 1987;125:133–139.

American Academy of Pediatrics, Committee on Infectious Diseases. Measles: reassessment of the current immunization policy. Pediatrics 1989;84:1110–1113.

American College of Surgeons [homepage on the Internet]. Chicago: American College of Surgeons; c. 1998–2004 [updated 2004 May 18; cited 2004 May 25]. Commission on cancer information. Available from: http://www.facs.org/cancer/index.html.

American Thoracic Society, Centers for Disease Control and Prevention. Treatment of tuberculosis and tuberculosis infection in adults and children. Am J Respir Crit Care Med 1994;149:1359–1374.

Barrows RC, Clayton PD. Privacy, confidentiality, and electronic medical records. JAMIA 1996;3:139–148.

Bell BP, Goldoft, M, Griffin PM, et al. A multistate outbreak of *Escherichia coli* O157:H7–asssociated bloody diarrhea and hemolytic uremic syndrome from hamburgers. The Washington experience. JAMA 1994;272:1349–1353.

Bellows MT. Case registers. Conference of Public Health Statistics. University of Michigan, School of Public Health, June 15, 1948.

Birkhead G, Chorba TL, Root S, Klaucke DN, Gibbs NJ. Timeliness of national reporting of communicable diseases: the experience of the National Electronic Telecommunications System for Surveillance. Am J Public Health 1991;81:1313–1315.

Broome CV, Horton HH, Tress D, Lucido SJ, Koo D. Statutory basis for public health reporting beyond specific diseases. J Urban Health: Bull NY Acad Med 2003:80(2)suppl 1:i14–i22.

Campos-Outcalt D, England R, Porter B. Reporting of communicable diseases by university physicians. Public Health Rep 1991;106:579–583.

Cancer Registries Amendment Act of 1992, Pub. L. No. 102-515, 106 Stat. 3372 (October 24, 1992) [cited 2003 Jul 21]. Available from: http://www.cdc.gov/cancer/npcr/npcrpdfs/publaw.pdf.

Centers for Disease Control and Prevention. Measles prevention. MMWR 1989;38(suppl 9):1–18.

Centers for Disease Control and Prevention. Case definitions for public health surveillance, 1990. MMWR 1990;39(no. RR-13):1–43.

Centers for Disease Control and Prevention. Initial therapy for tuberculosis in the era of multidrug resistance: recommendation of the Advisory Council for the Elimination of Tuberculosis. MMWR 1993a;42(no. RR-7):1–8.

Centers for Disease Control and Prevention. Summary of notifiable diseases, United States, 1993b. MMWR 1993b;42(53):iii.

Centers for Disease Control and Prevention. State cancer registries: status of authorizing legislation and enabling regulations—United States, October 1993. MMWR 1994;43(4): 71–75.

Centers for Disease Control and Prevention. Case definitions for infectious conditions under public health surveillance. MMWR 1997;46(no. RR-10):1–55.

Centers for Disease Control and Prevention. 1998 Guidelines for treatment of sexually transmitted diseases. MMWR 1998a;47(no. RR-1):1–111.

Centers for Disease Control and Prevention. Working Toward Implementation of HL7 in NAACCR Information Technology Standards: Meeting Summary Report. Atlanta: Centers for Disease Control and Prevention; 1998b [cited 2004 May 21]. Available from: http://www.cdc.gov/cancer/npcr/archives/npcr-archive-000426-1.htm.
Centers for Disease Control and Prevention. Summary of notifiable diseases, United States, 2000. MMWR 2000;49(53):v.
Centers for Disease Control and Prevention. Cancer Registries: The Foundation for Cancer Prevention and Control 2001. Atlanta: Centers for Disease Control and Prevention; 2001 [cited 2004 Nov 9]. Available from: http://www.cdc.gov/cancer/npcr/npcrpdfs/npcaag01.pdf.
Centers for Disease Control and Prevention. Cancer Registries: The Foundation for Cancer Prevention and Control. Atlanta: Centers for Disease Control and Prevention; 2003a [cited 2004 May 21]. Available from: http://www.cdc.gov/cancer/npcr/register.htm.
Centers for Disease Control and Prevention. National Program of Cancer Registries Research and Evaluation Activities. Atlanta: Centers for Disease Control and Prevention; 2003b, p. 1 [cited 2004 May 21]. Available from: http://www.cdc.gov/cancer/npcr/scienceinbrief-registries2003.htm.
Centers for Disease Control and Prevention [homepage on the Internet]. Atlanta: Centers for Disease Control and Prevention [updated 2004 May 12; cited 2004 May 21]. National Program of Cancer Registries. Available from: http://www.cdc.gov/cancer/npcr.
Centers for Disease Control and Prevention [homepage on the Internet]. Atlanta: Centers for Disease Control and Prevention [updated 2004 Apr 7; cited 2004 May 20]. Nationally notifiable infectious diseases. Available from: http://www.cdc.gov/epo/dphsi/phs/infdis.htm.
Centers for Disease Control and Prevention [homepage on the Internet]. Atlanta: Centers for Disease Control and Prevention [cited 2004 May 25]. National Electronic Disease Surveillance System. Available from: http://www.cdc.gov/nedss.
Centers for Disease Control and Prevention [homepage on the Internet]. Atlanta: Centers for Disease Control and Prevention [updated 2004 May 20; cited 2004 May 20]. Public health information network. Available from: http://www.cdc.gov/phin.
Chamblee RF, Evans MC. TRANSAX: The NCHS system for producing multiple cause-of-death statistics, 1968–1978. Vital and Health Statistics Series 1, No. 20. DHHS Publication No. (PHS) 86-1322. Washington, DC: GPO; 1986. Available from: http://www.cdc.gov/nchs/data/series/sr_01/sr01_020acc.pdf.
Clive RE, Miller DS. Introduction to cancer registries. In: Hutchison CL, Roffers SD, Fritz AD, eds. Cancer Registry Management: Principles and Practice. Lenexa, KS: National Cancer Registrars Association; 1997, pp. 1–8.
Collaborative Staging Task Force of the American Joint Committee on Cancer. Collaborative Staging Manual and Coding Instructions, Version 1.0. Chicago: American Joint Committee on Cancer; Bethesda, MD: U.S. Department of Health and Human Services; 2004. NIH Publication No. 04-5496 [cited 2004 May 21]. Available from: http://www.cancerstaging.org/collab.html.
Deapen D. Impact of privacy and confidentiality concerns. Presentation at C-Change summit on cancer surveillance and information: the next decade; Jan 30, 2004, Pointe Hilton Squaw Peak Resort, Phoenix, AZ [cited 2004 May 21]. Available from: http://www.ndoc.org/about_ndc/calendar_of_events/summitjan04/DEAPEN.pdf.
Fox J, Stahlsmith L, Remington P, Tymus T, Hargarten S. The Wisconsin Firearm-Related Injury Surveillance System. Am J Prev Med 1998;15(suppl 3):101–108.
Hampton, B. Collection of morbidity data and other sanitary information by the United States Public Health Service. Public Health Rep 1923;38:2817–2830.
Hankey BF, Ries LA, Edwards BK. The Surveillance, Epidemiology, and End Results Program: a national resource. Cancer Epidemiol Biomarkers Prev 1999;8(12):1117–1121.
Health Canada [homepage on the Internet]. Ottawa: Health Canada; [updated 2003 Dec 11;

cited 2004 May 21]. National notifiable diseases for 2000. Available from: http://dsol-smed.hc-sc.gc.ca/dsol-smed/ndis/list_e.html.
Health Level Seven [homepage on the Internet]. Ann Arbor, MI: Health Level Seven, Inc. c. 1997–2004 [cited 2004 Mar 3]. Available from: http://www.hl7.org.
Hetzel AM. U.S. Vital Statistics System: Major Activities and Developments, 1950–95. Hyattsville, MD: National Center for Health Statistics; 1997 [cited 2004 May 21]. Available from: http://www.cdc.gov/nchs/data/misc/usvss.pdf.
Hotes JL, Wu XC, McLauglin CC, Lake A, Firth R, Roney D, et al. Cancer in North America, 1996–2000. Vol. 1: Incidence. Springfield, IL: North American Association of Central Cancer Registries; 2003.
Howe HL. Conclusions of the Workgroup for High Quality Criteria for Data Use: The NAACCR Narrative. Springfield, IL: North American Association of Central Cancer Registries; 2001.
Hulstrom D. Extent of disease and cancer staging. In: Hutchison CL, Roffers SD, Fritz AD, eds. Cancer Registry Management: Principles and Practice. Lenexa, KS: National Cancer Registrars Association; 1997, pp. 83–100.
Hultstrom D. Standards for Cancer Registries. Vol. 2: Data Standards and Data Dictionary, version 10, 7th ed. Springfield, IL: North American Association of Central Cancer Registries; 2002.
Hutton MD, Simpson LD, Miller DS, Weir HK, McDavid K, Hall HI. Progress toward nationwide cancer surveillance: an evaluation of the National Program of Cancer Registries, 1994–1999. J Registry Manag 2001;28(3):113–120.
Kimball AM, Thacker SB, Levy ME. Shigella surveillance in a large metropolitan area: assessment of a passive reporting system. Am J Public Health 1980;70:164–166.
Kirsch T, Shesser R. A survey of emergency department communicable disease reporting practices. J Emerg Med 1991;9:211–214.
Konowitz PM, Petrossian GA, Rose DN. The underreporting of disease and physicians—knowledge of reporting requirements. Public Health Rep 1984;99:31–35.
Koo D, Wetterhall SF. History and current status of the National Notifiable Diseases Surveillance System. J Public Health Manag Pract 1996;2:4–10.
Langmuir AD. The surveillance of communicable diseases of national importance. N Engl J Med 1963;268:182–192.
LOINC [homepage on the Internet]. Indianapolis: Regenstrief Institute; ©2002–2004 [cited 2004 May 21]. Available from: http://www.loinc.org.
Marier R. The reporting of communicable diseases. Am J Epidemiol 1977;105:587–590.
Mathews TJ, Menacker F, MacDorman MF. Infant mortality statistics from the 2001 period linked birth/infant death data set. Natl Vital Stat Rep 2003;52(2):1–27. [cited 2004 May 4]. Available from: http://www.cdc.gov/nchs/data/nvsr/nvsr52/nvsr52_02.pdf.
Menck HR, West DW. Central cancer registries. In: Hutchison CL, Roffers SD, Fritz AD, eds. Cancer Registry Management: Principles and Practice. Lenexa, KS: National Cancer Registrars Association; 1997, pp. 395–422.
Mercy JA, Ikeda R, Powell KE. Firearm-related injury surveillance. an overview of progress and the challenges ahead. Am J Prev Med 1998;15(Suppl 3):6–16.
Meyer PA, Pivetz T, Dignam TA, Homa DM, Schoonover J, Brody D. Surveillance for elevated blood lead levels among children—United States, 1997—2001. MMWR CDC Surveill Summ 2003;52(SS10):1–21.
Minino AM, Arias E, Kochanek KD, Murphy SL, Smith BL. Deaths: Final Data for 2000. Natl Vital Stat Rep 50(15). Hyattsville, MD: National Center for Health Statistics; 2002.
Morris G, Snider D, Katz M. Integrating public health information and surveillance systems. J Public Health Manag Pract 1996;2:24–27.
Mullan F. Plagues and Politics: The Story of the United States Public Health Service. New York: Basic Books; 1989.

National Association for Public Health Statistics and Information Systems. Amendments to the Model State Vital Statistics Act. Resolution 2000-5. Enacted at the annual meeting of the National Association for Public Health Statistics and Information Systems, Austin, TX; June 18, 2000.

National Association for Public Health Statistics and Information Systems [homepage on the Internet]. Silver Spring, MD: National Association for Public Health Statistics and Information Systems [cited 2004 May 7]. About NAPHSIS. Available from: http://www.naphsis.org.

National Cancer Act of 1971, Pub. L. No. 92–218, 85 Stat. 1828 (Dec. 23, 1971) [accessed 2003, July 21]. Available from: http://www3.cancer.gov/legis/1971canc.html.

National Cancer Registrars Association [homepage on the Internet]. Washington, DC: National Cancer Registrars Association; c. 2003 [cited 2004 May 21]. Available from: http://www.ncra-usa.org.

National Center for Health Statistics. Model State Vital Statistics Act and Regulations, 1992 Revision. Hyattsville, MD: National Center for Health Statistics; 1995 [cited 2004 May 20]. Available from: http://www.cdc.gov/nchs/data/misc/mvsact92aacc.pdf.

National Center for Health Statistics. Current Legislative Authorities of the National Center for Health Statistics. Hyattsville, MD: National Center for Health Statistics; 2000a [cited 2004 May 7]. Available from: http://www.cdc.gov/nchs/data/misc/legis99.pdf.

National Center for Health Statistics, Division of Vital Statistics. Report of the Panel to Evaluate the U.S. Standard Certificates. Hyattsville, MD: National Center for Health Statistics; 2000b (Addendum November 2001) [cited 2004 May 7]. Available from: http://www.cdc.gov/nchs/vital_certs_rev.htm.

National Center for Health Statistics. Specifications for Collecting and Editing the United States Standard Certificates of Birth and Death—2003 revisions. Hyattsville, MD: National Center for Health Statistics; 2001a [cited 2004 May 7]. Available from: http://www.cdc.gov/nchs/vital_certs_rev.htm.

National Center for Health Statistics [monograph on the Internet]. Vital Statistics of the United States, 1999. Vol. I: Natality. Hyattsville, MD: National Center for Health Statistics; 2001b [cited 2004 May 7]. Available from: http://www.cdc.gov/nchs/datawh/statab/unpubd/natality/natab99.htm.

National Center for Health Statistics. Guide to Completing the Facility Worksheets for the Certificate of Live Birth and Report of Fetal Death (2003 Revision). Hyattsville, MD: National Center for Health Statistics 2003a [cited 2004 May 7]. Available from: http://www.cdc.gov/nchs/vital_certs_rev.htm.

National Center for Health Statistics. 1995–98 matched multiple birth data set. CD-ROM Series 21, No. 13A. Hyattsville (MD): National Center for Health Statistics; 2003b.

National Center for Health Statistics. 2001 Perinatal Mortality Data File. CD-ROM Series 20, No. 22. Hyattsville, MD: National Center for Health Statistics; 2004.

National Center for Health Statistics [homepage on the Internet]. Hyattsville, MD: National Center for Health Statistics [updated 2004 Apr 14; cited 2004 Nov 15]. 2003 revisions of the U.S. standard certifcates of live birth and death and the fetal death report. Available from: http://www.cdc.gov/nchs/vital_certs_rev.htm.

National Center for Health Statistics [homepage on the Internet]. Hyattsville, MD: National Center for Health Statistics [updated 2004 Apr 28; cited 2004 May 7]. HIST290A: Deaths for selected causes by 10-year age groups, race, and sex; death registration states, 1900–32, and United States, 1933–98. Available from: http://www.cdc.gov/nchs/datawh/statab/unpubd/mortabs/hist290a.htm.

National Center for Health Statistics [homepage on the Internet]. Hyattsville, MD: National Center for Health Statistics [updated 2004 May 4; cited 2004 May 7]. National Vital Statistics System. Available from: http://www.cdc.gov/nchs/nvss.htm.

National Electronic Disease Surveillance System Working Group. National Electronic Disease

Surveillance System (NEDSS): a standards-based approach to connect public health and clinical medicine. J Public Health Manag Pract 2001;7:43–50.

National Institute for Occupational Safety and Health [homepage on the Internet]. Atlanta: Centers for Disease Control and Prevention [cited 2004 May 21]. Health hazard evaluations. Available from: http://www.cdc.gov/niosh/hhe.

National Institute for Occupational Safety and Health [homepage on the Internet]. Atlanta: Centers for Disease Control and Prevention [cited 2004 May 21]. The Adult Blood Lead Epidemiology and Surveillance Program (ABLES). Available from: http://www.cdc.gov/niosh/ables.html.

North American Association of Central Cancer Registries. NAACCR 2002 Workshop Report: Data Security and Confidentiality. Springfield, IL: North American Association of Central Cancer Registries; 2002 [cited 2004 May 21]. Available from: http://www.naaccr.org/index.asp?Col_SectionKey=10&Col_ContentID=40.

North American Association of Central Cancer Registries [homepage on the Internet]. Springfield, IL: North American Association of Central Cancer Registries, Inc.; c. 2003 [cited 2004 May 21]. Available from: http://www.naaccr.org.

North American Association of Central Cancer Registries [homepage on the Internet]. Springfield, IL: North American Association of Central Cancer Registries, Inc.; c. 2003 [cited 2004 May 21]. Data standards and data dictionary. Available from: http://www.naaccr.org/standards.

North American Association of Central Cancer Registries [homepage on the Internet]. Springfield, IL: North American Association of Central Cancer Registries, Inc.; c. 2003 [cited 2004 May 21]. Registry certification. Available from: http://www.naaccr.org/index.asp?Col_SectionKey=12&Col_ContentID=54.

Office of Management and Budget. Revisions to the standards for the classification of federal data on race and ethnicity. Fed Reg 1997; 62(210):58782–58790 [cited 2002 July 10]. Available from: http://www.whitehouse.gov/omb/fedreg/ombdir15.html.

O'Malley C, Hu K, West D. North American Association of Central Cancer Registries: Race and Ethnicity Identifier Assessment Project. Springfield, IL: North American Association of Central Cancer Registries; 2002, pp. 2–55 [cited 2003 Jul 21]. Available from: http://www.naaccr.org/stats/EpiReports.html.

Percy C, Van Holten V, Muir C. International Classification of Diseases for Oncology, 2nd ed. Geneva: World Health Organization; 1990.

Potts M, Hafterson J, Wacker FF, Serbent J. Case ascertainment. In: Hutchison CL, Roffers SD, Fritz AD, eds. Cancer Registry Management: Principles and Practice. Lenexa, KS: National Cancer Registrars Association; 1997, pp. 53–62.

Public Health Service, National Office of Vital Statistics. Vital Statistics of the United States 1950: History and Organization of the Vital Statistics System. Washington, DC: U.S. Department of Health, Education, and Welfare; 1954. Reprinted in: Hetzel AM. U.S. Vital Statistics System: Major Activities and Developments, 1950–95. Hyattsville, MD: National Center for Health Statistics; 1997 [cited 2004 May 7]. Available from: http://www.cdc.gov/nchs/data/misc/usvss.pdf.

Reingold A. If syndromic surveillance is the answer, what is the question? Biosecur Bioterror 2003;1(2):1–5.

Roche LM, Skinner R, Weinstein RB. Use of a geographic information system to identify and characterize areas with high proportions of distant stage breast cancer. J Public Health Manag Practice 2002;8:26–32.

Rosenberg ML, Marr JS, Gangarosa EJ, Pollard RA, Wallace M, Brolnitsky O. Shigella surveillance in the United States, 1975. J Infect Dis 1977;136:458–460.

Rothwell CJ. Rejuvenating vital statistics. Presentation at the annual meeting of the National Association of Health Data Organizations; Baltimore, Nov 9, 2003.

Rotz LD, Koo D, O'Carroll PW, Kellogg RB, Lillibridge SR. Bioterrorism preparedness: planning for the future. J Public Health Manag Pract 2000;6(4):45–49.

Roush S, Birkhead G, Koo D, Cobb A, Fleming D. Mandatory reporting of diseases and conditions by health care professionals and laboratories. JAMA 1999;282:164–170.

Simpson DM. Improving the reporting of notifiable diseases in Texas: suggestions from an ad hoc committee of providers. J Public Health Manag Pract 1996;2:37–39.

Smillie WG. Public Health: Its Promise for the Future. New York: Macmillan; 1955.

SNOMED International [homepage on the Internet]. Northfield, IL: College of American Pathologists; c. 2000–2003 [updated 2003 Jan 3; cited 2004 Mar 3]. Available from: http://www.snomed.org.

Sosin DM. Syndromic surveillance: the case for skillful investment. Biosecur Bioterror 2003;1(4):1–7.

Stroup NE, Zack MM, Wharton M. Sources of routinely collected data for surveillance. In: Teutsch SM, Churchill RE, eds. Principles and Practice of Public Health Surveillance. New York: Oxford University Press; 1994, pp. 31–85.

Surveillance, Epidemiology, and End Results Program. The SEER Program Code Manual, 3rd ed. NIH Publication No. 98-1999. Bethesda, MD: National Cancer Institute; 1998.

Surveillance, Epidemiology, and End Results [homepage on the Internet]. Bethesda, MD: National Cancer Institute [cited 2004 May 21]. Available from: http://seer.cancer.gov.

Teutsch SM, Churchill RE, eds. Principles and Practice of Public Health Surveillance, 2nd ed. New York: Oxford University Press; 2000.

Thacker SB, Berkelman RL. Public health surveillance in the United States. Epidemiol Rev 1988:10:164–190.

Thacker SB, Stroup DF. Future directions for comprehensive public health surveillance and health information systems in the United States. Am J Epidemiol 1994:140:383–397.

Trask, JW. Vital statistics: a discussion of what they are and their uses in public health administration. Public Health Rep 1914;12:30–34.

Tucker TC, Howe HL. Measuring the quality of central cancer registries: the NAACCR perspective. J Registry Manag 2001;28:41–44.

Tucker TC, Howe HL, Weir HK. Certification of population-based cancer registries. J Registry Manag 1999;26(1):24–27.

U.S. Cancer Statistics Working Group. United States Cancer Statistics: 2000 Incidence. Atlanta: Centers for Disease Control and Prevention and Bethesda, MD: National Cancer Institute; 2003.

U.S. Consumer Product Safety Commission [homepage on the Internet]. Washington, DC: Consumer Product Safety Commission [cited 2004 May 20]. Report unsafe products. Available from: http://www.cpsc.gov/talk.html.

U.S. Department of Health and Human Services. Tracking Healthy People 2010. Washington, DC: GPO [cited 2004 May 7]. 2000. Available from: http://www.cdc.gov/nchs/hphome.htm.

U.S. Department of Health and Human Services [homepage on the Internet]. Washington, DC: U.S. Department of Health and Human Services [cited 2004 May 20]. The National Health Information Infrastructure. Available from: http://aspe.hhs.gov/sp/nhii.

U.S. Food and Drug Administration [homepage on the Internet]. Rockville, MD: Food and Drug Administration [updated 2003 Jul 29; cited 2004 May 20]. Reporting adverse reactions and medical product problems to the FDA. Available from: http://www.fda.gov/medwatch/how.htm.

U.S. Public Health and Marine Hospital Service. Transactions of the First Annual Conference of State and Territorial Health Officers with the United States Public Health and Marine-Hospital Service. Public Health Bull 1903;11.

Vaccine Adverse Event Reporting System [homepage on the Internet]. Atlanta: Centers for

Disease Control and Prevention and Rockville, MD: U.S. Food and Drug Administration [cited 2004 May 20]. Available from: http://www.vaers.org.
Weddell JM. Registers and registries: a review. Int J Epidemiol 1973;2:221–228.
Williams W. Population-based cancer registration: working with industry standards to improve reporting. Testimony to the National Committee of Vital and Health Statistics, Chicago; Jul 24, 2002, Chicago [cited 2004 May 20]. Available from: http://aspe.hhs.gov/sp/nhii/Agenda/020724mn.htm.
World Health Organization [homepage on the Internet]. Geneva: World Health Organization; c. 2004 [cited 2004 May 20]. International health regulations. Available from: http://www.who.int/csr/ihr/en.

CHAPTER 5

Health Surveys: A Resource to Inform Health Policy and Practice

Jennifer H. Madans and Steven B. Cohen

Surveys are a critical source of information for the development, implementation, and evaluation of policies and practices addressing health and health care. When properly designed, surveys can provide accurate, unbiased, and generalizable information on population characteristics, risk factors, health status, health-care access, use and insurance coverage, and the health-care system itself. To be most useful, surveys must be designed according to sound statistical and methodological principles.

Health surveys are data collection efforts designed to acquire information on a population's health and health-care characteristics. The general uses of health survey data include identifying public health problems; program planning and evaluation; health education and health promotion; epidemiologic, biomedical, and health services research; measuring the extent and impact of illness; and measuring the use of health-care services, related medical expenditures, and sources of payment for care.

Generally, surveys are defined by the structured and systematic gathering of information from a representative sample of the population or universe of interest (though a census would still be considered a survey) in order to describe the target population in quantitative terms (Groves et al. 2004). The target of interest is often a population, but it can be any identifiable group of individual units such as health-care providers or events such as health-care contacts. If the sample is selected as a probability sample, in which a frame exists for sample enumeration and every unit selected from the frame has a known probability of selection, the findings from the sample are generalizable to the population. This is a powerful attribute that enhances the integrity of the data collected. Surveys can have relatively simple or extremely complex designs, but the basic principles of sample design and data collection methodology remain the same. The complexity of the survey often reflects the complexity of the subject under study. As health and health care encompass a wide arrange of phenomena and relate directly and indirectly to many other domains, it is necessary to develop a range of health surveys to respond to differing needs for information. Each of these surveys is often based on complex designs and sophisticated data collections mechanisms.

In this chapter, we will review the various kinds of health surveys that are used to support the development, implementation, and evaluation of health policies and practices and will characterize each by its strengths and weaknesses. We will also discuss the current status of health surveys in the United States and address some major policy issues that affect how well these surveys meet the needs of the user community. Although the examples used are primarily from the United States, surveys conducted in other countries are similar in design.

TYPES OF HEALTH SURVEYS

There are three main types of health surveys: population-based surveys that obtain information directly from the subject (or a suitable proxy); surveys that obtain information about entities such as health-care providers; and surveys that are based on administrative records. Population-based surveys do not need to be geographically restricted, as in requiring representation of the entire U.S. population, the population of a specific state, or the population of a specific city. The target population could be defined to consist of all individuals with a given sociodemographic characteristic such as age; it could be limited to individuals with a medical condition such as diabetes; or it could consist of only those individuals with specific encounters with the health-care system such as hospitalizations. Purposive or convenience samples are occasionally used to obtain information about a target population of interest when it is difficult to identify all members of that population but means are available to reach those with characteristics of interest. For example, there is no national listing of persons who have arthritis from which to draw a sample. If an investigator were interested in this condition, information could be obtained from those attending arthritis support groups in the local area. But as random selection is not used to identify the sample, sampling theory cannot be applied to support any generalizations made from the sample findings.

The absence of a universal health-care system with a centralized administrative database limits the extent to which administrative records can be used in health surveys, particularly those that are national in scope. While there are many administratively based surveys in the United States, these types of surveys are more difficult to conduct here than in other countries with centralized health-care systems. Even when administrative databases are readily available, there are questions of policy relevance that cannot be addressed without directly contacting the individual. Often surveys are designed by using a combination of components from both approaches, often enhancing the quality of the resulting outputs.

Population-Based Surveys

Population-based surveys are used when it is essential to describe the characteristics of a defined population. Often the population of interest is the general U.S. population and specific subpopulations as defined by such characteristics as age, sex, race/ethnicity, or socioeconomic status. However, a population may also be defined by occupation or other well-defined characteristics. More specifically, physicians could also be the ultimate sample units of a population-based survey if the information sought related directly to the physician and his or her practice characteristics. Population-based surveys are most frequently adopted when it is best to obtain the required information directly from the subject or an informant. This would be a model to adopt when information is needed about the experience of pain or the ability to perform certain tasks. Population-based surveys are also adopted when there are gains in efficiency or data accessibility through this approach, even when alternate sources of data are available.

When a well-developed sample frame is available, samples for population-based surveys can be selected from lists of all eligible subjects. For example, surveys of Medicare or health plan beneficiaries can be drawn from a list of enrollees (Centers for Medicare and Medicaid Services [hp] Medicare Current Beneficiary Survey). When such lists are not available, other methods such as area-based probability samples are used. Whatever method is adopted, it is important that the sample be selected as a probability sample, and it may be evaluated for potential coverage and response biases. Once a sample is selected, different data collection modes can be used to collect the necessary information, including mail, phone, Web-based, and in-person. The nature of the content and the sample will affect the mode chosen.

Of critical importance is the survey instrument itself. The questionnaire or other data collection instruments need to be developed so that accurate and valid information is obtained. The identification of the respondent is also an important step in the process. In general, obtaining information directly from the survey subject provides more reliable and valid health data. This information can be obtained either through in-person or telephone interviews or mail questionnaires. However, this is not universally true, and depends on the nature of the information sought and the characteristics of the subject (Moore 1988). For example, while accurate information on risk behaviors among adolescents can probably be obtained only from adolescents in a private environment, adolescents are not good reporters of health-care use or household income. Similarly, information on diagnosed conditions and health services use is often also obtained through subject interviews, but the quality of information obtained in this way is questionable. Individuals may occasionally misreport diagnoses or may never have been given the information by their providers. Reporting of health-care encounters is also prone to recall errors. Bias can also be introduced if the reporting of health status in terms of disease prevalence is dependent on receiving health care. Individuals would have to have visited a health-care provider and received the appropriate tests before they can report that a condition exists.

Supplemental information in the form of medical records is often added to the information obtained from subjects to enhance completeness and quality. For example, with authorization from participants, it is possible to obtain records from Medicare or directly from providers and to incorporate these records with the information obtained from interviews. To obtain objective standardized information on health characteristics including undiagnosed conditions, surveys rely on direct examination of populations. These surveys are extremely complex and expensive to undertake but are of added value to accurately describe the health status of the population, particularly for those subpopulations who lack medical care.

Even in cases where direct reporting by subjects is important, it is not always possible, for example when a health condition does not permit a subject to respond personally. Since eliminating the subject from the survey would seriously bias the results, a proxy respondent is often used. While this strategy may reduce the bias in survey estimates attributable to nonresponse, the use of proxy respondents may introduce additional sources of error into the final survey estimates.

Many health surveys limit their population of interest. For example, it is common for health surveys to only include the noninstitutionalized population. The dramatic differences in the living conditions of the institutionalized and noninstitutionalized populations make it difficult to design survey methodologies that would apply in all situations. The military population is also often excluded from general health surveys. The scope of the universe needs to be clearly defined, especially if populations that differ in their health status are omitted, such as persons residing in nursing homes.

The National Health Interview Survey (NHIS) conducted by the National Center for Health Statistics (NCHS) is a good example of a large, nationally representative, general-purpose health survey (National Center for Health Statistics [hp] National Health Interview Survey). Information on a range of health-related issues such as demographics, socioeconomic status, health behaviors, health status, and health care use is collected from a large sample of the U.S. population. It is possible to use this survey to make estimates for the entire population and for subpopulations such as those defined by age, race/ethnicity, sex, and geography. The National Health and Nutrition Examination Survey, also collected by NCHS, complements the NHIS by collecting objective information through standardized medical exams on a probability sample of the U.S. population (National Center for Health Statistics [hp] National Health and

Nutrition Examination Survey). Similarly, other countries conduct major multipurpose health surveys, such as the Canadian Community Health Survey (Statistics Canada [hp] Canadian Community Health Survey).

General-purpose surveys are also designed to obtain estimates for most or all geographic subregions. For example, in the Behavioral Risk Factor Surveillance System (BRFSS), a partnership between the Centers for Disease Control and Prevention (CDC) and individual states, states collect information through telephone surveys in accordance with common core questionnaire modules, but they can also add state-specific content (National Center for Chronic Disease Prevention and Health Promotion [hp] Measuring behaviors that endanger health). Studies can also be done in one geographic area. An example of a more elaborate state effort is the California Health Interview Survey (CHIS), conducted by the UCLA Center for Health Policy Research in collaboration with the California Department of Health Services and Public Health Institute (California Health Interview Survey [hp]). Like the NHIS, the BRFSS and the CHIS are multipurpose but are conducted using a random-digit-dial telephone methodology rather than in person.

Other surveys focus on specific population groups or specific issues. The Youth Risk Behavior Survey, conducted by the CDC's National Center for Chronic Disease Prevention and Health Promotion, is an example of another kind of population-based survey (National Center for Chronic Disease Prevention and Health Promotion [hp] Assessing health risk behaviors among young people). In this case, information is required about a specific population group, youth. It is costly to identify this population using household surveys, as not all households contain individuals in the target group. In the case of youth, it is efficient to identify the target population by sampling schools and conducting the interviews in schools. The universe in this case is youth who are attending school rather than all youth.

Surveys of Providers

Surveys of the components of the health-care system provide information on the structure, capacity, and functioning of that system. These components range from private physicians' offices to hospitals, nursing homes, and home health-care agencies. To fully understand the system, it is necessary to cover all components. In order to select representative samples of these components, it is necessary to have sampling frames, equivalent to the population list frames mentioned above, that identify each member of each type of health-care provider. While lists are available for many of the more established providers, this is not the case for all providers. This diminishes the capacity to accurately characterize and understand the entire health-care system. As is the case for population-based studies, different collection modes are used for provider surveys. Internet surveys of these respondents seem to hold some promise, and research in this area is underway.

Surveys of providers can provide information on different aspects of the health-care system. Questions can be targeted at describing the number of components in a sector, as well as their organizational, legal, or financial characteristics. Information can be obtained on the individual provider, or on the interactions among related providers or between providers and patients. Interactions with patients can focus on the delivery of care or on how care is paid for. The National Nursing Home Survey conducted by the NCHS is one example of a survey that collects information on providers, in this case nursing homes (National Center for Health Statistics [hp] National Nursing Home Survey). A random sample of all nursing homes is selected, and information is obtained on the characteristics of the institutions' staff and on the services provided. Similarly, the NCHS surveys physicians, emergency departments, hospitals, home health-care providers, and hospices (National Center for Health Statistics [hp] National Health Care Survey). State-based provider data are also available (Wisconsin Department of Health and Family Services [hp] Health Care Information).

Surveys Based on Administrative Records

Sometimes the most accurate source of information comes from an administrative record that was generated as part of the routine operation of a system. This clearly would be the case when the objective of the research is the system producing the records. For example, use of Medicare services is most easily obtained from Medicare administrative records. The entire census of records is usually available for these purposes, but often samples of records are taken when the entire universe is not needed. While administrative records of contacts with the health-care system are usually created, they are often not stored in a uniform, standardized manner that makes them suitable for research (for further detail, see Chapter 6). This limitation occurs for both hospital financial records and insurance claims data. When there are several different record systems for hospital- or claims-related data, it is difficult to directly form an analytical data file to support desired analyses due to the lack of uniformity and standardization across systems. However, it may still be possible to take advantage of these record systems for obtaining provider-specific data through the selection of representative samples from these record systems, followed by the collection of standardized information via a survey.

As noted above, it is possible to obtain information about encounters with the health-care system directly from the patient. However, patients are often not reliable reporters of relevant information about the encounter. There is considerable misreporting of medical and nonmedical information. Obtaining information from the provider's records provides data of much higher quality at a much lower cost than obtaining the information from the patient. This is also true for other types of information such as the characteristics of insurance plans. When possible, information from administrative records is often sought as a way to improve the accuracy of information available from the subject in population-based surveys.

Health-care or provider surveys offer an independent assessment of disease prevalence by approaching the problem from the provider side rather than the patient side. Health-care surveys of providers are particularly important since they obtain information on rare conditions that would not be picked up in population-based surveys. While information is collected on all conditions for which health care is obtained, the nature of the information available is limited to that which would routinely be obtained from records. In addition, the event (e.g., the discharge), rather than the person, is the primary unit of analysis. An enhancement to health-care surveys of providers would be to follow patients after the health-care encounter.

An example of a survey of administrative records is the National Hospital Discharge Survey (National Center for Health Statistics [hp] National Hospital Discharge and Ambulatory Surgery data). This survey first samples hospitals and then obtains information about a sample of stays in the sampled hospitals by reviewing the discharge records.

SURVEY SPONSORSHIP

The basic requirements for survey design and implementation apply to all survey sponsors, although areas of emphasis may vary, depending on the sponsor. However, different sponsors have somewhat different roles in providing health information from surveys. Governments at all levels are responsible for developing and maintaining a statistical infrastructure, including health surveys, that provides the basic information needed to develop policies and administer programs. The scope of the surveys sponsored by public entities varies over time and across jurisdictions, but there is a particular emphasis on the ability to monitor trends over time, especially at the federal level. The core publicly sponsored health surveys collect information on key indicators of health and health care. While policies and programs may change, these basic indicators provide information on the health of the nation. Governments also sponsor surveys in particular areas of policy or programmatic concerns and to evaluate the effectiveness of these activities. As opposed to the core surveys, these data collections are often conducted intermittently. These surveys can also focus on an issue in more depth than can be done in a core program. For example, many states conduct surveys of tobacco use to monitor tobacco control programs, such as those funded by the settlement of a lawsuit pursued by states against tobacco companies (Social Sciences Data Collection [hp] California Tobacco Survey [CTS] Reports).

Privately sponsored surveys tend to be even more focused on specific issues. Often these surveys attempt to fill gaps in publicly sponsored activities, and they can often be more flexible and more responsive to changing conditions. Examples of surveys conducted by private organizations are the Community Tracking Study sponsored by the Robert Wood Johnson Foundation, the Commonwealth Fund's International Health Policy Survey, and the Kaiser Family Foundation's Survey of People with Disabilities. The Community Tracking Study is a set of periodic surveys of households, physicians, and employers that allows researchers to analyze information about local markets and the nation as a whole (Strouse et al. 2003). The Kaiser Family Foundation's Survey of People with Disabilities (permanent mental or physical disabilities) explores their health-care experiences and challenges in accessing and paying for care (Hanson et al. 2003). The Commonwealth Fund's International Health Policy Survey compares the health-care experiences of adults in Australia, Canada, New Zealand, the United Kingdom, and the United States. The data determine which of these countries have the highest proportion of residents facing access problems, often driven in large part by the difficulty many may face in paying for care (Schoen et al. 2002).

Publicly sponsored surveys, especially those carried out by government agencies, see the dissemination of data and the documentation of the survey process as key parts of the enterprise. Considerable resources are devoted to ensuring public access to data. This involves developing and documenting public use files, providing access to these files, and providing technical assistance in their use. Resources are also devoted to providing descriptive information on all aspects of the data collection activity so that the quality of the data can be evaluated. Privately funded surveys are not under the same obligation to make their data available or to document their collection procedures, although some privately sponsored surveys do follow these procedures.

POPULATIONS AND SUBPOPULATIONS

In order to be useful for policy and program development, data must be available on appropriate population groups. While national data for the total population form the core of the data systems, information is generally needed on subpopulations as defined by geographic and sociodemographic characteristics. As many health and health-care programs are delivered at the local level, data for political jurisdictions are particularly important. There are several basic models through which health surveys can be conducted at the state, county, and local levels. Surveys designed to produce national estimates (such as the NHIS, described earlier) would have to be extremely large to also produce estimates even at the state level. It is possible to develop designs for national data collection efforts that can produce data for local areas, but the more local the area, the harder and more expensive this is to do. This centralized approach produces highly standardized data, maximizing the comparability of data across areas, but it is by definition less flexible and less able to respond to local data needs. If information for an area cannot be obtained directly from the survey, it is possible to use statistical models to approximate results. An alternative approach is to conduct independent surveys in each area. This approach maximizes flexibility and relevance to local needs but at the expense of comparability. It is possible to increase comparability if some aspects of the data collections at the local area are standardized. Such standardization can take the form of sharing questionnaires and methods or can involve more formal relationships among data collectors. The BRFSS, described earlier, is an example of a state-based survey with agreements for standardization of many elements across states. However, the tension between comparability and flexibility is always a factor when planning health surveys for different geopolitical areas.

Health-care surveys also serve to provide essential information to inform program development requirements for specific population subgroups with specific needs. A first step in the process is to identify where there is variation in health and health care in the population. Samples then need to be designed so that the necessary information is collected for policy-relevant population subgroups that require special attention. Often these groups are defined by race/ethnicity and socioeconomic status. Unless national samples are very large, it is usually necessary to oversample these groups, and unless the groups are highly clustered geographically, oversampling will involve screening. Moreover, the residence pattern of the groups of interest might suggest a sampling scheme that is inconsistent with producing state- or county-level data.

For each of the modes of survey data collection employed to acquire the necessary information for population subgroups of analytic interest, the underlying costs for survey implementation may often be high. The increased costs cover the larger samples needed, the more complex sample designs required, and population screening. If the data collection is decentralized, this effort will require a larger number of survey statisticians and result in duplication of effort relative to a more centralized approach. While this may not be a problem for some state and local governments, it could be a strain for others. An alternative approach to conducting surveys on multiple population groups is to develop a more integrated approach where careful consideration is given to the type and specificity of information needed for each subgroup and surveys are designed to reflect these differing needs. Surveys at different levels of geography that provide data for different subgroups can be designed so that they reinforce each other. To the extent possible, standardized information could be collected using a centralized approach but allowing for flexible, locally relevant collections linked to the larger activities. To be most efficient, a range of data collection modes could be used (in-person, phone, Web) but, again, with an eye toward integration so that the strengths of each mode can be maximized and the limitations minimized.

OBJECTIVES AND CONTENT

Health surveys used for policy and program development can be either focused on a particular health or health-care issue or can be multipurpose in nature. The latter surveys tend to be conducted by public entities, are designed to provide ongoing descriptive information on a range of topics, and tend to be based on larger samples. While the information from these surveys can track changes in the population, they are less effective in obtaining detailed information on a particular subject or in evaluating the success of a survey. Such information is more appropriately obtained from focused surveys.

Information collected on health surveys can be divided into three general types: (*1*) health status; (*2*) determinants or correlates of health including health behaviors; and (*3*) health-care access, use of health-care services, and cost. In addition, information is collected on demographic and socioeconomic factors that affect health.

Health Status and Health Determinants

The multidimensional nature of health status requires that surveys include multiple indicators such as single summary measures, measures of disease incidence, prevalence, and symptoms, and measures of physical, cognitive, emotional, and social functioning. As noted previously, information on health status can be obtained directly from the subject through an interview process, via examination processes, or by a combination of the two approaches. Many of the interview-based indicators not only measure aspects of objective health status but also are affected by the social aspects. An individual's conceptualization of health in general and of his or her own health is conditioned by other sociodemographic characteristics. For example, self-assessed health status is a popular summary indicator of health status that has been shown to be highly correlated with other measures of health status and is predictive of mortality and admission to long-term care facilities. However, in responding to this question, individuals must evaluate their health status against an unstated standard. This standard will be defined by societal norms that vary across populations and over time, making it difficult to interpret observed changes or differentials in this measure.

Interview information collected on disease incidence and prevalence includes diagnosis by a health-care provider, symptomatology, medication use, date of onset, use of health-care services, and the impact of the condition on functional ability. In examination surveys, direct physical exams and diagnostic testing provide more objective measures, particularly for previously undiagnosed conditions and for the identification of biomarkers that indicate risks for disease.

Health surveys face a major challenge in covering all aspects of health status in sufficient depth, and difficult decisions are made about how to limit the scope of any given survey. Some surveys provide very limited information on a wide range of health status dimensions, while others focus on selected aspects. Ongoing surveys face the additional challenge of maintaining consistency in data collection so that trends can be monitored. Many ongoing surveys adopt a modular approach whereby some basic information is collected each time the survey is administered but other survey components are administered only periodically.

Another challenge for health surveys is to be comprehensive in capturing all health conditions of interest, a task complicated by the fact that there is no universal, standard lay language for describing health. To ensure that respondents will report on all relevant characteristics, some surveys use very broad wording. This has the disadvantage of including very minor conditions that are not of interest. Some surveys also include information on the consequences of health conditions such as the receipt of medical care or limiting usual activities in an attempt to standardize responses. However, these consequences also have a social component that can affect the interpretation of variations across groups, especially when these groups are defined along socioeconomic dimensions, as is often the case in health surveys.

In addition to obtaining information on conditions from interviews or examinations, this information can be obtained from surveys of health-care providers (hospitals, private physicians, hospital outpatient departments, emergency departments, ambulatory surgery centers, and long-term care settings). The information from these surveys can be used to study conditions that are associated with medical care and are particularly important, since the surveys obtain information on rare conditions that would not be picked up in population-based surveys. The available information is limited to that which would routinely be obtained from records, but this information is collected on all conditions for which health care is obtained. Cause-of-death statistics obtained from a vital statistics system also provides essential information on medical conditions.

An additional aspect of health status covered by many health surveys is physical, cognitive, emotional, and social functioning. While information on some aspects of functional status can be ascertained through objective tests, it is most often obtained through direct reporting by the individual or a proxy and is probably the most challenging of all the aspects of health status. The information needed encompasses a wide range of activities, and performance is a function of physiologic abilities as well as the environment. Aspects of the environment, including assistive devices, can serve as barriers or as facilitators and change over time. For some purposes, functional ability should be measured without the use of assistance of any type, but for other objectives, the interest is in usual performance. The lack of a standard vocabulary also affects the collection of information on functioning. Questions often do not include an explicit referent against which respondents compare their own functioning. This lack of a reference standard increases the chances that responses will be affected by external nonhealth factors.

The definition of the population covered by the survey will also affect the content. Surveys that are limited to the noninstitutionalized population will exclude nursing home residents who are in the poorest health and have the highest level of functional limitations. Special studies of these populations are often conducted but are viewed as distinct efforts. To obtain a comprehensive summary of the health of the entire population, it is necessary to combine results from the noninstitutionalized and long-term care populations. Distinguishing specific populations covered by health surveys will be affected by changes in the delivery of long-term care, particularly with the expansion of transitional establishments.

In addition to health status, health surveys generally include measures of determinants of health such as risk factors, health behaviors, and socioeconomic status. As is the case for health status, the range of potential measures is wide and not all dimensions are covered by all surveys. Most surveys include basic demographic and socioeconomic variables. Common risk factors included in health surveys are tobacco use, alcohol use, poor diet, and insufficient physical exercise.

Health-Care Access, Use of Health Services, and Cost

For comprehensive studies of the current health-care system, information is needed on the population's access to health care, their use of and expenditures for health-care services, and their health insurance coverage. Similarly, an evaluation of the system requires an understanding of the patterns and trends in the use of health-care services and their associated costs and sources of payment. To effectively address these issues, researchers and policymakers need accurate nationally representative data to permit a better understanding of how individual characteristics, behavioral factors, and financial and institutional arrangements affect health-care use and expenditures in a rapidly changing health-care market. Health surveys are often designed to acquire this information at both the national and subnational levels and for policy-relevant population subgroups of interest.

The population's access to health-care services is an important factor that may influence patterns of health-care use and associated health outcomes. Measures of access to care have also been used as indicators of the quality of the nation's health-care delivery system. In addition to facilitating determinations of the availability of a usual source of care for the provision of necessary medical care, access-to-care measures serve to identify barriers to care, which include shortages of health-care providers, financial restrictions, limitations in proximity to services, and constraints associated with waiting times. Measures of satisfaction with the usual source of health care are also obtained in health surveys. It is also of interest to make comparisons of access measures by age, race/ethnicity, sex, perceived health status, health insurance coverage, and place of residence to identify potential disparities in access to care. Evaluation of the effects of changes in the U.S. health-care system on access to care for at-risk or vulnerable populations will remain a critical issue for policymakers in the next few years.

An understanding of the patterns and trends in the use of health-care services is essential to facilitate evaluations of the current health-care system, in addition to informing proposals for modification. Assessments of the degree of equity in the distribution of health-care services and the identification of health-care disparities require an examination of health-care use across vulnerable population subgroups and how it has changed over time. These investigations are essential to discern how service use varies according to the characteristics of the population, their health plans, and their providers, and to identify other behavioral and institutional factors associated with disparities in service use.

An examination of the variations in the use of health-care services also helps determine the adequacy of access to care across the population. Underuse of health-care services may be attributable to limitations in access to care as a consequence of the lack of adequate health insurance, financial resources, or limited availability of services in certain areas. Detailed comparisons of patterns of use by subpopulations presumed to require more care (e.g., the elderly, those in poor health, or the terminally ill) relative to their less vulnerable counterparts help determine whether those most in need of care are receiving it.

The use measures that are required for these analyses typically consist of counts of the number of visits or events for specific health-care services that occur in a given calendar year. More specifically, health-care services include office-based visits, ambulatory hospital-based visits, inpatient hospital stays, dental visits, home health visits, and prescribed medicine purchases. This information is acquired through each of the survey venues discussed in this chapter: population-based surveys, surveys of providers, and surveys based on administrative records. Health-care surveys are designed to acquire this information at both the national and subnational levels and for policy-relevant population subgroups of interest.

Health-care expenditures represent nearly one-seventh of the U.S. gross domestic product, exhibit a rate of growth that exceeds that of other sectors of the economy, and constitute one of the largest components of federal and state budgets. Although the rate of growth in health-care costs slowed in the mid-1990s, it has recently begun to rise again, fueled primarily by increasing costs for hospital care and prescription medications. To effectively address these issues, researchers and policymakers need accurate nationally representative data to better permit an understanding of how individual characteristics, behavioral factors, financial incentives, and institutional arrangements affect health-care use and expenditures in a rapidly changing health-care market.

The continuing rise in the number of persons without private health insurance has made access to health insurance coverage a critical public policy issue. Informed public policy requires precise estimates of the size and composition of the insured and uninsured populations, as well as information on how demographic characteristics, economic factors, and health status affect health plan eligibility and decisions to enroll in health insurance plans (see Agency for Healthcare Research and Quality [hp] Medical Expenditure Panel Survey and National Center for Health Statistics [hp] National Health Interview Survey for the most current information on health insurance).

Population-based national health-care surveys, such as the Medical Expenditure Panel Survey (MEPS), cosponsored by the Agency for Healthcare Research and Quality (AHRQ) and the NCHS, collect information on several dimensions of access to health care in America (Agency for Healthcare Research and Quality [hp] Medical Expenditure Panel Survey). The MEPS, which uses the NHIS as its sample frame, provides extensive information on the population's access to, use of, and expenditures and sources of payment for health care; the availability and costs of private health insurance in the employment-related and nongroup markets; the population enrolled in public health insurance plans and those without health-care coverage; and the role of health status in health-care use, expenditures, and household decision making, and in health insurance and employment choices. These data are used in economic models to make projections concerning health-care expenditures and use and to answer questions about the impact of changes in financing, coverage, and reimbursement policy.

STANDARDIZATION OF DESIGN AND CONTENT TO IMPROVE COMPARABILITY ACROSS SURVEYS

The potential for an integrated approach to health surveys is enhanced by the use of data standards. There is considerable overlap in content across health surveys. Major health indicators will be collected in a variety of survey settings, either as the primary survey objective or because the information is needed to understand the primary survey outcomes. For example, a survey may be designed to obtain information on smoking prevalence, but since smoking status can affect the relationships between other variables of interest, smoking is included in many health surveys. Estimates of smoking prevalence can also be made from these surveys. Often the estimates from various surveys are not consistent, causing great confusion on the part of users and a lack of confidence in survey findings, especially among policymakers. A good example of this is health insurance, where estimates from different surveys can vary widely. There are many reasons why these estimates differ, including differences in how the concept is defined, difference in question wording, variations in how responses are coded and missing data handled, and different populations of interest. While it will not be possible or advisable to obtain complete consistency across all surveys, well-developed data standards can greatly improve comparability of estimates and facilitate understanding of the remaining variation. (See Chapter 8 for a more comprehensive treatment of the general topic of data standards.)

TECHNOLOGICAL ADVANCES

Advances in technology have affected the conduct of all surveys. Computer-assisted telephone interviewing (CATI) and personal interviewing (CAPI) have allowed for increasing levels of complexity of survey administration (Couper et al. 1998). Errors associated with keying and coding have been replaced by errors associated with programming. The use of these technologies has resulted in the need for longer lead times prior to fielding a study but has reduced the time from the end of data collection to the availability of results.

The increase in electronic as opposed to paper files has greatly expanded the opportunities for linking data from various sources. Ecological or contextual information about the geographic area in which survey respondents live can now be linked to the survey data. This has the advantage of allowing researchers to address different levels of analysis. Survey data can also be augmented with administrative data from mortality files and from health-care providers. In addition to reducing survey costs, this often leads to data of improved quality. The NHIS and the National Health and Nutrition Examination Survey (NHANES) obtain information on vital status by linking mortality records to the survey files. These surveys also obtain Medicare records for survey respondents.

More recent advances and technological changes associated with the Internet, mobile telephones, and handheld computers offer great potential for increased efficiency in data collection and data dissemination. These potential gains in cost efficiency need to be balanced by attention to maintaining standards for survey data quality, sample representativeness, and accuracy.

The use of mobile telephones is growing in the United States, and the advantages of including this technological advance as a component of data collection efforts are becoming more evident. This data collection tool is being used more conventionally to improve coverage in national surveys conducted via telephone. National telephone surveys can now be supplemented with area probability surveys that identify households without telephones, who are given a mobile phone with which to participate in the survey. On a related front, new innovations with respect to the capacity of handheld computers to support wireless transmissions are greatly expanding the environments in which computerized data collection can occur.

Data collection as well as dissemination efforts are currently being influenced by the Internet. These activities will increase as Internet access continues to grow over time (Research Triangle Institute [hp] RTI Teams with Knowledge Networks). Data collection efforts via this venue allow for more flexibility in questionnaire design and personalization, in a manner similar to that of CATI or CAPI, with greater potential for cost efficiency. Health surveys conducted through this venue must pay careful attention to control for sources of error attributable to sampling, coverage, nonresponse, and instrument and Web page design, in addition to visual layout. Internet-based surveys often devote more attention to programming tasks and Web page design than to traditional survey methodology. Given the high level of variation in access to the Internet across diverse population subgroups identified by distinct sociodemographic characteristics, the representative nature of the results derived from these surveys is often called into question. As more people gain access to the Internet over time, this modality will also serve as a more widely used source for advice or information about health or health care (Baker et al. 2003). More attention will need to be given to the inclusion of clear descriptions of the limitations of survey results obtained through the Internet when the samples are not representative of the target population of interest.

ANALYTICAL ENHANCEMENTS ACHIEVED THROUGH LINKAGE OF SURVEYS TO OTHER SOURCES OF DATA

The analytical capacity of health surveys can be dramatically enhanced through linkage to existing secondary data sources at higher levels of aggregation (both geographic and organizational), as well as through direct matches to additional health and socioeconomic measures acquired for the same set of sample units from other sources of survey-specific or administrative data (see Chapter 9 for a broader discussion of linking and combining data from multiple sources and Chapter 7 for a discussion of nonhealth sources for some of these data). One of the more pervasive uses of existing administrative databases is to serve as a sampling frame to facilitate a cost–efficient identification of an eligible survey population for purposes of sample selection, such as the use of Medicare administrative records as a sampling frame for a survey of Medicare beneficiaries. Health surveys that are so linked to administrative records from their inception benefit by this capacity for data supplementation that permits enhanced and more extensive analyses that are beyond the scope of the core health survey. Establishing similar connections to existing data sources that will substantially enhance a survey's capacity to address specific research questions is often more difficult after a survey has been administered. This is primarily a consequence of confidentiality restrictions that require the respondent's permission to link patient records to administrative data sources, in addition to problems with the availability of the necessary identifiers from survey respondents.

The large majority of the nationally representative population-based health surveys sponsored by the U.S. Department of Health and Human Services have benefited by the capacity to link survey data to county-level data on health service resources and health manpower statistics available on the Area Resources File (ARF). More specifically, the ARF is a county-specific health resources information system containing information on health facilities, health professions, measures of resource scarcity, health status, economic activity, health training programs, and socioeconomic and environmental characteristics. Geographic codes and descriptors are provided to enable linkage to health surveys to expand analyses conducted by planners, policymakers, researchers, and other professionals examining the nation's health-care delivery system and factors that may impact health status and health care in the United States. Comparable enhancements to health surveys for supplementation of economic indicators are achievable through linkage of survey data to the socioeconomic indicators made available by the U.S. Bureau of the Census through the County and City Data Book and public use files from the decennial census.

The quality and data content of household-specific health surveys are often enhanced through the conduct of follow-back surveys to medical providers and facilities that have provided care to household respondents. In terms of data quality, household-reported medical conditions can be evaluated for accuracy relative to provider-specific records on medical conditions of the same patient and specific health events. With respect to health-care expenditures collected from household respondents for their reported health-care events, available linked medical provider-level data are a more accurate source of information. The availability of such supplemental data on use and expenditures allows for the conduct of methodological studies to evaluate the accuracy of household-reported data and informs adjustment strategies to household data in the absence of provider-specific data to reduce bias attributable to response error.

CROSS-SECTIONAL AND LONGITUDINAL SURVEY DESIGNS

National health-care sample surveys are generally characterized by cross-sectional or longitudinal designs. The cross-sectional surveys are designed to provide a snapshot of population characteristics that relate to a fixed point or interval in time. By contrast, longitudinal surveys collect data on more than one occasion from the sample members of the population of interest in order to measure change and to obtain data for time periods too long to recall accurately in a single interview. Longitudinal observations are essential for characterizing variations in the population attributes that are sensitive to changes in time.

Longitudinal survey designs are adopted primarily when the objective is to assess changes in the behavior of the population over a specific time period or to relate risk characteristics measured at one point in time to outcomes measured at a future date. Designs to measure change are often referred to as *panel designs*; they permit measurement of seasonal and annual variations in population characteristics and behavior. They permit, for example, the investigation of the impact of changes in health status over time for individuals with respect to their use of health-care services and related expenditures. This type of survey design also allows for the development of economic models designed to produce national and regional estimates of the impact of changes in financing, coverage, and reimbursement policy over time, as well as estimates of who benefits and who bears the cost of such changes in policy.

Longitudinal designs are also used to relate characteristics obtained at a baseline with outcomes measured at one or multiple points in the future. These surveys are often called *follow-up studies.* They make it possible to study causal associations by clarifying the time link between independent and dependent variables and to study the natural history of disease. In many cases, cross-sectional surveys are used as the baseline cohorts for future active longitudinal follow-ups. The generation and analysis of such longitudinal data are greatly facilitated in countries (e.g., Sweden) where various governmental information systems and surveys can be linked.

CONFIDENTIALITY AND DATA RELEASE

As discussed in Chapter 14, information is often collected within ethical and legal frameworks that assure respondents that the confidentiality of their information will be protected. This is deemed necessary for ethical reasons as well as to ensure high response rates and valid information. Recent developments in technology and methods have complicated the already complex intersection of data access and release with the protection of confidentiality. For example, technological advances in data collection methodologies and in data linkage techniques have expanded the amount of information that can be obtained in health surveys. This has increased efficiency and has expanded the analytic utility of information for researchers and policy analysts. However, the amount and detail of the information collected has created challenges for data dissemination.

Health statistics organizations are providing greater electronic access (e.g., CD-ROMs, the Internet) to increasingly detailed data files, while other information on individuals and institutions is now routinely made available electronically. The capacity of users to combine multiple files increases the risk of disclosure of sensitive health information. As a result, and because of a general increase in sensitivity to issues of privacy, survey data files must undergo extensive disclosure reviews to minimize such risks before being made available to researchers. It has also been necessary to continue to develop methods for identifying disclosure risks and to modify files so that the risks no longer exist. For the data producer, data release activities have become more expensive and time-consuming. For the data user, in some cases there may be a decrease in the amount of data that can be accessed in public use files (e.g., detail on variables such as geography, income, and so on may be limited). In order to satisfy data needs, other mechanisms are being developed so that access to data can be maximized while protecting confidentiality. The employment of special use agreements, licensing, and research data centers are examples of these approaches (Special issue 1998).

CONCLUSION

Health surveys provide critical information for tracking the health status of populations and for studying the relationships between demographic and socioeconomic characteristics, risk factors, health care, and health status. Data from surveys are used by the research community, by policy and program officials, by the media, and by the public to improve the health of the population. Health surveys can be population based or can obtain information from business (health-care providers) or administrative records. They can focus on the total population or can be designed to obtain information on subpopulations defined by geography or by individual characteristics such as race or ethnicity. Surveys can be multipurpose or can be limited to specific health issues. Surveys are also constantly changing to take advantage of new methodologies and to increase the utility of the information collected. However, despite the variability in survey design and conduct, surveys must conform to high standards for their sample design and selection, collection instrumentation, field methods, analysis, documentation, dissemination, and the protection of survey participants if the data are to be credible.

REFERENCES

Agency for Healthcare Research and Quality [homepage on the Internet]. Rockville, MD: Agency for Healthcare Research and Quality [cited 2004 Mar 17]. Medical expenditure panel survey [about one screen]. Available from: http://www.ahrq.gov/data/mepsix.htm.

Baker L, Wagner T, Singer S, Bundorf M. Use of the Internet and e-mail for health care information: results from a national survey. JAMA 2003;289:2400–2406.

California Health Interview Survey [homepage on the Internet]. Berkeley: The Regents of the University of California; c. 2003 [cited 2004 Mar 17]. Available from: http://www.chis.ucla.edu.

Centers for Medicare and Medicaid Services [homepage on the Internet]. Baltimore: Centers for Medicare and Medicaid Services [updated 2003 Jul 24; cited 2004 Mar 17]. Medicare Current Beneficiary Survey [about one screen]. Available from: http://www.cms.hhs.gov/MCBS/default.asp.

Couper MP, Baker RP, Bethlehem J, Clark CZF, Martin J, Nicholls WL, O'Reilly JM, eds. Computer Assisted Survey Information Collection. New York: Wiley; 1998.

Groves RM, Fowler FJ, Couper MP, Lepkowski J, Singer E, Tourangeau R. Survey Methodology. New York: Wiley; 2004.

Hanson K, Neuman T, Voris M. Understanding the Health-Care Needs and Experiences of People with Disabilities: Findings from a 2003 Survey. Menlo Park, CA: Kaiser Family Foundation; 2003 [cited 2004 Mar 17]. Available from: http://www.kff.org/medicare/6106.cfm.

Madans J. Health surveys. In: Smelser NJ, Baltes PB, eds. International Encyclopedia of the Social and Behavioral Sciences. Amsterdam and New York: Elsevier; 2001.

Moore J. Self/Proxy response status and survey response quality: a review of the literature. J Off Stat 1988;4(2):155–172.

National Center for Chronic Disease Prevention and Health Promotion [homepage on the Internet]. Atlanta: Centers for Disease Control and Prevention [updated 2004 Mar 9; cited 2004 Mar 17]. Assessing health risk behaviors among young people: Youth Risk Behavior Surveillance System [about 10 screens]. Available from: http://www.cdc.gov/nccdphp/aag/aag_yrbss.htm.

National Center for Chronic Disease Prevention and Health Promotion [homepage on the Internet]. Atlanta: Centers for Disease Control and Prevention [updated 2003 Mar 3; cited 2004 Mar 17]. Measuring behaviors that endanger health [about 8 screens]. Available from: http://www.cdc.gov/nccdphp/bb_brfss_yrbss/index.htm.

National Center for Health Statistics [homepage on the Internet]. Hyattsville, MD: National Center for Health Statistics [updated 2002 Oct 9; cited 2004 Mar 17]. National health care survey [about 3 screens]. Available from: http://www.cdc.gov/nchs/nhcs.htm.

National Center for Health Statistics [homepage on the Internet]. Hyattsville, MD: National Center for Health Statistics [updated 2004 Mar 17; cited 2004 Mar 17]. National health interview survey (NHIS) [about 3 screens]. Available from: http://www.cdc.gov/nchs/nhis.htm.

National Center for Health Statistics [homepage on the Internet]. Hyattsville, MD: National Center for Health Statistics [updated 2003 Oct 30; cited 2004 Mar 17]. National health and nutrition examination survey [about 3 screens]. Available from: http://www.cdc.gov/nchs/nhanes.htm.

National Center for Health Statistics [homepage on the Internet]. Hyattsville, MD: National Center for Health Statistics [updated 2004 Feb 6; cited 2004 Mar 17]. National hospital discharge and ambulatory surgery data [about 3 screens]. Available from: http://www.cdc.gov/nchs/about/major/hdasd/nhds.htm.

National Center for Health Statistics [homepage on the Internet]. Hyattsville, MD: National Center for Health Statistics [updated 2002 Sep 27; cited 2004 Mar 17]. National nursing home survey [about 3 screens]. Available from: http://www.cdc.gov/nchs/about/major/nnhsd/nnhsd.htm.

Research Triangle Institute [homepage on the Internet]. Research Triangle Park, NC: Research Triangle Institute; c. 2004 [cited 2004 Mar 17]. RTI Teams with Knowledge Networks for Population Projectable Web-Enabled Survey Research [about 6 screens]. Available from: http://www.rti-knowledgenetworks.org/news_rel.htm.

Schoen C, Blendon R, DesRoches C, Osborn R. Comparison of health care system views and experiences in five nations, 2001: findings from The Commonwealth Fund 2001 International Health Policy Survey. Issue Brief (Commonwealth Fund) 2002; (542):1–6.

Social Sciences Data Collection [homepage on the Internet]. La Jolla: University of California at San Diego; c. 2000 [updated 2003 Aug 21; cited 2004 Mar 17]. California Tobacco Survey (CTS) Report [about 5 screens]. Available from: http://ssdc.ucsd.edu/tobacco/reports.

Statistics Canada [homepage on the Internet]. Ottawa: Statistics Canada [updated 2004 Mar 17; cited 2004 Mar 17]. Canadian Community Health Survey [about 5 screens]. Available from: http://www.statcan.ca/english/sdds/3226.htm.

Strouse R, Carlson B, Hall J. Community Tracking Study: Household Survey Methodology Report, 2000–01 (Round Three). Technical Publication No. 46. Washington, DC: Center for Studying Health System Change; 2003 [cited 2004 Mar 17]. Available from: http://www.hschange.org/index.cgi?file=pubs.

Special issue: disclosure limitation methods for protecting the confidentiality of statistical data. J Off Stat 1998;14(4):337–573 [cited 2004 Mar 17]. Available from: http://www.jos.nu/Contents/issue.asp?vol=14&no=4.

Wisconsin Department of Health and Family Services [homepage on the Internet]. Madison: Department of Health and Family Services [updated 2004 Mar 12; cited 2004 Mar 17]. Health Care Information [about 2 screens]. Available from: http://dhfs.wisconsin.gov/healthcareinfo/index.htm.

CHAPTER 6

Administrative Health Data

Lisa I. Iezzoni, Michael Shwartz, and Arlene S. Ash

Administrative data result from running the health-care system—enrolling people in health plans, paying claims, certifying coverage and approving expenditures, tracking service use, and monitoring payments and quality. While not produced explicitly to examine the health or health care of populations, administrative data nevertheless offer important advantages for such purposes:

- They represent large groups of people, sometimes entire populations (e.g., all persons hospitalized in a state).
- They derive from care practiced throughout the community rather than care rendered in specialized research settings.
- When linked at the individual level, they can track persons over time and across settings of care.
- Their large numbers help hide personal identities, thus protecting confidentiality after data are stripped of individual identifiers.
- They already exist, are relatively inexpensive to acquire, and are computer-readable.

Despite their administrative origins, these data have provided profound insights into health care practices. More than three decades ago, Wennberg and Gittlesohn (1973) used hospital discharge data to expose wide variations in rates of expensive medical interventions across small geographic areas with ostensibly similar populations. In the late 1980s, these and other unexplained variations (e.g., in hospital mortality rates, also identified using administrative data) precipitated an "era of assessment and accountability" in American health care (Relman 1988; Roper 1988). Administrative data figured prominently in plans to assess the effectiveness and outcomes of care rendered in communities. The 1989 legislation (P.L. 101-239) authorizing the federal Agency for Health Care Policy and Research (AHCPR, now the Agency for Healthcare Research and Quality or AHRQ) stipulated the use of large administrative databases to examine the "outcomes, effectiveness, and appropriateness" of health care services. The AHCPR's flagship projects, the Patient Outcomes Research Teams (PORTs), began with administrative data (Clancy and Eisenberg 1997; Lave et al. 1994; Mitchell et al. 1994).

Administrative data, however, inherit two significant limitations from the fragmented American health-care delivery system. First, to produce claims or encounter records, people typically must have public or private health insurance. Almost 98% of elderly people have Medicare (Medicare Payment Advisory Commission 1999, 5). In contrast, working-age adults and their children depend either on voluntary, employer-based, private health insurance or public "safety net" programs, Medicare and Medicaid. In 2002, 61.3% of persons had employer-based insurance, down 1.3 percentage points from 2001 (Mills and Bhandari 2003, 1). In 2001, 84.7% of employers offered health insurance to their full-time employees, but only 26.9% offered it to persons working less than 21 hours weekly (Rice et al. 2002, 191). With health care costs rising again at double-digit rates, "some notable employers are beginning to question their roles as purchasers of health insurance" (Trude et al. 2002, 67).

Most person-level administrative databases do not include uninsured individuals, estimated at 43.6 million (15.2% of the population) in 2002, up from 14.6% in 2001 (Mills and Bhandari 2003, 1). Uninsured individuals face a higher risk of experiencing poor health outcomes than do insured persons (Institute of Medicine 2004). In addition, lack of continuous coverage presents major problems for tracking persons across needs-based public insurance (Medicaid) and private, employment-based plans. High turnover, as often experienced by Medicaid recipients and rapidly changing workforces, impedes efforts to create longitudinal, population-based databases.

Second, health insurance must cover specific services for claims or encounter records (and their associated diagnosis codes) to be recorded. However, many important services for chronic conditions are not covered, especially by private health plans and Medicare (Fox 1993). Insurers often set annual limits on mental health services or "carve out" their coverage to other organizations (Gitterman et al. 2001). Reimbursement is especially restrictive for chronic, function-related items and services for persons with physical or sensory impairments (Cassel et al. 1999; Iezzoni 2003a; Pope and Tarlov 1991). Even with insurance, many people spend thousands of dollars annually out of pocket on health-related services (Foote and Hogan 2001). Thus, the services and medical conditions represented by claims or encounter records do not reflect fully the health needs of people with mental health problems and chronic diseases.

Administrative data have other limitations. Most importantly, their primary clinical insight derives from diagnoses coded with questionable accuracy, completeness, clinical scope, and meaningfulness (Hsia et al. 1988, 1992; Iezzoni 1997,

2003b; McCarthy et al. 2000; Romano 1993; Romano and Mark 1994). Furthermore, administrative data can be cumbersome to handle and may not be fully current. These and other problems led the former Office of Technology Assessment (1995, 6) to conclude:

> Contrary to the expectations expressed in the legislation establishing AHCPR and the mandates of the PORTs, administrative databases generally have not proved useful in answering questions about the comparative effectiveness of alternative medical treatments. Administrative databases are very useful for descriptive purposes (e.g., exploring variations in treatment patterns), but the practical and theoretical limitations of this research technique usually prevent it from being able to provide credible answers regarding which technologies, among alternatives, work best.

Despite these problems, administrative data provide important information about health services use, expenditures, selected clinical outcomes, and quality of care. This chapter examines U.S. administrative databases, briefly discusses data systems internationally, and explores their utility for population-based studies of health and health care.

OVERVIEW OF ADMINISTRATIVE DATABASES IN THE UNITED STATES

Administrative data are the by-product of operating and overseeing the health-care system. In some administrative databases, the unit of observation is specific services, typically hospitalizations. At least 36 states systematically collect information about hospital discharges—the hospital *discharge abstract*, containing demographic and administrative information, diagnosis and procedure codes, and discharge disposition (Donaldson and Lohr 1994). With some exceptions (e.g., California, New York), individuals do not have unique identification numbers, preventing tracking of hospitalizations at the person level. Hospital discharge databases generally cannot link with other settings of care.

In health insurance databases, individual persons are usually the unit of observation. Individuals are assigned unique identifiers, allowing tracking of services across settings covered by the insurer. Most health insurance databases contain two types of files: enrollment files, indicating eligibility for the health plan and demographic information, and claims (in fee-for-service plans) or encounter records (in capitated plans), representing individual services or sets of services. We focus here on person-level administrative data produced by public (e.g., Center for Medicare and Medicaid Services, or CMS, known as the Health Care Financing Administration, or HCFA, before 2001) and private health insurers. Persons outside these insurance plans can sometimes gain access to their data after meeting specified confidentiality and security requirements.

Clinical Content of Administrative Data

Clinical insights from administrative data mostly derive from records for individual services: claims submitted when billing for care (fee-for-service) or reports on health-care encounters submitted by providers to capitated plans (Hornbrook et al. 1998; Iezzoni 2003b). On claims and encounter records, clinical information generally includes:

Diagnoses coded using the International Classification of Diseases, Ninth Revision, Clinical Modification (ICD-9-CM);

Procedures or services coded using ICD-9-CM for claims submitted by institutional providers such as hospitals; the American Medical Association's *Current Procedural Terminology* (CPT-4) for individual physician services; or *HCFA's Common Procedure Coding System* (HCPCS) for nonphysician services not in CPT-4, including durable medical equipment; and

Prescription drugs coded using the Food and Drug Administration's National Drug Codes (NDC) on pharmacy claims from insurance plans (including Medicaid) offering drug coverage.

Medicare managed care organizations (MCOs) currently must report encounter records only for hospitalizations and limited clinical information on all health encounters, such as office visits. Major administrative records throughout the entire health-care system must now comply with transaction standards specified pursuant to the 1996 Health Insurance Portability and Accountability Act (HIPAA, P.L. 104-191). The HIPAA mandates standardized content, formats, and code sets for various computerized records. These requirements should make the content of standard administrative databases comparable across public and private payers.

Other Programmatic Reporting Requirements

In specified care settings, insurers can require providers to routinely report additional clinical information beyond the diagnosis, procedure, and drug codes. The best known examples come from Medicare, including

The Minimum Data Set (MDS), administered quarterly in nursing homes and containing more than 350 items (e.g., cognitive, sensory, and physical functioning) (Hawes et al. 1997; Morris et al. 1995) and

The Outcome and Assessment Information Set (OASIS), collected during home health-care visits, with over 125 items (e.g., functional status, equipment management) (Health Care Financing Administration 1997; Shaughnessy et al. 1995, 1997).

The MDS provides the basis for nursing home prospective payment using Resource Utilization Groups (RUGs) (Fries et al. 1994; Schneider et al. 1988; Swan and Newcomer 2000), while OASIS underlies home care prospective payment (Home Health Resource Groups or HHRGs). Rehabilitation hospitals also collect clinical information, primarily using the Functional Independence Measure (FIM, an 18-item scale) (Stineman 1997; Stineman et al. 1994, 1997; Williams et al. 1997).

The multiplicity of data-gathering tools for populations with roughly similar clinical concerns prompted the Medicare Payment Advisory Commission (2001, 94) to recommend development of a single "patient classification system that predicts costs within and across post-acute settings." These reporting requirements may therefore change over the years ahead. Our discussion below concentrates on standard, coded administrative data from claims or encounter records.

EXAMPLES OF PERSON-LEVEL ADMINISTRATIVE DATABASES

Medicare

Medicare insures eligible beneficiaries 65 years of age and older and younger persons with disabilities or end-stage renal disease (ESRD). Medicare includes two distinct parts: Part A, hospital insurance (coverage for care from institutions, including hospitals, skilled nursing facilities, hospices, and some home health services), and Part B, supplemental medical insurance (covering physician services, outpatient hospital services, certain medical equipment, and other services). While all qualified persons receive Part A, Part B is voluntary. In 2002, Medicare covered 40.6 million persons, including 34.6 million elderly people (Centers for Medicare and Medicaid Services 2003). With the aging population, Medicare enrollment is expected to exceed 77 million by 2030, with almost 69 million elderly (De Lew 2000, 88).

In administering Medicare, CMS processes massive quantities of beneficiary, institutional, billing, and other administrative data. In fiscal year (FY) 1999, Medicare received over 850 million claims, processing 97% of Part A and 80% of Part B claims electronically (De Lew 2000, 84). Medicare's administrative records are compiled into huge, computerized data files, reflecting CMS's three primary functions: (*1*) enrolling and tracking beneficiaries, each of whom receives a unique identification number; (*2*) designating and monitoring providers and institutions approved to accept Medicare payments; and (*3*) reimbursing health plans and individual services. Since 1991, all institutional provider and physician/supplier claims have been entered weekly into the National Claims History (NCH) file, containing approximately 160 variables and billions of records. Researchers inside and outside CMS have used NCH extracts linked with other administrative databases (e.g., beneficiaries' dates of deaths) to investigate the experiences of Medicare beneficiaries.

Because of its nationwide scope, Medicare's administrative files have yielded important insights into the health and health care of a significant fraction of the U.S. population (Virnig and McBean 2001). These data have explored such topics as persistent variations in service use across geographic regions (Burns et al. 1996a; Dartmouth Medical School 1996), racial differences in cardiac procedures (Ayanian et al. 1993) and mammography (Burns et al. 1996b), hospitalization outcomes (Riley et al. 1993), and expenditures in the last year of life (Lubitz and Riley 1993). Sometimes the government has used these data to address policy concerns, such as hospital mortality rates for Medicare beneficiaries meant to provide clues about quality (Sullivan and Wilensky 1991). The HCFA administrator Bruce Vladeck rescinded publication of these figures in 1993, arguing that administrative data unfairly penalized public hospitals by not accounting fully for health risks of medically indigent patients (U.S. General Accounting Office 1995).

Medicare's health maintenance or managed care organizations (MCOs) have heretofore produced little administrative data. While over 80% of Medicare beneficiaries remain in traditional fee-for-service plans, 6.2 million were enrolled in MCOs in 2000 (De Lew 2000, 101). To limit the data-gathering burdens on MCOs, HCFA did not require them to report any information about enrollees' health-care encounters until 1999. Since then, MCOs have had to submit hospitalization encounter records, which are used to set capitation payments as mandated by the 1997 Balanced Budget Act (BBA) (Iezzoni et al. 1998; Pope et al. 2000). Without information, MCO enrollees—possibly a healthier subset of Medicare beneficiaries (Morgan et al. 1997; Riley et al. 1996)—are thus excluded from studies using Medicare administrative data. New reporting requirements for Medicare MCOs have started recently, involving selected diagnoses regardless of treatment setting. How this reporting will proceed and the quality and accuracy of the diagnostic data should become clearer with time, as MCOs begin submitting this information.

Medicaid

Medicaid is a joint state and federal, means-tested program covering three major areas: (*1*) health insurance for low-income families and persons with disabilities; (*2*) long-term care for older persons and those with disabilities; and (*3*) supplemental coverage for low-income Medicare beneficiaries for services not covered by Medicare (such as outpatient prescription drugs) and costs of Medicare premiums and deductibles. In 2002, roughly 12% of the U.S. population under 65 years had Medicaid coverage (National Center for Health Statistics 2004). The number of Medicaid recipients with disabilities is growing at roughly twice the rate of other eligible populations, with approximately

6.6 million people in FY 1998. The Personal Responsibility and Work Opportunity Act of 1996 "effectively decoupled Medicaid from cash assistance for low-income families," with early evidence suggesting that "many such families did not retain their Medicaid benefits" (Klemm 2000, 110).

Details of Medicaid eligibility, benefits, and coverage vary across states, as do the databases (Ku et al. 1990). Medicaid administrative databases are currently available for 31 states, containing claims for all services (including prescription drugs) in the form of State Medicaid Research Files (SMRFs) (Research Data Assistance Center [hp] Medicaid). Enrollment information on SMRFs can be linked to claims, creating person-level records. Because of the huge volume of claims and fluctuations in eligibility of many Medicaid recipients, these files are generally massive and cumbersome to manipulate (Bright et al. 1989).

In addition, as for Medicare, Medicaid MCOs have only recently been required to submit encounter information. Managed care penetration varies across states, with two states having no and 12 states having 76% to 100% MCO enrollment (Provost and Hughes 2000, 150). Some states link the State Children's Health Insurance Program (SCHIP), created by the 1997 BBA, directly to their Medicaid programs (Hakim et al. 2000). In FY 1999, 2 million children were enrolled in SCHIP, with almost 700,000 in Medicaid expansion plans (Provost and Hughes 2000, 152). Plans for generating comprehensive data about SCHIP enrollees and experiences are evolving.

Inconsistencies across states in how populations are defined, large size and complexity, and lower visibility than Medicare files "may have caused some analysts to despair and decide that Medicaid data are hopeless" (Ku et al. 1990, 35). Despite this, Medicaid data offer important opportunities. One particularly important area involves Medicaid pharmacy data (Bright et al. 1989; Gerstman et al. 1990; Soumerai et al. 1987, 1991). Another area concerns children, 51% of FY 1998 Medicaid recipients (Provost and Hughes 2000, 162). Few other publicly available data sets contain large numbers of children; given the nature of Medicaid recipients, these studies often emphasize effects of poverty and chronic illness (Ettner et al. 2000; Kuhlthau et al. 1998; Perrin et al. 1998a, 1998b, 1999). Although Medicaid findings generalize to only a subset of the population, they provide important information about persons who are potentially vulnerable because of poverty and disability.

Private Insurance Files

Private health insurers also create administrative databases from their claims and encounter records (Garnick et al. 1996; Hornbrook et al. 1998; Iezzoni 2003b). These files are structured for insurers' business purposes, not outside investigators, and they can be complicated. Nonetheless, certain companies have produced files for analytic use, including use by outside investigators. Some insurers submit their data sets to companies (e.g., Mercer and Medstat) that produce physician practice profiles or other comparative reports. These businesses sometimes sell large, multiorganizational databases to external parties after ensuring confidentiality.

Private insurance claims offer information on services used by younger employed adults and their children—populations not represented in public administrative databases. Insurance files typically include details about plan enrollment and each covered service; some include interesting additional information, such as worker attendance and specifics of plan design. Apart from significant technical and logistical hurdles of using private insurance claims files for population-based studies, however, questions arise concerning the scope and content of these databases (Garnick et al. 1996; Hornbrook et al. 1998). Claims or encounter files do not reflect use of services for which enrollees do not submit bills. Some insurers retain information only on paid claims, deleting data on services below the deductible or above the maximum benefit levels. Information on prescription drugs and mental health care is often incomplete. Private insurers frequently require fewer diagnoses on claims than do public programs, and insurers sometimes assign their own idiosyncratic procedure codes for certain services. Private insurers typically do not collect information on race or ethnicity. Some inconsistencies across private insurers may disappear when HIPAA-mandated transaction standards take effect.

CLINICAL INFORMATION IN ADMINISTRATIVE DATABASES

Virtually all public and private organizations use their administrative databases for program management, oversight, and policymaking. For examining population health and analyses of physical or mental functioning or overall disease burden, however, administrative data have important limitations, relating primarily to their clinical information.

Diagnosis Codes

American clinicians and coding experts tailored ICD-9-CM explicitly to suit numerous administrative needs beyond vital statistics reporting, its original purpose. ICD-9-CM contains codes for many conditions that are technically not diseases (Table 6.1). Creatively combining diverse codes can yield plausible clinical stories encompassing physical, emotional, and even selected social dimensions. Diagnosis codes in administrative databases, however, aim not to tell stories but to generate reimbursement. Physicians (or their office staffs) list codes for outpatient office visits, while hospital medical record departments assign discharge diagnoses for hospitalizations. Extensive guidelines, posted on the Web site of the National Center for Health Statistics and published by the American

TABLE 6.1
Examples of ICD-9-CM Codes

Type of Information	*Number*	*Description of Code*
Clinical diagnosis	250.53	Type I diabetes mellitus with ophthalmic manifestations, uncontrolled
	410.01	Acute myocardial infarction of anterolateral wall, initial episode of care
Pathological process	414.01	Coronary atherosclerosis of native coronary artery
	324.0	Intracranial abscess
Symptoms	569.42	Anal or rectal pain
	780.4	Dizziness or giddiness
Physical findings	342.0	Flaccid hemiplegia
	611.72	Lump or mass in breast
Laboratory or other test findings	794.31	Abnormal electrocardiogram
	790.2	Abnormal glucose tolerance test
	793.8	Nonspecific abnormal findings on radiologic and other examination of breast (includes abnormal mammogram)
Acuity or severity indicator	427.5	Cardiac arrest
	518.81	Respiratory failure
	V46.1	Dependence on respirator
Potential quality indicator	964.7	Poisoning by natural blood and blood products
	998.7	Acute reaction to foreign substance accidentally left during a procedure
Psychological factors and mental health	308.0	Acute reaction to stress, predominant disturbance of emotions
	296.54	Bipolar affective disorder, depressed, severe, specified as with psychotic behavior
Cognitive factors	290.0	Senile dementia, uncomplicated
	318.2	Profound mental retardation (IQ under 20)
Substance abuse	304.21	Continuous cocaine dependency
	303.93	Chronic alcoholism in remission
Social factors	V61.1	Marital problems
	V60.0	Lack of housing
Physical functional impairments	344.1	Paraplegia
	V53.8	Wheelchair
External environmental factors	E900.0	Excessive heat due to weather conditions
	E965.0	Assault by a handgun

ICD-9-CM = International Statistical Classification of Diseases and Health Related Problems, Ninth Revision, Clinical Modification.

Hospital Association in its quarterly *Coding Clinic for ICD-9-CM*, govern the assignment of codes. Medicare pays for some services only when certain codes are listed, thus significantly affecting coding practices. Numerous studies document significant problems with the accuracy, completeness, clinical scope, and meaningfulness of diagnosis codes (Hsia et al. 1988, 1992; Iezzoni 1997, 2003b; McCarthy et al. 2000; Romano 1993; Romano and Mark 1994).

ICD-9-CM codes and coding practices present special problems for examining health and the functional consequences of disease. First, ICD-9-CM works best for specific medical conditions, such as heart attacks, cancer, or pneumonia. Nevertheless, one must list multiple codes to depict fully the extent of these conditions (e.g., coding not only primary lung cancer but also metastatic tumors and complications, such as respiratory failure or hepatic coma). Individual codes rarely indicate the severity of conditions or their pace of progression, but physicians rarely code more than one diagnosis, especially for outpatient visits.

Second, incomplete coding is especially problematic for chronic conditions. Good evidence suggests that hospitals undercode chronic diseases, such as diabetes mellitus and hypertension, particularly for acutely ill patients (Iezzoni et al. 1992; Jencks et al. 1988; Jollis et al. 1993; Malenka et al. 1994). Of Medicare beneficiaries coded with either an inpatient or outpatient diagnosis of dementia in 1994, only 59% had dementia coded in 1995; of patients coded with paraplegia or quadriplegia in 1994, only 52% had these codes in 1995 (Medicare Payment Advisory Commission 1998, 17). Using Medicaid data from seven states, the percentages of people coded with specific diagnoses in a second year who had the code the previous year were: 80% for schizophrenia, 68% for diabetes, 58% for multiple sclerosis, 57% for quadriplegia, and 34% for cystic fibrosis (Kronick et al. 2000, 60). None of these conditions disappear. Their absence in the subsequent year highlights the incompleteness of coding.

Third, unless a condition is actively treated, physicians and hospitals rarely code it. Although codes exist for blindness, deafness, and hard of hearing, for example, they are infrequently listed on claims for services unrelated to the eyes or ears. Mental retardation is rarely coded for adults or children, perhaps because few health interventions directly target this condition (Ettner et al. 2000; Kronick et al. 2000). Sometimes physicians intentionally avoid coding potentially stigmatizing diagnoses (e.g., mental health disorders, acquired immunodeficiency syndrome) when other conditions can be listed legitimately. V codes, a supplementary classification of factors influencing health status and contact with health services, are coded infrequently; insurers rarely pay based on V codes.

Fourth, coding practices are heavily influenced by payment procedures and other policies. Medicare's diagnosis related group (DRG)-based payment system fundamentally altered the context of coding for hospitalizations (Hsia et al. 1988, 1992; Simborg 1981). Local initiatives using hospital diagnosis data in comparing mortality rates across facilities also potentially affect diagnosis coding, as happened in California (Romano et al. 1997). The quality of outpatient coding has been less studied but is suspect (Fowles et al. 1995).

Finally, no codes adequately capture functional status. Code 344.9, paralysis unspecified, for example, depicts conditions ranging from complete paralysis to generalized weakness. No codes indicate performance of activities of daily living or basic physical actions, such as walking or climbing stairs. Without valid information about physical, sensory, cognitive, or emotional functioning, one cannot accurately identify people with potentially disabling conditions or track meaningful outcomes of care. Although the *International Classification of Functioning, Disability, and Health* (ICF), promulgated by the World Health Organization (2001), classifies functional abilities and social and environmental contexts, this coding scheme is not used routinely for administrative data collection in the United States (Iezzoni and Greenberg 2003).

Procedure Codes

Because health-care providers are paid for specific procedures, procedures are generally coded more accurately and completely than diagnoses (Fisher et al. 1992; Iezzoni 2003b; Romano and Luft 1992). Procedure coding is especially good for high-risk or costly services, such as chemotherapy and mechanical ventilation (Romano and Luft 1992). Medicare, Medicaid, and private insurers generally pay for acute care services without demur, sometimes requiring proof of medical necessity or appropriateness. Because of high costs, patients are unlikely to obtain such services without insurance coverage. Therefore, administrative databases should represent virtually all covered procedures or treatments obtained within a given time period.

Some procedures imply chronic debilitating conditions. Examples include amputation of a limb, hip arthroplasty, major organ transplantation, tracheostomy tube insertion, or gastrostomy tube placement. Certain treatments, such as chemotherapy, also suggest important chronic illness. However, relying on procedure codes to identify people with specific conditions or functional limitations raises important questions.

First, even for potentially life-prolonging interventions (e.g., tracheostomy tube placement), significant variations in procedure use are likely because of differing preferences for care, practice styles, and availability of services across patients, physicians, institutions, and geographic regions. Second, people may have received the service during a time period previous to that covered by the administrative database. Although certain V codes (ICD-9-CM diagnoses) indicate selected prior procedures (e.g., *transplant status*), pertinent V codes are not always listed. Third, restrictive payment policies limiting some services (such as mental health care or physical therapy) mean that some services are missing from administrative files. Finally, procedure codes reveal little about outcomes. Presumably appendectomies universally cure appendicitis, for example, but a hip replacement may or may not restore a person's mobility.

Pharmacy Data

Administrative databases from insurers offering prescription drug benefits, including Medicaid, generally contain pharmacy claims. Pharmacy data represent prescriptions that were filled (instead of prescriptions written but never obtained). Obviously, administrative files do not indicate whether people took medications as prescribed. Pharmacy data can identify people with specific conditions, such as diabetes, bipolar disorder, asthma, and acquired immunodeficiency syndrome (Fishman and Shay 1999; Johnson et al. 1994; Lamers 1999). These data suggest the severity of some medical conditions. For example, people receiving insulin presumably have more intractable diabetes mellitus than those taking oral hypoglycemic agents. Certain drugs suggest the pace of illness or the course of a disease. People with multiple sclerosis taking interferon-beta, for instance, presumably have relapsing-remitting rather than secondary progressive disease. However, like procedure codes, pharmacy data identify only selected subgroups of people, varying practice patterns compromise the generalizability of findings, and drugs not covered by insurance plans escape detection.

MERGING ADMINISTRATIVE DATA WITH OTHER DATA SOURCES

Merging administrative data with other data sources can efficiently enrich administrative files (Lillard and Farmer 1997; U.S. General Accounting Office 2001). Using aggregate information collected by the decennial census, for example, researchers have linked person-level information with data on population characteristics (e.g., poverty level, racial distribution) within small geographic areas. Linking information from the American Hospital Association's annual survey allows insight into the institutions providing services (e.g., teaching status, number of beds). These examples involve merging information about individuals with aggregate contextual information (e.g., census tracts, hospitals).

Linking two or more data sources containing information on individuals provides considerable additional insight. Most such merges include Medicare data because of their huge size and nationwide scope. Merging Medicare data with population-based data sources produces hybrid data sets—conflating representative samples with Medicare participation, especially fee-for-service Medicare (remembering that Medicare MCOs have not previously supplied comprehensive encounter records).

One example merges two different sources from within Medicare itself—the Medicare Current Beneficiary Survey (MCBS) with the National Claims History file. The MCBS is an ongoing longitudinal survey of a representative panel of roughly 12,000 Medicare beneficiaries, with oversampling of persons under age 65 and 85 years of age and older (Adler 1994, 1995). Respondents typically remain empaneled in the MCBS for 4 years, with in-person interviews conducted three times annually. Two types of surveys (based on residence within communities or institutions) solicit information about physical and sensory functioning, satisfaction with and access to care, out-of-pocket payments, and numerous other topics. Merging MCBS survey responses with Medicare claims facilitates varied analyses, such as examining screening and preventive services (Chan et al. 1999); satisfaction with care (Adler 1995; Hermann et al. 1998; Iezzoni et al. 2003; Rosenbach 1995); access to care (Foote and Hogan 2001; Rosenbach 1995); and out-of-pocket expenditures by ability to perform activities of daily living (Foote and Hogan 2001).

Surveys derived from national sampling have been merged with Medicare data, notably the Longitudinal Survey of Aging (LSOA) and the National Long-Term Care Survey, both of which contain extensive functional status information. Prior to linking these files, survey respondents must consent; 80% typically do, but consent rates vary across surveys (Lillard and Farmer 1997, 694). These linked survey files have been used extensively to study patterns of service use, especially among elderly persons with functional deficits (Culler et al. 1995; Manton et al. 1993; Mor et al. 1994; Stearns et al. 1996). Plans are proceeding to merge NHIS responses with Medicare claims files, allowing wide-ranging analyses of service use associated with personal attributes and health-related attributes captured by the NHIS. To protect confidentiality, the content of these files and access to these data may be carefully regulated.

A prominent interagency linkage involves merging Medicare claims files with the National Cancer Institute's (NCI) Surveillance, Epidemiology, and End Results (SEER) Program data (Potosky et al. 1993). The SEER Program gathers information from 11 population-based cancer registries and 3 supplemental registries covering about 14% of the U.S. population (National Cancer Institute [hp] About SEER). Started in 1973, the SEER database contains information on over 2.5 million cancer cases, with about 160,000 new cases added annually. SEER routinely collects data on patients' demographics, primary tumor site, morphology, stage at diagnosis, first course of treatment (followed for up to 4 months), and vital status.

Data elements from the SEER Program (Social Security number, name, sex, dates of birth and death) facilitate linkage with Medicare claims files. Using a deterministic matching algorithm, the first merge (for patients diagnosed from 1973 to 1989) matched 93.8% of persons diagnosed at 65 years of age or older (Potosky et al. 1993). Although information on Medicare beneficiaries younger than 65 (disabled, ESRD) is also merged, these linkages have not been validated. The most recent linkage, completed in December 1999, included SEER cases through 1996 and their Medicare claims through 1998. The NCI and CMS plan to update the merge every 3 years, adding Medicare claims during intervening years (National Cancer Institute [hp] SEER-Medicare Database). The database also contains a 5% random sample of Medicare beneficiaries not in the SEER registry but residing in SEER areas (so-called noncancer cases) to allow comparisons.

Researchers have typically used the clinical detail of the SEER database to enrich analyses of cancer care conducted with Medicare claims. Riley and colleagues (1995) examined Medicare costs between diagnosis and death using merged files from 1984 through 1990, finding unexpectedly low costs for lung cancer, presumably because of short life spans. Studies have used merged SEER-Medicare data to compare early detection of cancer for fee-for-service versus MCO insurance (Riley et al. 1994a, 1999), outcomes of care by insurance type (Potosky et al. 1997, 1999), and mammogram experience by race (McCarthy et al. 1998) and age (McCarthy et al. 2000).

Some researchers leverage the broad reach of Medicare to enhance SEER analyses. For instance, using Medicare claims to identify incident cases, McBean, Babish, and Warren (1993) found that 1986–1990 age-adjusted lung cancer incidence rates among Medicare beneficiaries residing outside nine SEER areas were 8% to 13% higher than rates for residents of the SEER regions. The researchers urged complementing SEER cancer incidence data with Medicare claims–derived rates, since Medicare covers the entire country and SEER sites may not be nationally representative.

Since the Social Security Administration (SSA) determines Medicare eligibility, for persons with disabilities in particular, one useful interdepartmental data merge links SSA and Medicare records. To examine Medicare costs for newly entitled disabled persons, for example, analysts at SSA and HCFA merged SSA's Master Beneficiary Record (records of entitlement and cash payments for all persons who ever received Social Security benefits); the Continuous Disability History Sample (a 20% sample of SSA disability determinations); and Medicare claims files (Bye et al. 1987). With this merged file, they examined long-term Medicare costs for disabled beneficiaries (Bye et al. 1987) and the potential costs to Medicare of eliminating the 2-year waiting period between SSA disability determination and Medicare eligibility (Bye and Riley 1989; Bye et al. 1991).

Merging SSA disability and Medicare files required careful interdepartmental negotiations, primarily to ensure strict privacy and security of the resulting database. With detailed information on SSA's disability determinations linked with Medicare claims, even files stripped of specific identifiers (name, Social Security number) could present potential privacy risks. Merged SSA and Medicare databases are not generally released to outside investigators.

EXAMPLES OF ADMINISTRATIVE DATA FROM OTHER COUNTRIES

To a large extent, the fragmented nature of administrative data systems in the United States reflects its fragmented health-care delivery system. In countries and regions where central authorities deliver health care to well-defined populations, comprehensive administrative data systems could facilitate monitoring of health and health-care delivery (Nerenz 1996). The POPULIS data system in

Manitoba, Canada, offers a good example (Roos and Shapiro 1995a; Roos et al. 1995). POPULIS interconnects various data sets, tying factors affecting a population's need for health care to its use of health-care services, to the supply of health care resources within defined geographic areas, to the health status of the population (see Chapters 9 and 18).

At POPULIS's core is a population registry (e.g., births, deaths, geographic mobility) for defined geographic areas. Linked to this core are data sets containing indicators of socioeconomic status (derived from census tract–level information on household income, employment, education, and cultural diversity); indicators of health (e.g., all-cause and cause-specific mortality rates, various indicators derived from hospital discharge abstracts and physicians' claims); and use of health care (e.g., payments to hospitals, nursing homes, physicians) (Roos et al. 1995). POPULIS also includes data on immunizations, prescription drugs, and home health care and other community-based services (Chapter 18). Researchers have used POPULIS to investigate "premature" mortality (Cohen and MacWilliams 1995), the association of socioeconomic factors with health status and service use (Mustard and Frolich 1995), and the effect of hospital bed closures (Roos and Shapiro 1995b). POPULIS is evolving into "a true system of population health information, of which health care services are only a part" (Evans and Mustard 1995, DS5).

Several other developed nations are building data systems similar to POPULIS (Chapter 17). Examples of current trends include:

- Collection of data beyond acute, short-term hospitalizations and physicians' services (e.g., Australia, Canada, and New Zealand have started gathering mental health and home care information).
- Increased linkage and sharing of data definitions across information systems (e.g., Australia is exploring linkage of person-level census data with health care data. In Canada, respondents to the National Population Health Survey are asked permission to link their responses with data from administrative data sets; most agree. Denmark uses civil registration numbers to link information on various health-care services for individuals).
- Efforts to protect individual confidentiality and privacy in linked data sets using consistent strategies across countries.
- Making health information more accessible, including reports on overall health and health system performance and international comparisons. Six of 18 European countries track progress against health targets, and another 8 are expanding their systems to permit such tracking. Many countries are developing user-friendly Web-based systems to share health statistics.

In Great Britain, the National Health Service (NHS) has committed by 2005 to create lifelong electronic health records; offer 24 hour on-line access to patient records and information about best clinical practices; share information across delivery sites, including community-based services; and provide information for planners and managers (National Health Service Information Authority [hp] Information for Health). The NHS views administrative data as flowing from clinical practices rather than being produced primarily for administrative purposes.

FUTURE ISSUES

Merging databases and constructing person-level files highlight concerns about individual privacy, an issue that could significantly affect the creation and use of administrative databases in the future. In its report, *Record Linkage and Privacy*, the U.S. General Accounting Office (2001, 70) suggests that "reidentification risks may be higher for datasets with person-by-person linkages than for their component parts," largely because of the greater depth of information on individuals. They describe strategies for protecting the privacy and security of linked data files, but even stand-alone administrative databases generate privacy concerns among some observers (U.S. General Accounting Office 1999).

In Chapter 14, Fanning examines privacy issues in greater detail, including the HIPAA-mandated federal health information privacy rules implemented in 2001. Here, however, questions about individual informed consent are especially pertinent. Unlike clinical trials, where informed consent theoretically protects the safety and rights of research subjects, studies using administrative databases are generally absolved from requiring consent. This exemption recognizes that obtaining consent is burdensome and infeasible given the size and composition of administrative databases; requiring consent could yield biased subsamples of participants (Gostin and Hadley 1998).

Organizations may release private health information in administrative databases without individuals' permission, but only if recipients obtain a waiver from their institutional review board or privacy board. The waiver criteria include findings that (*1*) the use or disclosure involves no more than minimal risk; (*2*) the research could not practicably be conducted without the waiver; (*3*) the privacy risks are reasonable in relation to the anticipated benefits, if any, to individuals and the importance of the research; (*4*) a plan to destroy the identifiers exists unless there is a health or research justification for retaining them; and (*5*) there are written assurances that the data will not be reused or disclosed to others, except for research oversight or additional research that would qualify for a waiver (Gostin 2001, 3018–3019). Organizations like CMS, which release administrative data for "public use," routinely remove personal identifiers and require researchers to adhere to privacy and security standards. These public use files therefore meet the waiver criterion of posing minimal if any risk of breaching privacy.

One potential future development will likely heighten privacy concerns—the merging of detailed clinical data (e.g., laboratory, radiology, and other diagnostic test results) with administrative claims files. As hospitals and other health-care providers increasingly capture clinical information electronically, linking these data to administrative files offers tremendous opportunities (Pine et al. 1997). Access to detailed clinical information overcomes the reservations described above about the limited clinical content of administrative data. Merging clinical and administrative files would facilitate quality measurement, practice profiling, and health system monitoring. Research on large populations could potentially account for clinical factors that only painstaking chart reviews allow today. Yet, as with other merged data sets, the potential for identifying individuals might expand with more detailed clinical data.

Fortunately, methods exist to address most privacy concerns. But these strategies need to be applied systematically throughout the health-care system, from the ground up (U.S. General Accounting Office 2001). Unlike research trials or even population-based surveys, where parties generating and responsible for data are easily identified, administrative data, by definition, result from the messy public-private U.S. health care system. Persons producing data range from billing clerks in physicians' offices to health information systems managers within massive bureaucracies such as CMS. Attention to data quality and privacy protection is critical at all points. Although today's administrative data have significant limitations, future data sets could offer a rich source of information about the health of insured populations.

REFERENCES

Adler GS. A profile of the Medicare Current Beneficiary Survey. Health Care Finan Rev 1994;15(4):153–163.

Adler GS. Medicare beneficiaries rate their medical care: new data from the MCBS. Health Care Finan Rev 1995;16(4):175–187.

Ayanian JZ, Udvarhelyi IS, Gatsonis CA, Pashos CL, Epstein AM. Racial differences in the use of revascularization procedures after coronary angiography. JAMA 1993;269:2642–2646.

Bright RA, Avorn J, Everitt DE. Medicaid data as a resource for epidemiologic studies: strengths and limitations. JAMA 1989;42:937–945.

Burns RB, McCarthy EP, Freund KM, et al. Variability in mammography use among older women. J Am Geriatr Soc 1996a;44:922–926.

Burns RB, McCarthy EP, Freund KM, et al. Black women receive less mammography even with similar use of primary care. Ann Intern Med 1996b;125:173–182.

Bye BV, Dykacz JM, Hennessey JC, Riley GF. Medicare costs prior to retirement for disabled-worker beneficiaries. Soc Secur Bull 1991;54:2–23.

Bye BV, Riley GF. Eliminating the Medicare waiting period for Social Security disabled-worker beneficiaries. Soc Secur Bull 1989;52:2–15.

Bye BV, Riley GF, Lubitz J. Medicare utilization by disabled-worker beneficiaries: a longitudinal analysis. Soc Secur Bull 1987;50:13–28.

Cassel CK, Besdine RW, Siegel LC. Restructuring Medicare for the next century: what will beneficiaries really need? Health Aff 1999;18:118–131.

Centers for Medicare and Medicaid Services. Table I.C1—Medicare data for calendar year

2002 [cited 12 Sep 2003]. Available from: www.cms.hhs.gov/publications/trusteesreport/2003/table1.asp.

Chan L, Doctor JN, MacLehose RF, Lawson H, Rosenblatt RA, Baldwin LM, Jha A. Do Medicare patients with disabilities receive preventive services? A population-based study. Arch Phys Med Rehabil 1999;80:642–646.

Clancy CM, Eisenberg JM. Outcomes research at the Agency for Health Care Policy and Research. Disease Manag Clin Outcomes 1997;1:72–80.

Cohen MM, MacWilliams L. Measuring the health of the population. Med Care 1995;33(suppl):DS21–DS42.

Culler SD, Callahan CM, Wolinsky FD. Predicting hospital costs among older decedents over time. Med Care 1995;33:1089–1105.

Dartmouth Medical School, Center for Evaluative Clinical Studies. The Dartmouth Atlas of Health Care. Chicago: American Hospital Association; 1996.

De Lew N. Medicare: 35 years of service. Health Care Finan Rev 2000;22(1):75–103.

Donaldson MS, Lohr KN. Health Data in the Information Age: Use, Disclosure, and Privacy. Washington, DC: National Academy Press; 1994.

Elixhauser A, Andrews RM, Fox S. Clinical Classifications for Health Policy Research: Discharge Statistics by Principal Diagnosis and Procedure. AHCPR Publication no. 93-0043. Division of Provider Studies Research Note 17. Rockville, MD: Agency for Health Care Policy and Research; 1993.

Ettner SL, Kuhlthau K, McLaughlin TJ, Perrin JM, Gortmaker SL. Impact of expanding SSI on Medicaid expenditures of disabled children. Health Care Financ Rev 2000;21:185–201.

Evans RG, Mustard JF. Forward. Med Care 1995;33(suppl):DS5–DS6.

Fisher ES, Whaley FS, Krushat WM, Malenka DJ, Fleming C, Baron JA, Hsia DC. The accuracy of Medicare's hospital claims data: progress has been made, but problems remain. Am J Public Health 1992;82:243–248.

Fishman PA, Shay DK. Development and estimation of a pediatric chronic disease score using automated pharmacy data. Med Care 1999;37:874–883.

Foote SM, Hogan C. Disability profile and health care costs of Medicare beneficiaries under age sixty-five. Health Aff 2001;20(6):242–253.

Fowles JB, Lawthers AG, Weiner JP, Garnick DW, Petrie DS, Palmer RH. Agreement between physicians' office records and Medicare part B claims data. Health Care Financ Rev 1995;16(4):189–199.

Fox DM. Power and Illness: The Failure and Future of American Health Policy. Berkeley: University of California Press; 1993.

Fries BE, Schneider DP, Foley WJ, Gavazzi M, Burke R, Cornelius E. Refining a case-mix measure for nursing homes: resource utilization groups (RUGS-III). Med Care 1994; 32:668–685.

Garnick DW, Hendricks AM, Cornstock CB, Pryor DB. A guide to using administrative data for medical effectiveness research. J Outcomes Manag 1996;3:18–23.

Gerstman BB, Lundin FE, Stadel BV, Faich GA. A method of pharmacoepidemiologic analysis that uses computerized Medicaid. J Clin Epidemiol 1990;43:1387–1393.

Gitterman DP, Strum R, Scheffler RM. Toward full mental health parity and beyond. Health Aff 2001;20(4):68–76.

Gostin LO. National health information privacy. Regulations under the Health Insurance Portability and Accountability Act. JAMA 2001;285:3015–3021.

Gostin LO, Hadley J. Health services research: public benefits, personal privacy, and proprietary interests. Ann Intern Med 1998;129:833–835.

Hakim RB, Boben PJ, Bonney JB. Medicaid and the health of children. Health Care Finan Rev 2000:22(1):133–140.

Hawes C, Mor V, Phillips CD, et al. The OBRA-87 Nursing home regulations and implementation of the Resident Assessment Instrument: effects on process quality. J Am Geriatr Soc 1997;45:977–985.

Health Care Financing Administration, Department of Health and Human Services. Medicare and Medicaid programs; revision of conditions of participation for home health agencies and use of Outcome Assessment Information Set (OASIS); proposed rules. 42 CFR Part 484. Fed Reg 1997;62:11004–11064.

Hermann RC, Ettner SL, Dorwart RA. The influence of psychiatric disorders on patients' ratings of satisfaction with health care. Med Care 1998;36:720–727.

Hornbrook MC, Goodman MJ, Fishman PA, Meenan RT, O'Keefe-Rosetti M, Bachman DJ. Building health plan databases to risk adjust outcomes and payments. Int J Qual Health Care 1998;10:531–538.

Hsia DC, Ahern CA, Ritchie BP, Moscoe LM, Krushat WM. Medicare reimbursement accuracy under the prospective payment system, 1985 to 1988. JAMA 1992;268:896–899.

Hsia DC, Krushat WM, Fagan AB, Tebbutt JA, Kusserow RP. Accuracy of diagnostic coding for Medicare patients under the prospective-payment system. N Engl J Med 1988;318:352–355.

Iezzoni LI. Assessing quality using administrative data. Ann Intern Med 1997;127:666–674.

Iezzoni LI. When Walking Fails. Mobility Problems of Adults with Chronic Conditions. Berkeley: University of California Press; 2003a.

Iezzoni LI. Coded data from administrative sources. In Iezzoni LI, ed. Risk Adjustment for Measuring Health Care Outcomes, 3rd ed. Chicago: Health Administration Press; 2003b, pp. 83–138.

Iezzoni LI, Ayanian JZ, Bates DW, Burstin H. Paying more fairly for Medicare capitated care. N Engl J Med 1998;339:1933–1938.

Iezzoni LI, Davis RB, Soukup J, O'Day B. Quality dimensions that most concern people with physical and sensory disabilities. Arch Intern Med 2003;163:2085–2092.

Iezzoni LI, Foley SM, Daley J, Hughes J, Fisher ES, Heeren T. Comorbidities, complications, and coding bias. Does the number of diagnosis codes matter in predicting in-hospital mortality? JAMA 1992;267:2197–2203.

Iezzoni LI, Greenberg MS. Capturing and classifying functional status information in administrative databases. Health Care Fin Rev 2003;24:61–76.

Institute of Medicine, Committee on the Consequences of Uninsurance. Insuring America's Health: Principles and Recommendations. Washington, DC: National Academy Press; 2004.

Jencks SF, Williams DK, Kay TL. Assessing hospital-associated deaths from discharge data: the role of length of stay and comorbidities. JAMA 1988;260:2240–2246.

Johnson RE, Hornbrook MC, Nichols GA. Replicating the chronic disease score (CDS) from automated pharmacy data. J Clin Epidemiol 1994;47:1191–1199.

Jollis JG, Ancukiewicz M, DeLong ER, Pryor DB, Muhlbaier LH, Mark DH. Discordance of databases designed for claims payment versus clinical information systems. Implications for outcomes research. Ann Intern Med 1993;119:844–850.

Klemm JD. Medicaid spending: a brief history. Health Care Finan Rev 2000;22(1):105–112.

Kronick R, Gilmer T, Dreyfus T, Lee L. Improving health-based payment for Medicaid beneficiaries: CDPS. Health Care Financ Rev 2000;21:29–64.

Ku L, Ellwood MR, Klemm J. Deciphering Medicaid data: issues and needs. Health Care Finan Rev 1990(ann suppl):35–45.

Kuhlthau K, Perrin JM, Ettner SL, McLaughlin TJ, Gortmaker SL. High-expenditure children with Supplemental Security Income. Pediatrics 1998;102:610–615.

Lamers LM. Pharmacy Cost Groups. A risk-adjuster for capitation payment based on the use of prescription drugs. Med Care 1999;37:824–830.

Lave JR, Pashos CL, Anderson GF, et al. Costing medical care: using Medicare administrative data. Med Care 1994;32:JS77–JS89.

Lillard LA, Farmer MM. Linking Medicare and national survey data. Ann Intern Med 1997;127(8 part 2):691–695.

Lubitz JD, Riley GF. Trends in Medicare payments in the last year of life. N Engl J Med 1993;328(15):1092–1096.

Malenka DJ, McLerran D, Roos N, Fisher ES, Wennberg JE. Using administrative data to describe casemix: a comparison with the medical record. J Clin Epidemiol 1994;47:1027–1032.
Manton KG, Corder L, Stallard E. Changes in the use of personal assistance and special equipment, from 1982 to 1989: Results from the 1982 and 1989 NLTCS. Gerontologist 1993; 33(2):168–176.
McBean AM, Babish JD, Warren JL. Determination of lung cancer incidence in the elderly using Medicare claims data. Am J Epidemiol 1993;137:226–234.
McCarthy EP, Burns RB, Coughlin SS, et al. Mammography use helps to explain differences in breast cancer stage at diagnosis between older black and white women. Ann Intern Med 1998;128(9):729–736.
McCarthy EP, Burns RB, Freund KM, et al. Mammography use, breast cancer stage at diagnosis, and survival among older women. J Am Geriatr Soc 2000;48:1226–1233.
McCarthy EP, Iezzoni LI, Davis RB, Palmer RH, Cahalane M, Hamel MB, Mukamal K, Phillips RS, Davies DT Jr. Does clinical evidence support ICD-9–CM diagnosis coding of complications? Med Care 2000;38:868–876.
Medicare Payment Advisory Commission. Report to the Congress: Medicare Payment Policy. Vol. II: Analytical Papers. Washington, DC: Medicare Payment Advisory Commission; 1998.
Medicare Payment Advisory Commission. Report to the Congress. Selected Medicare Issues. Washington, DC: Medicare Payment Advisory Commission; 1999.
Medicare Payment Advisory Commission. Report to the Congress: Medicare Payment Policy. Washington, DC: Medicare Payment Advisory Commission; 2001.
Mills R, Bhandari S. Health Insurance Coverage in the United States: 2002. Current Population Reports. P60-223. Washington, DC: U.S. Census Bureau; 2003.
Mitchell JB, Bubolz T, Paul JE, et al. Using Medicare claims for outcomes research. Med Care 1994;32:JS38–JS51.
Mor V, Wilcox V, Rakowski W, Hiris J. Functional transitions among the elderly: patterns, predictions, and related hospital use. Am J Public Health 1994;84:1274–1280.
Morgan RO, Virnig BA, DeVito CA, Persily NA. The Medicare-HMO revolving door—the healthy go in and the sick go out. N Engl J Med 1997;337:169–175.
Morris JN, Murphy K, Nonemaker S. Long Term Care Resident Assessment Instrument User's Manual, version 2.0. Baltimore: Health Care Financing Administration; 1995.
Mustard CA, Frohlich N. Socioeconomic status and the health of the population. Med Care 1995;33(suppl):DS43–DS54.
National Cancer Institute [homepage on the Internet]. Bethesda, MD: NCI [cited 2004 Mar 8]. About SEER [about 2 screens]. Available from: http://seer.cancer.gov/about.
National Cancer Institute [homepage on the Internet]. Bethesda, MD: NCI [cited 2004 Mar 8]. SEER-Medicare Database [about 2 screens]. Available from: http://dccps.nci.nih.gov/bb/seer_medicare.html.
National Center for Health Statistics. Health, United States, 2004. Hyattsville, MD; 2004.
National Health Service Information Authority [homepage on the Internet]. Birmingham, UK: NHS Information Authority; c. 2004 [updated 2001 Jul 24; cited 2004 Mar 8]. Information for Health—1. An information strategy for the modern NHS [about 10 screens]. Available from: http://www.nhsia.nhs.uk/def/pages/info4health/1.asp.
Nerenz DR. Who has responsibility for a population's health? Milbank Q 1996;74:43–49.
Office of Technology Assessment, U.S. Congress. Bringing Health Care Online: The Role of Information Technologies. OTA-ITC-624. Washington, DC: GPO; 1995.
Perrin JM, Ettner SL, McLaughlin TJ, Gortmaker SL, Bloom SR, Kuhlthau K. State variations in Supplemental Security Income enrollment for children and adolescents. Am J Public Health 1998b;88:928–931.
Perrin JM, Kuhlthau K, Ettner SL, McLaughlin TJ, Gortmaker SL. Previous Medicaid status of children newly enrolled in Supplemental Security Income. Health Care Fin Rev 1998a:19:117–127.

Perrin JM, Kuhlthau K, McLaughlin TJ, Ettner SL, Gortmaker SL. Changing patterns of conditions among children receiving Supplemental Security Income disability benefits. Arch Pediatr Adolesc Med 1999;153:80–84.

Pine M, Norusis M, Jones B, Rosenthal GE. Predictions of hospital mortality rates: a comparison of data sources. Ann Intern Med 1997;126:347–354.

Pope AM, Tarlov AR. Disability in America: Toward a National Agenda for Prevention. Washington, DC: National Academy Press; 1991.

Pope GC, Ellis RP, Ash AS, et al. Principal inpatient diagnostic cost group model for Medicare risk adjustment. Health Care Fin Rev 2000;21:93–118.

Potosky AL, Merrill RM, Riley GP, Taplin SH, Barlow W, Fireman BH, Ballard-Barbash R. Breast cancer survival and treatment in health maintenance organizations and fee-for-service settings. J National Cancer Inst 1997;89:1683–1691.

Potosky AL, Merrill RM, Riley GP, Taplin SH, Barlow W, Fireman BH, Lubitz JD. Prostate cancer treatment and ten-year survival among group/staff HMO and fee-for-service Medicare patients. Health Serv Res 1999;34:525–546.

Potosky AL, Riley GF, Lubitz JD, Mentnech RM, Kessler LG. Potential for cancer related health services research using a linked Medicare-tumor registry database. Med Care 1993;31:732–748.

Provost C, Hughes P. Medicaid: 35 years of service. Health Care Fin Rev 2000:22(1):141–174.

Relman AS. Assessment and accountability: the third revolution in medical care. N Engl J Med 1988;319:1220–1222.

Research Data Assistance Center [homepage on the Internet]. Minneapolis: Regents of the University of Minnesota; c. 2003 [cited 2004 Mar 8]. Medicaid [about 2 screens]. Available from: http://www.resdac.umn.edu/Medicaid/index.asp.

Rice T, Gabel J, Levitt L, Hawkins S. Workers and their health plans: free to choose? Health Affairs 2002;21:182–187.

Riley G, Lubitz J, Gornick M, Mentnech R, Eggers P, McBean M. Medicare beneficiaries: adverse outcomes after hospitalization for eight procedures. Med Care 1993;31:921–949.

Riley GF, Potosky AL, Klabunde CN, Warren JL, Ballard-Barbash R. Stage at diagnosis and treatment patterns among older women with breast cancer: an HMO and fee-for-service comparison. JAMA 1999;281:720–726.

Riley GF, Potosky AL, Lubitz JD, Brown ML. Stage of cancer at diagnosis for Medicare HMO and fee-for-service enrollees. Am J Public Health 1994a;84:1598–1604.

Riley GF, Potosky AL, Lubitz JD, Kessler LG. Medicare payments from diagnosis to death for elderly cancer patients by stage at diagnosis. Med Care 1995;33:828–841.

Riley G, Tudor C, Chiang YP, Ingber M. Health status of Medicare enrollees in HMOs and fee-for-service in 1994b. Health Care Fin Rev 1996;17:65–76.

Romano PS. Can administrative data be used to compare the quality of health care? Med Care 1993;50:451–477.

Romano PS, Luft HS. Getting the most out of messy data: problems and approaches for dealing with large administrative data sets. In: Grady ML, Schwartz HA, eds. Medical Effectiveness Research Data Methods. AHCPR Publication No. 92-0056. Rockville, MD: Agency for Health Care Policy and Research; 1992, pp. 57–75.

Romano PS, Luft HS, Rainwater JA, Zach AP. Report on Heart Attack 1991–1993. Vol. Two: Technical Guide. Sacramento: California Office of Statewide Health Planning and Development; 1997.

Romano PS, Mark DH. Bias in the coding of hospital discharge data and its implications for quality assessment. Med Care 1994;32:81–90.

Roos NP, Black CD, Frolich N, Decoster C, Cohen MM, et al. A population-based health information system. Med Care 1995;33(suppl):DS12–DS20.

Roos NP, Shapiro E. A productive experiment with administrative data. Med Care 1995a; 33(suppl):DS7–DS12.

Roos NP, Shapiro E. Using the information system to assess change: the impact of downsizing the acute sector. Med Care 1995b;33(suppl):DS109–DS126.
Roper WL, Winkenwerder W, Hackbarth GM, Krakauer H. Effectiveness in health care: an initiative to evaluate and improve medical practice. N Engl J Med 1988;319:1197–1202.
Rosenbach ML. Access and satisfaction within the disabled Medicare population. Health Care Fin Rev 1995;17(2):147–167.
Schneider DP, Fries BE, Foley WJ, Desmond M, Gormley WJ. Case mix for nursing home payment: Resource Utilization Groups, Version II. Health Care Fin Rev 1988 Dec; Spec No:39–52.
Shaugnessy PW, Crisler KS, Schlenker RE, Arnold AG. Outcomes across the care continuum: home health care. Med Care 1997;35:NS115–NS123.
Shaugnessy PW, Schlenker RE, Hittle DF. Case mix of home health patients under capitated and fee-for-service payment. Health Serv Res 1995;30:79–113.
Simborg DW. DRG creep: a new hospital-acquired disease. N Engl J Med 1981;304:1602–1604.
Soumerai SB, Avorn J, Ross-Degnan D, Gortmaker S. Payment restrictions for prescription drugs under Medicaid. Effects on therapy, cost and equity. N Engl J Med 1987;317:550–556.
Soumerai SB, Ross-Degnan D, Avorn J, McLaughlin TJ, Choodnovskiy I. Effects of Medicaid drug-payment limits on admission to hospitals and nursing homes. N Engl J Med 1991;325:1072–1077.
Stearns SC, Kovar MG, Hayes K, Koch GG. Risk indicators for hospitalization during the last year of life. Health Serv Res 1996;31:49–69.
Stineman MG. Measuring casemix, severity, and complexity in geriatric patients undergoing rehabilitation. Med Care 1997;35:JS90–JS105.
Stineman MG, Escarce JJ, Goin JE, Hamilton BB, Granger CV, Williams SV. A case-mix classification system for medical rehabilitation. Med Care 1994;32:366–379.
Stineman MG, Goin JE, Tassoni CJ, Granger CV, Williams SV. Classifying rehabilitation inpatients by expected functional gain. Med Care 1997;35:JS90–JS105.
Sullivan LW, Wilensky GR. Medicare Hospital Mortality Information 1987, 1988, 1989. Washington, DC: U.S. Department of Health and Human Services, Health Care Financing Administration; 1991.
Swan J, Newcomer R. Residential care supply, nursing home licensing, and case mix in four states. Health Care Fin Rev 2000;21:203–229.
Trude S, Christianson JB, Lesser CS, Watts C, Benoit AM. Employer-sponsored health insurance: pressing problems, incremental changes. Health Aff 2002;21:66–75.
U.S. General Accounting Office. Employers and Individual Consumers Want Additional Information on Quality. GAO/HEHS-95-201. Washington, DC: U.S. General Accounting Office; 1995.
U.S. General Accounting Office. Medical Records Privacy: Access Needed for Health Research, But Oversight of Privacy Protections Is Limited. GAO/HEHS-99-55. Washington, DC: U.S. General Accounting Office; 1999.
U.S. General Accounting Office. Record Linkage and Privacy. Issues in Creating New Federal Research and Statistical Information. GAO-01-126SP. Washington, DC: U.S. General Accounting Office; 2001.
Virnig BA, McBean M. Administrative data for public health surveillance and planning. Annu Rev Pub Health 2001;22:213–229.
Wennberg J, Gittelsohn A. Small area variations in health care delivery. Science 1973;182: 1102–1108.
Williams BC, Li Y, Fries BE, Warren RL. Predicting patient scores between the Functional Independence Measure and the Minimum Data Set: development and performance of a FIM-MDS "Crosswalk." Arch Phys Med Rehabil 1997;78:48–54.
World Health Organization. International Classification of Functioning, Disability and Health. Geneva: World Health Organization; 2001.

CHAPTER 7

Health Statistics from Nonhealth Sources

Walter Phillip Bailey, Amy Brock Martin, Elizabeth H. Corley,
Daniel J. Friedman, and R. Gibson Parrish II

> Many factors influence the health of a population, and to be useful, health statistics must provide a comprehensive and coherent picture of them all. Gathering and presenting data on diseases alone limits understanding of the complex interactions that affect health and encourages concentration on the prevention and management of disease instead of a more broadly integrated approach to maximizing health and reducing illness.
>
> —*Friedman et al. 2002, vii*

Traditional health statistics provide a baseline of information that helps characterize the health of a population or population subgroup. Where health statistics often fall short is in their ability to identify factors that affect population health but fall outside the traditional purview of public health agencies or health care providers. Figure 1.3 identifies a broad range of community and contextual factors that influence a population's health. As illustrated in Table 7.1, this chapter uses the term *complementary data* to refer to data on those factors that affect population health and yet are not generally collected by, or analyzed within, U.S. public health agencies.[1] Examples include data on air and water quality monitoring, transportation, employment, crime, abuse and neglect, tax revenues from the sale of tobacco and alcohol, and housing characteristics.

Understanding variation in access to health care provides an example of the usefulness of complementary data. Traditional sources of data for health statistics, such as hospital discharge data, can reveal geopolitical and demographic variation in preventable hospitalizations. However, these indicators do little to

TABLE 7.1
Data Topics Important for Understanding Influences on Health by Whether They Are Typically Collected by, or Analyzed within, U.S. Public Health Agencies

Data Topics Typically Collected by, or Analyzed within, U.S. Public Health Agencies	*Data Topics* Not *Typically Collected by, or Analyzed within, U.S. Public Health Agencies*
Biological characteristics	Built environment
Disease	Cultural context
Functional status	Economic resources
Health services	Natural environment
Lifestyles and health practices	Political context
Population-based health programs	Social attributes
Well-being	

identify causal or other factors related to variations in access, such as inability to pay for services, household composition, availability of transportation, and environmental factors. Policymakers interested in reducing preventable hospitalizations will be unsatisfied by investigations limited to traditional health statistics data unless those data are supplemented by complementary data that can address causal or related factors. A study conducted by Shi et al. (1999), using South Carolina inpatient hospital discharge data, identified relationships among income, ambulatory care, and inpatient hospitalization rates by linking the latter two to census income characteristics at the zip code level. This study further quantified the cost of potentially avoidable hospitalizations by estimating costs from charges data contained in hospital discharge data sets, supplemented by hospital cost-to-charge ratios found in Medicare cost reports.

This chapter describes the major types of complementary data and presents examples of the use of such data. The examples will give the reader an understanding of the variety of ways in which complementary data can be used. When both traditional health data and complementary data contain sufficient detail to enable linkage, powerful tools for assessing communities, designing and targeting programs, evaluating programs, creating knowledge, and informing the public emerge.

TYPES OF COMPLEMENTARY DATA

The types of complementary data are many and varied. Such data can pertain to individual people, their community, the environment, or the social and political contexts in which they live. National, state, and local governments, as well as private sector and nonprofit programs, gather these data. Table 7.2 categorizes and provides examples of the main types of complementary data and

TABLE 7.2

Major Types of Complementary Data, Typical Approaches for Gathering These Data, and Systems That Gather These Data in the United States at the National and State Levels

Type of Complementary Data	*Typical Approaches for Gathering Complementary Data*	*Examples—Systems That Gather Complementary Data: National Level*	*Examples—Systems That Gather Complementary Data: State Level*
Context			
Natural Environment			
Climate and weather (atmosphere)	Weather monitoring stations; satellite data	National Oceanographic and Atmospheric Administration and National Weather Service data files; private companies	National Oceanographic and Atmospheric Administration and National Weather Service data files; private companies
Air quality; water quality; environmental contaminants	Environmental monitoring systems; sentinel surveys and special studies of vectors	U.S. Environmental Protection Agency: Aerometric Information Retrieval System; STORET	State environmental protection departments; state air quality control boards; state health departments
Geology; topography; vegetative cover; water resources	Land surveys; satellite images; aerial photographs	U.S. Geological Survey; U.S. Department of Agriculture; U.S. Environmental Protection Agency	State geology departments; state agriculture departments; state environmental protection departments
Animal vectors (biosphere)	Field surveys		State health departments; state agriculture departments
Cultural Context			
Norms and values		General Social Survey	
Racism		General Social Survey	

(*continued*)

TABLE 7.2
Continued

Type of Complementary Data	*Typical Approaches for Gathering Complementary Data*	*Examples—Systems That Gather Complementary Data: National Level*	*Examples—Systems That Gather Complementary Data: State Level*
Political Context			
Public policies and laws (social, economic, health, environmental)	Compilations and indexes	Thomas—U.S. Congress on the Internet	National Conference of State Legislatures
Political culture		General Social Survey	
Community Resources			
Built Environment			
Land use (deforestation, farming)	Land surveys; satellite images; aerial photographs; population surveys	U.S. Department of Agriculture; decennial census	State agriculture departments
Urbanization (type, location, and extent); housing		Department of Housing and Urban Development	Decennial census
Workplaces	Surveys of the U.S. population; business and employer surveys; workplace regulatory inspections	Bureau of Labor Statistics; Occupational Safety and Health Administration; Mine Safety and Health Administration; Census Bureau	Current Population Survey; County Business Patterns; Census of Industrial Sectors; Census of Agriculture; state labor departments

Transportation infrastructure	Land surveys; satellite images; aerial photographs	U.S. Department of Transportation	State transportation departments
Communication infrastructure (access to health information)	Surveys of population; government regulatory activities; mandated reporting by private organizations	Federal Communications Commission; Census Bureau; private telecommunication companies	Private telecommunication companies
Economic Context			
Economic development and equity (e.g., income distribution, employment, access to material resources)	Population surveys; national financial records; World Bank	Department of Commerce; Department of Labor, Bureau of Labor Statistics	State economic development departments
Work environment	Population surveys; business and employer surveys; workplace regulatory inspections	Bureau of Labor Statistics; Occupational Safety and Health Administration; Mine Safety and Health Administration; Census Bureau; National Council on Compensation; National Agricultural Workers Survey	Current Population Survey; County Business Patterns; Census of Industrial Sectors; Census of Agriculture; state labor departments

their sources in the United States. While many of the sources are maintained by federal or state government agencies, they sometimes do not provide the geopolitical specificity needed to understand population health at substate, regional, or community levels.

Untapped resources exist in data systems used to administer and manage government programs, especially at the state level. Virtually all areas of human services can provide data that support a better understanding of population health. Table 7.3 delineates some sources of health services data not commonly used by public health agencies and sources of complementary data typically available at the state level, and provides examples of the types of information that these sources can add to characterize influences on health.

THE POTENTIAL FOR USING COMPLEMENTARY DATA SOURCES

Delving More Deeply into Health Issues

The value of using complementary data to elucidate community and contextual attributes influencing population health often arises from comparative analysis or from delving more deeply into a known health issue. For example, one state may compare itself with others relative to infant mortality based on data from national sources. Identifying factors that stand out in a state with a high infant mortality rate, such as level of poverty, household structure, Medicaid penetration, percentage of primary and specialty care physicians accepting Medicaid reimbursement, use of family planning services, and parental demographic characteristics will result from gathering data from several sources. These complementary data will not identify the etiology of infant mortality in the particular state, but they can more fully reveal the context of high infant mortality and uncover associated factors that could be addressed by state policymakers. For example, in South Carolina's Pee Dee Healthy Start project, locations of the residence of mothers of infants who died in the first year of life were geocoded using a geographic information system (GIS) tool and mapped at the census block level. Two demographically and economically similar census blocks with different infant mortality experience were identified. After these results were presented to a local coalition, coalition members canvassed the local areas in an effort to determine differences (Bailey 1996). Their findings of differences in faith-based resources and in social culture yielded contextual knowledge for shaping proposed interventions.

Linkage and Geographic Information Systems

As more fully explained by Black and Roos in Chapter 9, data linkage occurs when two or more data records are combined. Complementary data containing iden-

TABLE 7.3

Sources of State-Level Health Services Data Not Commonly Used by Public Health Agencies, Sources of State-Level Complementary Data, and Examples of the Types of Information That These Sources Can Add to Characterize Influences on Health

Data Type	*Specific Source*	*Examples of Information Obtained from Data Source*
Health Care and Health Resources	Ambulance records	Emergency services provided prior to arrival at hospital, including run times, destination, and trauma severity
	Licensed health professions databases (state licensing boards)	Number of practicing health-care providers by location, type of practice, specialty, setting, educational background, and hours worked; annual rates of change of health-care providers by reason
	Annual hospital financial data (state surveys and Medicare cost reports)	Charity care, expenses by type, cost-to-charge ratios by department
	Federally qualified health centers, community health centers, and free clinics	Client information, such as diagnosis and services used for individuals using government-sponsored and free clinics
	Vocational rehabilitation	Disability determination, vocational training, employment for children and adults with special health-care needs
	Mental health	Number and characteristics of clients receiving inpatient and outpatient state mental health services by diagnosis and type of service
	Elder programs, including community long-term care	Number and characteristics of clients with meals delivered to their place of residence ("Meals on Wheels") or receiving assistance with transportation, respite care, or other alternatives to skilled nursing care
	Substance abuse services	Client information on individuals receiving treatment for substance abuse or addiction
Social Services	Child care reimbursement programs	Number and characteristics of clients receiving assistance by type of child care
	Temporary Assistance to Needy Families (TANF) and supporting data systems on work history and wages	Number and characteristics of clients who are on welfare and their time limit for receiving welfare; information on current employment, barriers to employment, and participation in training programs, as well as availability of a personal automobile for transportation

(*continued*)

TABLE 7.3
Continued

Data Type	*Specific Source*	*Examples of Information Obtained from Data Source*
	Food stamps	Number and characteristics of clients who receive food stamps, including information on their income level and household structure
	Foster care	Number and characteristics of children who are in the foster care system
	Child protective services	Number and characteristics of children who are confirmed cases of abuse and/or neglect, by abuse type
	Adult protective services	Number and characteristics of adults who are "founded" cases of abuse and/or neglect, by abuse type
	Child support system	Information on the children affected, as well as the adults, in a family where child support is a source of income
Public Safety	Motor vehicle crash data systems and driver citations	Time and location of crash, road conditions, use of restraint by driver and occupant, severity of crash, probable cause
Criminal Justice	Juvenile justice	Referrals to the juvenile justice system, including prior offense(s) and type of offense, as well as related information on family, truancy rates, and education
	Criminal history file and crime incident reports	Criminal histories for criminal justice offenders; type, date and location of previous crimes
Education	Public education files, kindergarten through grade 12	Demographic information, participation in free and reduced-cost lunch programs, achievement test scores, first-grade readiness, graduation rates, educational handicaps, alternative school participation, individual education plans

tifiers can be linked to other complementary or health data containing the same identifying variables. Linkage and subsequent analysis can occur in three ways. First, data can be linked at the individual person level, either linking data about the person from two or more different data sets or linking data about the same person at different points in time from within the same data set (Armstrong and Kricker 1999). For example, the Western Australia Road Injury Database links traditional health statistics data sources such as death records and hospital discharge records with such complementary data as drunk driving arrests and police crash reports (Rosman 1996, 2001; Rosman et al. 2001).

When complementary data contain some form of addresses, GIS tools enable each address to be assigned numeric codes that identify census tracts, census block groups and blocks, or even specific latitude and longitude. This geocoding then enables a second form of linkage: linking individual person records to records pertaining to the person's geographical or geopolitical area. Typical examples of the use of complementary data for linking individual person data to geopolitical-level data have been in studies of the relationship between income and infant outcomes. In the United States, birth certificates contain data on low birth weight, congenital anomalies, and other infant outcomes but have no directly measured data on parental income. Studies relating birth outcomes to parental income have typically geocoded parental residential addresses to census tracts and then linked complementary data from the U.S. Census on census tract level median household income to birth certificate data (Fang et al. 1999; Gould and LeRoy 1988; Pearl et al. 2001; Wegner et al. 2001). Stated simplistically, these studies have generally indicated that mothers living in lower-income neighborhoods are more likely to deliver low birth weight infants than mothers living in higher-income neighborhoods.

A third form of linkage, also enabled by geocoded addresses or some form of location identifiers, entails linking data at a geographical or geopolitical level to other data at that same level. These data could be aggregated from individual person data to the geographic level, or the data could exist only at that geographic level. Interesting examples of linkage at a geopolitical level using complementary data aggregated from the individual person level involve investigations of the relationship between income inequality, social capital, crime, and mortality in U.S. states. One group of researchers linked complementary data on interpersonal trust and civic engagement from the National Opinion Research Center's General Social Survey to data on income inequality (from the U.S. Census), mortality (from death certificates), and crime (from the Federal Bureau of Investigation and the U.S. Department of Justice's Uniform Crime Reports) (Kawachi and Kennedy 1997; Kawachi et al. 1997; Kennedy et al. 1998; Wilkinson et al. 1998). Although the original General Social Survey, mortality, and crime data were all initially collected at the individual person and event levels, the researchers aggregated these data to the state level and then linked them. These investigations revealed relationships between greater state-level income inequality and less social capital, on the one hand, and higher mortality and crime, on the other hand.

In addition, GIS tools enable the spatial display of statistical indicators, incorporating complementary data (Lee and Irving 1999). A traditional example of this type of display incorporates the mapping of air quality or water quality with a specific health condition through either dot or choropleth maps (Cromley and McLafferty 2002; McLafferty and Cromley 1999; Melnick 2002). Using complementary data on all waterborne disease outbreaks from 1948 to 1994 from the U.S. Environmental Protection Agency's Office of Research and Development, on U.S. watersheds from the U.S. Geological Survey, and on precipitation from the National Climactic Data Center, researchers created a dot map of the United States to display the relationship between extreme precipitation and waterborne disease outbreaks in U.S. watersheds (Curriero et al. 2001). Choropleth maps, which are segmented by subareas, such as neighborhoods, census tracts, or zip codes, with the subareas then given varying colors or patterns to depict different levels of variables, are especially attractive if used appropriately. Choropleth maps are also useful in "overlaying" two or more variables to visually demonstrate relationships, as well as in overlaying locations of health-care providers, waste sites, and so forth on represented health outcome data. For example, North Carolina officials used choropleth maps to demonstrate the relationship between poverty status and the location of family day-care providers in substate areas (Hanchette 1999).

Defining Subpopulations

A powerful use of linkage is in defining subpopulations, such as the *safety net population*, and then identifying subpopulation characteristics. In South Carolina, Medicaid, food stamps, school free and reduced-cost lunch data, and uninsured emergency room visit files were linked and deduplicated, which enabled state policymakers to determine the size and geographic locations of poor subpopulations dependent on government programs and solutions. One use of this information was in the state's efforts to locate children eligible for enrollment in the State Children's Health Insurance Program (SCHIP), the expanded Medicaid program covering children up to 150% of the poverty level, in partnership with the Robert Wood Johnson Foundation's "Covering Kids" program (Covering Kids & Families [hp]).

Comparing Subpopulations

Traditional health statistics data can provide the ability to compare subpopulations on common indicators such as age, race, and sex. Because of the confounding factor of poverty, conclusions about population health drawn from data stratified only by age, race, and sex can be misleading. Complementary data can further define the characteristics of subpopulations. Using the safety net example above, linking Medicaid enrollment data to population-based data such as hospital discharges or birth certificates enables analysis of hospital use and birth outcomes by poverty status as well as by age and race. This adds a new dimension to our understanding of the relationships of age or race and poverty. For example, researchers have linked North Carolina Medicaid enrollment data, Medicaid paid claims data, and Women, Infants, and Children (WIC) data to birth certificate data to measure the use of health services by race for children enrolled in Medicaid (Buescher et al. 2003). After controlling for numerous factors that affect use of health-care services, most of which were obtained from birth certificates, the researchers found that African-American children enrolled in Medicaid used fewer services than white children enrolled in Medicaid.

USES OF COMPLEMENTARY DATA

Complementary data can be used for multiple purposes in public health. This section illustrates uses of complementary data for six different purposes: monitoring health status and outcomes; assessing community health; designing public health programs and targeting interventions; evaluating programs; creating knowledge; and informing the public. Chapter 12 provides fuller explanations of five of these purposes, and Chapter 10 provides a fuller explanation of using health statistics to create knowledge.

Monitoring Health Status and Outcomes

Largely through the leadership of the World Health Organization (WHO), ongoing international and national efforts to monitor health status and outcomes have focused increasingly on a broad range of factors that may influence population health. This breadth has resulted from the WHO definition of health as "a state of complete physical, mental, and social well-being, and not merely the absence of disease or infirmity" (World Health Organization [hp] Constitution of the World Health Organization 1946). The World Health Organization has emphasized that health is affected not only by health programs and health services, but also by a wide variety of other community and contextual influences. Some of these influences are represented in Figure 1.3.

The growing acceptance of a broad conceptualization of population health has led to the use of indicators for monitoring health status and outcomes that reflect the wide variety of influences on population health. Just as the influences on population health extend far beyond the factors traditionally included within the purview of health statistics, the complementary data needed to monitor those influences extend well beyond those data traditionally used in health statistics. The health statistics armamentarium of registries and notifiable diseases and conditions, health surveys, and administrative health data are insufficient to monitor many influences on the health of populations, including community attributes such as the built environment (e.g., housing, workplaces, schools, transportation), economic resources, and contextual attributes such as the political context and the natural environment.

At the international level, the Conference Board of Canada's *Performance and Potential 2003–2004* benchmarks Canada's performance against the 12 top-performing Organisation for Economic Co-operation and Development (OECD) countries in six domains: health, economy, innovation, environment, education and skills, and society (Barrett et al. 2003). The Conference Board's health domain includes multiple measured determinants of health, including income and social status, social support networks, education, employment/working conditions, social environments, physical environments, personal health practices and coping skills, healthy child development, and health services prevention and treatment, as well as the unmeasured domains of biology and genetic environment, gender, and culture. Measured determinants include indicators drawn from a wide variety of complementary data sources. For example, the social environments determinant is measured by three indicators: corruption perceptions index, people victimized by property crime, and people victimized by assaults and threats. The social supports networks determinant is also measured by three indicators: group membership, net social expenditures as a percentage of gross domestic product, and divorces per 100 marriages.

In addition to their use in monitoring population health and its determinants, complementary data are used in monitoring social health. Social health can be conceptualized as one aspect of population health or as an influence on population health. Social indicator reports have been published in a wide variety of nations, as well as internationally (Miringoff and Miringoff 1999; Noll 1996). A good example of national social health reports is New Zealand's *Social Health Report*, which includes such domains as health; knowledge and skills; safety and security; paid work; civil, political, and human rights; culture and identity; economic standard of living; social connectedness; and environment (Ministry of Social Development 2002). As with *Promise and Performance 2003–2004*, each domain in the New Zealand report is measured by multiple indicators relying heavily upon complementary data. For example, the social connectedness domain includes such indicators as telephone and Internet access in the home, participation in family activities and regular contact with family/friends, membership and involvement in groups, and unpaid work outside the home.

Assessing Community Health

Complementary data are useful for conducting needs assessments and defining policy issues. Table 7.4 provides examples of indicators not routinely used in health statistics, which are useful for needs assessments. Because of the categorical nature of many complementary data sets, indicators in Table 7.4 often can be

TABLE 7.4
Examples of Indicators Useful for Conducting Needs Assessments That Are Available from Complementary Data Sets

Health and other service use	Doctor's office visit rates and reasons, emergency room visit rates and reasons, prescription drug use rates, cost of health care by type of care, mental health service use and rates by type, type of specialist used in care, EPDST visits, and number and percentage of clients using multiple agencies' services
Education	Four-year-old kindergarten attendance, school readiness, test scores, number and rate of children in alternative schools, percentage of students with individual education plans; Head Start participation, school readiness programs
Home and family life	Household structure, availability of child care by type, marriage and divorce rates, abuse and neglect rates by type, rates of children in foster care, free and reduced-cost lunch rates, information on family resources, housing or rental costs, transportation availability, educational levels
Quality-of-life indicators	Children with special health-care needs by type, disability rates by type, accident and injury rates by type, fire injuries; death rates by type, disparity analyses, urban–rural comparisons, prevalence of health conditions, vocational rehabilitation rates, air and water quality

EPDST = Early and Periodic Screening, Diagnosis, and Treatment.

applied to specific populations of interest, whether they are demographic, geographic, program-specific, or disease-specific.

Just as population health concepts have led to the extensive use of complementary data sources in national and international reports that measure health status and outcomes, they have also led to the extensive use of complementary data sources in local community health assessments. An excellent example is the *Local Basket of Inequality Indicators* published by the London Health Observatory in conjunction with the Association of Public Health Observatories and the Health Development Agency within the National Health Service (Fitzpatrick and Jacobson 2003). The *Local Basket of Inequality Indicators* was developed in response to recommendations included in the Department of Health's report *Tackling Health Inequalities: A Programme for Action*, which called for actions to be taken across a broad spectrum of government departments and for "local health organizations . . . to make tackling health inequalities a central part of achieving their nationally set targets and standards of care" (Department of Health 2003, 31). The local basket of inequalities indicators includes such domains as health and mental health, as well as employment, poverty, and deprivation; housing and homelessness; education; crime; pollution and the physical environment; and community development. As with the reports cited earlier, these indicators derive from complementary data sources, including the Annual Local Area Labour Force Survey, the Land Registry/New Earnings Survey, national curriculum assessment tests, and notifiable offenses recorded by police.

Another example of the use of complementary data for community assessment is *The Wisdom of Our Choices: Boston's Indicators of Progress, Change and Sustainability 2000* (Boston Foundation 2000). This community assessment includes a public health domain, as well as civic health, cultural life and the arts, economy, education, environment, housing, public safety, technology, and transportation domains. As an example, the civic involvement domain includes indicators of volunteer activity in the Read Boston program, percentage of youth who feel connected to the community, charitable donations by neighborhood, voter participation, stability and investment within neighborhoods, and others. Although *The Wisdom of Our Choices* is not explicitly built around a population health model, its domains fit well within the model of the influences on population health presented in Chapter 1. The emphasis in *The Wisdom of Our Choices* on using complementary data to develop asset-based measures to identify the strengths of Boston neighborhoods is fully consistent with the WHO Healthy Cities measurement approach cited in Chapter 12 (Doyle et al. 1997).

Designing Public Health Programs and Targeting Interventions

Complementary data can be crucial in designing public health programs and targeting interventions. One typical example of the use of complementary data is a Jefferson County, Kentucky, study focusing on the relationships among pediatric blood lead levels, on the one hand, and housing value and age, on the other hand (Kim et al. 2002). This study combined county lead screening registry data with housing value and age data from a county tax assessor database. Results indicated that children living in lower-valued houses are at greater risk of lead poisoning, pointing to the importance of targeting deleading and lead poisoning screening programs based both on housing valuation and on housing age.

Another example of the potential use of complementary data to target interventions is a study of the relationship between food store location and dietary intake in Maryland, North Carolina, Mississippi, and Minnesota (Morland et al. 2002). The study obtained data from local health departments and state departments of agriculture on the number and types of food stores and food service places by census tract. Data on dietary intake were obtained from participants in the Atherosclerosis Risk in Communities study. Results indicated that African Americans living in census tracts with supermarkets and full-service restaurants had healthier diets. These results point to the need for targeting interventions for increasing adherence to dietary guidelines in census tracts with high proportions of African Americans and few supermarkets and restaurants.

Evaluating Programs

A wide variety of public policies and programs are intended to improve the population's health, focusing on diverse proximate and more distal influences on population health. In evaluating policies and programs, it is often necessary to move beyond traditional health statistics data. Excellent examples of program evaluation using complementary data can be found in tobacco control programs. Meier and Licari (1997), focusing on states as the unit of analysis, conducted a time series analysis of the relationship between state excise taxes on cigarettes and cigarette consumption. Data on the number of cigarette packs per capita consumed annually in each state and on state cigarette excise taxes were derived from the Tobacco Institute's annual historical compilation. Meier and Licari's evaluation revealed that increases in cigarette excise taxes were associated with decreased cigarette consumption.

Another example of tobacco control program evaluation using complementary data focuses on the impact of the Massachusetts Tobacco Control Program (MTCP) funding of local boards of health on the enactment of local tobacco control policies (Bartosch and Pope 2002). Data on local tobacco control policies were obtained from multiple complementary data sources, including a Massachusetts Association of Health Boards survey, an MTCP ordinance database, and review of local policy documents. This evaluation demonstrated a relationship between MTCP funding and passage of local tobacco control policies and ordinances, such as youth access policies and environmental tobacco smoke policies.

Evaluations of automobile injury prevention programs also provide interesting examples of the use of complementary data for evaluating programs. Employing National Automotive Sampling System Crashworthiness Data System data from 1993 to 1996, an evaluation revealed that air bag deployment in frontal crashes reduced the probability of fatal and near-fatal injuries, while air bag deployment in less severe crashes actually increased the probability of injuries, especially for women (Segui-Gomez 2000). Another example of the use of complementary data to evaluate automobile injury prevention programs is a study of the impact of a California red light camera law, which enabled cities to implement local red light camera enforcement programs by installing cameras at traffic lights to identify automobiles running red lights (Retting and Kyrychenko 2002). Using data from the California Statewide Integrated Traffic Records System, this evaluation compared crash data for 29 months before and for 29 months after red light camera implementation in Oxnard and three control cities. Results indicated that greater reductions in injury crashes occurred in Oxnard compared to the control cities, and that the Oxnard reductions occurred throughout the city and not only at those intersections with cameras installed.

Creating Knowledge

Complementary data can also be used to create basic knowledge about population health and the influences on population health, with studies of the relationship between the environment and population health providing excellent examples. Several investigations have related air pollution data to hospital discharges. Combining hospital discharge data from the New South Wales Health Department's inpatient statistics database with New South Wales Environment Protection Authority daily air pollution data on levels of ozone, nitrogen dioxide, and particulates from 1990 to 1994, one study revealed that increased air pollution in Sydney, Australia, was associated with increased hospital admissions for asthma, heart disease, and chronic obstructive pulmonary disease (Morgan et al. 1998). Another study employed air pollution measurements by Helsinki municipal district authorities and data from a registry of all illnesses requiring hospitalization, finding that hospital admissions for cardiac and cerebrovascular diseases were related to specific types of air pollution, sometimes at lower levels than specified in WHO guidelines (Ponka and Virtanen 1996). Other researchers combined blood pressure data obtained during a WHO survey in Augsburg, Germany, with air pollution data from the Bavarian Air Quality Network, finding increases in blood pressure associated with temporary increases in air pollution (Ibald-Mulli et al. 2001).

Informing the Public

Complementary data can be used to inform the public about population health through a variety of mechanisms. As indicated in Chapter 12, several international, national, and subnational Web sites focusing on population health now provide free public interactive access to multiple types of traditional health statistics and complementary data (ORC Macro 2000). In the United States, these interactive Web sites include such complementary data sets as food stamps, WIC enrollment, unemployment compensation, the Crash Outcome Data Evaluation System, and numerous social programs. Community assessment reports, discussed earlier in this chapter as well as in Chapter 12, often provide the public with access to complementary data in easily understandable formats. Franklin County, Maine's, community assessment report contains social capital/environment as a domain, with indicators relating to youth mentoring and volunteer programs, neighborhood attachment, and environmental risks affecting social capital (Healthy Community Coalition 2003). San Antonio, Texas's, community assessment contains an environment domain with zip code and census tract level maps and tables, including such indicators as air quality health alert days, heat/cold exposure-related illness emergency medical service calls, and estimated extent of chlorinated solvents in groundwater (San Antonio Metropolitan Health District 2001). Reports in the popular media focusing on local health status and outcomes also often use complementary data sources as well as more traditional health statistics data. For example, *Boston Magazine*'s article "The Healthiest Towns" supplemented traditional health statistics data such as breast and other cancer incidence rates with complementary data on per pupil spending, public safety spending per capita, liquor licenses, population density, smoking bans, and presence of health clubs (Blanding 2003).

CASE STUDY: LESSONS FROM SOUTH CAROLINA IN USING COMPLEMENTARY DATA SETS

Complementary data allow the researcher to reach beyond traditional scopes of inquiry. Complementary data, especially when linked and integrated with other data sets, can portray events across a fuller range of factors that influence population health. Complementary data, again when linked and integrated, can also portray health across the life span, enabling longitudinal analyses of the delivery and impact of health and human services. It is even possible to follow a cohort from birth to death and the life events in between. The challenge is educating a community of public health practitioners and researchers to think in such broad, comprehensive ways. Having the technology and data is only half of the equation; public health practitioners and researchers with conceptual skills and commitment to new analytic processes are needed to complete it.

The South Carolina experience has demonstrated that one successful method of maximizing the use of complementary data is the formation of an organization dedicated to bringing data together from the multiple sources described in this chapter. For decades, South Carolina has invested in sharing complementary data and building an integrated data system based upon these data. The South Carolina model represents a comprehensive integration of traditional health data sets (inpatient hospital discharge, emergency room visits, ambulatory surgery, home health visits), state agency health and human services administrative data sets (such as Medicaid claims, clients served, and services received by clients of a multitude of state agencies), census data, and health resources data sets. For a full description, the reader should refer to Table 7.3. Data sets that are maintained at the individual person level are fully linkable at the individual level, while other data sets, such as census data and health facilities data, may be linked with individual level data sets at aggregate levels. These data and the resulting integrated data system are housed in a neutral agency, the Office of Research and Statistics (ORS). Based upon the South Carolina experience, several guidelines in developing the capacity to use complementary data follow.

Organizational Structure

A sound organizational structure is essential. Locating analyses of complementary data and any associated integrated data systems in a neutral organization may allow data to be used in a noncompetitive and apolitical environment. A neutral organization—whether governmental, quasi-governmental, or nongovernmental—further allows for the development of analytic partnerships with government agencies and researchers by placing data experts on analytic and research project teams.

Tips for Fostering Partnerships

- *Develop expertise in dealing with complementary data sets by establishing key agency contacts.* No one knows the data better than the programmatic personnel who work with the data sources on a daily basis. It is important that those working with complementary data maintain an ongoing relationship with key agency data staff.
- *Understand the complexities surrounding complementary data sources.* It is not enough to understand the complementary data that agencies and organizations produce. It is equally important to understand the policies and data use practices of each contributing organization. This knowledge will enrich the analyst's ability to fully use complementary data and to avoid the unknowing misuse of data because of a lack of understanding.
- *Build trust.* Depending on the environment, one of the most challenging components of sharing complementary data is establishing trust among the various data sources. Data can personify power to many, and sharing data in a hostile environment can create resistance among potential data partners. For example, decades of building trusting relationships with data partners have resulted, for South Carolina, in an integrated data organization that houses data from virtually every state agency, the private health care sector, many not-for-profit organizations, and medical clinics.

Principles for Building Trust

The following eight principles can serve well for building the trust necessary for sharing complementary data.

1. Secure support for data sharing and linkage first. Do not attempt to work out all the issues at the beginning.
2. Do not try to replace existing agency functions.
3. Do not duplicate or compete with agency statistical offices.
4. Treat all contributing organizations equally.

5. Tread carefully around political issues.
6. Make the extraction process as nonintrusive as possible.
7. Before dealing at the executive level, gain support from statistical and information system offices.
8. Put it in writing. Execute memoranda of understanding and agreements establishing rules of data sharing and assuring agency control. Nothing demonstrates trust more than a written commitment. The partners should retain control over their own data and should provide direction on what types of linkages should occur. Putting these commitments in writing ensures trust.

Supporting Legislation

The South Carolina ORS has been supported by state legislation that has two intents: first, to put decisions about data release in the hands of appropriate stakeholders, enabling ORS to maintain its neutral position; and second, to ensure that any shared individual person data are treated with the utmost confidentiality and privacy.

The original legislation (S.C. Code of Laws, Section 44-6-170, 1993 and subsequent amendments) addressed only private health-care sector data and established the South Carolina Data Oversight Council, composed of representatives from the private sector (hospitals, physicians, and nursing homes), the public sector (governor's office, health department, health and human services department), third-party payers, and the business community. Release of the private health-care sector data occurs at the Council's direction. This policy reinforces the guideline of treating all participating organizations equally.

Second, a legislative proviso (S.C. Code of Laws, Proviso 72.21, 2002) was passed in 2002 that solidified data sharing among South Carolina's state agencies. Key requirements of the proviso include the following: Agencies collect and provide client data to the ORS as a neutral organization, and ORS establishes a memorandum of understanding with each agency that specifies all procedures relating to maintaining confidentiality, including data release. Agencies retain ownership of their data. No data are released by ORS without the express permission of the agency contributing the data. The key linker system, which deidentifies individuals, fosters adherence to all federal and state laws and regulations pertaining to confidentiality and privacy.

A third legislative thrust is a statutory environment that facilitates the sharing of data with selected programs. South Carolina laws permit the sharing of data, with identifiers, from the integrated system with selected disease registries. The sharing of integrated data for this purpose ensures more accurate registries and ultimately strengthens the services provided to individuals with these conditions. This also makes possible opportunities for expanded research, such as identifying a cohort of individuals diagnosed with cancer in order to ascertain pharmaceutical use or local air quality.

NOTE

1. Although we use the term *complementary* to refer to data not generally collected by, or analyzed within, U.S. public health agencies, other terms such as *alternative*, *nontraditional*, and *intersectoral* also describe these data. The WHO uses *intersectoral* to refer to the interaction of the health and nonhealth sectors to promote health (Kreisel and von Schirnding 1998).

REFERENCES

Armstrong BK, Kricker A. Record linkage—a vision renewed. Aust NZ J Public Health 1999;23(5):451–452.

Bailey WP. The Pee Dee Healthy Start MIS. Presentation to the Williamsburg County Healthy Start Coalition; September 1996.

Barrett C, Bussiere L, Darby P, Lafleur B, MacDuff D, Vail S. Performance and Potential 2003–2004. Ottawa: Conference Board of Canada; 2003.

Bartosch WJ, Pope GC. Local enactment of tobacco control policies in Massachusetts. Am J Public Health 2002;92(6):941–943.

Blanding M. The healthiest towns. Boston Magazine. April 2003; 78–85.

Boston Foundation. The Wisdom of Our Choices: Boston's Indicators of Progress, Change and Sustainability 2000. Boston: The Boston Foundation; 2000.

Buescher PA, Horton SJ, Devaney BL, Roholt SJ, Lenihan AJ, Whitmire JT, Kotch JB. Differences in use of health services between White and African American children enrolled in Medicaid in North Carolina. Matern Child Health J 2003;7(1):45–52.

Covering Kids & Families [homepage on the Internet]. Columbia, SC: Covering Kids and Families National Program Office [updated 2003; cited 2004 Mar 10]. Covering Kids and Families. Available from: http://coveringkidsandfamilies.org/about.

Cromley EK, McLafferty SL. GIS and Public Health. New York: Guilford Press; 2002.

Curriero FC, Patz JA, Rose JB, Lele S. The association between extreme precipitation and waterborne disease outbreaks in the United States, 1948–1994. Am J Public Health 2001;91(8):1194–1199.

Department of Health. Tackling Health Inequalities: A Programme for Action. London: Department of Health; July 2003.

Doyle Y, Brunning D, Cryer C, Hedley S, Hodgson CR. Healthy Cities Indicators: Analysis of Data from Cities Across Europe. Copenhagen: World Health Organization, Regional Office for Europe; 1997.

Fang J, Madhavan S, Alderman MH. Low birth weight: race and maternal nativity—impact of community income. Pediatrics 1999;103(1):E5.

Fitzpatrick J, Jacobson B. Local Basket of Inequalities Indicators. London: London Health Observatory; October 2003.

Friedman DJ, Hunter EL, Parrish RG, eds. Shaping a Health Statistics Vision for the 21st Century. Final report, November 2002. Hyattsville, MD: Centers for Disease Control and Prevention, National Center for Health Statistics; Washington, DC: U.S. Department of Health and Human Services Data Council, National Committee on Vital and Health Statistics; 2002.

Gould JB, LeRoy S. Socioeconomic status and low birth weight: a racial comparison. Pediatrics 1988;82(6):896–904.

Hanchette CL. GIS and decision making for public health agencies: childhood lead poisoning and welfare reform. J Public Health Manag Pract 1999;5(4):41–47.

Healthy Community Coalition. Community Health Assessment and Visioning 2003. Wilton, ME: Healthy Community Coalition; 2003.

Ibald-Mulli A, Stieber J, Wichmann H-E, Koenig W, Peters A. Effects of air pollution on blood pressure: a population-based approach. Am J Public Health 2001;91(4):571–577.

Kawachi I, Kennedy BP. Health and social cohesion: why care about income inequality? Br Med J 1997;314:1037–1040.

Kawachi I, Kennedy BP, Lochner K, Prothrow-Stith D. Social capital, income inequality, and mortality. Am J Public Health 1997;87(9):1491–1498.

Kennedy BP, Kawachi I, Prothrow-Stith D, Lochner K, Gupta V. Social capital, income inequality, and firearm violent crime. Soc Sci Med 1998;47(10):7–17.

Kim DY, Staley F, Curtis G, Buchanan S. Relation between housing age, housing value, and childhood blood lead levels in children in Jefferson County, KY. Am J Public Health 2002;92(5):769–770.

Kreisel W, von Schirnding Y. Intersectoral action for health: a cornerstone for health for all in the 21st century. World Health Stat Q 1998;51(1):75–78.

Lee CV, Irving JL. Sources of spatial data for community heath planning. J Public Health Manag Pract 1999;5(4):7–33.

McLafferty S, Cromley EK. Your first mapping project on your own: from A to Z. J Public Health Manag Pract 1999;5(2):76–82.

Meier KJ, Licari MJ. The effect of cigarette taxes on cigarette consumption, 1955 through 1994. Am J Public Health 1997;87(7):1126–1130.

Melnick AL. Introduction to geographic information systems in public health. Gaithersburg, MD: Aspen, 2002.

Ministry of Social Development. The Social Health Report 2002. Auckland, NZ: Ministry of Social Development; 2002.

Miringoff M, Miringoff M-L. The Social Health of the Nation: How America Is Really Doing. New York: Oxford University Press; 1999.

Morgan G, Corbett S, Wlodarczyk J. Air pollution and hospital admissions in Sydney, Australia, 1990 to 1994. Am J Public Health 1998;88(12):1761–1766.

Morland K, Wing S, Diez-Roux A. The contextual effect of the local food environment on residents' diets: the Atherosclerosis Risk in Communities study. Am J Public Health 2002;92(11):1761–1767.

Noll H. Social indicators reporting: the international experience. Presentation to the Symposium on Measuring Well-being and Social Indicators, Oct. 4, 1996. Ottawa: Canadian Council on Social Development; 1996.

ORC Macro. Evaluation of State-Based Integrated Health Information Systems: Summary of Abstracts. Atlanta: ORC Macro; 2000.

Pearl M, Braveman P, Abrams B. The relationship of neighborhood socioeconomic characteristics to birth weight among 5 ethnic groups in California. Am J Public Health 2001; 91(11):1783–1789.

Ponka A, Virtanen M. Low-level air pollution and hospital admissions for cardiac and cerebrovascular diseases in Helsinki. Am J Public Health 1996;86(9):1273–1280.

Retting RA, Kyrychenko SY. Reductions in injury crashes associated with red light enforcement in Oxnard, California. Am J Public Health 2002;92(11):1822–1825.

Rosman DL. The feasibility of linking hospital and police road crash casualty records without names. Accid Anal Prev 1996;28(2):271–274.

Rosman DL. The Western Australia road injury database (1987–1996): ten years of linked police, hospital and death records of road crashes and injuries. Accid Anal Prev 2001; 33(1):81–88.

Rosman DL, Ferrante AM, Marom Y. A linkage study of Western Australia drink driving arrests and road crash records. Accid Anal Prev 2001;33(2):211–220.

San Antonio Metropolitan Health District. Health Profile 2001. San Antonio, TX: San Antonio Metropolitan Health District; 2001.

Segui-Gomez M. Driver air bag effectiveness by severity of the crash. Am J Public Health 2000;90(10):1575–1581.

Shi L, Samuels ME, Pease M, Bailey WP, Corley EH. Patient characteristics associated with hospitalizations for ambulatory care sensitive conditions in South Carolina. South Med J 1999;92(10):989–998.

Wegner EL, Loos GP, Onaka AT, Crowell D, Li Y, Zheng H. Changes in the association of low birth weight with socioeconomic status in Hawaii: 1970–1990. Soc Biol 2001;48(3–4):196–211.

Wilkinson RG, Kawachi I, Kennedy BP. Mortality, the social environment, crime, and violence. Sociol Health Illn 1998;20(5):578–597.

World Health Organization [homepage on the Internet]. Geneva: World Health Organization [cited 2004 Mar 11]. Constitution of the World Health Organization, 1946. Available from: http://whqlibdoc.who.int/hist/official_records/constitution.pdf.

CHAPTER 8

Standards and Their Use in Health Statistics

Marjorie S. Greenberg and R. Gibson Parrish II

We use standards every day to carry out a multitude of tasks efficiently. A carpenter could not function without standards of measurement (e.g., feet, inches, and meters), and trade would be stymied without standards of monetary exchange (e.g., the dollar and the euro). Similarly, widely accepted standards facilitate the efficient operation of the health statistics enterprise and the health information systems that it relies upon. Standards are the common language that allows the exchange of data between disparate data systems, the comparison of data contained in different systems, and the presentation of data in ways that can be understood and used. Standards are one of the fundamental building blocks of effective health information systems that are the source of health statistics. When producers of health information use common standards for collecting, classifying, and displaying data, data can be compared and combined to examine trends, tease out causal relations, and evaluate programs.

At the same time, developing and ensuring the use of widely agreed-upon standards can be time-consuming and difficult. Frequently organizations develop their own standards for collecting or exchanging information without reference to broader national or international standards. This may be due to lack of knowledge, to inadequacy of current standards, or to unwillingness to invest the effort required to achieve consensus across organizations, states, and even countries. In these circumstances, the health statistics enterprise faces a multiplicity of standards without agreement on which should be used. If data are to become more comparable and interchangeable, a process of education, communication, and negotiation is needed so that agreement can be reached on migration toward more common standards. The challenge is for people in the health statistics enterprise to understand and appreciate the importance of standards and the processes for defining, changing, and adopting them, including the identification of new standards that are needed to facilitate the work of the health statistics enterprise.

In this chapter we first discuss briefly the history of standards, their definition, and the classification of their purposes and types.[1] Then we describe the types of standards used by the health statistics enterprise and the process for developing national standards. In this context, we provide numerous examples of standards in current use.

HISTORY OF STANDARDS

One of the earliest known standards was the use of cylindrical stones as units of weight in Egypt in 7000 B.C. (Breitenberg 1987). An early attempt to establish a standard in the Western world occurred in 1120 A.D. when King Henry I of England ordered that the ell, the ancient yard, be used as the standard unit of length throughout his kingdom. The ell, which is now 45 inches, was originally derived from the length of King Henry's arm. The specification of standardized materials, dimensions, and routines (i.e., processes) has been critical to the development of faster, more efficient, and more uniform methods of manufacturing, all the way from the trading ships and galleys of war in Venice in the fifteenth and sixteenth centuries to muskets at the end of the eighteenth century and automobiles in the early twentieth century. Standards have also played a critical role in allowing the interchange and use of manufactured goods by different groups. Examples include the compulsory use of a standard size for bricks (9 × 4 × 4 inches) in Boston in the late seventeenth century; standard gage for railroad tracks in Britain, the United States, Canada, and most of Europe; and establishment in 1948 of standard pitches and dimensions for screw threads manufactured in the United States, Britain, and Canada.

Standards have also played an important role in improving health and safety. In 1914 the American Society of Mechanical Engineers issued its first boiler code, which the American Standards Association cited in 1952 as having "done more for national safety" than any other single standard in America. Finally, recognizing the universal importance of standards, representatives from 19 nations held the first formal conference on international standards, the International Conference on Weights and Measures, in Paris in 1875 and signed a convention that established a permanent International Bureau of Weights and Measures (American Standards Association 1972).

Florence Nightingale, the founder of modern nursing in the mid-nineteenth century, is often considered the mother of health data standards and the modern medical record. Her skills as a statistician in gathering standardized data won her election to the Royal Statistical Society and honorary membership in the American Statistical Association (Miller 1992, 1029). Two centuries earlier, John Graunt's work on the London Bills of Mortality may have been the first effort at the systematic classification or statistical study of disease (World Health Organization 1993). In 1837 William Farr, the first medical statistician for the General Register's Office of England and Wales, advanced this work considerably, noting in his first annual report that a uniform statistical nomenclature was as important for the Bills of Mortality "as weights and measures in the physical sciences" (Registrar General of England and Wales 1839, 99). The formal structure of the International Statistical Classification of Diseases and Health Related Problems was established in 1893 with the Bertillon Classification or International List of Causes of Death. In the United States, the Census Bureau produced the first standard certificates used to register live births and deaths in 1900, and the first Model State Vital Statistics Act was published in 1907 (National Center for Health Statistics 1997). The current field of health-care informatics standards dates to the late 1960s with the development over the next several decades of a variety of health-care message standards and uniform data sets (Kanaan 2001). The Administrative Simplification (AS) provisions (Health Insurance Portability and Accountability Act of 1996, Subtitle F) of the Health Insurance Portability and Accountability Act of 1996 (HIPAA) are moving the health-care industry toward standardized electronic transmission of certain administrative and financial transactions previously carried out manually on paper or in nonstandard electronic formats. These provisions have served as a major stimulus to bring a variety of groups to the table to work together on standards for health data.

DEFINITION

In 1978 the National Standards Policy Advisory Committee defined a standard as "a prescribed set of rules, conditions, or requirements concerning definition of terms; classification of components; specification of materials, performance or operations; delineation of procedures; or measurement of quantity and quality in describing materials, products, systems, services or practices"(National Standards Policy Advisory Committee 1978, 6). The International Organization for Standardization (ISO) defines a standard as "documented agreements containing technical specifications or other precise criteria to be used consistently as rules, guidelines, or definitions of characteristics, to ensure that materials, products, processes, and services are fit for their purpose" (International Organization for Standardization [hp] ISO Introduction). Both definitions emphasize that a standard is clearly described, can cover a broad range of topics, and is meant to be followed to be effective.

PURPOSES AND TYPES OF STANDARDS

As suggested in the definitions above, standards serve a number of purposes. ISO Guide 2 differentiates eight types of standards based on purpose (International

Organization for Standardization 1996). These categories are not meant to be comprehensive or mutually exclusive; a given standard may fit under two or more categories.

1. *Basic* standards cover topics with either a broad range of application or with general application to a particular field. An example might be a standard for plastics, which affects a range of products from cups to portable toilets.[2]
2. *Terminology* standards define words, phrases, or other terms to permit different parties to use a common, clearly understood language. Terminology standards may be supplemented with notes, diagrams, or examples.
3. *Testing* standards specify the test methods to be used to evaluate the performance or other characteristics of a product. Test methods may include methods of sampling, statistical analysis of data, and the order in which testing should be conducted.
4. *Product* standards establish characteristics or requirements for a product or groups of products to ensure that it will serve its purpose.[3]
5. *Process* standards establish requirements to be met by a process, such as an assembly line's operation, to ensure that it will serve its purpose.
6. *Service* standards establish requirements to be met by a service, such as serving a client of a financial institution, to ensure that it will meet its purpose.[4]
7. *Interface* standards, such as the point of connection between a telephone and telephone wiring, establish requirements to ensure the compatibility of products or systems at their points of connection.
8. *Data to be provided* standards specify a list of "characteristics for which values or other data are to be stated for specifying the product, process, or service."[5]

Standards may differ in the extent of their application. Local standards may be developed and used by a specific business or industry in a particular geographic area to facilitate the manufacture of a particular product. National standards are usually embraced by a country. For example, the United States uses the English, as opposed to the metric, system of measuring distance (e.g., miles and feet versus kilometers and meters). International standards are intended to be worldwide in their scope and application, such as the ISO international standard for the optimal thickness of the plastic used to manufacture credit cards.

Some standards may be voluntary, whereas others may be mandatory. The use of Accredited Standards Committee (ASC) X12F (Finance) standards for the exchange of financial information between financial institutions in the United States is voluntary, whereas the use of the dollar as the standard currency in the United States is mandatory. Finally, there are different ways in which standards may be developed. Standards may be developed and maintained by officially sanctioned national organizations that follow prescribed procedures to ensure openness and consensus (see "Developing and Maintaining Standards" below).

In contrast, businesses, organizations, or even governments and international organizations may develop guidelines or standards to serve the needs of their own customers or constituents. Because of their usefulness, other businesses or organizations or governmental entities may subsequently adopt these standards so that they come to be common practice.[6] Standards developed in this way are known as *de facto* standards.[7] Thus, a de facto standard is a "standard that is widely accepted and used, but lacks formal approval by a recognized standards organization." (Secretariat, Alliance for Telecommunications Industry Solutions 2001). The development and maintenance of standards is discussed later in this chapter.

PURPOSES AND TYPES OF STANDARDS USED IN HEALTH STATISTICS AND OTHER HEALTH INFORMATION SYSTEMS

Data are central to the health statistics enterprise. They are collected, processed, stored, analyzed, interpreted, disseminated, shared, and evaluated over time and in different locations. To ensure comparable high-quality data, it is critical that data-related activities and the methods they employ, wherever possible and appropriate, follow recognized standards. These standards enhance data quality and consistency over time, make possible direct comparison and linkage of data sets, promote interoperability between computer and information systems, and facilitate training and supervising the staff that process and maintain these data. By moving away from proprietary or nonstandard approaches and toward standards-based methods, the health statistics enterprise can increase the quality and utility of the data that it produces and reduce the time and resources spent in obtaining, processing, and disseminating these data. Five of the eight types of ISO Guide 2 standards described above are particularly applicable to the health statistics enterprise. The remainder of this chapter will focus on the application of these to the health statistics enterprise.

- *Terminology* standards are needed so that the definition and classification of health-related terms are clearly understood by all who use them. Examples of terminology standards include the Systematized Nomenclature of Medicine (SNOMED) and the International Statistical Classification of Diseases and Health Related Problems (ICD).
- *Product* standards are needed to establish qualities or requirements for products of the health statistics enterprise to ensure that they will serve their purpose. For example, health statistics reports that include specific information on mortality should use standard methods of calculating mortality rates and standard classification schemes for diseases and injuries, such as the monthly and annual reports on mortality issued by the

National Center for Health Statistics (NCHS) (NCHS 1996, 2002) or the World Health Organization (WHO) (WHO 2003). Because product standards in health statistics have so much overlap with processing standards, we have combined them in our discussion of these standards later in this chapter.

- *Process* standards are needed to ensure that the collection and processing of health data are efficient, complete, protective of confidentiality, and of high quality, with no loss or corruption of data during the process. Examples of de facto process standards are the methods used by the U.S. Census and the National Health Interview Survey to collect and process their data, including the use of standardized, field-tested, and validated questions and questionnaires to obtain information.
- *Interface* standards are needed to ensure that the exchange of data between different health statistics or other health information systems maintains the quality, integrity, security, and usability of the data. Examples of interface standards include the message format standards developed by ASC X12N (Insurance) and Health Level Seven (HL7), the mapping of various health-related terminologies and classifications into each other by the Unified Medical Language System (UMLS), and the Federal Information Processing Standards (FIPS) for geopolitical entities in the United States developed by the National Institute of Standards and Technology (NIST) (NIST 1987, 1990).
- *Data to be provided* standards specify a listing of data requirements for a product or service for which values need to be obtained. Examples of these standards are unique identifiers for health-care providers and the uniform or core data sets that have been developed for hospital discharge data, ambulatory care data, and vital records.

In 1997 NIST published *Healthcare Standards Needs for Using the NII* (Katz 1997), which included a draft list of "categories of health standards," the major categories of which are shown in Table 8.1. This report used the framework developed earlier by the American National Standards Institute (ANSI) for identifying requirements for standards for the National Information Intrastructure (NII) (ANSI 1995). Although these NIST categories address standards for health care rather than for health statistics or health information, several of the categories refer directly to standards needed for the collection and processing of health information. Although the NIST categories differ from those listed above for ISO, several categories share a conceptual relationship (e.g., *codes and terminology* and *information exchange and interface*). Both of these schemes for specifying types of health information standards suggest that a broad array of standards is needed to facilitate the work of the health statistics enterprise and other health information systems.

We now review specific standards of each type that are relevant to the health statistics enterprise. Our aim is to be illustrative rather than comprehensive.

TABLE 8.1
Categories of Health-Care Standards

1. Information exchange (shared with other industries)
    1.1. Electronic data interchange
    1.2. Network protocols
    1.3. Security
    1.4. Database and data management (including configuration management)
    1.5. Graphics
    1.6. Language processing
    1.7. Multimedia exchange
    1.8. Image processing
2. Information content
    2.1. Format (class)
        2.1.1. Identifiers
        2.1.2. Computer-based patient records
        2.1.3. Practice guidelines
        2.1.4. Claims
        2.1.5. Billing
        2.1.6. Clinical reports
        2.1.7. Procurement forms (for goods and services)
    2.2. Codes (instances)
        2.2.1. Diagnosis (e.g., ICD, SNOMED)
        2.2.2. Procedures (e.g., Current Procedural Terminology)
        2.2.3. Drugs (prescription and over-the-counter)
        2.2.4. Toxins
        2.2.5. Anatomic locations
        2.2.6. Units of measure (including standard proxy measurements)
        2.2.7. Symptoms
        2.2.8. Signs
    2.3. Quality assurance
        2.3.1. Prevention guidelines
        2.3.2. Practice guidelines
        2.3.3. Standards for conducting clinical trials
        2.3.4. Standards for conducting outcomes studies
        2.3.5. Standards for conducting interview and examination surveys

ICD = International Statistical Classification of Diseases and Health Related Problems; SNOMED = Systemized Nomenclature of Medicine.
Source: Katz (1997), pp. 2–3.

Terminology Standards

In health information, *terminology* is a collective term used to describe the continuum of code sets, classifications, and nomenclatures or vocabularies (Chute 2000). In the past 10 years, much work has been devoted to terminology standards, and a framework for health terminology systems in the United States was recently proposed (Chute et al. 1998). (See Table 8.2.) Below we present examples of terminologies important to the health statistics enterprise.

TABLE 8.2
Functional Characteristics That Must Be Achieved by Terminologies

1. General
   1.1. Completeness
   1.2. Comprehensiveness
   1.3. Characteristics of integration
      1.3.1. Nonoverlapping
      1.3.2. Integrated
   1.4. Nonredundant
   1.5. Mapping
2. Structure of the terminology model
   2.1. Atomic base
   2.2. Compositional
   2.3. Synonyms
   2.4. Attributes
      2.4.1. Inheritance
   2.5. Multiple hierarchies
      2.5.1. Consistency of view
   2.6. Explicit uncertainty
   2.7. Lexical rules
   2.8. Representation
3. Maintenance
   3.1. Context-free identifiers
   3.2. Unique identifiers
   3.3. Version control
      3.3.1. Dated
      3.3.2. Obsolete marking
   3.4. Definitions
   3.5. Language independence
   3.6. Responsiveness
4. Administration
   4.1. Coordination
   4.2. Access
   4.3. Funding

Source: Chute et al. (1998), p. 503.

Nomenclature

A nomenclature or vocabulary is a set of specialized terms that facilitates precise communication by eliminating ambiguity. A *controlled vocabulary* allows the use of only the set of terms in the vocabulary. A *structured vocabulary* or *reference terminology* relates terms to one another (with a set of relationships) and qualifies them (with a set of attributes) to promote precise and accurate interpretation (NCVHS 2000, 62).

- Medicine—SNOMED CT[8] is a concept-based reference terminology, including over 344,000 concepts linked to clinical knowledge, 913,000 synonym terms, and more than 1.3 million explicit relationships between terms. The nomenclature is used in electronic health records, clinical laboratory systems, and other applications (SNOMED [hp]). In 2003, the National Library of Medicine (NLM) signed an agreement with the College of American Pathologists to allow use of SNOMED CT by all U.S. organizations, without additional license fees. This is expected to enable wider incorporation of the terminology in electronic medical records. The National Committee on Vital and Health Statistics has recommended SNOMED CT (as licensed by NLM) as part of a core set of Patient Medical Record Information (PMRI) Terminologies (NCVHS 2002b).
- Geography—The Office of Management and Budget (OMB) defines metropolitan and micropolitan statistical areas, which are used by federal agencies for their data collections (OMB 2000, 2003). The Bureau of the Census defines the types of and terms for other geographic areas that are used in the census of the population (e.g., census block and tract) (U.S. Census Bureau 2000). Because geographic and population data collected by the U.S. government are used extensively in health statistics, these terms and definitions have been accepted as de facto standards by the health statistics enterprise in the United States.

Classification

A classification arranges or organizes like or related terms for easy retrieval and analysis. Classifications are a necessary adjunct to vocabularies for the standardized coding of information for statistical and related purposes. Vocabularies and classifications should be considered complementary (Madden et al. 2002). Below we describe several classification systems that are relevant to the health statistics enterprise.

- Disease and health problems—The ICD, now in its tenth revision, has become the international standard diagnostic classification for all general epidemiologic and many health management purposes. The formal structure of the ICD was established in 1893 with the Bertillon Classification or International List of Causes of Death. The ICD is the standard used throughout the world for classifying causes of mortality as recorded at the registration of death and for reporting these data nationally to WHO. Originally designed to classify causes of death, the scope of the ICD was extended at the Sixth Revision in 1948 to include nonfatal diseases. The application of the classification to morbidity statistics has expanded with each subsequent revision. Nonetheless, the United States and a number of other countries have found it necessary to develop clinical modifications of the ICD to meet the needs of their respective health-care systems for more detailed clinical information from hospital, clinic and physician records. The clinical modification of ICD-9 (ICD-9-CM) was adopted by the United States in 1979 for morbidity applications and will be replaced by the clinical modification of ICD-10 (ICD-10-CM). In addition to its use in records and surveys, ICD-9-CM is used to classify diseases and health conditions on health-care claims and is the basis for prospective payment to hospitals.

- Functional status—In 1972 WHO started developing a preliminary conceptual framework for classifying the "consequences of disease . . . and of their implications for the lives of individuals" (WHO 2001). This evolved into the International Classification of Impairments, Disabilities, and Handicaps (ICIDH), first published by WHO in 1980. The United Nations Disability Statistics Database (DISTAT) has used ICIDH as the framework for collecting statistics from member countries on persons with disability (UN [hp] Disability statistics). In 1993 WHO began a lengthy and intensive process for revising ICIDH, resulting in approval by the World Health Assembly of the International Classification of Functioning, Disability and Health (ICF) in May 2001. The ICF includes a classification of environmental factors, which interact with the other dimensions of body functions and structures, activities, and participation. The National Committee on Vital and Health Statistics (NCVHS) has recognized the ICF as the only viable comprehensive code set for classifying functional status in clinical and administrative records and as a promising approach for providing the common language that is needed for this critical information (NCVHS 2001a). The DISTAT is migrating to the new ICF framework, and ICF is guiding a variety of other activities in disability statistics, both in the United States and internationally (NCHS [hp] ICF).
- Procedures—In the United States, two classifications are used for capturing diagnostic, therapeutic, and preventive services (e.g., measurement of blood glucose level, tonsillectomy, immunizations). Volume 3 of ICD-9-CM is used for hospital inpatient reporting and billing and for statistics, and the Current Procedural Terminology (CPT-4) is used for professional services billing.
- Drugs and medications—Drugs can be coded with the Healthcare Common Procedure Coding System J codes or National Drug Codes. The Food and Drug Administration is working with the NLM to develop a common terminology for medications (RxNorm) based on active ingredients. The NCVHS has recommended several Federal Drug Terminologies, including RxNorm, as part of the core set of PMRI terminologies (NCVHS 2002b).
- Occupation and industry—Various schemes for classifying industries and occupations have been employed in the United States over the past 30 years. These include the Standard Industrial Classification and the

Standard Occupational Classification, both developed by the OMB, and the *Dictionary of Occupational Titles*, developed by the U.S. Bureau of the Census. In 1997—with a major revision in 2002—the U.S. Bureau of the Census, in collaboration with Canada and Mexico, developed a new classification for industries, known as the North American Industry Classification System (OMB 2002). For international use, the International Labour Organization publishes the International Standard Industrial Classification of All Economic Activities, which is currently in its third revision (ILO [hp] ILO Statistics).

- Geographic areas—The NIST has developed a number of FIPS, which are used to classify and code geographic areas within the United States. These include classifications for metropolitan areas (NIST 1995), counties (NIST 1990), and states (NIST 1987). These FIPS are used extensively by the health statistics enterprise to ensure geographic comparability of data collected by different data systems and to facilitate the exchange of electronic information between systems. In addition to being classification standards, these standards are processing and interface standards.

Process and Product Standards

There are many important de facto standards that have been developed for the collection, processing, and analysis of health-related data. These standards are critical to ensure that the data are accurate and can be compared across different populations, geopolitical areas, or time periods. Examples of these standards are presented below.

Collecting and Processing Data

- Guidelines for information quality—The OMB heads the Interagency Council on Statistical Policy (ICSP), which is composed of the heads of the U.S. government's 10 principal statistical agencies plus the heads of the statistical units of 4 nonstatistical agencies. The ICSP coordinates statistical work across organizations, enabling the exchange of information about organization programs and activities, and provides advice and counsel to the OMB on statistical activities. The statistical activities of these agencies are predominantly the collection, compilation, processing or analysis of information for statistical purposes. Within this framework, NCHS functions as the federal agency responsible for the collection and dissemination of the nation's vital and health statistics. Its mission is to provide statistical information that will guide actions and policies to improve the health of the American people. The OMB has issued guidelines for ensuring the quality of information disseminated by U.S. government agencies and has required all of these agencies to develop their own guidelines to ensure the quality of the data that they collect and disseminate (OMB [hp] Agency Info Quality), including the NCHS (NCHS [hp] Quality). Additionally, the OMB periodically issues guidelines or standards on the collection of specific types of data (OMB [hp] Stat Programs). One of these standards, which addresses the collection and classification of data on race and ethnicity, is described below. Professional organizations also develop guidelines and standards for information quality that are in common practice.[9]

- Questionnaire and survey design—The U.S. National Laboratory for Collaborative Research in Cognition and Survey Measurement was established in 1985 to apply cognitive methods to questionnaire design research. In collaboration with other NCHS programs, the Laboratory develops and tests NCHS data collection instruments. It also supports a questionnaire design research program in collaboration with university scientists by means of research contracts (NCHS [hp] Research).
- Race and ethnicity—The OMB first issued standards for collecting, maintaining, and presenting federal data on race and ethnicity in 1977. These standards were revised in 1997, requiring for the first time that agencies provide the opportunity for individuals to choose more than one racial category if they wish to reflect multiple racial heritages. The standards also specify that ethnicity should be asked for before race (OMB 1997). The NCHS has developed methods to bridge the Census 2000 multiple-race resident population to single-race categories (Ingram et al. 2003).
- Medical certification of cause of death—The international standard for medical certification of cause of death was approved by the World Health Assembly in 1948 and continues to be followed worldwide. This standard includes the format for certification and the rules for selecting the underlying cause of death, which is the cause that is tabulated for most mortality statistics. The United States has taken the lead in developing and standardizing automated systems for processing mortality data, including causes of death (NCHS [hp] ICE).
- Disease registries—The North American Association of Central Cancer Registries (NAACCR) is a professional organization of state, provincial, territorial, and local health departments; American and Canadian government agencies; private nonprofit and for-profit organizations; and individuals that develops and promotes uniform data standards for cancer registration. In doing so, it uses both international standards (HL7) and consensus standards agreed to by its members to ensure uniformity and comparability of data. The NAACCR also provides education and training; certifies population-based registries; aggregates and publishes data from central cancer registries; and promotes the use of cancer surveillance data and systems for cancer control and epidemiologic research, public health programs, and patient care to reduce the burden of cancer in North America (NAACCR [hp]).

Analyzing, Presenting, and Comparing Data

In some instances, conventions have been developed regarding analytic practices that facilitate uniformity and allow the comparison of information for different populations and geographic areas (see Table 8.3 for some examples). These conventions often reflect the consensus of a field and become ubiquitous in their application. Definitions of rates for various population-related events are good examples. Birth and death rates may be related to the entire population (crude rate), or they may be restricted to subpopulations of a specific age, sex, race, or marital status. All of these rates may be further restricted to a specific geographic area or jurisdiction. In addition to these crude and specific rates, consensus approaches have been developed for adjusting some of these rates to allow comparison of the rates for two or more populations that differ in the distribution of one or more attributes (e.g., age adjustment of the birth rate or the death rate; Klein and Schoenborn 2001). Uniform methods were developed for these calculations, including direct and indirect methods, in the nineteenth century (Curtin and Klein 1995). When an age-adjusted rate is calculated using the direct method, age-specific rates are multiplied by the number of persons in age-specific strata of a standard population. Both NCHS (Anderson and Rosenberg 1998) and WHO (Ahmad et al. 2000) have defined standard populations for the age adjustment of death rates (see Tables 8.4 and 8.5). Rates can be similarly adjusted for race, sex, income, or any other population characteristic. The periodic issuance of a standard reference population (a published de facto standard), and the consensus on how to apply analytic techniques across geographic areas to calculate rates provide examples of the standards and conventions that are needed to facilitate the comparison of statistical information across geographic areas.

Several states, the U.S. Centers for Disease Control and Prevention, the National Association of Public Health Statistics and Information Systems, the U.S. Health Resources and Services Administration, and the National Association of Health Data Organizations have collaborated on the development of de facto standards for analyzing and displaying health statistics collected by state and local health departments in the United States. Examples of systems to display health statistics and other information that have been developed by individual states and are being used as standard templates by other state and local health departments include the Missouri Information for Community Assessment (MDHSS [db] MICA), the Massachusetts Community Health Information Profile (MDPH [db] MassCHIP), and Utah's Indicator-Based Information System for Public Health (UDH [db] IBIS).

Ensuring Privacy and Confidentiality of Data

The Privacy Act of 1974 provides a code of fair information practices to regulate the collection, maintenance, use, and dissemination of personal information by federal government agencies. Federal policy for the protection of human subjects

TABLE 8.3

Definitions of Various Rates Developed to Facilitate Comparison of Events in Different Populations

Birth rate is calculated by dividing the number of live births in a population in a year by the midyear resident population. Birth rates are expressed as the number of live births per 1000 population.

Fertility rate is the total number of live births, regardless of age of mother, per 1000 women of reproductive age, 15–44 years.

Death rate is calculated by dividing the number of deaths in a population in a year by the midyear resident population. Death rates are expressed as the number of deaths per 100,000 population.

Fetal death rate is the number of fetal deaths with stated or presumed gestation of 20 weeks or more divided by the sum of live births plus fetal deaths, stated per 1000 live births plus fetal deaths.

Late fetal death rate is the number of fetal deaths with stated or presumed gestation of 28 weeks or more divided by the sum of live births plus late fetal deaths, stated per 1000 live births plus late fetal deaths.

Infant mortality rate is the number of infant deaths per 1000 live births and is calculated by dividing the number of infant deaths during a calendar year by the number of live births reported in the same year.

Neonatal mortality rate is the number of deaths of children under 28 days of age per 1000 live births.

Postneonatal mortality rate is the number of deaths of children that occur between 28 days and 365 days after birth per 1000 live births.

Perinatal mortality rate is the sum of late fetal deaths plus infant deaths within 7 days of birth divided by the sum of live births plus late fetal deaths, stated per 1000 live births plus late fetal deaths. (Perinatal relates to the period surrounding the birth event. Rates and ratios are based on events reported in a calendar year.) Perinatal mortality ratio is the sum of late fetal deaths plus infant deaths within 7 days of birth divided by the number of live births, stated per 1000 live births.

Maternal mortality rate is defined as the number of maternal deaths per 100,000 live births. The maternal mortality rate is a measure of the likelihood that a pregnant woman will die from maternal causes. The number of live births used in the denominator is a proxy for the population of pregnant women who are at risk of a maternal death. Maternal death is defined as the death of a woman while pregnant or within 42 days of termination of pregnancy, irrespective of the duration and site of the pregnancy. Maternal death is one for which the certifying physician has designated a maternal condition as the underlying cause of death. Maternal conditions are those assigned to complications of pregnancy, childbirth, and the puerperium, ICD-10 codes O00–O99.

Source: National Center for Health Statistics [hp; updated 2002 Sep 13; cited 2004 Mar 3].

TABLE 8.4
Projected Year 2000 U.S. Population and Proportion Distribution by Age

Age Group (years)	*Standard Million*
Under 1	13,818
1–4	55,317
5–14	145,565
15–24	138,646
25–34	135,573
35–44	162,613
45–54	134,834
55–64	87,247
65–74	66,037
75–84	44,842
85+	15,508
Total	1,000,000

Source: Anderson and Rosenberg (1998, p. 4).

in research conducted or supported by the federal government, known as the Common Rule,[10] was first published in 1991 by the U.S. Department of Health and Human Services (USDHHS) (Protection of human subjects 1991). In 2000, the Department, in response to a mandate under the HIPAA (HIPPA 1996, Subtitle F), issued the first-ever U.S. national standards to protect patients' personal medical records. These standards define appropriate and inappropriate disclosures of individually identifiable health information and how patients' rights are to be protected (USDHHS [hp] Admin Simp). The NCHS develops—with state participation—a model law for state vital registration systems, which includes guidance on definitions, registration practices, disclosure, and issuance procedures.

Interface Standards

Providing standards for the electronic exchange of data is becoming increasingly important, as data prepared by the health statistics enterprise in an electronic form are of growing interest to public health practitioners, researchers, and the private sector. The development of standards for the electronic or computerized patient record and for the administrative transactions related to health care has been particularly active in the United States over the past 5 years. Because of the sensitivity of these records and transactions, much work has also been applied to the development of standards to ensure their security during processing, storage, and transmission.

TABLE 8.5
World Health Organization World Standard Population Distribution (%), Based on World Average Population, 2000–2025

Age Group (years)	*World Standard*
0–4	8.86
5–9	8.69
10–14	8.60
15–19	8.47
20–24	8.22
25–29	7.93
30–34	7.61
35–39	7.15
40–44	6.59
45–49	6.04
50–54	5.37
55–59	4.55
60–64	3.72
65–69	2.96
70–74	2.21
75–79	1.52
80–84	0.91
85–89	0.44
90–94	0.15
95–99	0.04
100+	0.005
Total	100

Source: Ahmad et al. (2000), p. 12.

- Administrative transactions—Electronic transaction formats have been developed to exchange data for specific administrative and financial functions in health care. The claim or encounter transaction standard is of most relevance to health statistics because of the information it contains on patient demographics, providers, diagnoses, services, and expenditures. More detailed clinical information may be requested by an insurer or health plan in an attachment, which supports the information on the claim. The USDHHS released the standards for administrative transactions under the HIPAA in August 2000, specifying the message formats for submitting electronic claims and other administrative transactions. These standards used format standards developed by ASC X12N for all of the specified transactions with the exception of retail pharmacy transactions, which used standards developed by the National Council for Prescription Drug Programs. Other regulations will cover identifiers for health-care providers, health plans, and employers, as well as standards for claims attachments. As directed by the U.S. Congress, work on the HIPAA requirement for a unique health identifier for individuals has been suspended.

- Electronic patient records—The HIPAA statute also directed the NCVHS to "study the issues related to the adoption of uniform data standards for patient medical record information and the electronic exchange of such information." In July 2000, the NCVHS issued its report, *Uniform Data Standards for Patient Medical Record Information* (NCVHS 2000), and in February 2002 the NCVHS provided specific recommendations on standards for formatting electronic messages that contain information from the patient medical record (NCVHS 2002a). Recommendations on vocabulary standards were issued in 2003 (NCVHS 2001a, 2002b). Health Level Seven is developing a functional outline for the Electronic Health Record in response to guidance from the Institute of Medicine (IOM [LR] 2003). The availability of standardized electronic patient records holds considerable promise for health statistics as well as clinical care. Aggregated data from these records could enrich the information available for research and policy development on quality and outcomes of care, patient safety, and health disparities.
- Security and electronic signature standards—The HIPAA also required the adoption of standards for the security of individual health information. A report from the National Research Council (1997) found poor practices in health-care organizations in the handling of paper-based health information and explored ways of protecting health information that increasingly is collected, used, and stored in electronic form. Confidentiality potentially is threatened not only by the risk of improper access to electronically stored information, but also by the risk of interception during electronic transmission of the information. The USDHHS found that there was no recognized single standard that integrates all the components of security (administrative procedures, physical safeguards, technical security services, and technical mechanisms) that could be adopted. This required designating a new comprehensive standard, which was published as a final rule in 2003 (USDHHS 2003a).

Data to Be Provided Standards

Standards that specify the content[11] of forms and questionnaires ensure that critical information is collected in a consistent and comparable manner.

- Vital registration—The U.S. Standard Certificates and Reports for births, deaths, fetal deaths, marriages, divorces, and abortions are one of the principal means by which uniformity of data collection and processing is achieved in the U.S. National Vital Statistics System (NCHS 2000). To ensure that the standard certificates and reports and the items they contain meet health information and administrative needs, they are evaluated and revised every 10 to 15 years by the NCHS and the states, which operate the vital registration systems. In the 1970s, the Cooperative Health Statistics System envisioned similar federal-state partnerships concerning encounter, facility, and manpower data. However, the only component with sustained federal funding has been the Vital Statistics Cooperative Program.

- Reporting of clinical and other encounter data—Since the late 1960s, the U.S. government has been engaged in extensive development of de facto standards for minimum data sets[12] and core health data elements (McCormick et al. 1997). The NCVHS has been a partner in these activities. The Uniform Hospital Discharge Data Set (UHDDS) is the best known and most widely used of these data sets. The UHDDS was first presented in a 1972 report of the NCVHS and underwent a number of revisions over a 20-year period. Although the official data set was last promulgated in a July1985 *Federal Register* notice, it has been incorporated into the Uniform Bill for Hospitals (UB-82, UB-92, and UB-04, forthcoming), which defines the data content for the institutional claim under the HIPAA. Approximately 42 states require hospitals to report data on all discharges using the UB-92 or other specialized forms. The UHDDS is also the basis for the data collected in the National Hospital Discharge Survey, which has been conducted continuously by the NCHS since 1965.[13] The Agency for Healthcare Research and Quality has developed the Healthcare Cost and Utilization Project, building on the hospital discharge data systems in approximately half of the U.S. states.

The USDHHS never officially promulgated the Uniform Ambulatory Care Data Set (UACDS), a companion data set to the UHDDS for ambulatory care, but the Health Insurance Claim Form for professional services (known as the HCFA-1500) has served as a de facto standard for collecting many of the data elements specified in the UACDS and defines the content for the professional claim under the HIPAA. Many of the UACDS elements are collected in the NCHS National Ambulatory Medical Care Survey. In 1996, the NCVHS updated its recommendations on data elements for hospital and ambulatory care in a milestone report that identified 42 data elements for standardization, including demographic, socioeconomic, and health status information about a person, and data specific to a person's encounter with the health-care system as either an inpatient or an outpatient (NCVHS 1996). Another data set, which has been recognized in the HIPAA process, is Data Elements for Emergency Department Systems (DEEDS), developed by the National Center for Injury Prevention and Control in 1997. The DEEDS is the basis for the claim attachment standard for emergency departments.

- Health interview surveys—An excellent example of a collaborative effort among public and private sector organizations to develop standards for collecting comparable information across multiple health interview surveys is the U.S. Food Security Measurement Project. This project developed standardized questionnaires and methods to define and obtain data on the prevalence of food insufficiency in the United States. These standardized approaches are used in a variety of national and subnational surveys, including the National Health and Nutrition Examination Survey, the Survey of Program Dynamics, and the Early Childhood Longitudinal Study (Economic Research Service [hp]). In the international arena, the Washington Group (NCHS [hp] WG) hopes to develop a small set of general disability measures suitable for use in censuses, sample-based national surveys, or other statistical formats, which will provide needed information on disability throughout the world.
- Administrative reporting—The HIPAA regulations specify the content of electronic transactions between health-care providers and payers for health-care enrollment, eligibility, claims, and remittances. A consortium of organizations, referred to as Designated Standards Maintenance Organizations, maintains the content (Designated Standards Maintenance Organizations [hp]).
- Electronic patient record—Several organizations have done work to identify the content of an electronic patient record. The American Society for Testing and Materials has a committee (E31) that develops standards for health record content, structure, functionality, privacy, security, vocabularies, and selected health-care information message standards (ASTM [hp]). The initial claims attachment standards proposed under the HIPAA would standardize clinical content to support health-care claims data in the following areas: ambulance, emergency department, laboratory results, clinical reports, medications, and rehabilitation services.

DEVELOPING AND MAINTAINING STANDARDS

More than 175 distinct entities are accredited in the United States to develop standards, and there are almost 15,000 approved American National Standards that cover a broad range of services, products and tests (ANSI [hp]). Founded in 1918, the American National Standards Institute (ANSI) is a private, non-profit organization that administers and coordinates the U.S. voluntary standardization and conformity assessment system. The ANSI does not itself create standards; rather, it accredits organizations to create standards. To obtain accreditation, organizations agree to adhere to a set of guiding principles—consensus, due process and openness—developed by the ANSI. These accredited organizations are referred to by the ANSI as Accredited Standards Developer(s) or Standards Development Organization(s) (SDOs). In addition to overseeing the development of national standards in the United States, the ANSI is the official U.S. representative to the ISO.

The ISO, a nongovernmental organization established in 1947, is a worldwide federation of national standards bodies from some 100 countries, one from each country. Its mission is to promote the development of standardization and related activities in the world with a view to facilitating the international exchange of goods and services and to developing cooperation in the spheres of intellectual, scientific, technological, and economic activity (ISO [hp] About ISO). The ISO standards are developed according to three principles, which differ somewhat from those of the ANSI: (*1*) consensus, which ensures that the "views of all interests are taken into account"; (*2*) industrywide, which strives to "satisfy industries and customers worldwide"; and (*3*) voluntary. The ISO process for developing standards consists of three phases: (*1*) defining the technical scope of the proposed standard; (*2*) building consensus, in which countries negotiate the detailed specifications of the standard; and (*3*) approving the standard, which requires formal approval of the draft International Standard by two-thirds of the ISO members that have participated in the standards development process and by three-quarters of all members that vote (ISO [hp] About ISO). A U.S. Technical Advisory Group develops recommendations to the ISO Technical Committee on Health Informatics (TC 215), which develops international standards for health information to ensure compatibility and interoperability among different health information systems (ISO [hp] TC 215).

Many of the standards used in health statistics, especially those for processing data, are de facto standards that have been developed over the past 100 years by various government statistical agencies, academic centers, or the private sector. In the United States the NCHS has played a prominent role in developing standard methods for collecting, processing, analyzing, and presenting health statistics. Recommendations for several de facto standards have also been developed by the NCVHS, which was established by the U.S. Surgeon General in 1949 in response to a WHO recommendation that "such national committees study broadly the problem of producing satisfactory national and international statistics in the fields of health" (USNCVHS 1949). In addition to de facto standards, several dozen organizations that are accredited by the ANSI develop and maintain standards for health information in the United States. Health-care providers, health plans, vendors, state and federal employees, and researchers participate in the standards development process. Increasingly, these standards are being evaluated and adopted by the public and private sectors to enhance the interoperability[14] of information systems in the United States and abroad. Health statistics that rely on or interact with data from the health-care system are necessarily influenced by these standards. The administrative simplification provisions of the HIPAA gave prominence and preference to standards "developed, adopted or modified by a standard setting organization" that is accredited by ANSI (HIPAA 1996, Sect. 1172).

It is important to know the principal players in the development of health information standards in the United States because these organizations are responsible not only for developing standards but also for maintaining and modifying those standards. Some of the key organizations are described in Table 8.6.

In addition to the organizations that develop and maintain health data standards, other organizations have been established to coordinate and promote the development and implementation of standards.

- ANSI Healthcare Informatics Standards Board (HISB) (ANSI [hp] HISB) —The HISB provides an open public forum for the voluntary coordination of health-care informatics standards among all U.S. SDOs. The organization is supporting the U.S. Health Information Knowledgebase (USHIK), a metadata registry to catalog and harmonize data elements across organizations. The USHIK is based on ISO and ANSI standards, as well as the Australian Knowledgebase (AIHW [hp]).
- USDHHS Data Council (USDHHS [hp] Data Council)—The USDHHS Data Council was created in 1996 to coordinate all health and nonhealth data collection and analysis activities of the USDHHS. It oversees survey integration and the HIPAA standards-setting process.
- National Library of Medicine (NLM [hp])—The NLM, a component of the U.S. National Institutes for Health, has designed the UMLS to help researchers in investigating knowledge representation and retrieval questions. The ULMS Metathesaurus contains information about biomedical concepts and terms from many controlled vocabularies and classifications. It will be the vehicle for distributing SNOMED CT.
- Consolidated Health Informatics (CHI) Initiative—The CHI was established in 2002 as the health-care component of the President's eGov initiatives to make it easier for citizens and businesses to interact with the U.S. government. Led by the Centers for Medicare and Medicaid Services and including involvement of numerous other federal agencies, the CHI recommends message and vocabulary standards for the exchange of clinical information between and among these agencies (USDHHS 2003b). These standards are considered part of the National Health Information Infrastructure.
- Public Health Data Standards Consortium (NCHS [hp] PHDSC; PHDSC [hp] Resource Center)—The Consortium was established in 1999 in response to recommendations of a 1998 workshop that explored the implications of HIPAA administrative simplification provisions for public health and health services research. The Consortium, a voluntary confederation of federal, state, and local health agencies; national and local professional associations; and public and private sector organizations, serves as a mechanism for ongoing representation of public health and health services research interests in data standards setting processes, including HIPAA implementation. U.S. federal and state representatives

TABLE 8.6
Developers and Maintainers of Health Data Standards

Organization	*Type of Standard*	*Standard*	*Uses*
ASC X12 (ASC X12 [hp])	Interface and data to be provided	Message format and content standards for electronic interchange	Administrative and financial data exchange
American Medical Association (AMA [hp] CPT)	Terminology	CPT	Classification of physician services, reimbursement
Centers for Medicare and Medicaid Services (CMS [hp] HIPAA)	Terminology	ICD-9-CM, Vol. 3, HCPCS	Procedure statistics, reimbursement
College of American Pathology (SNOMED [hp])	Terminology	SNOMED CT	Clinical vocabulary for electronic medical records
Health Level Seven (HL7 [hp])	Interface and data to be provided	Message format and content standards for electronic interchange	Clinical data exchange
National Center for Health Statistics (NCHS [hp] Classif)	Terminology	ICD-9-CM, Vols. 1 and 2; ICD-10-CM	Disease statistics, reimbursement
National Center for Health Statistics (NCHS [hp])	Data to be provided	Standard certificates Questionnaires	Vital statistics Surveys
National Uniform Billing Committee (NUBC [hp])	Data to be provided	Standardized data set and uniform bill for hospitals	Institutional claims and encounter data exchange
National Uniform Claim Committee (NUCC [hp])	Data to be provided	Standardized data set and uniform bill	Noninstitutional claims and encounter data exchange
World Health Organization (WHO [hp] Classif)	Terminology	ICD, ICF	Statistical classification and related purposes

CPT = Current Procedural Terminology; ICD = International Statistical Classification of Diseases and Health Related Problems; ICD-9-CM = ICD, Ninth Revision, Clinical Modification; ICF = International Classification of Functioning, Disability, and Health; SNOMED CT = Systemized Nomenclature of Medicine Clinical Terms.

serve on the National Uniform Billing Committee and the National Uniform Claim Committee and participate in ASC X12N and HL7, where they advocate for data content of importance to public health and research.

STANDARDS THAT ARE NEEDED

In 1997 the NIST published *Healthcare Standards Needs for Using the NII* (Katz 1997), which listed new standards that are needed to facilitate the collection, processing, exchange, and use of health data. The titles of these needs are listed in Table 8.7. Several of these standards (e.g., usability of health encounter data for population health studies, limits for level of detail to maintain confidentiality, unique identifiers and their allowed uses) could contribute to more robust and comparable health statistics. Consensus standards for clinical vocabularies are a high-priority need for achieving electronic exchange of detailed health-care information. In the area of vital statistics, consensus standards are needed for electronic birth and death registration.

Identification of important areas for standards development should be guided by the view articulated by the NCVHS in a 1996 report about its roles and functions (Coltin and Iezzoni 1999). This view emphasized that the policy and programmatic questions that one is trying to answer must drive the development and content of standards. If standards development is isolated from the purposes for which the standards are needed, the standards will not meet those needs and are unlikely to be adopted. In the NCVHS report, this view of the role of standards in health information "unfolds as does an old-fashioned camera, starting at the top with the 'viewfinder' through which the customer or user of information . . . poses questions about the health and health care of the American people." These

TABLE 8.7
Health-Care Standards Needs for Using the National Information Infrastructure

A11.	Usability of health encounter data for population health studies
A21.	Environmental–health interface
A31.	Timely availability of patient information during health-care encounters
A4.	Reporting and assessment from supporting medical services data
B.1.a.	Spoken language processing
B.1.b.	Written language processing
B.1.c.	Natural language understanding
B.1.d.	Human language translation
B.2.	Graphics and image processing
B.2.1.	Limits for level of detail to maintain confidentiality
B.2.2.	Unique identifiers and their allowed uses
C.1.	Response time and ease of use in critical clinical situations

Source: Katz (1997).

questions are increasingly focused to identify the specific standards (e.g., data elements, identifiers, classifications, data transmission formats) that are needed to answer the questions for individuals, populations, and events. In the words of the NCVHS report, specific technical standards "cannot be considered without addressing each of the preceding levels. Otherwise, the camera is unaimed and may transmit useless images to the user" (Coltin and Iezzoni 1999). Several of the other chapters in this volume address the broader questions about health and health care for which standards have been and must continue to be developed.

Conceptual data models and concept dictionaries can also serve as guides for identifying standards that are needed for health statistics and health information systems. The HL7 Reference Information Model (HL7 [hp] Data Model) and the Public Health Conceptual Data Model, developed by the U.S. Centers for Disease Control and Prevention (CDC 2000), provide overall frameworks for information used in health care and public health. As such, they identify areas in which standards are needed and show the relationship among different classes of information. The Australian Institute of Health and Welfare's Knowledgebase (AIHW [hp]), the Manitoba Centre for Health Policy's Concept Dictionary (MCHP [hp]), and the USHIK (USHIK [hp]) provide detailed definitions of terms and concepts used in health information systems and can provide the basis for terminology and processing standards.

CONCLUSION

The twentieth century saw tremendous growth in the health statistics enterprise and in the development of standards for collecting, processing, analyzing, and exchanging data. The challenge in the twenty-first century is to overcome barriers to migrating to common standards and to improve the health statistics enterprise's ability to take advantage of standards in the electronic age. Collaboration is needed at the national and international levels to enhance existing standards for the broadest use and to develop new standards to facilitate analyses of determinants of health that have been inadequately addressed by the health statistics enterprise. The emerging U.S. National Health Information Infrastructure needs full participation by health statistics practitioners to ensure that the health statistics enterprise will reap the benefits of more standardized and timely clinical and population-based information (NCVHS 2001b).

NOTES

1. Three good overviews of standards are Breitenberg (1987), International Organization for Standardization (hp), and American Standards Association (1972).
2. The ISO Guide 2 notes that a basic standard "may function as a standard for direct application or as a basis for other standards."

3. The ISO Guide 2 notes that a product standard may also include requirements related to "terminology, sampling, testing, packaging and labeling and, sometimes, processing" and that "a product standard can be either complete or not, according to whether it specifies all or only a part of the necessary requirements."

4. The ISO Guide 2 notes that "service standards may be prepared in fields such as laundering, hotel-keeping, transport, car-servicing, telecommunications, insurance, banking, trading."

5. The ISO Guide 2 notes that some standards require data to be provided by suppliers, whereas other standards require data to be provided by purchasers.

6. Governments may require, through regulation, businesses or organizations to use guidelines or standards developed by the government even though they have not been developed by officially sanctioned national organizations that follow prescribed procedures to ensure openness and consensus. Such official organizations may not develop standards that are needed or used in health statistics and, in some cases, may not be the most appropriate approach for developing a statistical standard (e.g., terminology standards).

7. Two well-known de facto standards are the architecture for the personal computer originally developed by the International Business Machines Corporation, and the PostScript page description language developed by Adobe.

8. The Systematized Nomenclature of Medicine Clinical Terms (SNOMED CT) combines the content and structure of the SNOMED Reference Terminology with the U.K. National Health Service's Clinical Terms Version 3.

9. As an example, the American Association for Public Opinion Research has articulated standards for professional ethics and practices in the field of survey research (AAPOR [hp]).

10. A prominent feature of the Common Rule is the informed consent requirement.

11. Data to be provided standards are often referred to as *content* standards because they may specify the data content to be provided in a form or other data collection instrument.

12. A minimum data set is "a minimum set of items of information with uniform definitions and categories concerning a specific aspect or dimension of the health care system which meets the essential needs of multiple users" (USDHHS 1983).

13. The items collected in the survey include birth date* or age, sex, race, ethnicity, marital status, ZIP code,* expected sources of payment, admission and discharge dates, discharge status, medical record number,* up to seven diagnoses, as many as four surgical and nonsurgical operations, and procedures and dates of surgery. The starred items are confidential, as are the hospital identities.

14. The ability of one computer system to exchange information with another computer system.

REFERENCES

Accredited Standards Committee X12 [homepage on the Internet]. Falls Church, VA: Data Interchange Standards Association; c. 2003 [cited 2004 Mar 3]. Available from: http://www.x12.org.

Ahmad OB, Boschi-Pinto C, Lopez AD, Murray CJL, Lozano R, Inoue M. Age standardization of rates: a new WHO standard. Global Programme on Evidence Discussion Paper Series: No. 31. Geneva: WHO; 2000 [cited 2004 Mar 3]. Available from: http://www3.who.int/whosis/discussion_papers/discussion_papers.cfm#.

American Association for Public Opinion Research [homepage on the Internet]. Lenexa, KS: AAPOR; c. 2002 [cited 2004 Feb 8]. AAPOR. Code of professional ethics and practices [about 3 screens]. Available from: http://www.aapor.org/codeofethics.html.

American Medical Association [homepage on the Internet]. Chicago: AMA; c. 1995–2004 [updated 2004 Jan 20; cited 2004 Mar 3]. CPT (Current Procedural Terminology) [about 1 screen]. Available from: http://www.ama-assn.org/ama/pub/category/3113.html.

American National Standards Institute, International Infrastructure Standards Panel. Framework for Identifying Requirements for Standards for the National Information Infrastructure. IISP document no. 95-0056. Washington, DC: American National Standards Institute; 1995 [cited 2002 May 23]. Available from: http://www.ansi.org/public/iisp/docs/fram4nii.html.

American National Standards Institute [homepage on the Internet]. Washington, DC: ANSI; [cited 2004 Mar 3]. ANSI Healthcare Informatics Standards Board (HISB) [about 5 screens]. Available from: http://www.ansi.org/standards_activities/standards_boards_panels/hisb/overview.aspx?menuid=3.

American National Standards Institute [homepage on the Internet]. Washington, DC: American National Standards Institute (ANSI) [cited 2004 Mar 3]. Available from: http://www.ansi.org.

American Standards Association. Through history with standards. In: Glie R, ed. Speaking of Standards. Boston: Cahners Books; 1972, pp. 36–71.

Anderson RN, Rosenberg HM. Age Standardization of Death Rates: Implementation of the Year 2000 Standard. National Vital Statistics Reports. Vol. 47, no. 3 Hyattsville, MD: National Center for Health Statistics; 1998 [cited 2004 Mar 3]. Available at http://www.cdc.gov/nchs/data/nvsr/nvsr47/nvs47_03.pdf.

ASTM International [homepage on the Internet]. West Conshohocken, PA: ASTM International; c. 1996–2004 [cited 2004 Mar 3]. Committee E31 on Healthcare Informatics. Committee overview [about 1 screen]. Available from: http://www.astm.org/cgi-bin/SoftCart.exe/COMMIT/COMMITTEE/E31.htm?L+mystore+eivx5500+1029402264.

Australian Institute of Health and Welfare [homepage on the Internet]. Canberra: AIHW [updated 2002 Jun 20; cited 2004 Mar 3]. The knowledge base [about 3 screens]. Available from: http://www.aihw.gov.au/knowledgebase.

Breitenberg MA. The ABC's of Standards-Related Activities in the United States. Gaithersburg, MD: National Institute of Standards and Technology; 1987 [cited 2004 Mar 3]. Available from: http://ts.nist.gov/ts/htdocs/210/ncsci/stdpmr.htm.

Centers for Disease Control and Prevention. Public Health Conceptual Data Model. Atlanta: CDC; 2000 [cited 2004 Mar 3]. Available from: http://www.cdc.gov/nedss/DataModels/phcdm.pdf.

Centers for Medicare and Medicaid Services [homepage on the Internet]. Baltimore: CMS [updated 2003 May 30; cited 2004 Mar 3]. HIPAA Administrative simplification—regulations and standards [about 2 screens]. Available from: http://www.cms.hhs.gov/hipaa/hipaa2/default.asp.

Chute CG. Clinical classification and terminology: some history and current observations. J Am Med Inform Assoc 2000;7(3):298 [cited 2004 Mar 3]. Available from: http://www.pubmedcentral.gov/articlerender.fcgi?tool=pubmed&pubmedid=10833167.

Chute CG, Cohn SP, Campbell JR; the Healthcare Informatics Standards Board Vocabulary Working Group, the Computer-based Patient Records Institute Working Group on Codes and Structures. A framework for comprehensive health terminology systems in the United States: development guidelines, criteria for selection, and public policy implications. J Am Med Inform Assoc 1998;5(6):503 [cited 2004 Mar 3]. Available from: http://www.pubmedcentral.gov/articlerender.fcgi?artid=61331.

Coltin K, Iezzoni L. Appendix II: thoughts on the functions and form of the National Committee on Vital and Health Statistics. In: National Committee on Vital and Health Statistics. Report to Secretary Shalala for the Period 1996–1998. Hyattsville, MD: National Center for Health Statistics; 1999, pp. 31–32 [cited 2004 Mar 3]. Available from: http://www.ncvhs.hhs.gov/90727nv.htm.

Curtin LR, Klein RJ. Direct Standardization (Age-Adjusted Death Rates). Healthy People Statistical Notes No. 6 (revised). Hyattsville, MD: National Center for Health Statistics; 1995 [cited 2004 Mar 3]. Available at http://www.cdc.gov/nchs/data/statnt/statnt06rv.pdf.

Economic Research Service [homepage on the Internet]. Washington, DC: Economic Research Service; [updated 2003 Oct 28; cited 2004 Mar 3]. ERS. Food security in the United States: history of the food security measurement project [about 3 screens]. Available from: http://www.ers.usda.gov/briefing/FoodSecurity/history/index.htm.

Health Insurance Portability and Accountability Act of 1996, Pub. L. 104-191, Subtitle F (1996 Aug 21). Available from: http://aspe.os.dhhs.gov/admnsimp.

Health Insurance Portability and Accountability Act of 1996, Pub. L. No. 104-191, Subtitle F, Sect. 1172 (Aug. 21, 1996).

Health Level Seven [homepage on the Internet]. Ann Arbor, MI: Health Level Seven, Inc. c. 1997–2004 [cited 2004 Mar 3]. HL7 Data Model Development [about 3 screens]. Available from: http://www.hl7.org/library/data-model/index.cfm.

Health Level Seven [homepage on the Internet]. Ann Arbor, MI: Health Level Seven, Inc. c. 1997–2004 [cited 2004 Mar 3]. Available from: http://www.hl7.org.

Designated Standards Maintenance Organizations [homepage on the Internet]. Washington, DC: Washington Publishing Company; c. 2000 [cited 2004 Nov 11]. Available from: http://www.hipaa-dsmo.org.

Ingram DD, Parker JD, Schenker N, et al. United States Census 2000 Population with Bridged Race categories. Hyattsville, MD: National Center for Health Statistics. Vital Health Stat 2, No. 135; 2003 [cited 2004 Mar 3]. Available from: http://www.cdc.gov/nchs/data/series/sr_02/sr02_135.pdf.

Institute of Medicine, Board on Health Care Services, Committee on Data Standards for Patient Safety. Key Capabilities of an Electronic Health Record System, Letter Report. Washington, DC: National Academies Press; 2003 [cited 2004 Mar 3]. Available from: http://books.nap.edu/html/ehr/NI000427.pdf.

International Labour Organization (ILO) [homepage on the Internet]. Geneva: International Labour Organization; c. 1996–2004 [updated 2000 Mar 8; cited 2004 Mar 3]. ILO Statistics. International standard industrial classification of all economic activities, 3rd rev. [about 5 screens]. Available from: http://www.ilo.org/public/english/bureau/stat/class/isic.htm.

International Organization for Standardization. Standardization and Related Activities—General Vocabulary, ISO/IEC Guide 2. Geneva: International Organization for Standardization; 1996 [cited 2004 Jan 15]. Available from: www.iso.org or www.ansi.org.

International Organization for Standardization [homepage on the Internet]. Geneva: International Organization for Standardization; [cited 2002 May 22]. ISO Introduction [about 20 screens]. Available from: http://www.iso.ch/iso/en/aboutiso/introduction/index.html.

International Organization for Standardization [homepage on the Internet]. Geneva: International Organization for Standardization; c. 2002 [updated 2004 Feb 16; cited 2004 Mar 3]. About ISO [about 10 screens]. Available from: http://www.iso.ch/iso/en/aboutiso/introduction/index.html.

International Organization for Standardization [homepage on the Internet]. Geneva: International Organization for Standardization; c. 2002 [cited 2004 Mar 3]. ISO, TC 215. Health informatics [about 2 screens]. Available from: http://www.iso.ch/iso/en/stdsdevelopment/tc/tclist/TechnicalCommitteeDetailPage.TechnicalCommitteeDetail?COMMID=4720.

Kanaan SB. The National Committee on Vital and Health Statistics, 1949–99: a history. In: NCVHS 50th Anniversary Symposium. Hyattsville, MD: Department of Health and Human Services; 2001, pp. 13–47 [cited 2004 Mar 3]. Available from: http://www.ncvhs.hhs.gov/ncvhs50th.pdf.

Katz SB. Healthcare Standards Needs for Using the NII: An Application of the IISP Framework Method. Gaithersburg, MD: National Institute of Standards and Technology; 1997.

Klein RJ, Schoenborn CA. Age adjustment using the 2000 projected U.S. population. Healthy People Statistical Notes. No. 20. Hyattsville, MD: National Center for Health Statistics;

2001 [cited 2004 Mar 3]. Available from: http://www.cdc.gov/nchs/data/statnt/statnt20.pdf.
Madden RC, Üstün TB, Ashley J, Hirs WM, Schiøler G, Sykes CR. The WHO family of international classifications. Unpublished; March 2002.
Manitoba Centre for Health Policy (MCHP) [homepage on the Internet]. Winnipeg: MCHP; c. 2003 [updated 2003 Oct 24; cited 2004 Mar 3]. MCHP's Concept Dictionary [about 2 screens]. Available from: http://www.umanitoba.ca/centres/mchp/concept/concept.frame.shtml.
Massachusetts Department of Public Health [database on the Internet]. Boston: Massachusetts Department of Public Health; c. 1995–2002 [updated 2003 Feb 28; cited 2004 Mar 3]. Massachusetts Community Health Information Profile (MassCHIP) [about 1 screen]. Available from: http://masschip.state.ma.us.
McCormick K, Renner A, Mayes R, Regan J, Greenberg M. The federal and private sector roles in the development of minimum data sets and core health data elements. Comput Nurs 1997;15(2):523–532.
Miller BF. Encyclopedia and Dictionary of Medicine, Nursing and Allied Health, 5th ed. Philadelphia: W.B. Saunders; 1992, p. 1029.
Missouri Department of Health and Senior Services [database on the Internet]. Springfield: MDHSS [cited 2004 Mar 3]. Missouri information for community assessment (MICA) [about 1 screen]. Available from: http://www.health.state.mo.us/MICA/nojava.html.
National Center for Health Statistics. Vital Statistics of the United States, 1992. Vol. II: Mortality Part B. PHS Publication No. 96-1102. Hyattsville, MD: National Center for Health Statistics; 1996 [cited 2002 May 23]. Available from: http://www.cdc.gov/nchs/products/pubs/pubd/vsus/vsus.htm.
National Center for Health Statistics. U.S. Vital Statistics System, Major Activities and Developments, 1950–95. Hyattsville, MD: National Center for Health Statistics; 1997.
National Center for Health Statistics. Report of the Panel to Evaluate the U.S. Standard Certificates. Hyattsville, MD: National Center for Health Statistics; 2000 [cited 2004 Mar 3]. Available from: http://www.cdc.gov/nchs/data/dvs/panelreport_acc.pdf.
National Center for Health Statistics. Births, marriages, divorces, and deaths: provisional data for August 2001. National Vital Statistics Reports. Vol. 50, No. 7. DHHS Publication No. 2002-1120. Hyattsville, MD: National Center for Health Statistics; 2002 [cited 2002 May 23]. Available from: http://www.cdc.gov/nchs/products/pubs/pubd/nvsr/nvsr.htm.
National Center for Health Statistics [homepage on the Internet]. Hyattsville, MD: NCHS [updated 2004 Mar 1; cited 2004 Mar 3]. Available from: http://www.cdc.gov/nchs/default.htm.
National Center for Health Statistics [homepage on the Internet]. Hyattsville, MD: NCHS [updated 2003 Sep 25; cited 2004 Mar 3]. Classifications of diseases and functioning and disability [about 3 screens]. Available from: http://www.cdc.gov/nchs/icd9.htm.
National Center for Health Statistics [homepage on the Internet]. Hyattsville, MD: NCHS [updated 2004 Feb 25; cited 2004 Mar 3]. International Classification of Functioning, Disability and Health (ICF) [about 5 screens]. Available from: http://www.cdc.gov/nchs/about/otheract/icd9/icfhome.htm.
National Center for Health Statistics [homepage on the Internet]. Hyattsville, MD: NCHS [updated 2002 Oct 21; cited 2004 Mar 3]. NCHS guidelines for ensuring the quality of information disseminated to the public [about 8 screens]. Available from: http://www.cdc.gov/nchs/about/quality.htm.
National Center for Health Statistics [homepage on the Internet]. Hyattsville, MD: NCHS [updated 2004 Jan 5; cited 2004 Mar 3]. Public Health Data Standards Consortium [about 5 screens]. Available from: http://www.cdc.gov/nchs/otheract/phdsc/phdsc.htm.
National Center for Health Statistics [homepage on the Internet]. Hyattsville, MD: NCHS

[updated 2002 Sep 13; cited 2004 Mar 3]. Rate [about 3 screens]. Available from: http://www.cdc.gov/nchs/datawh/nchsdefs/rates.htm.

National Center for Health Statistics [homepage on the Internet]. Hyattsville, MD: NCHS [updated 1999 Nov 5; cited 2004 Mar 3]. Research and methods [about 2 screens]. Available from: http://www.cdc.gov/nchs/r&d/rm.htm.

National Center for Health Statistics [homepage on the Internet]. Hyattsville, MD: NCHS [updated 2004 Jan 28; cited 2004 Mar 3]. Washington Group on Disability Statistics. Current objectives, as modified at first meeting [about 2 screens]. Available from: http://www.cdc.gov/nchs/about/otheract/citygroup/objectives.htm.

National Center for Health Statistics [homepage on the Internet]. Hyattsville, MD: NCHS [updated 2003 Sep 3; cited 2004 Mar 3]. What is ICE on automating mortality? [about 4 screens]. Available from: http://www.cdc.gov/nchs/about/otheract/ice/automort/automort.htm.

National Committee on Vital and Health Statistics. Core Health Data Elements. Hyattsville, MD: National Center for Health Statistics; 1996 [cited 2004 Mar 3]. Available from: http://www.ncvhs.hhs.gov/ncvhsr1.htm.

National Committee on Vital and Health Statistics. Uniform Data Standards for Patient Medical Record Information. Washington, DC: National Committee on Vital and Health Statistics; 2000 [cited 2004 Mar 3]. Available from: http://www.ncvhs.hhs.gov/hipaa000706.pdf.

National Committee on Vital and Health Statistics. Classifying and Reporting Functional Status. Washington, DC: NCVHS; 2001a.

National Committee on Vital and Health Statistics. Information for Health: A Strategy for Building the National Health Information Infrastructure. Washington, DC: U.S. Department of Health and Human Services; 2001b [cited 2004 Mar 3]. Available from: http://ncvhs.hhs.gov/nhiilayo.pdf.

National Committee on Vital and Health Statistics. Letter to Tommy G. Thompson, Secretary, U.S. Department of Health and Human Services; 2002a Feb 27 [cited 2004 Mar 3]. Available from: http://www.ncvhs.hhs.gov/020227lt.htm.

National Committee on Vital and Health Statistics. NCVHS Patient Medical Record Information Terminology Analysis Reports. Washington, DC: National Committee on Vital and Health Statistics; 2002b [cited 2003 Dec 24]. Available from: http://www.ncvhs.hhs.gov/031105rpt.pdf.

National Institute of Standards and Technology. Federal Information Processing Standards Publication 5-2—Codes for the Identification of the States, the District of Columbia and the Outlying Areas of the United States, and Associated Areas. Gaithersburg, MD: NIST; 1987 [cited 2004 Mar 3]. Available at http://www.itl.nist.gov/fipspubs/fip5-2.htm.

National Institute of Standards and Technology. Federal Information Processing Standards Publication 6-4—Counties and Equivalent Entities of the United States, Its Possessions, and Associated Areas. Gaithersburg, MD: NIST; 1990 [cited 2004 Mar 3]. Available from: http://www.itl.nist.gov/fipspubs/fip6-4.htm.

National Institute of Standards and Technology. Federal Information Processing Standards Publication 8-6—Metropolitan Areas (including MAs, CMSAs, PMSAs, and NECMAs). Gaithersburg, MD: NIST; 1995 [cited 2002 July 10]. Available from: http://www.itl.nist.gov/fipspubs/fip8-6-0.htm.

National Library of Medicine [homepage on the Internet]. Bethesda, MD: NLM [cited 2004 Mar 3]. Available from: http://www.nlm.nih.gov.

National Research Council; Commission on Physical Sciences, Mathematics, and Applications; Computer Science and Telecommunications Board; Committee on Maintaining Privacy and Security in Health Care Applications of the National Information Infrastructure. For the Record: Protecting Electronic Health Information. Washington, DC: National Academies Press; 1997 [cited 2004 Mar 3]. Available from: http://books.nap.edu/openbook/0309056977/html/index.html.

National Standards Policy Advisory Committee. National Policy on Standards for the United States and a Recommended Implementation Plan. Washington, DC: National Standards Policy Advisory Committee; 1978, p. 6.

National Uniform Billing Committee [homepage on the Internet]. Chicago: American Hospital Association; c. 2004 [cited 2004 Mar 3]. Available from: http://www.nubc.org.

National Uniform Claim Committee [homepage on the Internet]. Chicago: American Medical Association; c. 2003 [cited 2004 Mar 3]. Available from: http://www.nucc.org.

North American Association of Central Cancer Registries [homepage on the Internet]. Springfield, IL: North American Association of Central Cancer Registries, Inc.; c. 2003 [cited 2003 Apr 7]. Available from: http://www.naaccr.org/. Chen V, President North American Association of Central Cancer Registries. Personal communication. 2003 Apr 10.

Office of Management and Budget. Revisions to the standards for the classification of federal data on race and ethnicity. Fed Reg 1997;62(210):58782–58790 [cited 2002 July 10]. Available from: http://www.whitehouse.gov/omb/fedreg/ombdir15.html.

Office of Management and Budget. Standards for defining metropolitan and micropolitan statistical areas; notice. Fed Reg 2000;65(249): 82228–82238 [cited 2004 Mar 3]. Available from: http://www.whitehouse.gov/omb/fedreg/metroareas122700.pdf.

Office of Management and Budget. North American Industry Classification System—United States, 2002. Springfield, VA: National Technical Information Service; 2002 [cited 2004 Mar 3]. Available from: http://www.census.gov/epcd/www/naics.html.

Office of Management and Budget. Revised Definitions of Metropolitan Statistical Areas, New Definitions of Micropolitan Statistical Areas and Combined Statistical Areas, and Guidance on Uses of the Statistical Definitions of These Areas. Washington, DC: Office of Management and Budget; 2003 [cited 2004 Jan 14]. Available from: http://www.whitehouse.gov/omb/bulletins/b03-04.html.

Office of Management and Budget [homepage on the Internet]. Washington, DC: OMB [cited 2004 Mar 3]. Agency Information Quality Guidelines [about 5 screens]. Available from: http://www.whitehouse.gov/omb/inforeg/agency_info_quality_links.html.

Office of Management and Budget [homepage on the Internet]. Washington, DC: OMB [cited 2004 Mar 3]. Statistical Programs and Standards [about 3 screens]. Available from: http://www.whitehouse.gov/omb/inforeg/statpolicy.html.

Protection of human subjects, 45 C.F.R. 46 Sect. 46.102 (1991) [cited 2004 Feb 8]. Available from: http://ohrp.osophs.dhhs.gov/humansubjects/guidance/45cfr46.htm#46.102.

Public Health Data Standards Consortium [homepage on the Internet]. Hyattsville, MD: National Center for Health Statistics [updated 2003 Jun 6; cited 2004 Mar 3]. Public Health Data Standards Consortium Web-based Resource Center [about 1 screen]. Available from: http://phdatastandards.info.

Registrar General of England and Wales. First Annual Report. London: Registrar General of England and Wales; 1839, p. 99.

Secretariat, Alliance for Telecommunications Industry Solutions. American national standard T1.523–2001. In: American National Standard for Telecommunications—Telecom Glossary 2000. New York: American National Standards Institute; 2001. Available from: http://www.its.bldrdoc.gov/projects/devglossary/t1g2k.html [cited 2004 Mar 3] or http://www.its.bldrdoc.gov/projects/devglossary/_de_facto_standard.html [cited 2004 Mar 3].

SNOMED International [homepage on the Internet]. Northfield, IL: College of American Pathologists; c. 2000–2003 [updated 2003 Jan 3; cited 2004 Mar 3]. Available from: http://www.snomed.org.

United Nations [homepage on the Internet]. New York: United Nations; c. 2003 [cited 2004 Mar 3]. Statistics Division. Disability statistic [1 screen]. Available from: http://unstats.un.org/unsd/disability.

United States Health Information Knowledgebase (USHIK) [registry on the Internet]. Washington, DC: ANSI Healthcare Informatics Standards Board [cited 2004 Mar 3].

Available from: http://156.40.135.128/registry/USHIKmain.html and http://www.ushik.org.

The United States National Committee on Vital and Health Statistics. October 1949. Cited in Kanaan 2001; p. 15.

U.S. Census Bureau. Appendix A. Census 2000 Geographic Terms and Concepts. Washington, DC: U.S. Census Bureau; 2000, pp. A1–A27 [cited 2004 Mar 3]. Available from: http://www.census.gov/geo/www/tiger/glossry2.pdf.

U.S. Department of Health and Human Services, Health Information Policy Council. Background paper: uniform minimum health data sets [unpublished]. Washington, DC: 1983.

U.S. Department of Health and Human Services. Health insurance reform: security standards. Fed Reg 2003a; 68(34):8334–8381 [cited 2004 Mar 3]. Available from: http://aspe.os.dhhs.gov/admnsimp/FINAL/FR03-8334.pdf.

U.S. Department of Health and Human Services [news release on the Internet]. Federal government announces first federal eGOV health information exchange standards. Washington, DC: USDHHS; 2003b Mar 21 [cited 2004 Mar 3]. Available from: http://www.hhs.gov/news/press/2003pres/20030321a.html.

U.S. Department of Health and Human Services [homepage on the Internet]. Washington, DC: USDHHS [updated 2001 Aug 9; cited 2004 Mar 3] Administrative simplification: privacy and security [about 3 screens]. Available from: http://aspe.os.dhhs.gov/admnsimp/bannerps.htm.

U.S. Department of Health and Human Services [homepage on the Internet]. Washington, DC: USDHHS [updated 2002 Oct 9; cited 2004 Mar 3]. The HHS Data Council [about 1 screen]. Available from: http://aspe.hhs.gov/datacncl/index.shtml.

Utah Department of Health [database on the Internet]. Salt Lake City: UDOH [cited 2004 Mar 3]. UDOH: Utah's Indicator-Based Information System for Public Health (IBIS-PH) [about 1 screen]. Available from: http://health.utah.gov/ibis-ph/index.html.

World Health Organization. International Statistical Classification of Diseases and Health Related Problems, vol. 2. Geneva: World Health Organization; 1993.

World Health Organization. International Classification of Functioning, Disability and Health. Geneva: World Health Organization; 2001.

World Health Organization. The World Health Report 2003—Shaping the Future. Geneva: World Health Organization; 2003 [cited 2004 Mar 3]. Available from: http://www.who.int/whr/en.

World Health Organization [homepage on the Internet]. Geneva: WHO; c. 2004 [cited 2004 Mar 3]. WHO family of international classifications [about 1 screen]. Available from: http://www.who.int/classification.

CHAPTER 9

Linking and Combining Data to Develop Statistics for Understanding the Population's Health

Charlyn Black and Leslie L. Roos

> Data are unlike other tools of the research endeavor. They provide the raw material from which information can be created. . . . [U]nlike printed tables which, like a postcard, provide a larger view of a larger phenomenon, data can act as a camera, allowing the researcher to manipulate the background, change the foreground and more fully investigate the object under study.
>
> —*Watkins (1994)*

This quote, from a Canadian initiative to make data more available to researchers, identifies data as the raw material of the research process, but speaks to a more complex process by which analysts can manipulate data to provide deeper understanding of important phenomena that we wish to understand more fully. It suggests that data collection is but one small component of the process of research and the production of health statistics—and that tremendous gains may come from paying attention to the processes by which we use data, especially in areas where we are seeking new understanding. To develop more compelling information about population health, we must therefore improve processes that will permit us to combine and use data to frame new perspectives.

Many U.S. states have recognized the need for reliable data-driven information to plan and implement health-care policy. However, these needs have been difficult to meet because data are typically gathered and stored in separate data systems geared to support distinct programs or applications. Despite having huge amounts of health data, few states have been able to leverage the data in their holdings to link information across databases and produce useful analyses. Such data linkages typically allow information on a particular person from one data system to be linked with information about that same person from another system. With linked data, it is possible to make use of information that already exists to gain a better, more comprehensive understanding of health status, service use, market patterns, expenditures, and health outcomes. In order to develop the next generation of health statistics, we must deliberately consider opportunities to link and combine data in powerful new ways to create a new generation of health statistics.

In its final report on developing a health statistics vision for the twenty-first century, the National Committee on Vital and Health Statistics (NCVHS) and its partners in the National Center for Health Statistics (NCHS) and the Department of Health and Human Services set out a bold new agenda for health statistics, one that was strongly influenced by a new model of the factors that influence the population's health (Friedman et al. 2002). This model is presented as Figure 1.3 of this book. The premise of the document was that the area of population health is one where there is a clear need to bring greater understanding; only recently have we identified some of the shortfalls in our frameworks for mapping factors that influence human health (Evans and Stoddart 1990; Friedman et al. 2002).

The health statistics vision document focused on developing a stronger approach to producing health statistics and identified the following processes as key elements in the health statistics cycle: (*1*) collecting, aggregating, and compiling data, (*2*) analyzing statistics, and (*3*) translating statistics, for users; the health statistics cycle is explicated in this book in Chapter 3 and in Figure 3.1. This chapter will review linkage and other ways of combining data, approaches that have enormous potential to enhance the portfolio of health statistics we create, to provide perspective on the health of populations and the factors that influence the patterns we observe, and to enhance dissemination of health statistics that will improve the approaches we use to make improvements in health.

WHAT IS LINKAGE?

What is record linkage? Simply stated, records from one database are somehow linked to records in another, separate database. Record linkage is accomplished in our daily lives, for instance when we review transactions in our bank statements and reconcile them with checkbooks, returned checks, and/or electronic transaction receipts. Sometimes the information is incorrect or incomplete, because we have written something down incorrectly, forgotten to write something down, or lost transaction slips. But we must use the less than perfect information we do have to draw conclusions about the accuracy of our bank statements. In essence, we must match (or link) multiple sources of data by examining transaction numbers and occasionally consulting other information, such as the amount of the payment, to ensure that our records are accurate (adapted from Dean and Olson 1999).

The use of linkage in research is not novel, although its popularity has increased significantly in recent years. The term *data linkage* has been used to refer to "the assembly of data in a common format from different sources but pertaining to the same unit of observation" such as a person, event or other unit (United Nations 1999). The more specific term *record linkage* was coined over 50 years ago in a paper describing the creation of individual "books of life" to be used for administrative and statistical purposes (Dunn 1946).

One classic work refers to record linkage as simply bringing together information from two records that are believed to relate to the same "entity" (Newcombe 1988). The same author suggested that for work in the area of health, the entities of interest are usually individual persons or families. Stated most simply, record linkage is a computer process that combines multiple sources of existing data at a common unit of analysis. It involves merging two or more files to ensure minimal misclassification so that records referring to the same entity are connected, while records without corresponding matches remain separate. In the realm of health, the term *linkage* typically refers to techniques that are used to identify and merge electronic records relating to the same person, encounter, or service provider. These techniques often involve personal identifiers and are therefore considered highly sensitive from a privacy perspective.

A recent report on record linkage and privacy published by the U.S. General Accounting Office (USGAO) extended the definition of record linkage beyond the concept of matching units of analysis to include "combining 1) existing person-specific data with 2) additional data that refer to the same persons, their family and friends, school or employer, area of residence or geographic environment" (USGAO 2001). This definition explicitly expands the definition of linkage as extending beyond matching of individual-level information to include information about contextual factors beyond the individual that are likely to influence health.

WHY LINK?

Record linkage has expanded markedly from the initial purposes imagined (Newcombe et al. 1959). Felligi and Sunter (1969), in a seminal publication, noted an expansion of interest in linkage techniques in the late 1960s. They attributed this increase to two factors: first, the creation (often as a by-product of administrative programs) of large files that require maintenance over long periods of time and that often contain important statistical information whose value could be increased by linkage of individual records in different files; and second, advances in electronic data processing equipment and techniques. These circumstances have only accelerated in the 36 years since publication of these observations, and linkage techniques now have many applications in government statistics, public administration, and the private sector, in addition to those in epidemiology and health services research (Felligi 1997; Howe 1998). Record linkage is also being used in research settings to maintain registries for longitudinal studies, to manage comprehensive multifile databases, and to link with external sources (Roos et al. 1998; Roos and Roos 2001). Some of the important factors that have driven the expanding use of record linkage approaches are described in recent reports from the National Academy of Sciences (Hewitt and Simone 2000; Institute of Medicine 2000; Mackie and Bradburn 2000). Benefits that relate to the production of health statistics are outlined below.

Answering New Questions and Providing New Perspectives

Since data are typically gathered and stored in separate data systems to support distinct programs or applications, one of the most compelling reasons for expanding the use of linkage techniques is to address questions that would be impossible to answer with a single data source. Linking records from two existing data files to form a new data file expands the power of the information beyond that contained in each separate file. Linking data from a variety of sources can enable decision makers to obtain analyses that would otherwise be impossible or prohibitively expensive.

Linked data that integrate health service use with demographic and lifestyle information can help answer key questions about health, health care, and public health issues. For example, linkage can be used to answer the question "What is the impact of seat belt use on the charges incurred in hospitals following motor vehicle crashes?" (Dean and Olson 1999). This relatively simple and important question is impossible to answer simply by consulting traffic records, crash records, or hospital records. Indeed, it cannot be answered unless one links crash records with hospital records.[1] In this example, linkage clearly advances understanding beyond the scope of the underlying data sources.

As another example, a state can link multiple sources of data to develop statistics about children's immunization status. For instance, information on immunizations received by one low-income child might be captured in any of the following data holdings: (*1*) public health clinic records; (*2*) physician, clinic, and outpatient hospital medical claims data; (*3*) Medicaid Early and Periodic Screening, Diagnosis, and Treatment (EPSDT) data systems; (*4*) managed care plan encounter data; (*5*) Medicaid enrollment files; and (*6*) school system records (Chu et al. 1998). Any single source of data, however, will provide incomplete information. A critical challenge for policymakers who want to track and improve immunizations in their states is to bring all these data together to determine whether children are adequately covered and that immunizations are not being missed or repeated unnecessarily.

Finally, linking and combining data can provide powerful new perspectives and understandings. A recent report on record linkage and privacy by the USGAO suggests that when researchers and statisticians link records, they are putting together "pieces of a puzzle" (USGAO 2001). Once linked, diverse data sources—that as individual data sets may be limited in breadth or depth—can generate more detailed, more comprehensive, and potentially more valuable information. Perhaps even more important, linkage can support the creation of new information that might not be obtainable in any other way. Since linkage is often applied to data collected in the course of delivering programs that represent important public investments, linkage techniques applied to the administrative files generated from such programs support increased and more appropriate use of empirical data in planning, evaluation, and policy formulation. Boruch et al. (1991) argued that linkage using existing data sources helps to support work that meets both scientific standards and requirements for policy relevance.

Achieving Efficiencies in Using Data

It is well recognized that U.S. states collect huge amounts of health data but have great difficulty answering questions that matter. In addition to answering important questions in scientifically valid ways, linkage strategies that use existing databases provide an efficient and relatively inexpensive approach, in contrast to approaches that would collect new information for each question identified for study. Reduced data collection costs are also associated with other benefits in the form of reduced information burdens for both respondents and care providers.

Over time, the production of health statistics has benefited from recognizing the value of large, representative samples, of replication of approaches, of longitudinal analysis, and of obtaining a broad array of measures—all factors that add to the cost of data collection. The consequence has been a growing recognition that a small number of well-planned, fully funded, multipurpose data collection strategies may serve the needs of health statistics better than a plethora of narrowly focused approaches. Linkage subsequently allows us to maximize the benefits of such investments by allowing us to bring information together. It also contributes to reducing data collection costs and reducing the burden on respondents over the longer term, perhaps therefore indirectly contributing to reduced sampling bias and a more "virtuous" cycle of data collection.

Validating Data Sources and Improving Data Quality

Many researchers have relied extensively on record linkage techniques to ensure data quality in the acquisition and development of data. In Canada, linkage has been used to generate population-based research registries from periodic snapshots of provincial health insurance registries (Chamberlayne et al. 1998; Roos and Nicol 1999). When two files are supposed to contain the same individuals, the degree of overlap between the files provides a measure of the quality of the information system. If the same individuals are supposed to be on both files, are they? And if not, why not? Such issues are important both for developing and maintaining registries (linking between registry and vital statistics) and for linking across other files (e.g., linking between hospital and physician files). Cross-sectional Canadian analyses typically find between 96% and 99+% percent agreement between files with regard to specifying individuals covered under provincial insurance systems (Chamberlayne et al. 1998; Howe 1998).

Comparing content across data sources presents other opportunities for data validation. With individuals specified as being on both files, individual items (date of death, presence of a procedure or diagnosis) can be compared to ascertain the degree of agreement (Roos et al. 1989) and used to provide important information about the validity of the data holdings. Linkage has also permitted the validation of administrative data through triangulation of items in relation to survey and clinical information (Roos and Nicol 1999).

Supporting Long-Term Follow-Up and Tracking of Outcomes

Just as linkage provides opportunities to link across data sets, it also provides opportunities to link events that occur at different points in time. For example, individuals who have experienced a past event such as a surgical procedure can be followed to study health outcomes such as risk of readmission to a hospital for complications and mortality. Many data sets (hospital, medical claims, pharmaceutical, nursing home, home care) can be used to track use of services, making it possible to compile comprehensive histories for individuals over time. Other studies have used record linkage techniques to conduct extensive longitudinal analyses (Havens and Hall 2001). This is a critically important feature to exploit if we are to develop health data and information that can measure the impact of factors that influence health, since the effects of many factors are not immediate but occur many years later.

Supporting Population-Based Approaches

Many data sets used in linkage are population based. As more medical information migrates to electronic systems in the future, population-based information will become the norm. Many states currently collect data on 100% of hospitalizations. Most states also collect information on births and deaths, contagious diseases, emergency medical services, and dozens of other areas of public health interest. Given the investment in collecting these population-based data, interest in linking databases will increase, enabling us to answer many more complex questions for entire state populations. Population-based approaches also support the study of rare outcomes, an important approach for public health.

Building Information-Rich Environments

Roos and Roos (2001) have argued that record linkage techniques combined with population-based insurance systems allow the creation of "information-rich" environments. They cite examples from around the world, including several Canadian provinces, western Australia, Scotland, and Oxfordshire in the United Kingdom (Chamberlayne et al. 1998; Holman et al. 1999; Kendrick et al. 1998). In these settings, the existence of population-based registers, often developed to maintain information about individuals who are eligible for publicly funded health insurance, provides a framework for the development of rich systems of data. Together with routine annual updates of substantive files (building on consistent data formats), they allow the creation of multifile data environments that span many years of observation and support many types of analysis, including cohort studies of outcomes and studies of variation over time. These innovations provide an epidemiologic perspective on health care, building on ideas introduced by White et al. (1961) over 40 years ago. Figure 9.1 provides an example of the data holdings of one such information-rich environment (Roos et al. 2003).

Creating and managing an information-rich environment can be conceptualized as a series of investments that build on one another. The first set of activities includes data acquisition, maintenance, and enhancement. A second set of activities represents the development of tools—specific measures of health and health-care use for various entities within the data holdings, many of which require linkage of various data sets (Burchill et al. 2000). Both of these activities—data maintenance and tool development—in turn, support more substantive research in specific fields such as epidemiology, clinical epidemiology, health services research, health economics, and health policy. For example, person-based and provider-based measures of service use can be developed across a constellation of data sets—hospital, physician, long-term care, home care, and pharmaceutical—to construct comprehensive patterns of service use over a defined time period. These, in turn, can be used to identify high users of care (Reid et al. 2003) or to study variations in population-based patterns of use across a variety of types of care (Black et al. 1999; Martens et al. 2003). Similarly, person-based and provider-based profiles of service use can be constructed over time to identify changing patterns of care (Watson et al. 2003, 2004). Record linkage plays a critical part in all three of the activities (i.e., data acquisition, maintenance, and enhancement; tool development; and substantive research) required to support an information-rich research environment. These environments maximize the value and richness of data sets that, by themselves, are subject to various limitations—

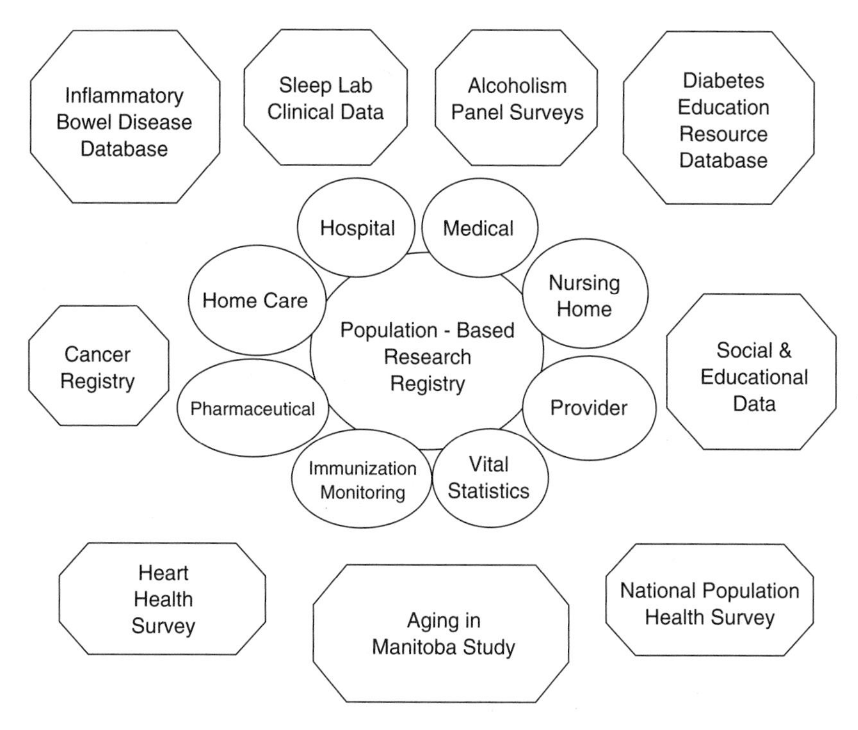

FIGURE 9.1
An example of data holdings and linkage in an information-rich environment: the Manitoba Population Health Research Data Repository and linkable databases. The inner ring of files represents administrative data that are routinely linked for updating and ongoing projects. The outer ring of files represents various external data sets that investigators have linked with the administrative data. (Source: Roos et al 2003.)

for areas such as health-care delivery and outcomes (USGAO 2001). They also provide opportunities to combine information from disparate data sets and address lacunae in single-source data holdings, using the most valid information available; such environments represent an important model for building future capacity to improve health statistics.

Supporting New Applications

Finally, data linkage can play a role in unforeseen applications in the development of health statistics. As an example, Winkler (1997, 1998) suggests that data collection agencies use linkage techniques to improve protection of confidentiality of public release data files. There is a substantially increased demand from researchers for large, general-purpose, public-use files that can be used for a variety of analyses. Balancing these analytic needs are requirements that agencies not release individually identifiable data. When a public-use file is created, agencies must determine if the file meets analytic needs and confidentiality requirements. Winkler has described the use of record linkage methods to assess privacy risks associated with the production of such public-use data files. Record linkage methods that employ new metrics for comparing somewhat related quantitative data provide a useful enhancement and yield higher reidentification rates than less sophisticated methods. If an agency can effectively use these techniques to determine that a small percentage of records might be reidentified, then it can take additional precautions to protect these public-use files.

WHY IS LINKAGE IMPORTANT FOR DEVELOPING POPULATION HEALTH STATISTICS?

Our increasing ability to develop, accumulate, store, retrieve, and use vast numbers of electronic records in an ever faster and more cost–efficient manner is widely recognized. To date, however, our use of this information to advance our understanding of population health has been limited to relatively small demonstrations of potential. The previous section identifies many advantages that linkage can provide to move us forward in improving health statistics.

The model of influences on the population's health presented in Chapter 1 identifies the broad set of factors that must be understood and brought into focus by a forward-looking health statistics enterprise (see Fig. 1.3). What is unique about this model is its focus on levels other than the level of the individual (i.e., individual health states and predictors of those states). In fact, all variables in the model are either aggregate or ecological, where aggregate measures represent those community attributes that can be derived from individual members of the community (e.g., community age structure, median household income) and ecological measures represent those community attributes that are not derivable from the attributes of individual members of the community (e.g., measured levels of water or air pollution, public health policies). This model clearly moves us beyond a focus on characteristics of individual health and its influences, but it also requires a shift in thinking about data sources and mechanisms to combine data to gain perspective on population health. MacIntyre et al. (2002) have recently argued for an agenda of increased conceptualization, operationalization, and measurement of *place effects* as a critically important agenda for population health. They suggest moving beyond treating place effects simply as a residual category of unexplained variation, focusing more explicitly on factors that underlie such effects, and developing robust theoretical frameworks to explain their mechanisms of influence. Consistent with Figure 1.3, they stress the importance of studying the effects of compositional or contextual data, which refer to area- or group-level variables, and urge us to expand our approaches beyond those that have driven our current data collection strategies.[2] Clearly, from a population health perspective, such suggestions have implications for how we develop our data systems. A focus on population health requires that we put the pieces together, see the bigger picture, and seek to understand new and important relationships that focus on factors that influence the health of groups of individuals—in ways that differ from the assumptions that have driven many of our individual data collection strategies. Models of data development to inform health statistics must clearly build in the capacity for measurement and linkages across individuals and context, as well as over time and across place.[3] The following section introduces a framework for linking and combining data that builds on this perspective.

A FRAMEWORK FOR LINKING AND COMBINING DATA WITHIN THE CONTEXT OF POPULATION HEALTH

Much of what we know about linking and combining data sources is derived from a perspective that operates at the level of the individual. While this perspective is relevant, in order to understand the levels at which data can and must be combined to further an understanding of population health, we require a data development framework that explicitly includes these multiple levels and perspectives. While important advances can be achieved by pursuing linkages at the individual level, we must link and combine data at other levels in order to advance our understanding of population health. A potential framework for describing the types of data development and linkage that underpin such a vision is outlined in Figure 9.2. This figure is consistent with the model for influences on population health outlined in Chapter 1 and builds on the framework for linkage advanced by the U.S. General Accounting Office (2001). It identifies data and linkage at the level of the individual (i.e., the person level) as an important part of the data and linkage terrain, and one that contributes important perspective about the health of populations. But Figure 9.2 also identifies data related to context as important information to be added and combined to better understand both individual and population health. New systems of health statistics must therefore consider opportunities for linkage of three different types: linkages of data at the individual or person level; linkages between person-level data with data about the contexts in which individuals live, work, and spend time; and linkages of data about contexts. Each of these is discussed below.

Person Level

Most of our deliberate and routine data collection strategies operate at the level of the individual and focus on aspects of individual perceptions, experiences,

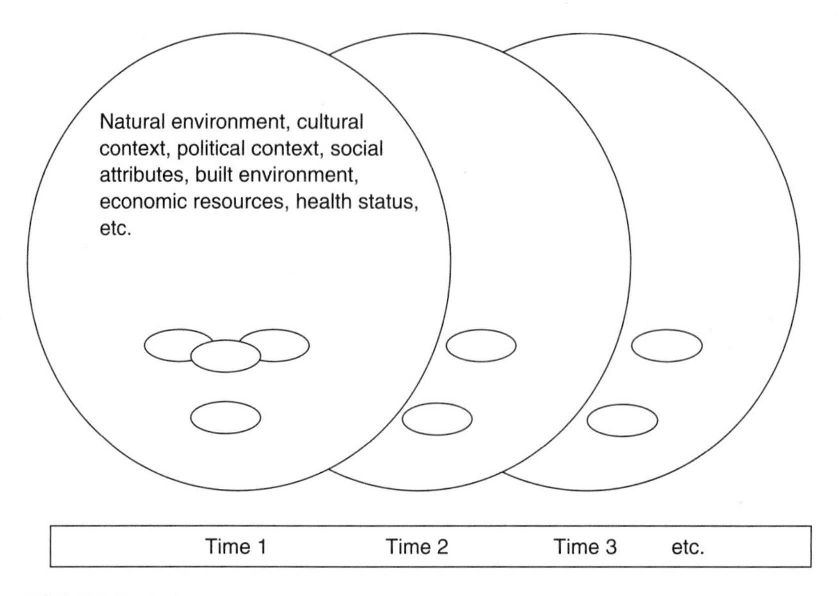

FIGURE 9.2
A framework for describing data development and linkage.
Context-Level Observations and Linkage
Provide information about the context in which person-level attitudes, behaviors, or other experiences take place. This level includes both aggregate (derived from individual-level observations) and ecological (attributes not derivable from attributes of individuals) observations, often related to specific populations or geographic locations.
Person-by-Context-Level Linkage
Provides information about the relationship between individuals and the contexts that influence their lives.
Person-Level Linkage
Multiperson observations requiring individual-level linkage
Provide information about groups based on a relationship between persons (e.g., spouses, best friends, families)
Person-level observations and linkage
Provide information about individuals (e.g., personal characteristics, behavior, service use, health status)
Linkage Across Time
Linkages for any level above can be made at a single point in time as well as across points in time.

health states, and service encounters—some of which are directly aimed at improving health (e.g., medical care) and others of which are aimed at other aspects of our lives that nonetheless have important effects on health (e.g., educational experience). The overwhelming majority of linkage activity has also taken place at this level. Person-level linkages represent the best fit with Newcombe's (1988) definition of record linkage and are the most extensively documented and used form of linkage activity. Data sources for this level of analysis include sample surveys and archival or registry data sets.[4] Linkage activities can occur for single persons, across persons who have some attribute in common (e.g., multiperson observations such as mothers and children, siblings, twins, friends), within single data sets, and across data holdings, as well as over time and place.

Examples of this type of linkage range from simple one-off studies to more complex and involved research programs.[5] As an example of a person-level linkage study across data sets and over time, Tsuji et al. (2003) published results based on linkage of a survey of National Health Insurance beneficiaries in rural Japan with their claims history files in order to study the relationship between time spent walking and costs of medical care. Baseline survey results from 1994 were used to identify a cohort of 27,431 Japanese men and women who had no functional limitation or conditions interfering with physical activity in order to characterize the amount of time they spent walking each day (less than or equal to 30 minutes, 30 minutes to 1 hour, or over 1 hour) and to measure important confounders. Survey results were linked with claims history files at a later point in time to measure hospitalizations, outpatient visits, and hospital costs. The study found that survey reports of time spent walking in 1994 were significantly associated with lower medical costs 1 to 4 years later after adjusting for potential confounders.

A more extensive program of individual-level linkage has been undertaken in California, where statewide hospital discharge data have been linked with three other types of data—birth records, death data, and cancer registry records for breast cancer—each owned by different state agencies or departments (Chu et al. 1998). Live birth records from the vital statistics system linked with hospital discharge data have allowed researchers to determine the general effects of morbidity, prenatal care, hospital care, and demographic factors on birth outcomes. Death data linked with hospital discharge data have facilitated the analysis of treatment patterns, effectiveness of treatment, costs of different illnesses, and causes of death. Finally, the linkage of breast cancer registry data has allowed study of the effectiveness of different treatments for cancer.

In the area of mother-child health, states have undertaken different approaches to developing programs of research that use extensive linkage infrastructure. For example, Hawaii's long-term perinatal data development strategy links birth certificate data with hospital discharge data, as well as with data from newborn screening programs for metabolic and hearing disorders (Prince 2001). The Massachusetts Pregnancy to Early Life Longitudinal Linkage (PELL) Project has been built on an extensive program of data development to assess the impact of prenatal environment on subsequent child (and maternal) health. This program draws on a collection of data that includes birth certificates, hospital discharge data for the mother and child, death records, and special program files. The data development program builds on three major sets of data linkage activities: (*1*) linkage of core data holdings (birth certificate, children's hospital discharge records, maternal hospital discharge records, and fetal death records);

(*2*) linkage with programmatic files (Women, Infants, and Children [WIC], early intervention, healthy start programs, and MassHealth data); and (*3*) longitudinal linkage involving maternal predelivery records and postdelivery linkage of service delivery information for both mother and child, as well as subsequent birth information for mothers (Kotelchuck et al. 2003). This program has extensive experience in applying probabilistic linkage techniques (i.e., linkage without unique identifiers that relies on using identifiers such as hospital number and medical record number, baby's date of birth, mother's date of birth, date of delivery, and zip code), in developing extensive processes for both validation and enhancement of linkage algorithms, and in addressing confidentiality and access issues associated with data linkage. The U.S. Health Resources and Services Administration's Maternal and Child Health Bureau provided funding under the State Systems Development Initiative (SSDI) to develop the state-level mother-child health data infrastructure. It focuses on establishing or improving data linkages between birth records and infant death certificates, Medicaid eligibility or paid claims files, WIC eligibility files, and newborn screening files, with additional support for improving access to additional data resources. The SSDI has stimulated considerable activity across states to link and use data to improve delivery of maternal and child health programming.

PERSON-BY-CONTEXT LEVEL

A second level of linkage and analytic activity moves beyond linkage at the individual level and focuses on linking individual-level data with data about the contexts, environments, or places in which individuals spend their time. This important emerging area recognizes that features beyond our individual-level experiences (e.g., the nature of our family situations, peer groups, working environments, the communities in which we live, the physical environments to which we are exposed, and the policies that affect our lives) profoundly influence the health of individuals, as well as the health states of the larger population groups to which we belong. Emerging work focuses on promoting understanding of the direct impacts of these contextual factors, as well as the mechanisms by which these contextual factors interact with our individual characteristics to produce variations in health. The USGAO (2001) referred to these larger influences as *context* and to this level of linkage as *person-by-context linkage.*

Person-by-context linkage brings together information about a person and information about a larger entity, context, or environment with which that person is associated (e.g., an individual and the characteristics of his or her work environment). These linkages do not fit with Newcombe's definition, but they represent an important and expanding area of investigation for the area of population health. The USGAO report identifies several examples of such work; for example, the National Institute of Child Health and Human Development has linked health survey data on teens with data about the neighborhoods and schools with which they are associated (USGAO 2001). Other work being supported by both the National Cancer Institute and the Centers for Medicare and Medicaid Services has linked Surveillance, Epidemiology, and End Results (SEER) clinical data and Medicare insurance records to census tract information based on patient address data. Other examples of person-by-context linkage are now appearing with increasing frequency in published research, to the point that one commentary declared that in less than 10 years, the field of epidemiology has been transformed by this activity (O'Campo 2003).

Multilevel studies assessing the effects of neighborhood residential environments (measured using aggregate-level measures of context, either as compositional or contextual variables) on health or health-care outcomes have been the most common type of study to date. For example, Merkin et al. (2002) examined the association between geographic socioeconomic status and advanced-stage breast cancer separately for whites and blacks by linking person-level breast cancer information to context-level measures of residential education and income. They found independent racial and socioeconomic differences in the risk of advanced-stage breast cancer in a large, diverse population in New York City. After adjusting for age and year at diagnosis, residence in areas with lower levels of education and income increased the odds of presenting with advanced-stage breast cancer by 50% for black women and by 75% for white women. In a more complex person-by-context linkage study, Pearl et al. (2001) studied relationships between neighborhood socioeconomic characteristics and birth weight, while accounting for individual socioeconomic characteristics, among five ethnic groups. Person-level birth records for women delivering infants at 18 California hospitals were linked to measures of neighborhood levels of poverty, unemployment, and education that were derived from census block (i.e., context-level) data. Additional person-level information on income and other factors was obtained from a survey of a subset of the women included in the study population. This study, involving both person-level and context-level measures for socioeconomic status, was able to adjust for mothers' individual socioeconomic characteristics as well as context-level measures of socioeconomic status and other risk factors. Less favorable neighborhood socioeconomic characteristics were associated with lower birth weight among blacks and Asians, but there was no consistent relationship between neighborhood socioeconomic characteristics and birth weight among other ethnic groups. These findings were not explained by measured individual-level behavioral or cultural factors, demonstrating the greater importance of contextual factors for health outcomes. The authors concluded that, in addition to individual socioeconomic characteristics, living in neighborhoods that are less socioeconomically advantaged may differentially influence birth weight, depending on women's ethnicity and nativity.

Some have suggested that person-by-context linkage will become more extensive in the future, given the greater use of geographic positioning systems in research and data collection activities and the development of statistical methods such as multilevel modeling that can simultaneously assess the impact of both individual and context-level effects on health (USGAO 2001). Others have argued for the development of appropriate theoretical and methodological foundations for this area of work, which are currently underdeveloped (e.g., MacIntyre et al. 2002; O'Campo 2003). We are clearly on a very early trajectory in using person-by-context linkages to understand health impacts and develop health statistics, but this area is likely to generate new information that will be useful for planning programs and policy decision making. As with person-level linkage, this type of linkage may also be very sensitive from a privacy perspective. In contrast to person-level linkages, there is relatively little experience with this level of linkage to date.

Context Level

Studies at the context level are aimed at better understanding the nature of the larger contexts of our lives, aspects that profoundly affect our health. The term *context* encompasses the two broad levels of influence identified as important influences on population health in the health statistics vision model, *context* and *community attributes*, and includes a vast array of influences that have received relatively little systematic attention in health research or health statistics to date. For example, Chapter 1 identifies context-specific influences as including aspects such as the natural environment (e.g., climate and weather, air quality, environmental contaminants, geology, water resources, and animal vectors); the cultural context (e.g., degree of competition or cooperation); and the political context (e.g., public policies and laws, political culture, and political participation). Community resource–specific influences are identified in several areas: biologic characteristics (e.g., population characteristics, biologic composition such as genetic endowment and immune status, fertility, and natality); characteristics of the built environment (e.g., land use, urbanization, transportation); social (e.g., level of social support, education); economic (e.g., economic development and equity, work environment); population health programs (e.g., water supply and disposal); personal health practices; and health services.

To date, we have missed important opportunities to understand the impact of contextual influences and their individual effects on health. It therefore goes without saying that we have also missed opportunities to understand how they combine and interact to produce health effects for both populations and individuals. Understanding the impact of these larger influences represents an important future agenda for health research and for the development of population health statistics, one that is desperately needed to provide more comprehensive understanding of the factors that influence both individual and population health. Putting together information about contexts to support the health statistics enterprise can be understood as context-by-context linkage. As an analogy to linking person-level data, we should consider opportunities to combine or bring together non-person-level information from different sources to more fully describe populations or areas. This area has received little attention to date, both from a theoretical and an analytical perspective.

Some public health research has used contextual information to study impacts on health. A study by Shi and Starfield (2001), based on a multivariate ecologic analysis of 1990 data from 273 U.S. metropolitan areas, provides an example of this type of research. This study assessed whether income inequality and primary care physician supply have a different effect on mortality among blacks compared with whites. Both income inequality and primary care physician supply were significantly associated with white mortality; conversely, while the effect of income inequality on black mortality was significant, the effect of primary care physician supply was not, particularly in areas with high levels of income inequality. As another example, Krieger et al. (2003) have argued that the use of multilevel frameworks and area-based socioeconomic measures for public health monitoring can potentially overcome the absence of socioeconomic data in most U.S. public health surveillance systems. They have geocoded and linked public health surveillance data from Massachusetts and Rhode Island to 1990 block group, tract, and zip code area-base socioeconomic measures to study health outcomes, including death, birth, cancer incidence, tuberculosis, sexually transmitted infections, childhood lead poisoning, and nonfatal weapons-related injuries. Measures of economic deprivation (e.g., percentage below the poverty level) were most sensitive to expected socioeconomic gradients in health, with the most consistent results and maximal geocoding linkage evident for census tract–level analyses.

Some have argued that there is an urgent need for studies to go beyond the use of census or administrative data. To date, however, few studies of context and health have simultaneously examined the role of economic, political, cultural, and institutional processes. The rich neighborhood-level data from the Project on Human Development in Chicago Neighborhoods ([hp] 2001) provides some understanding of the possibilities for providing richer data about context. For this project, data are derived not only from observational videos taken of block faces (i.e., videotaping environments and residences) but also from repeated surveys of several thousand randomly selected residents. Similar data collection efforts, perhaps on a smaller scale than this project, will have to be undertaken for future contextual research if information on domains that are not captured in census and administrative data are to be captured. Challenging issues such as spatial definitions, defining areas for study, and how to combine information to provide richer information about context will all need to be addressed to improve our ability to understand the impact of contextual influences on health.

Linking and Combining Over Time

A final dimension for understanding linkage is time. In the discussion above, it was clear that linkages and combinations of data take place *within* each of the three levels for a particular time and place. Another important dimension of understanding for population health involves the study of factors that influence health at each of these levels—person level, person-by-context level, and context level—over time. This is very important because of the temporal nature of influences on health: person-level and context-level influences are unlikely to have immediate effects on health and are more likely to exert their influence at much later points in time. Linkages at all three levels can be made over various time frames: short, long, life course, and even over generations.

Many published studies use linkage at the person level to examine the relationship between factors that influence health and temporally lagged measures of health outcomes. An example was described earlier in this chapter in the discussion of person level linkage (Tsuji et al. 2003). Examples at the context level exist in a series of studies that have been published by Brenner (e.g., Brenner 2002). Brenner examines the impact of contextual factors that relate to labor policy, employment rates, unemployment rates, and other factors on population-level health effects, such as mortality rate and life expectancy, using temporally lagged models. Similar opportunities exist to link data about longer-term health outcomes in person-by-context linkage activities, greatly expanding our ability to understand the temporal aspects of how contextual influences affect health outcomes at both the individual and population levels. However, the issue of measuring the impact of multiple contextual factors that may exert their effects on health over different periods of time will raise additional theoretical and methodical challenges for future research and production of health statistics.

TECHNICAL ASPECTS OF LINKAGE

Linkage involves bringing together information from two records that are believed to relate to the same individual or family. Record linkage involves combining two data sets that have some commonality in terms of the variables used to identify individuals. The fundamental operation at the core of all forms of record linkage is the comparison of partially identifying data from two (or more) sources. The comparison may be as simple as determining whether the values match exactly. Linkage is achieved by comparing a limited subset of the total available information for an individual, using specified *linkage variables* selected for their ability to identify an individual uniquely and reliably. These variables may include name, address (or geocode), date of birth (or death), and scalar quantities such as age, as well as other assigned identifiers (e.g., hospital number).[6] Linkage is much simpler if a reliably coded unique identifier (such as the Social Security number) is available. Where a unique common identifier is not available, the task is more difficult; typically, an ensemble of nonunique, partially identifying attributes such as name, date of birth, and address are used to infer probabilistically which records refer to the same entity. The accuracy of linkage varies because, for example, some names are very common, the digits in some key variables may be recorded with some degree of error, or many of the attributes used for linkage (such as address) vary over time.

Any variable that discriminates between records may act as a linkage variable, and different selections or combinations of linkage variables can be used in the process of integrating data sets. Actual implementation of record linkage typically involves an iterative process in which the cycle of matching and distinguishing linked pairs continues until no further links can be made. Each linkage step leads to a re-examination of earlier results and may influence the choice of linkage variables in a subsequent iteration. As a result, even in highly automated environments, record linkage processes benefit from extensive human involvement to examine the effect of different linkage variables, to scrutinize record pairs, to remove acceptable matches, and to plan the next linkage iteration.

Two main approaches to linkage—*deterministic* and *probabilistic*—have been described. Deterministic linkage generates candidate record pairs based on explicit instructions about the relative ability of each linkage variable to identify potential matches and the number of linkage variables in each pair. This approach provides a simple but subjective categorical assessment (i.e., yes, no, possible) of the likelihood that any candidate pair represents a match. Deterministic linkage is relatively simple and should be used primarily when data collections share a common, unique entity or identifier, or when the data are known to be complete and to have few coding errors. Probabilistic linkage uses information in the data to estimate the likelihood that the records represent a match and then uses that information in the decision-making process. Each method has advantages. Probabilistic linkage is more robust when relatively few linkage variables are available, data are incomplete, or coding errors are common. However, probabilistic linkage is more complex to implement than deterministic linkage, so accuracy versus simplicity often becomes an important trade-off (Newcombe et al. 1989a, 1989b; Roos and Wajda 1991).

Data linkage represents a complex and growing area of activity, and many resources can be currently accessed for a more in-depth discussion of technical issues (e.g., ANU Data Mining Group [hp] 2003; Newcombe 1988).

PRIVACY ISSUES ASSOCIATED WITH LINKAGE

Techniques to link and combine data for research and statistics, because of their power to shift the focus and increase the specificity of findings, raise privacy issues that go beyond the considerations of working with individual data sets. This section will outline some of the associated issues.[7] In Chapter 14, Fanning addresses broader issues in privacy and confidentiality.

Linkage may heighten the sensitivity of data sets that, separately, appear to be relatively innocuous. For example, if person-specific survey responses about health behavior are linked to reportable public health public information such as human immunodeficiency virus (HIV) status—and the results indicate that infected individuals are engaged in risky behavior that is likely to put others at risk of contracting the disease—the linked data would be even more sensitive than the original independent data. Even some person-to-context links could create sensitivity by, for example, making it possible to identify persons associated with residential areas, schools, or places of employment that have specific characteristics (e.g., high rates of stigmatized diseases). Although not all linkage activity increases the sensitivity of the resultant data, it is fair to say that sensitivity is potentially increased whenever the whole is greater than the sum of the parts. For a variety of reasons, certain questions—or linkages—may be perceived as sensitive by at least some data subjects even if there appears to be no risk of harm in the eye of the researcher or other outside observers.

Activities to link data may also raise privacy issues associated with the sharing of personal information beyond a single agency, with attendant risks to confidentiality and security. Traditionally, data have been kept separately and various statutes have been enacted to prohibit or control certain kinds of data sharing. In order to carry out record linkage, agencies must share identifiable person-specific data, and it is necessary for someone to be given access to the ensemble of identifying attributes for all of the relevant records in the data collections to be linked. Good practice dictates that substantive information contained in the records of each database should be removed before the record is passed to a person or organization undertaking the linkage process. In addition, some *trusted third party* should be selected as the agency or organization to undertake the record linkage function in order to safeguard the perceived as well as thé actual confidentiality of the linkage process. A number of protocols for this have been described (Boruch and Cecil 1979; Churches 2003; Kelman et al. 2002; Pommerening et al. 1996).

In general, data collected for research or statistical purposes should not be made available for administrative action toward a particular subject. According to this principle, information collected or compiled for research or statistical purposes may enter into administrative and policy decision making only in aggregate or completely anonymous form. Although it is generally agreed that research and statistical data should be protected from use in government actions taken with respect to specific individuals, record linkage sometimes involves sharing research and statistical data with specific individuals or units within program agencies. For such situations, data-sharing arrangements and agreements must be developed to protect against improper uses. The important features of any agency or organization undertaking record linkage include the creation of stringent ethical frameworks and processes that circumscribe the activity and provide for appropriate penalties if contravened.

In spite of these activities, data linkage increases the potential for reidentification of individuals. Federal agencies have a long history of creating public-use data sets with deidentified information. These deidentified data have provided researchers and members of the general public with maximum access to information; they have also helped agencies maximize the return on their data collection investments. Growing concerns about reidentification risks have led to considerable efforts to develop methods aimed at minimizing these risks, which are likely higher for linked data sets than for the component data.

Finally, issues of data linkage raise issues about the need for consent for data linkage. Although data subjects' consent for linkage is sometimes obtained, in other instances subjects may be unaware that, in essence, new information about them is being created. Some linkages require data sharing between agencies; when this occurs, certain laws and policies concerning disclosure and consent are relevant. The U.S. Privacy Act generally requires consent for disclosure from one agency to another, but there are exceptions. Moreover, perceptions about the need for consent may vary according to the type of linkage. For example, consent requirements have been advocated for multiarchive links (because full sets of existing records often do not have a voluntary component) and for linkages that are not closely related to the original purpose of the data collection. Consent requirements have also been advocated when vulnerable populations are involved or when risks appear to be higher. There is a spectrum of opinions as to whether data subjects' consent is needed for both person-level and person-by-context linkage (USGAO 2001).

PROVIDING ACCESS TO LINKED HEALTH DATA AND STATISTICS

While the benefit of linkage accrues to society in general, any risk associated with linkage applies to the individual. The USGAO review of record linkage and privacy suggested that opinions and values on information issues are often conceptualized as a one-dimensional spectrum, ranging from those who put the highest priority on privacy issues to those who put the highest priority on information gains. Instead, they interviewed some experts who felt that it is possible to develop systems and models that prioritize *both* privacy and information gains (USGAO 2001). In fact, most federal agencies are accountable for ensuring appropriate standards of privacy and confidentiality, as well as facilitating responsible dissemination to users.

Many publicly funded U.S. data collectors regard dissemination of data and information—ranging from linked person-specific micro data sets, through detailed place-specific health data, to aggregate health statistics—as important parts of their mission. For example, the NCHS regards the dissemination of data, together with collection and analysis of data, as one of its key roles; the data collected are disseminated using a wide range of mechanisms and formats.

Development of thoughtful data and information release policies is therefore an essential component of public database collection and analysis. Considerations of access to all types of data, including linked data, require the development of approaches to protect the privacy of individuals and confidentiality of information about them. Agencies face trade-offs between providing wider access and more detailed information against these privacy risks. Over time, privacy concerns associated with release of sensitive data have led to the development of innovations that work to protect the privacy of individuals while ensuring that the public benefits inherent in the broader use of linked data can be achieved. Many different models have been developed to achieve this balance; a small number of successful models are described below.

A model used by many organizations is to provide access to data only in less sensitive tabular or aggregate formats, rather than providing direct access to micro-data.[8] As an example, the Massachusetts Community Health Information Profile (MassCHIP) provides free online access to a variety of health and social indicators (Massachusetts Department of Public Health [db]). It draws from multiple data sources to create compilations of indicators that provide community-level data that can be used to assess health needs, monitor health status, and evaluate health programs. It uses two formats to make this information accessible to users. Predefined (standard) reports provide information on a variety of topics for a choice of geography and include notes about population data, limitations of small numbers, differences from previously published data, and time period. As an alternative, customized reports are created through user-defined queries. These reports provide a great deal of flexibility and a more in-depth look with user-selected choices of data sets, variables, and statistical measures. Mapping and charting features are also available.

Another model of data access involves the development of research data archives. The essential functions of a data archive are to identify and preserve the best data sets in a field of inquiry, to promote the secondary use of these data sets through increased accessibility, and to do so more efficiently that the alternative informal system of data sharing between individual investigators or data holders. As important by-products, a good archive may promote standards of data quality for data collection and documentation, improve the teaching of both substance and method, and broaden and strengthen the network of analysts working in the field (Card and Peterson 1991). An example of this model is the University of Michigan's Inter-university Consortium for Political and Social Research (ICPSR), established in 1962. The ICPSR maintains and provides access to a vast archive of social science data for research and instruction, and offers training in quantitative methods to facilitate effective data use. To ensure that data resources are available to future generations of scholars, the ICPSR preserves data, shifting them to new storage media as changes in technology warrant. It also provides user support to assist researchers in identifying relevant data for analysis and in conducting their research projects. In addition, the ICPSR hosts a number of topical archives, including a Health and Medical Care Archive.

Other models focus on providing more direct access to micro-data in ways that facilitate in-depth analysis while addressing privacy risks. The NCHS is legislatively mandated to ensure that data are made as widely available as is practical, but must balance this requirement against the need to protect respondent confidentiality and to ensure data quality. It relies on a variety of data release strategies to fulfill this obligation, ranging from general public release of less sensitive files, to creation of special use files, to more restrictive access within the NCHS data center. The NCHS has recently released a policy on micro-data dissemination that provides a detailed discussion of the approaches used (National Center for Health Statistics 2002).

Yet another model of access to sensitive data involves the development of research centers that provide a very high degree of security to sensitive data holdings and support a concentration of expertise about data custodianship, handling, documentation, and development. Examples of these models include the Research Data Centers (RDCs) that have been developed by the NCHS. The continuing demand for analyses that require data at lower levels of geography such as states, counties, and even smaller areas, but without confidential identifiers, has provided the impetus for the creation of the RDC located at the NCHS headquarters. Designed for researchers outside of the NCHS, the RDC allows access to data that would not otherwise be permissible to analyze because of confidentiality and disclosure rules and regulations. Similar pressures in Canada have led to the creation of university-based RDCs that facilitate access to the data holdings of Statistics Canada at a number of sites across the country. The RDC program is part of an initiative by Statistics Canada, research funders, and universities to strengthen Canada's social research capacity and to support the policy research community. The RDCs provide researchers with access, in a secure university setting, to micro-data from population and household surveys. The centers are staffed by Statistics Canada employees and are accessible only to researchers with approved projects who have been sworn in under the Statistics Act as *deemed employees.*

An emerging Canadian model is the equivalent of a data laboratory. This model is exemplified by a number of Canadian research centers, which are largely funded by provincial governments and use data from provincially funded health insurance programs to develop programs of research that focus on health and health care. These organizations house large banks of administrative data files and engage in extensive data development activities to enhance the utility of their holdings, as described in the previous section on "Building Information-Rich Environments." From a data access perspective, there are two versions of these data laboratories. The first is a *fortress* model, in which researchers must be affiliated with the custodial organization and work on site to access the data for approved research projects (e.g., the Manitoba Centre for Health Policy and the Institute for Clinical Evaluative Sciences). The second is a *public utility* model, which has legislative authority to provide customized linked micro-data files for approved research projects to researchers external to the organization under clearly delineated processes, for example the British Columbia Linked Health Database (Centre for Health Services and Policy Research 2003).

IMPROVING PROSPECTS FOR LINKING AND COMBINING DATA

In spite of large demonstrated benefits, and in relation to the potential they can provide to a population health agenda, linkage strategies remain underused. A number of factors contribute to this situation. Fragmented approaches to health problems, the categorical nature of funding for health-related programs, and program-specific data systems discourage more comprehensive approaches. Combined with data collection strategies that focus on the individual and a relative underinvestment in systematic collection of contextual level data, we have missed opportunities to link and combine data to understand some of the major influences on human health. To date, our use of techniques to link and combine data has been limited to relatively small demonstrations of potential. This chapter suggests that a more comprehensive strategy, one that realizes the potential to be gained from putting the pieces together in a more deliberate fashion, is likely to yield important benefits.

While linkage techniques have been most extensively used at the person level, person-by-context linkage approaches have emerged as an important area of study over the past 10 years. In spite of this, conceptual models that explain the pathways by which contextual factors may influence individual and population health are at a relatively early stage of development. Advancement of these models represents a critical step for the refinement of data collection priorities and linkage strategies, given the prominent role of contextual factors in Figure 1.3.

Linkage raises important privacy issues that must be addressed. At the same time, in an era of increasing concerns about privacy, we face increasing demands for data at finer levels of detail. The recent USGAO (2001) report on record linkage and privacy suggests that it is possible to implement strategies that *simultaneously* enhance both information gains and privacy. As we develop the potential to use linked data, we must continue to pay meticulous attention to privacy, confidentiality, and security issues, ensure that the best practices are adopted, and constantly strive to improve privacy protection with emerging innovations. The USGAO report outlines approaches to building a *privacy toolbox* that includes adopting the best practices for data sharing, procedures for reducing reidentification risks, and techniques to reduce data sensitivity, as well as strategies for enhancing data stewardship. New approaches have been developed that can provide the benefits of access to linked data and information derived from linked data while mitigating privacy risks. We must also seek to better inform the public about the benefits and risks of data linkage in environments where privacy is taken seriously.

Linkages can be conducted on existing data in ways that have not been anticipated. As the potential for linkage becomes ever more apparent, new data collection tools must be developed to anticipate future uses of this approach. Survey tools should explicitly anticipate future linkages and request permission to link to defined data resources or to provide general support for less defined future linkages. It is important to recognize that future uses of population-based databases are nearly impossible to predict. The myriad questions that may be answered 5 or 10 years from now have not yet been conceived: it would be preposterous for us as researchers or regulators to fail to recognize this. Databases should be viewed as valuable assets that will be applied to difficult problems in the future, even as we acknowledge that we cannot predict those problems. At the same time, we must anticipate future opportunities for linkage and work to fill gaps in the data being collected if we are to develop more useful information and statistics about the population's health.

NOTES

1. An alternative would be to initiate an entirely new data collection effort, interviewing every victim of every crash, following up with every medical bill, and so on—an approach that would be prohibitively expensive and would not provide historical data for the period of interest.
2. The terms *compositional* and *contextual*, as used by Macintyre et al., are consistent with the terms *aggregate* and *ecological*, as used in the health statistics vision document.
3. As with person-specific data, data about context, provided at the same unit of observation, can also be linked, but are considered less sensitive because they do not relate to specific individuals. To recognize that different approaches are required for contextual data (in relation to both technical issues and to levels of sensitivity from a privacy perspective), linkage at this level will be referred to as *combining* data. For the purposes of this chapter, the term *linkage* will be used inclusively to mean any approaches to combine data elements at any level. Where greater specificity is required, the term *record linkage* will be used to refer to linkage that involves matching of records at the individual level and *combining data* will be used to refer to activities to merge or compile contextual level data.
4. A recent report by the USGAO (2001) used the term *archive* to refer to "a full set of existing records . . . that is intended to cover all relevant individuals." The document stressed the crucial importance of archival data sources because they make linkage to a sample survey or to other existing records possible. A detailed discussion of U.S. archival data is provided in the report.
5. For an extensive bibliography of published research using linkage techniques, many of which involve person level linkage, see http://www.ncbi.nlm.nih.gov/entrez/query.fcgi?CMD=Pager&DB=PubMed.
6. Geocodes are location codes, ranging from postal codes (e.g., zip code plus four digits) to latitude and longitude measures, which can be determined by handheld Global Positioning System devices.
7. For a more detailed discussion, readers are directed to a recent publication from the USGAO entitled *Record Linkage and Privacy: Issues in Creating New Federal Research and Statistical Information* (2001).
8. *Micro-data* refers to data files in which each record provides information for the unit of data collection, for example, an individual person (NCHS 2002).

REFERENCES

ANU Data Mining Group [homepage on the Internet]. Canberra, Australia: ANU Data Mining Group [updated 2003 Nov 21; cited 2003 Nov 22]. Parallel techniques for high-performance record linkage [about 10 screens]. Available from: http://datamining.anu.edu.au/projects/linkage.html.

Black C, Roos N, Fransoo R, Martens P. Comparative Indicators of Population Health and Health Care Use for Manitoba's Regional Health Authorities: A POPULIS Project. Winnipeg: Manitoba Centre for Health Policy, University of Manitoba; 1999.

Boruch RF, Cecil JS. Assuring the Confidentiality of Social Research Data. Philadelphia: University of Pennsylvania Press; 1979.

Boruch RF, Reiss A, Garner J, Larntz K, Freels S. Sharing confidential and sensitive data. In: Sieber JE, ed. Sharing Social Science Data. Newbury Park, CA: Sage; 1991, pp. 61–86.

Brenner MH. Unemployment and Public Health: Interim Report [monograph on the Internet]. Proceedings of the seminar on the study "Unemployment and Public Health": scientific evidence and policy implications; Brussels; 2001 Oct 5. Brussels: European Commission, Directorate General for Employment and Social Affairs; 2002 [cited 2004 Mar 10]. Available from: http://europa.eu.int/comm/employment_social/news/2002/may/unempl_en.html.

Burchill C, Roos LL, Fergusson P, Jebamani L, Turner K [serial on the Internet]. Organizing the present, looking to the future: an online knowledge repository to facilitate collaboration. J Med Internet Res 2000; 2(2):e10 [cited 2004 Mar 10]. Available from: http://www.jmir.org/2000/2/e10/index.htm.

Card JJ, Peterson JL. Establishing and operating a social science data archive. In: Sieber JE, ed. Sharing Social Science Data: Advantages and Challenges. Newbury Park, CA: Sage; 1991, pp. 116–127.

Centre for Health Services and Policy Research [homepage on the Internet]. Vancouver, BC: Centre for Health Services and Policy Research [updated 2003 Dec 12; cited 2004 Mar 10]. About the BCLHD [about 3 screens]. Available from: http://www.chspr.ubc.ca/Bclhd/aboutbclhd.htm.

Chamberlayne R, Green B, Barer ML, Hertzman C, Lawrence WJ, Sheps SB. Creating a population-based linked health database: a new resource for health services research. Can J Public Health 1998;89(4):270–273.

Chu K, Cherlow A, Gold M, Heiser N. How to link data sets to support policy development. In: The Stein Group, ed. Health Data in Action: A Series on Using Data and Information for State Health Policy. Document No. PP98-14. Washington: Mathematica Policy Research; 1998.

Churches T [serial on the Internet]. A proposed architecture and method of operation for improving the protection of privacy and confidentiality in disease registers. BMC Med Res Meth 2003 Jan 6;3(1):e1 [cited 2004 Feb 2]. Available from: http://www.biomedcentral.com/1471-2288/3/1.

Dean JM, Olson L. Protecting confidentiality of linked datasets: don't throw the baby out with the bathwater. In: Workshop on Confidentiality of and Access to Research Data Files: Workshop Papers. Washington, DC: Committee on National Statistics; 1999.

Dunn H. Record linkage. Am J Public Health 1946;36:1412–1416.

Evans RG, Stoddart GL. Producing health, consuming health care. Soc Sci Med 1990;31(12):1347–1363.

Felligi IP. Record linkage and public policy—a dynamic evolution. In: Alvey W, Jamerson B, eds. Record Linkage Techniques, 1997. Washington, DC: Federal Committee; 1997, pp. 3–12.

Felligi IP, Sunter AB. A theory for record linkage. J Am Stat Assoc 1969;64(328):1183–1210.

Friedman DJ, Hunter EL, Parrish RG, eds. Shaping a Health Statistics Vision for the 21st Century. Final Report, November 2002. Hyattsville, MD: Centers for Disease Control and Prevention, National Center for Health Statistics; Washington, DC: U.S. Department of Health and Human Services Data Council, National Committee on Vital and Health Statistics; 2002 [cited 2004 Mar 17]. Available from: http://www.ncvhs.hhs.gov/reptrecs.htm.

Havens B, Hall M. Challenges of longitudinal research with older populations: aging in Manitoba over thirty-years. Gerontologist 2001;41(1):386.

Hewitt M, Simone JV, eds. Enhancing Data Systems to Improve the Quality of Cancer Care. Washington, DC: National Academy Press; 2000.

Holman CDJ, Bass AJ, Rouse IL, Hobbs MST. Population-based linkage of health records in Western Australia: development of a health services research linked database. Aust NZ J Public Health 1999;23(5):453–459.

Howe GR. Use of computerized record linkage in cohort studies. Epidemiol Rev 1998; 20(1):112–121.

Institute of Medicine. Protecting Data Privacy in Health Services Research. Washington, DC: National Academy Press; 2000.

Kelman CW, Bass AJ, Holman CD. Research use of linked health data—a best practice protocol. Aust NZ J Public Health 2002;26(3):251–255.

Kendrick SW, Douglas MM, Gardner D, Hucker D. Best-link matching of Scottish health data sets. Methods Inf Med 1998;37(1):64–68.

Kotelchuck M, Barger M, Declercq G, Lazar J, Richman A, Weiss J, Nannini A, Thomashek K. The Massachusetts Pregnancy to Early Life Longitudinal (PELL) Linkage Project: overview, challenges, and opportunities [presentation on the Internet]; 2003 Mar 5 [cited 2004 Mar 10]. Available from: http://www.uic.edu/sph/cade/mchepi/meetings/march2003/index.htm.

Krieger N, Chen JT, Waterman PD, Rehkopf DH, Subramanian SV. Race/ethnicity, gender, and monitoring socioeconomic gradients in health: a comparison of area-based socioeconomic measures—The Public Health Disparities Geocoding Project. Am J Public Health 2003:93(10):1655–1671.

MacIntyre S, Ellaway A, Cummins S. Place effects on health: how can we conceptualise, operationalise and measure them? Soc Sci Med 2002;55:125–139.

Mackie C, Bradburn N, eds. Improving Access to and Confidentiality of Research Data: Report of a Workshop. Washington, DC: National Academy Press; 2000.

Martens P, Fransoo R, The Need to Know Team, Burland E, Jebamani L, Burchill C, et al. The Manitoba RHA Indicators Atlas: Population-Based Comparisons of Health and Health Care Use. Winnipeg: Manitoba Centre for Health Policy, University of Manitoba; 2003.

Massachusetts Department of Public Health [database on the Internet]. Boston: Massachusetts Department of Public Health [cited 2004 Mar 16]. Massachusetts Community Health Information Profile (MassCHIP). Available from: http://masschip.state.ma.us.

Merkin SS, Stevenson L, Powe N. Geographic socioeconomic status, race, and advanced stage breast cancer in New York City. Am J Public Health 2002;92(1):64–81.

National Center for Health Statistics [monograph on the Internet]. Policy on Micro-Data Dissemination. Hyattsville, MD: National Center for Health Statistics; 2002 [cited 2004 Mar 10]. Available from: http://www.cdc.gov/nchs/data/NCHS%20Micro-Data%20Release%20Policy%204–02A.pdf.

Newcombe HB. Handbook of Record Linkage: Methods for Health and Statistical Studies, Administration, and Business. Oxford: Oxford University Press; 1988.

Newcombe HB, Fair ME, Lalonde P. Discriminating powers of partial agreements of names for linking personal records. Part I: the logical basis. Meth Inform Med 1989a;28:86–91.

Newcombe HB, Fair ME, Lalonde P. Discriminating powers of partial agreements of names for linking personal records. Part II: the empirical test. Meth Inform Med 1989b;28:92–96.

Newcombe HB, Kennedy JM, Axford SJ, James AP. Automatic linkage of vital records. Science 1959;130:954–959.

O'Campo P. Advancing theory and methods for multilevel models of residential neighborhoods and health. Am J Epidemiol 2003:157(1):9–13.

Pearl M, Braveman P, Abrams B. The relationship of neighborhood socioeconomic characteristics to birthweight among 5 ethnic groups in California. Am J Public Health 2001; 91(11):1808–1814.

Pommerening K, Miller M, Schidtmann I, Michaelis J. Pseudonyms for cancer registries. Methods Inform Med 1996,35:112–121.

Prince CB. Building a perinatal data system in Hawaii [presentation on the Internet]. Presentation given at the Seventh Annual Maternal and Child Health Epidemiology Conference, Dec. 12–13, 2001, Clearwater Beach, FL [cited 2004 Mar 10]. Available from: http://128.248.232.90/archives/mchb/mchepi2001/slides/prince2/frame.htm.

Project on Human Development in Chicago Neighborhoods [homepage on the Internet]. Boston: The Project on Human Development in Chicago Neighborhoods, Harvard University; c. 2004 [cited 2004 Mar 10]. PHDCN General Overview [about 1 screen]. Available from: http://www.hms.harvard.edu/chase/projects/chicago/about/about.html.

Reid RJ, Evans RG, Barer ML, Sheps S, Kerluke K, McGrail K, Hertzman C, Pagliccia N. Conspicuous consumption: characterizing high users of physician services in one Canadian province. J Health Serv Res Policy 2003;8(4):215–224.

Roos LL, Nicol JP. A research registry: uses, development, and accuracy. J Clin Epidemiol 1999;52(1):39–47.

Roos LL, Romano P, Fergusson P. Administrative data bases. In: Armitage P, Colton T, eds. Encyclopedia of Biostatistics. Chichester, UK: Wiley; 1998, pp. 62–73.

Roos LL, Roos N. Of space and time, of health care and health. J Health Serv Res Policy 2001;6(2):120–122.

Roos LL, Sharp SM, Wajda A. Assessing data quality: a computerized approach. Soc Sci Med 1989;28(2):175–182.

Roos LL, Soodeen R-A, Bond R, Burchill C. Working more productively: tools for administrative data. Health Serv Res 2003;38(5):1339–1357.

Roos LL, Wajda A. Record linkage strategies: Part I: estimating information and evaluating approaches. Meth Inform Med 1991;30:117–123.

Shi L, Starfield B. The effect of primary care physician supply and income inequality on mortality among blacks and whites in U.S. metropolitan areas. Am J Public Health 2001; 91(8):1246–1250.

Tsuji I, Takahaski TI, Nishino Y, Ohkubo T, Kuriyama S, Watanabe Y, et al. Impact of walking upon medical care expenditure in Japan: the Ohsaki cohort study. Int J Epidemiol 2003; 32(5):809–814.

United Nations Population Information Network. Dictionary of Demographic and Reproductive Health Terminology. New York: United Nations; 1999.

U.S. General Accounting Office. Record Linkage and Privacy: Issues in Creating New Federal Research and Statistical Information. Report No. GAO-01-126SP. Washington, DC: United States General Accounting Office; April 2001.

Watkins W [serial on the Internet]. The data liberation initiative: a new cooperative model. Government Information in Canada. 1994;1(2.5) [cited 2004 Feb 15; about 5 pages]. Available from: http://www.usask.ca/library/gic/v1n2/watkins/watkins.html.

Watson D, Bogdanovic B, Heppner P, Katz A, Reid R, Roos N. Supply, Availability and Use of Family Physicians in Winnipeg. Winnipeg: Manitoba Centre for Health Policy; May 2003.

Watson D, Katz A, Reid R, Bogdanovic B, Roos N, Heppner P. Family physician workloads and access to care in Winnipeg: 1991–2001. Can Med Assoc J 2004;171(4):339–342.

White KL, Williams TF, Greenberg BG. The ecology of medical care. N Engl J Med 1961; 265(18):885–892.

Winkler WE [serial on the Internet]. Producing public-use microdata that are analytically valid and confidential. Proceedings of the Survey Research Methods Section, American Statistical Association; 1997: 41–50 [cited 2004 Feb 15]. Available from: http://www.amstat.org/sections/srms/Proceedings/papers/1997_006.pdf.

Winkler WE. Re-identification methods for evaluating the confidentiality of analytically valid microdata. Res Off Stat 1998;1:87–104.

PART III

Using Health Statistics

Health statistics have three major uses (see Chapter 1). The first use is creating fundamental knowledge about the health of populations, influences on health, and interactions among those influences. The second use is developing information to guide health policy development, assessment, and evaluation. The third use is generating information to guide implementation, targeting, evaluation, and refinement of health programs and other interventions for populations and to guide personal health decisions. Each chapter in this part focuses on one of these three uses of health statistics.

In Chapter 10, Friedman et al. address health statistics in knowledge creation. Data, information, and knowledge are defined, and their relationship to each other and to health statistics is described. Knowledge creation is characterized as a process that includes knowledge development, dissemination and use, with an emphasis on pinpointing the definition of research and its connection to knowledge development. The uses of health statistics in each of the components of knowledge creation are then examined in greater detail, using research on smoking and low birth weight as a recurring example. Finally, challenges in knowledge creation and health statistics are delineated.

In Chapter 11, Feder and Levitt discuss health statistics in health policy. While Chapter 10 describes health statistics and knowledge use, including the use of health statistics in policymaking and in changing population health, Chapter 11 focuses on the use of health statistics through the use of a single major historical example of attempted health policymaking: the U.S. health reform debate of President Bill Clinton's first term. Feder and Levitt dissect the arguments for and promises of Clinton's Health Security Act, revealing "the potential for and limits to the use of statistics in policymaking." Drawing on the U.S. experience in the early 1990s, they offer suggestions for how health statistics practitioners inside and outside of government can contribute constructively to policymaking.

In the final chapter in this part, Oswald, Friedman, and Hargreaves explore health statistics in public health practice. The authors initially discuss models for public health practice and the roles that health statistics play in the core functions of public health practice and in the essential public health services. They then delineate five ways in which health statistics are employed in public health practice: monitoring health status and outcomes; assessing community health; designing public health programs and targeting interventions; evaluating programs; and informing the public. Examples of these uses in several countries are provided. The chapter concludes with two case studies of the uses of health statistics in state public health practice.

CHAPTER 10

Health Statistics and Knowledge Creation

Daniel J. Friedman, R. Gibson Parrish II, Adil Moiduddin,
and Alana E. Ketchel

> The learning and knowledge that we have, is, at the most, but little compared with that of which we are ignorant.
>
> —*Plato*

> Of the three ways in which men think that they acquire knowledge of things—authority, reasoning, and experience—only the last is effective and able to bring peace to the intellect.
>
> —*Roger Bacon*

> [I]t is only experience which teaches us the nature and bounds of cause and effect, and enables us to infer the existence of one object from that of another.
>
> —*David Hume*

Health statistics are both the background and foreground of decision making in health. They lay the groundwork by providing a basic description of health and its influences, but they also play a direct role in decision making by providing the quantitative basis for action. From explication of basic facts to use in sophisticated research models, health statistics contribute to our knowledge of health, the influences on health, and our understanding of potential solutions to health problems. The purpose of this chapter is to explore the ways in which raw data are translated into useful health information and, in turn, into knowledge that can be disseminated and used for a variety of purposes in advancing the population's health.

As described in Chapter 1, health statistics have three principal uses: (*1*) creating fundamental knowledge about the health of populations, influences on health, and interactions among those influences; (*2*) developing information to guide health policy development, assessment, and evaluation; and (*3*) generating information to guide implementation, targeting, evaluation, and refinement of health programs and other interventions for populations and to guide personal health decisions. In this chapter, we focus on the first of these uses—creating knowledge: defining key terms and their interrelationships; describing knowledge creation, its components, and its relationship to research; and discussing the central role of health statistics in the process of knowledge creation in the field of health. We explore ways in which knowledge derived from health statistics is disseminated and used in policy and practice, and conclude with an overview of key challenges. Throughout, we present various examples drawn from the health literature that illustrate the application of health statistics to knowledge creation, with a focus on the application of knowledge creation to the issue of tobacco use and low birth weight.

DEFINITIONS AND RELATIONSHIPS OF KEY TERMS RELATING TO KNOWLEDGE CREATION

Data, Information, and Knowledge

Data is defined as "factual information (as measurements or statistics) used as a basis for reasoning, discussion, or calculation" (Merriam-Webster Online Dictionary [hp]). Data are the basic, elemental facts on which information, knowledge, and health statistics are built; they may be numerical or nonnumerical (e.g., verbal or written descriptions). An example of numerical data is the statement "A total of 2,416,425 deaths occurred." An example of nonnumerical data is the statement "Cigarettes contain nicotine."

Information is defined as "knowledge obtained from investigation, study, or instruction" or, more simply, as "facts, data" (Merriam-Webster Online Dictionary [hp]). Although the meaning of information depends on the context of its use, it is interesting to note that *information* can be used synonymously with *data* or *knowledge.* Another way of thinking of information is to consider it as the imposition of a pattern on data. Wolfson (1994, 314) describes information as "the ordering and interpretation of data to impose or extract meaning. For example, . . . a hospital separation [discharge] record is a collection of descriptive data. Aggregated into an occupancy rate, or a population-based utilization rate, such data are transformed into information." An example of numerical information is the statement "In 2001 a total of 2,416,425 deaths occurred in the United States, which represented a crude death rate of 848.5 deaths per 100,000 population" (Arias et al. 2003, 3).

Knowledge is defined as "the fact or condition of knowing something with familiarity gained through experience or association" (Merriam-Webster Online Dictionary [hp]). The distinction between knowledge gained through experience (or observation) versus association (i.e., inferential knowledge based on reasoning using facts, observations, or other inferential knowledge) will be important later when we discuss the development of knowledge and its relationship to research. *Knowledge* is a comprehensive term and encompasses "descriptions, hypotheses, concepts, theories, principles and procedures which to a reasonable degree of certainty are either true or useful" (Wikipedia [en] Knowledge). Knowledge encompasses both the qualitative or quantitative description (observations) of populations or events gained through experience *and* an understanding of the factors that caused the observations. Thus, a description of the mortality experience of a population for a given year *and* a description of the factors that caused that observed mortality experience (i.e., how the mortality experience came about) constitute knowledge, whereas a description of the mortality experience alone is information.

Relationship of Data, Information, and Knowledge

The definitions of data, information, and knowledge are overlapping. In some situations, the terms may even be interchanged or used synonymously. Nevertheless, there have been attempts to distinguish them and to establish relationships among them[1] (see Fig. 10.1). Ackoff (1996, 28–29) defined the terms—and the term *understanding*—and compared and contrasted them by using the familiar interrogatives who, what, where, when, how many, how, and why:

?
INFORMATION...
...rabbits eat grass...
..grass grows in soil...
...rain falls from clouds..
...wolves eat rabbits...
etc...
etc...
KNOWLEDGE...
if I kill off all the wolves, the rabbits will eat up the grass, & the soil will all wash away!
...WISDOM!

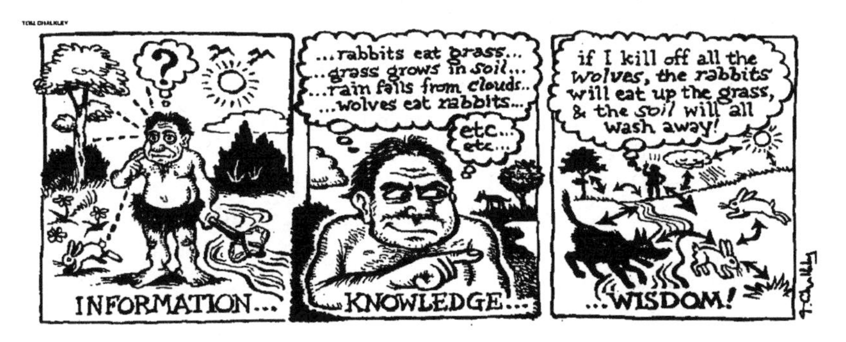

FIGURE 10.1
The relationship of information, knowledge, and wisdom. (Source: Chalkley T. Cartoon on information, knowledge, and wisdom. In: Cleveland H. Information as resource. The Futurist 1982;16:34–39; Chalkley T [homepage on the Internet]. Baltimore: Tom Chalkley c. 2004 [cited 2004 Apr 1]. Available from: http://www.tomchalk.com/contact.html. Used with permission.)

> **Data** *consists of symbols that represent objects, events, and/or their properties.* They are products of **observation**. . . . **Information** *is contained in descriptions, in answers to questions that begin with such words as who, what, where, when, and how many.* Information is usable in deciding **what** to do, not **how** to do it. . . . Answers to **how-to** questions constitute **knowledge**. . . . **Knowledge** *is contained in instructions.* Knowledge consists of **know-how**, for example, knowing how a system works or how to make it work in a desired way. It makes *maintenance* and *control* of objects, systems, and events possible. . . . **Understanding** is contained in explanations, answers to **why** questions.

Other authors have developed their own view of the hierarchy of data, information, and knowledge (Bellinger et al. 2004; Haeckel and Nolan 1993).

The hierarchical view of data, information, and knowledge is helpful in that it provides a framework and terminology for the process that starts with basic data, facts, and other observations; moves through the compilation of data within a context; continues with the analysis of observations for possible associations; and concludes with the development and testing of hypotheses, ultimately resulting in theories and laws about how things work. Health statistics, as the numerical data that characterize the health of populations and the influences that affect it, obviously play a central role in this process as it relates to health.

Relationship of Health Statistics to Data, Information, and Knowledge

In light of the above discussion, although health statistics are defined as *numerical data*, in many ways they more closely resemble information. Health statistics are usually developed and presented within a specific context, and they answer the questions typically answered by information. For example:

What happened: People died
Where did they die: London, England
When did they die: In the year 1636
How many died: 23,359
Who died: 12,377 males and 10,982 females

Thus, health statistics tell us that 12,377 males and 10,982 females—a total of 23,359 persons—died in London in 1636 (Graunt 1662, 76–77).

Health statistics can become knowledge. By further analyzing health statistics and introducing the *comparison* of statistics for different groups, for different time periods (Table 10.1), or for different places (Tables 10.1 and 2.1), they lead us toward knowledge, as the act of comparing statistics leads to the identification of possible *associations* of different factors. Thus, health statistics can suggest *how* events within the population occurred. By using previous observation and knowledge, one can characterize the causes of death (Tables 10.1 and

10.2). Differences between populations and differences in characteristics among populations suggest reasons (i.e., hypotheses) for the observed differences (Table 2.1; Box 10.1). In some instances, health statistics can be used to test the validity of a hypothesis. Even if health statistics alone are insufficient to test a hypothesis, they often provide valuable background information, sampling frames, or other contributions to studies that can do so.

By providing a basic foundation of data on which hypotheses and questions are formed, health statistics also play a role in identifying knowledge gaps or areas where further data, information, or knowledge is warranted. For example, an unusually high incidence of rare diseases such as Kaposi's sarcoma and pneumocystis pneumonia among homosexual men served as an early indicator of the rapid emergence of the human immunodeficiency virus/acquired immunodeficiency syndrome (HIV/AIDS) epidemic and highlighted our limited understanding of what was soon to be recognized as a global health concern of staggering proportions (CDC 1981). By defining areas where there is too limited an understanding of important issues for effective decision making, health statistics can often point the way to additional research or data collection activities that are necessary to advance our understanding and thus our capacity to address the issue.

Knowledge Creation

There is an extensive literature on knowledge creation, principally as it relates to business and other organizational innovation and management (Google directory [db] Knowledge creation; Nonaka and Takeuchi 1995; Thomas [mg]; Von Krogh et al. 2000; Wikipedia [en] Knowledge creation). In this context, knowledge creation is viewed as a process of transforming tacit knowledge, which is based in individual experiences and mental associations and, therefore, not easily shared, into explicit knowledge, which can be shared (i.e., communicated) and used.

For the purposes of this chapter, we define *knowledge creation* as the process by which knowledge is developed, disseminated, and used. It consists of three components: knowledge development (or production); knowledge dissemination (or sharing); and knowledge use, each of which is discussed in more detail below.

Definition of Research and Its Relationship to Knowledge Development

Most simply, *research* is defined as "the collecting of information about a particular subject." A more complex definition—and view—of research is "studious inquiry or examination; especially: investigation or experimentation aimed at the discovery and interpretation of facts, revision of accepted theories or laws

TABLE 10.1

Selected Years from *The Table of Burials, and Christnings*

Anno Dom.	*97 Parishes*	*16 Parishes*	*Out-Parishes*	*Buried in All*	*Besides of* the Plague	*Christned*
1629	2,536	3,992	2,243	8,771	0	9,901
1630	2,506	4,201	2,521	9,237	1,317	9,315
1631	2,459	3,697	2,132	8,288	274	8,524
1632	2,704	4,412	2,411	9,527	8	9,584
1633	2,378	3,936	2,078	8,392	0	9,997
1634	2,937	4,980	2,982	10,899	1	9,855
1635	2,742	4,966	2,943	10,651	0	10,034
1636	2,825	6,924	3,210	12,959	10,400	9,522
1637	2,288	4,265	2,128	8,681	3,082	9,160
1638	3,584	5,926	3,751	13,261	363	10,311
1639	2,592	4,344	2,612	9,548	314	10,150
1640	2,919	5,156	3,246	11,321	1,450	10,850
1641	3,248	5,092	3,427	11,767	1,375	10,670
1642	3,176	5,245	3,578	11,999	1,274	10,370
1643	3,395	5,552	3,269	12,216	996	9,410
1644	2,593	4,274	2,574	9,441	1,492	8,104
1645	2,524	4,639	2,445	9,608	1,871	7,966
1646	2,746	4,872	2,797	10,415	2,365	7,163
1647	2,672	4,749	3,041	10,462	3,597	7,332
1648	2,480	4,288	2,515	9,283	611	6,544
1649	2,865	4,714	2,920	10,499	67	5,825
1650	2,301	4,138	2,310	8,749	15	5,612
1651	2,845	5,002	2,597	10,804	23	6,071
1652	3,293	5,719	3,546	12,553	16	6,128
1653	2,527	4,635	2,919	10,081	6	6,155
1654	3,323	6,063	3,845	13,231	16	6,620
1655	2,761	5,148	3,439	11,348	9	7,004
1656	3,327	6,573	4,015	13,915	6	7,050
1657	3,014	5,646	3,770	12,430	4	6,685
1658	3,613	6,923	4,443	14,979	14	6,170
1659	3,431	6,988	4,301	14,720	36	5,690
1660	3,098	5,644	3,926	12,668	13	6,971
1661	3,804	7,309	5,532	16,645	20	8,855

Advertisements for the better understanding of the several Tables:

IT is to be noted, that in all the several Columns of the *Burials* those dying of the *Plague* are left out, being reckoned all together in the sixth Column. Whereas in the original Bills the *Plague*, and all other diseases are reckoned together, with mention how many of the respective totals are of the *Plague*.

Secondly, From the year 1642 forwards the accompt of the Christnings is not to be trusted, the neglects of the same beginning about that year: for in 1642 there are set down 10370, and about the same Number several years before, after which time the said Christnings decreased to between 5000 and 6000 by omission of the greater part.

Source: Graunt (1662).

TABLE 10.2
Selected Casualties (i.e., Causes of Death) for London, 1629–1636

Year	*1629*	*1630*	*1631*	*1632*	*1633*	*1634*	*1635*	*1636*
Livergrown, Spleen, and Rickets	94	112	99	87	82	77	98	99
Lunatique	6	11	6	5	4	2	2	5
Meagrom			24					22
Measles	42	2	3	80	21	33	27	12
Mother	1							3
Murdered			3	7		6	5	8
Overlayd, and starved at Nurse	4	10	13	7	8	14	10	14
Palsy	17	23	17	25	14	21	25	17
Plague		1317	274	8		1		10400
Plague in the Guts								
Pleurisy	26	24	26	36	21		45	24
Poysoned					2			2
Purples, and spotted Fever	32	58	58	38	24	125	245	397
Quinsy, and Sore-throat	1	8	6	7	24	4	5	22
Rickets						14	49	50
Mother, Rising of the Lights	44	72	99	98	60	84	72	104
Rupture	2	6	4	9	4	3	10	13
Scal'd-head								
Scurvy	5	7	9		9			25

Source: Graunt (1662).

in the light of new facts, or practical application of such new or revised theories or laws" (Merriam-Webster Online Dictionary [hp]). The first definition aligns research with the process of developing data or information; the second is much more closely aligned with the process of developing knowledge. The second definition, which we will adopt for this chapter, also hints at the distinction between basic and applied research.[2] In adopting this definition, we view knowledge development, which is discussed in greater detail below, and research as synonymous. Knowledge creation, however, extends beyond research to include the dissemination and use of knowledge.

BOX 10.1

The First Three General Observations Made on the Bills of Mortality by John Graunt

Having premised these general Advertisements, our first Observation upon the *Casualties* shall be, that in twenty Years there dying of all diseases and *Casualties*, 229250. that 71124. dyed of the *Thrush*, *Convulsion*, *Rickets*, *Teeth*, and *Worms*; and as *Abortives*, *Chrysomes*, *Infants*, *Liver-grown*, and *Over- laid*; that is to say, that about 1/3. of the whole died of those Diseases, which we guess did all light upon Children under four or five Years old.

There died also of the *Small-Pox*, *Swine-Pox*, and *Measles*, and of *Worms* without *Convulsion*, 12210. of which number we suppose likewise, that about 1/2. might be Children under six Years old. Now, if we consider that 16. of the said 229 thousand died of that extraordinary and grand *Casualty* the *Plague*, we shall finde that about thirty six *per centum* of all quick conceptions, died before six years old.

The second Observation is; That of the said 229250. dying of all Diseases, there died of acute Diseases (the *Plague* excepted) but about 50000, or 2/9 parts. The which proportion doth give a measure of the state, and disposition of this *Climate*, and *Air*, as to health, these *acute*, and *Epidemical* Diseases happening suddenly, and vehemently, upon the like corruptions, and alterations in the *Air*.

The third Observation is, that of the said 229. thousand about 70. died of *Chronical* Diseases, which shews (as I conceive) the state, and disposition of the Country (including as well it's *Food*, as *Air*) in reference to health, or rather to *longævity*: for as the proportion of the *Acute* and *Epidemical* Diseases shews the aptness of the *Air* to suddain and vehement Impressions, so the *Chronical* Diseases shew the ordinary temper of the Place, so that upon the proportion of *Chronical* Diseases seems to hang the judgment of the fitness of the Country for *long Life*. For, I conceive, that in Countries subject to great *Epidemical* sweeps men may live very long, but where the proportion of the *Chronical* distempers is great, it is not likely to be so; because men being long sick and alwayes sickly, cannot live to any great age, as we see in several sorts of *Metal-men*, who although they are less subject to acute Diseases then others, yet seldome live to be old, that is, not to reach unto those years, which *David* saies is the age of man.

Source: Graunt (1662), pp. 15–16.

Rules for Establishing Causation and Its Place in the Research Process

Knowledge development and research refer to knowing something, either through observation (i.e., collection of information about a particular subject) or through the association of observations, which may ultimately lead to understanding the cause of the observations. Association is necessary but not sufficient to establish a causal relationship. Recent efforts to establish criteria for causal relationships include the efforts of the Advisory Committee to the U.S. Surgeon General concerning the relationship of smoking to lung cancer (U.S. Department of Health, Education, and Welfare 1964) and Hill's (1965) nine "aspects" of causal association, which form the basis of most current lists of causal criteria.[3]

Research with the goal of identifying associations or causal relationships—the more commonly used definition of research—typically follows a well-ordered, time-honored process that involves the following steps: formulation of the topic for study, generation of a hypothesis(es) through review of existing observations and knowledge, selection of an approach (method) to test the hypothesis, collection of data, processing and analysis of data, and interpretation of the findings (data and associations), including assessment of the validity of the hypothesis in light of the findings (Abramson and Abramson 1999).

KNOWLEDGE DEVELOPMENT AND HEALTH STATISTICS

Uses of Health Statistics for Knowledge Development

Health statistics are related to knowledge development because they contribute to the creation of knowledge about population health through the collection, compilation, analysis, and interpretation of numeric data about population health and the influences that affect it. Health statistics may be a source of observations (in other words, facts or measures) about population health and its influences, generally referred to as *descriptive health statistics* (e.g., the number of live births with low birth weight; the proportion of pregnant women who smoke cigarettes), or of potential associations between observations (e.g., smoking more than 30 packs of cigarettes during pregnancy is associated with low birth weight among live births). In descriptive statistics, the measures used to report findings are typically counts, rates, and proportions (e.g., total number of live births; total number of live births with low birth weight; rate of low birth weight; proportion of live births with low birth weight). In analyses for association, measures of association are used: rate ratio and difference, relative risk, odds ratio, and correlation and regression coefficients. In both situations, health statistics contribute directly to the development of knowledge.

Whether a given set of health statistics can be used as a source of observations, associations, or both depends on the information that it contains, the way in which it was collected, and the ways in which it can be analyzed. Many health statistics are collected solely to provide a description of population health, with no attempt to identify associations or correlations between one or more influences and observed health outcomes. Some descriptive statistics may, however, be used to generate hypotheses for separate studies of association and, in this way, can be an important motivator of knowledge development. Other health statistics contain sufficient information to allow analysis for associations between different observations. When the analysis of observations can be performed at the level at which influences on health operate and when the rules for establishing causation are met, the analysis is known as *etiologic.* Linking individual-level data from two or more health statistics data sets can facilitate such an analysis (see Chapter 9 for a detailed discussion of linkage). Health statistics data sets can also be used as sampling frames for, or provide other significant contributions to, separate etiologic studies.

Sometimes, two or more data sets can be used to look at the possible association between an observed effect and an observed factor hypothesized as an influence on that effect, but the analysis proceeds at the population or subpopulation level rather than at the individual level for either of two reasons. The first reason is that the data sets cannot be linked *at the individual level* because of privacy concerns, data incompatibility, or data limitations. The second reason is that the hypothesis under consideration relates to population rather than individual phenomena and relationships. Analyses at the population, subpopulation, or group level are known as *ecological* analyses. An example would be examining the association between the state- or country-level rate of cigarette smoking during pregnancy (obtained from health behavior surveys) and the rate of low birth weight (obtained from birth certificates) for different states of the United States or different countries. Ecological analyses can identify associations, but these associations, if imputed to the individual level, could be spurious because it is not known whether those with the adverse observed outcome (e.g., women giving birth to low weight infants) also had the risk factor (e.g., cigarette smoking).[4]

Examples of Health Statistics in Knowledge Development

This section illustrates how health statistics are used for knowledge development, drawing on research literature dealing with smoking and low birth weight as a common example. The section demonstrates how researchers from many countries have applied both descriptive statistics and measures of association to the three traditional types of health statistics data sources to investigate the relationship between smoking and low birth weight. The section is not intended as a summary or an integration of research findings.

The National Library of Medicine's PubMed database includes 709 articles, published since 1990, with both *smoking* and *low birth weight* as key words, in the title, or in the abstract.[5] To circumscribe the analysis of this literature, only articles referring to the three traditional health statistics data sources were selected: registries (in this case, birth registries or birth certificates); administrative health data (in this case, hospital discharge, encounter, or claims data); and surveys (in this case, surveys or questionnaires). After additional simple selection criteria were employed, 168 articles published since 1990 were selected as the population of articles on smoking and low birth weight citing traditional health statistics data sources.[6] The 168 selected articles represent a wide range of topics and hypotheses. Some articles focus directly on the relationship between active smoking, passive smoking, or former smoking and low birth weight. Others examine the relationship between other hypothesized influences on infant outcomes, but include smoking and low birth weight as control variables. The variety of countries and U.S. states used as sites for the sampled studies demonstrates the broad international basis for health statistics, health statistics data sources, and typical health statistics approaches for identifying influences on population health.

Health Statistics for Knowledge Development—Reports and Registries

Of the 168 selected PubMed articles meeting the search criteria, 37 referred to birth registries or birth certificates. The birth registries used in the subset of these articles focusing on smoking and low birth weight were located in several countries and U.S. states, including Finland and Sweden (Gissler et al. 2003a, 2003b), Denmark (Olsen and Frische 1993), the United States as a whole (Mathews 2001; Ventura et al. 2003), Quebec City (Fortier et al. 1994), Contra Costa, California (Chen and Petitti 1995), and the states of Alabama, Alaska, Georgia, Maine, South Carolina, West Virginia (Dietz et al. 1998), Massachusetts (Cohen et al. 1993), Missouri (Land and Stockhauser 1993), New Jersey (Berry and Bove 1997), Washington (Fox et al. 1994; Li and Daling 1991), and Wisconsin (Aronson et al. 1993).

Employing the birth certificate as a data source for knowledge development, the authors of these articles reached a wide range of conclusions. For example:

- Maternal smoking explained up to half of the excess risk of adverse perinatal outcomes, including low birth weight, among Finns of lower socioeconomic status (Gissler et al. 2003a).
- The incidence of low birth weight among infants of smoking mothers was approximately twice that of nonsmoking mothers (Aronson et al. 1993; Ventura et al. 2003).
- Passive smoking did not increase the likelihood of delivering a small for gestational age infant (Chen and Petitti 1995; Fortier et al. 1994), but it was related to low birth weight (Windham et al. 2000).

Birth certificates were used for several different purposes in the sampled articles. Most typically, secondary analysis of birth certificate data was conducted, tapping the availability of birth weight and additional perinatal outcome information in birth certificates. Examples include:

- A comparative study of women born in Finland who gave birth in Sweden from 1987 to 1998, all Finnish women delivering in Finland during the same years, and a 10% sample of Swedish women delivering in Sweden during those years explored differences in perinatal outcomes of Finnish mothers in Finland and those in Sweden (Gissler et al. 2003b).
- National U.S. studies demonstrated an almost 40% decrease from 1989 to 2000 in the percentage of mothers who smoked during pregnancy (Ventura et al. 2003) and decreases in all racial/ethnic groups (Mathews 2001).
- A New Jersey study of births from 1961 to 1988 in four towns hypothesized low birth weight differences associated with proximity to a hazardous waste landfill (Berry and Bove 1997).

Some researchers also linked interview data to birth certificates, using interviews to obtain information on maternal characteristics and behaviors, and birth certificates to obtain data on perinatal outcomes available from the birth certificate. For example, Windham and colleagues (2000) conducted a prospective study of active smokers, nonsmoking mothers environmentally exposed to tobacco smoke, and nonsmoking mothers not environmentally exposed, and Chen and Petetti (1995) conducted a case control study of the relationship of passive smoking and small for gestational age births among nonsmoking women. Other studies used birth registries to establish a sampling frame, such as for case control studies of passive smoking and small for gestational age births in Contra Costa and Quebec City (Chen and Pettiti 1995; Fortier et al. 1994).

None of the studies discussed here actually established causal relationships between smoking and low birth weight. Some studies employed descriptive statistics such as the percentage of mothers delivering low birth weight infants, as when comparing the percentage of low birth weight infants born to Finnish mothers in Sweden and in Finland (Gissler et al. 2003b), or the incidence of low birth weight infants born to smoking and nonsmoking mothers in 49 U.S. states (Ventura et al. 2003). Other studies used measures of association such as odds ratios or adjusted odds ratios, as when examining relationships between environmental tobacco smoke and low birth weight (Chen and Petitti 1995; Windham et al. 2000), or relative risk or adjusted relative risk, as in a study of the effect of mother's age on the relationship between smoking and birth weight (Fox et al. 1994).

Health Statistics for Knowledge Development—Surveys

Of the 168 articles in the PubMed database meeting the specified search criteria, 126 referred to surveys or questionnaires. The survey- and questionnaire-based studies that deal directly with smoking and low birth weight were conducted in many countries, including invidual states and cities in the United States, as well.

The sampled survey- and questionnaire-based studies were essentially of three main types. One type relied on large, ongoing population-based surveys and employed secondary analyses to investigate smoking and low birth weight. Secondary analyses were conducted of such ongoing U.S. surveys as the National Health and Nutrition Examination Survey (Okosun et al. 2000), the Hispanic National Health and Nutrition Examination Survey (Wolff and Portis 1996; Wolff et al. 1993), the National Health Interview Survey (Hueston et al. 1994; Mainous and Hueston 1994), the National Longitudinal Survey of Youth (Faden and Graubard 1994), the National Maternal and Infant Health Interview Survey (Wu et al. 1998), the Pregnancy Risk Assessment Monitoring System (Dietz et al. 1998; Ramsey et al. 1993), and the Canadian National Longitudinal Survey of Children and Youth (Millar and Chen 1998). A second type of sampled study relied on specially conducted, population-based surveys, usually directed to a relatively narrow range of topics. For example, Bonati and Fellin (1991) studied changes in smoking and drinking behavior before and during pregnancy among Italian mothers, using 1989–1990 survey data from the World Health Organization Drug Use in Pregnancy Study. Visscher and colleagues (2003) studied the impact of smoking and additional substance use on birth weight, using survey data from the 1992 District of Columbia Metropolitan Area Drug Survey. A third type of study involved the administration of questionnaires to samples of clinical patients. For example, the Auckland Birthweight Collaborative Study, using maternal interview data from three Auckland birth hospitals, was used to investigate risk factors in small for gestational age births (Thompson et al. 2001).

Health Statistics for Knowledge Development—Administrative Health Data

Of the 168 sampled PubMed articles, 15 referred to claims, encounter, or hospital discharge data. Those few articles meeting the search criteria and focusing more specifically on smoking and low birth weight employed administrative health data to investigate smoking-related costs (Miller et al. 2001; Phillips et al. 1992; Reichman and Pagnini 1997). For example, Miller and colleagues used claims data to develop a model to estimate the magnitude of excess costs attributable to smoking during pregnancy, and discovered that the largest smoking attributable cost was low birth weight (Miller et al. 2001).

Health Statistics for Knowledge Development—Complementary Data

In addition to the 168 sampled PubMed articles using the three traditional health statistics data sources in investigations relevant to smoking and low birth weight, another search was conducted that identified 8 articles relating to smoking and low birth weight and also referring to a complementary data source (in this case, a census). In the most relevant articles, census data were linked at the individual (Ericson et al. 1993; Olausson et al. 1997) or area (Bell and Lumley 1992) level in order to obtain measures of maternal socioeconomic status. For example, in a study of low birth weight and socioeconomic status in Victoria, Australia, census data at the postal code level were linked to birth data (Bell and Lumley 1992).

KNOWLEDGE DISSEMINATION AND HEALTH STATISTICS

As indicated earlier, knowledge creation consists of three steps: knowledge development, knowledge dissemination, and knowledge use. This section focuses on the knowledge dissemination process, or the mechanisms through which research findings are shared. Two general routes are identified for the sharing of research findings: professional routes and popular media routes. The two routes are neither mutually exclusive nor independent of each other.

Knowledge dissemination can be conceptualized as a continuum (Central West Health Planning Information Network 2000). At one end of the continuum is knowledge diffusion: researchers conduct research and release their findings only through professional routes. No other route(s) for sharing research findings are employed, and no special attempts are made to share their research findings with audiences beyond the researchers' professional peers. At the other end of the knowledge dissemination continuum is effective dissemination, in which researchers recognize that the characteristics of the prospective users and the contexts in which prospective users work and live must be actively taken into account in sharing research findings. Empirical research on social science knowledge use in Canada (Landry et al. 2001) and the United States (Lester 1993) has employed knowledge use scales; while the specifics of the scales vary, they range along a continuum including such steps as transmission, cognition reference, adoption, influence, and application (Landry et al. 2001). The use of health statistics research findings as knowledge is discussed in a later section, which focuses especially on the use of knowledge in policymaking and in changing population health.

Professional Routes for Knowledge Dissemination

The most typical professional routes for knowledge dissemination are journals, professional meetings, and advisory boards. These routes typically overlap, and the same research findings are often disseminated through all three routes.

Professional Journals

Using the example of research on smoking and low birth weight, the 168 sampled articles using traditional health statistics data sources appeared in 95 different journals. One journal (*American Journal of Epidemiology*) published 15 of the sampled articles, 3 journals each published 5 to 8 of the sampled articles (*Obstetrics and Gynecology*, *Pediatrics*, and *Epidemiology*), 3 journals each published 4 (*American Journal of Public Health*, *International Journal of Epidemiology*, *Paediatric and Perinatal Epidemiology*), 27 journals each had 2 or 3 articles, and 61 journals each had a single article. This dispersion of publication of research findings on smoking and low birth weight among 95 different journals indicates the extent to which health statistics practitioners can rely on multiple professional journals for disseminating research findings.

The health statistics enterprise disseminates its research findings through several different types of journals published in many different countries. Some journals that serve as dissemination routes for health statistics pertain to public health as a broad field, such as the *American Journal of Public Health*, the *Australian and New Zealand Journal of Public Health*, the *Canadian Journal of Public Health*, *Morbidity and Mortality Weekly Report*, *Public Health*, and *Public Health Reports*. Other journals that serve as dissemination routes for health statistics focus on epidemiology, such as the *American Journal of Epidemiology*, *Journal of Epidemiology and Community Health*, *International Journal of Epidemiology*, *Paediatric and Perinatal Epidemiology*, and *Epidemiology*. Yet other journals through which health statistics research findings are disseminated are more topical, either in medicine (such as *British Medical Journal*, *Journal of the American Medical Association*, the *New England Journal of Medicine*, and *Social Science and Medicine*), health services research (such as *Health Affairs* and *Health Services Research*), or other fields closely related to public health (such as *Environmental Health Perspectives*, *Family Planning Perspectives*, *Maternal and Child Health Journal*, and *Early Human Development*).

Professional Conferences

In addition to professional journals, professional conferences also serve as major routes for disseminating health statistics research findings. Typically, each health statistics or related professional association holds an annual meeting. These range from large annual conferences with several thousand attendees and hundreds of presentations (such as the American Public Health Association or the AcademyHealth Annual Research Meeting) to moderate-sized and small conferences with several hundred attendees or even fewer (such as the American Epidemiological Society). The academically based professional associations invite presentations, with abstracts being competitively peer reviewed prior to acceptance. Often, presentations at these professional conferences precede publication of research findings in a professional journal.

Advisory Boards

A third route for dissemination of health statistics research findings is advisory boards. Some of the best-known advisory boards are ongoing, such as the

National Committee on Vital and Health Statistics, which since 1949 has advised the Secretary of the U.S. Department of Health and Human Services on the health information policy. Other advisory boards are assembled to address specific topical issues and then disbanded, such as the Committee to Assess the Science Base for Tobacco Harm Reduction of the Institute of Medicine's Board on Health Promotion and Disease Prevention, which produced the 2001 report *Clearing the Smoke: Assessing the Science Base for Tobacco Harm Reduction* (Stratton et al. 2001), and the U.S. Surgeon General's Advisory Committee on Smoking and Health, which produced *Smoking and Health*, the initial Surgeon General's report on the deleterious impacts of smoking (U.S. Department of Health, Education, and Welfare 1964).

Popular Media

Health statistics are regular staples in newspapers, magazines, and electronic media (television, radio, and the Web). The uses of statistics in the popular media cover a wide spectrum of the continuum of knowledge from data to information to knowledge. At their most simple, statistical data are presented as points of interest, as in *USA Today*'s daily front page graphic (see, for example, USA Today [hp] USA Today snapshot). Newspapers, in particular, frequently report the results of health surveys, such as trends in obesity, smoking, or health insurance, as matters of public interest (see, e.g., Chong 2003 for reporting on smoking rates in California). As such, basic facts about health find their way into more general public discourse.

Media also frequently use health statistics to provide context for stories on health-related issues, providing a factual basis for further investigation. For example, stories reporting on the controversy over whether different diets are effective often highlight statistics on obesity and overweight, as well as statistics on exercise and caloric or fat consumption from national surveys (Taubes 2002). News reporting on public policy debates or political campaigns frequently uses statistics on trends or health problems to illustrate the nature of the issue or to frame the positions of advocates (as in debate over health insurance policy, described in Chapter 11).

Similarly, public education campaigns organized by advocacy organizations or associations use popular media in several forms to disseminate health statistics that are meant to provoke thought and, in so doing, promote a certain health behavior or policy choice. In its recent campaign for preventing teenage smoking, the American Legacy Foundation used television ads, grassroots events, Web sites, and other media to communicate trends on morbidity and mortality associated with cigarette smoking (American Legacy Foundation [hp] truth campaign).

Finally, the findings of research based on health statistics are frequently highlighted in the popular press, which often draws on articles published in professional journals or on the *gray literature* (reports from government agencies or private foundations). Articles in major peer-reviewed journals often generate substantial media attention. For example, an article published in the *New England Journal of Medicine* documenting deficits in the quality of health care in the United States and their health consequences was carried as a major news story in national newspapers, including the *Washington Post* (Brown 2003; McGlynn 2003). We note that there is substantial content overlap between dissemination through various channels. For example, media accounts of information derived from health statistics will often summarize and reference the publication of results in a peer-reviewed journal or another scientific forum.

The widespread reporting of health statistics in the popular media is the product of multiple forces: (*1*) the public's large appetite for information about their own health; (*2*) the desire of media outlets to feed this appetite and the need for a factual basis for reporting; and (*3*) the existence of often sophisticated efforts to gain media attention for the products of individual researchers, agencies, and institutions. Although those in the health statistics enterprise often overlook the last element, increasing efforts are being made to place statistics and research findings in the popular media. The relationship between the media and the producers of statistics and research is cultivated in several ways. Professional associations such as AcademyHealth (health services research) and the American Statistical Association encourage their membership to become media-savvy through training (AcademyHealth [ma] Annual research meeting), and make efforts to help media locate experts in the field (American Statistical Association [hp]). Professional journals, research institutions, and individual researchers increasingly employ sophisticated strategies (press releases, media visits, events) to draw media attention to the results of research, thereby extending the audience for such studies well beyond the readership of the professional literature (deSemir et al. 1998; Entwistle 1995). The extent of popular reporting of health research results has even generated debate over whether research results *should* be so widely disseminated to the public, particularly those that are presented in preliminary form traditionally to inform other researchers (Schwartz 2002). In this way, widespread reporting can add to public knowledge about facts, context, and analysis, but can also contribute to information overload.

Similarly, the popular media report only a small percentage of scientific findings on health, and the selection of stories is based on what is judged newsworthy rather than on a systematic selection of a representative range of findings on health. As a result, public perceptions of health and health risks are potentially skewed by the nature of the news and other information that reaches them. Singer and Endreny (1993, 1994), for example, note that sampled newspapers, weekly news magazines, and television news programs issue a disproportionately large number of news stories relating to sensational hazards and disasters compared to illnesses and especially chronic illnesses, given actual death rates for each.

KNOWLEDGE USE AND HEALTH STATISTICS

Use of Knowledge in Policymaking

In 1601, James Lancaster prevented scurvy on the largest ship of the first East India Company fleet to sail from Torbay, England, to India by requiring sailors to drink 3 teaspoons of lemon juice each day (Mosteller 1981). Between 1768 and 1779, Captain James Cook imposed a strict antiscorbutic diet on sailors who shipped on the *Endeavor* and the *Resolution*, and even submitted a paper to the Royal Society's Philosophical Transactions on the health of seamen (Hough 1994). Yet it was not until 1865 that the British Board of Trade introduced citrus juice as a routine preventive for scurvy in the mercantile marine. This simple example is illustrative of the myriad issues involved in trying to understand the role of knowledge in policymaking generally and the role of knowledge derived from health statistics in policymaking more specifically. These issues include what is policy; what is the policymaking process; who makes policy; what factors and conditions support or impede the use of knowledge in policymaking; how is knowledge used during policymaking; and how can the use of knowledge in policymaking be increased?

A substantial body of literature, both domestic and international, has emerged on defining policy, understanding the policymaking process, and identifying the relationship that research as knowledge development does and should have to policymaking. Much of this literature has been theoretical. Some of it has been empirical, based on case studies or surveys of policymakers and researchers. Empirical research about the use of research in making health policy has also been conducted through comparative meta-analyses of studies conducted in individual countries (Innvaer et al. 2002). This section provides a brief overview of some major perspectives from the theoretical and empirical literature, and leaves to the reader further investigation of the points raised.

Defining Policy

The most basic issue in understanding the role of knowledge in policymaking is defining *policy*. Subtly different definitions of policy exist in standard dictionaries. The difference between the definitions lies in whether policy necessitates (*1*) conscious choice of a course or method of action among (*2*) alternative courses or methods of action. In this chapter, we will consider policy broadly as an institutionalized "plan or course of action . . . intended to influence and determine decisions, actions, and other matters" (American Heritage 2000).

Health policy should be conceived of as consisting of different types, each relevant for different types of research findings. Webb and Wistow (1982, 14; see also Web and Wistow 1986, 82–83) and Black (2001) conceptualize *policy streams* as consisting of *service* (*or output*) *policies* ("concerned with meeting social needs and include the allocation of priority to particular client groups or the specification of preferred ways of responding to need"), *resource policies* ("concerned with desired levels and combinations of financial, manpower and capital inputs"), and *governance policies* ("concerned with perceptions of the proper role of the state in general and of central government in particular; the structuring of relationships between governmental and non-governmental bodies; and the organization and management of such bodies"). Lomas (1990) describes three levels of health policymaking as clinical (roughly corresponding to practice), administrative (roughly corresponding to service), and legislative (roughly corresponding to governance). Different types of research findings, differently presented, will be relevant for the making of different types of health policy (Hanney et al. 2003).

Defining Policymaking

Within the health context, we can consider policy to be made within many different types of organizations and by different types of professionals. Most obviously, policy can be made through national and state legislative decisions, as in passage of new laws affecting health or health programs, regulations, and budgets. Policies can also be made through purely administrative decisions in state and local health agencies or in health-care provider organizations such as hospitals or neighborhood health centers, as in decisions about how to implement health programs. Finally, policies can be made through *street-level bureaucracy*, via decisions of individual service providers, whether public or private, about what specific services to provide in given situations and to whom those services should be provided (Lipsky 1983).

Recent attempts to understand the relationship of research findings to policymaking have stressed the need for a nuanced understanding of the process through which policies are made. Kingdon (2003) defined public policymaking as "a set of processes, including at least 1) the setting of the agenda, 2) specification of alternatives from which a choice is to be made, 3) an authoritative choice among those specified alternatives, and 4) implementation of the decision." In Chapter 11, Feder and Levitt build on Kingdon's model to examine the role of health statistics in the Clinton health reform debate. Others have emphasized the less planned and more random aspects of policymaking. Cohen, March, and Olsen (1972) described the *garbage can* process of decision making in which "problems are worked upon in the context of some choice, but choices are made only when the shifting combinations of problems, solutions, and decision makers happen to make action possible." Lindblom (1959) described the science of muddling through, in which decisions and policies are made through a series of "successive limited comparisons" of alternatives and "analysis is drastically limited." Health policymaking does not necessarily follow a simple, linear path; indeed, paths to the making of policy are often unpredictable (Pestieau 2003). In all likelihood, health policymaking occurs differently at different times, in different organizations, and on different topics. Thus, the manner in which health statistics impact on policy may vary, depending on the specifics of the policymaking in question.

Research as Evidence in Policymaking

To understand how health statistics can influence policymaking, idealized conceptions of the potential influence of research findings on policy should be abandoned (Davis and Howden-Chapman 1996). Research findings, and by implication health statistics, need to be recognized as only one type of evidence employed in the policymaking process (Weiss 1980). Other evidence typically used in making policy includes personal experiences, media reports, anecdotes, and quasi-scientific information sources (Canadian Research Transfer Network 2002; Day 1997). As Day indicated, "we must accept that no single source of information is perfect; that research findings, on the one hand, are neither finite nor definitive" (Day 1997, 66; see also Lindblom and Cohen 1979, 72–85).

Research plays multiple roles with respect to policymaking. It may be used as evidence in policymaking when decisions are made about what to do (adoption), when the decisions are actually implemented (use), or when "actions . . . become part of the expected and customary routines for doing things" (institutionalization) (Beyer and Trice 1982). Research can also help identify options or prioritize policy decision making based on agreed-on metrics. Knowledge can be used during adoption, use, or institutionalization. Health statistics as knowledge may play a particularly important role in overcoming what Stone described as the *implementation gap*, or the differences between intentions at adoption, on the one hand, and actual implementation and institutionalization, on the other hand (Stone 2002). In Chapter 12, Oswald, Friedman, and Hargreaves focus on specific uses of health statistics in public health practice; many of these uses are intended to overcome the implementation gap and the fractionalization within implementation by increasing the uses of health statistics as knowledge in public health practice.

Research can be used in various modes in policymaking: as general ideas, as substantive knowledge, or as analyses of the implications of alternative courses of action (Bulmer 1987). A range of models of research use in policymaking have been posited. At one extreme is Thomas's *limestone model*, in which researchers largely assume that research findings will seep into policymaking, just as water seeps through limestone. The key assumption of the limestone model is that researchers can rely "on indirect or cumulative interest and requires no action other than the research itself and the presentation of the findings in a readable way" (Thomas 1987, 57). Weiss (1977, 1979, 1980) delineated multiple models of research use in policymaking, based both on her review of the literature and on her interviews about the usefulness of social science research with senior officials in federal, state, and local mental health agencies. These models of research use include the *knowledge-driven model*, in which basic research leads to applied research, which leads to development of techniques to apply the findings of applied research, which leads to application of techniques in policy. At the same extreme of greater usefulness of the substantive results of research, Weiss (1979) also described the *problem-solving model*, which "involves the direct application of the results of a specific . . . study to a pending decision." At the other extreme are Weiss's *political model*, in which research "becomes ammunition for the side that finds its conclusions congenial and supportive," and the *tactical model*, in which "it is not the content of the findings that is invoked but the sheer fact that research is being done" (see also Buxton and Hanney 1996).

Ascertaining whether and how research findings have actually been used in and affected policymaking can be difficult. Smoking and low birth weight can serve as an example. In 1964, the U.S. Department of Health, Education, and Welfare released *Smoking and Health: Report of the Advisory Committee to the Surgeon General of the Public Health Service*, the first of the 31 Surgeon General's reports on smoking to be released between 1964 and 2001 (U.S. Department of Health, Education, and Welfare 1964). The 1964 report reviewed research findings about smoking and its impact on birth weight, concluding that "women smoking during pregnancy have babies of lower birth weight than non-smokers of the same social class. . . . [However,] it is not known whether this decrease in birth weight has any influence on the biological fitness of the newborn" (U.S. Department of Health, Education, and Welfare 1964, 343). Thirteen of the subsequent 30 Surgeon General's reports on the health impacts of smoking also summarized research findings relating to smoking and low birth weight. Yet it is difficult to conclude how the reviews and invocations of research findings on smoking and low birth weight in the Surgeon General's reports specifically affected subsequent tobacco control policies and programs.

Factors Affecting the Use of Research in Policymaking

Contributors to the theoretical and empirical literature have recognized that a variety of factors affect whether, how, and the extent to which research is used in policymaking. Different authors have conceptualized these factors, and the relationships among them, in different ways. For example, Lomas (1991), in summarizing the literature, described a process of "interaction between characteristics of the receiver, the source, the message, and the channel of the information." Klein (1990) emphasized that the characteristics of the research evidence (the message) can be viewed as either ambiguous or unambiguous. The interaction among the characteristics of the receiver, the source, the message, and the channel occurs within a specific context for the individual policy being made, including the institutional structures and societal and personal values surrounding the decision, which affects the relationship between health statistics as knowledge and policymaking (Lomas 2000). The characteristics of the receiver include both core values and beliefs. As Lomas (1990, 527) indicated, "values are like enzymes. They are used to digest and transform information but in the process may be transformed themselves. They are both the screening through which information must pass and the target to be changed by the information." Finally, it is important to recognize that the relationship between research and policy making is mutual and bidirectional. As Tighe and Biersdorff (1993) indicate in a somewhat different context, "the traditional view of research informing practice without any sense that practice also can inform research has driven a wedge between researchers and potential consumers of research."

Use of Knowledge in Changing Population Health—Reducing Tobacco Use

This section illustrates how knowledge developed from health statistics is used to improve the population's health. To make the task manageable, this section is limited to a single example of the application of knowledge to change population health: recent efforts to reduce smoking and other tobacco use and, thereby, to reduce the adverse health effects of tobacco use. Throughout, we rely heavily on the U.S. Surgeon General's 2000 report on smoking and health, which focused on reducing tobacco use (USDHHS 2000). First, we present a summary of the influences on the decision to use tobacco and the approaches to reducing its use. We then provide examples of the applications of research, including intervention trials at the individual and community levels, simulation models, and other individual and population-based approaches to reduce tobacco use. The section demonstrates how researchers, policymakers, clinicians, public health workers, and others from many countries have applied knowledge about tobacco use and its causes—often obtained from direct analyses or other uses of health statistics—to this vexing but important population health problem.

Influences on Tobacco Use

Chapter 1 presented an overview of the influences on population health (see Fig. 1.3 and the accompanying discussion). It emphasized the diversity of these influences and the importance of taking a broad-minded approach when considering any particular health problem. This point is well illustrated by the diverse influences that bear on the use of tobacco products, as shown in Figure 10.2.

Approaches to Reducing Tobacco Use

Given these diverse influences, a variety of interventions have been developed and used to reduce tobacco use. These approaches include educational strategies, management of nicotine addiction, multiple regulatory efforts (including antitobacco advertising and promotion, mandatory warning labels on cigarette packs, tobacco product regulation, clean indoor air regulation, limiting minors' access to tobacco, and litigation against the tobacco industry), economic approaches (including taxation, tariffs, trade restrictions, and support of tobacco

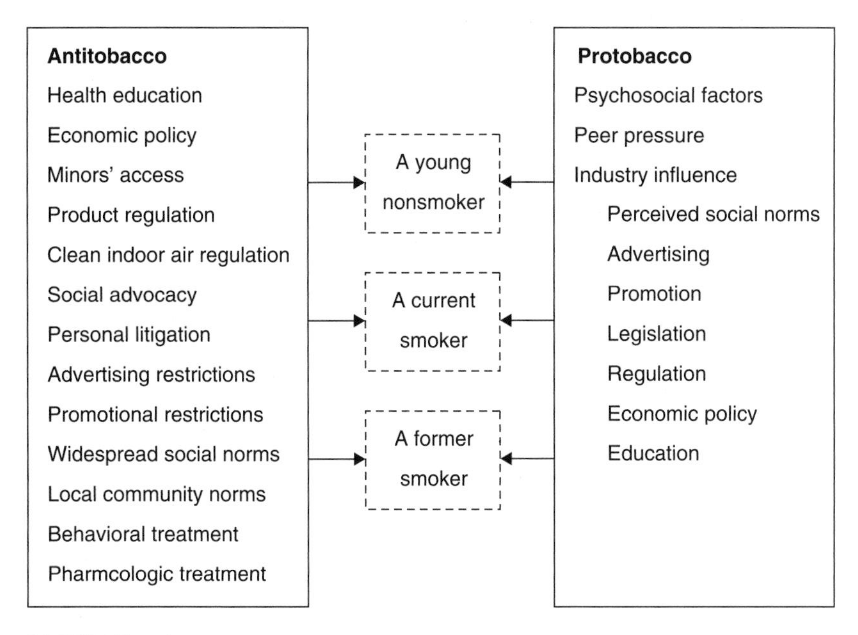

FIGURE 10.2
Influences on the decision to use tobacco. (Source: U.S. Department of Health and Human Services 2000, p. 7.)

growers), and comprehensive programs that combine two or more of these strategies. These interventions vary in their target audiences (e.g., current smokers and nonsmoking adolescents), tools used, breadth or span of impact, and size of impact (Table 10.3).

Role of Health Statistics in Reducing Tobacco Use

The role of health statistics in these interventions varies. For most interventions, health statistics provide information on the prevalence of smoking over time and within different population subgroups, the extent and nature of the morbidity and mortality from smoking, and how different groups have been affected (e.g., increased mortality among men initially, followed by increased mortality among women; increased mortality from cardiovascular disease, lung cancer, and other lung diseases). This information can be used as (*1*) background for policy development (discussed earlier in this chapter) and for the planning and implementation of specific interventions; (*2*) factual material presented in education strategies to inform the public and specific groups about the dangers of tobacco use; and (*3*) a means to evaluate the effectiveness of specific interventions (e.g., data from surveys on smoking prevalence among teenage girls in a community before and after implementation of a comprehensive educational

TABLE 10.3

Characteristics of Interventions and an Example of a Qualitative Assessment of Their Impact

Type of Intervention	*Targets*	*Tools*	*Study Approaches*	*Example of Qualitative Assessment of Intervention Impact*		
				Specific Intervention Modality	*Span of Impact of Intervention*	*Size of Impact of Intervention*
Educational	Children and adolescents, usually in school Administrative groups (e.g., members of health maintenance organizations) General population Health-care providers	School curricula Interactive training Targeted services Mass media	Epidemiologic and behavioral Usually a comparison of treatment and no-treatment groups Control of confounding by behavioral and social variables	School curriculum Mass media	Large Large	Moderate Small
Clinical	Persons who smoke, usually in a health-care setting General population of smokers in a commercial or quasi-commercial setting	Pharmacologic methods Behavioral modification Reinforcing environment	Epidemiologic and behavioral Usually a comparison of treatment and no-treatment groups Control of confounding by behavioral and demographic variables	Pharmacologic Behavioral (alone)	Small Small	Moderate Very small

Regulatory	Product manufacture Product sale Vendors and buyers Public venues Public transportation Worksites Health-care sites	Local ordinance State regulation Federal regulation Federal law Nongovernment action (e.g., joint commission accreditation of hospital organization)	Observational Knowledge/attitude/practice studies Surveillance Case study	Product manufacture Product sale Worksites	Very large Large Large	Very large Large Small
Economic	Taxes Tariffs and trade Price supports	Local ordinance State regulation Federal regulation Federal law International agreements	Econometric analysis Trend analysis Multivariate models	Taxation Tariffs and trade	Very large Very large	Very large Very large
Social/Comprehensive	Legislators Media Communication networks Case-by-case strategy State/local programs	Media advocacy Direct advocacy Community interventions Countermarketing Regulation Policy formation	Observational Case study General epidemiologic methods Trend analysis Knowledge/attitude/practice studies	Statewide programs Case-by-case strategy	Large Unpredictable	Large Unpredictable

Source: Adapted from U.S. Department of Health and Human Services (2000), Tables 1.1 and 1.2, pp. 9 and 11, respectively.

program to reduce smoking initiation; average blood cotinine levels of a nonsmoking population before and after implementation of clean indoor air regulations). A broader view of health statistics, similar to that advocated in Chapter 1, would add to the above uses of health statistics the use of quantitative data on the amount of tobacco products purchased before and after increases in tobacco excise taxes in selected U.S. states, or the relationship of tobacco consumption to price in different countries in order to evaluate the effectiveness of different economic approaches.

When used in conjunction with concepts and findings from other fields, health statistics have been especially useful in attempts to inform the public and reduce tobacco use. For example, social psychological research about attitudes and behavior change has been applied to the design of cigarette pack warning labels, including content principles (the wording of the warning label) and process principles (the style of the warning label) (Strahan et al. 2002). At the same time, health statistics are applied to develop the factual contents of warning labels by guiding the focus to specific research findings, such as the relationship of smoking to adverse pregnancy outcomes.

The same research findings from health statistics are sometimes used both as background for policy development and for the planning and implementation of specific interventions, on the one hand, and as factual material presented in education strategies to inform the public and specific groups, on the other hand. Cigarette warning labels, particularly those that warn about the association between smoking and infant low birth weight, can serve as an example. Despite active opposition from the tobacco industry (Kluger 1996; see also Aftab et al. 1999), the United States has required warning labels on cigarette packs since the passage of the Federal Cigarette Labeling and Advertising Act of 1965 (Centers for Disease Control and Prevention [hp] Warning label fact sheet). By the early 1990s, 77 countries required cigarette pack warning labels of various types (World Bank 1999), including Australia (Lewis 1993), Canada (Mahood 1999), France (CBSNews.com [hp]), India (Shimkhada and Peabody 2003), and the United Kingdom (Tobacco Manufacturers' Association [fs]). Starting with the passage of the Comprehensive Smoking Education Act of 1984, the United States required warning labels that specifically mention low birth weight: "Surgeon General's Warning: Smoking by Pregnant Women May Result in Fetal Injury, Premature Birth, and Low Birth Weight" (warning introduced in 1984) and "Surgeon General's Warning: Tobacco Use Increases the Risk of Infertility, Stillbirth and Low Birth Weight" (warning introduced in 2000) (Centers for Disease Control and Prevention [hp] Warning label fact sheet). The warning labels targeted to pregnant women, and specifically mentioning the risks of low birth weight, are intended as *information shocks* and reflect the substantial body of research findings relating smoking to low birth weight. Research has also focused on evaluating the efficacy of warning labels for smokers and nonsmokers and has demonstrated mixed results, depending on such factors as whether the warning labels are used in developed or developing countries (Aftab et al. 1999), the ages of the target audience (Cecil et al. 1996; Crawford et al. 2002), and the size and graphic presentation of the warning labels (Borland 1997; Hammond et al. 2003; Kaiserman 1993).

Two challenges in the use of health statistics as knowledge in reducing tobacco use are the complexity of the influences on, and the diversity of interventions to reduce, tobacco use and, as a result, the need to select appropriate (and comparable) metrics to assess the effectiveness of different interventions. Various metrics have been used to evaluate program effectiveness, and these metrics have often not been comparable. Furthermore, complex analyses may be necessary to tease out the respective contributions of different interventions, and many evaluations have not addressed this need (USDHHS 2000, 8, 10). Nevertheless, health statistics as knowledge have had, and will continue to have, a central role in society's attempts to reduce tobacco use, as well as in its attempt to effect positive change in other aspects of population health.

CONCLUSIONS: CHALLENGES IN KNOWLEDGE CREATION AND HEALTH STATISTICS

The discussion in this chapter of the role of health statistics in knowledge creation highlights the contributions of health statistics but also the remaining challenges. Several challenges are summarized below.

First, there is a continuing need to emphasize the translation (i.e., dissemination and use) of health statistics. As described in Chapter 3, there are gaps in performance in the health statistics cycle, especially where statistics are not fully translated into usable form. Furthermore, feedback from use of statistics is not systematically compiled and applied to making improvements in data collection. As the performance of the health statistics enterprise in this translation function improves, the contribution of health statistics to overall knowledge creation will increase. Similarly, knowledge gained from data collection will improve as the enterprise moves from a primary focus on data gathering to adding value through analysis and interpretation.

Second, with the increasing quantity of readily available health statistics, those who seek straightforward answers to specific questions face the prospect of information overload. For example, information about health insurance coverage is collected in multiple health surveys in different ways (e.g., uninsured at a point in time, for part of the past year, for a full year) (Cohen et al. 2004). While each estimate is useful in understanding different elements of a multifaceted health issue, the existence of multiple and sometimes conflicting estimates contributes to confusion among policymakers and the public. Efforts to explain differences among estimates, place different estimates in context, and help educate users on appropriate uses are time-consuming and complex, and not clearly in the mandate of any single element of the health statistics enterprise as currently organized.

BOX 10.2
Conclusion

IT may be now asked, to what purpose tends all this laborious buzzling, and groping? To know,

1. The number of the People?
2. How many *Males*, and *Females?*
3. How many Married, and single?
4. How many *Teeming* Women?
5. How Many of every *Septenary*, or *Decad* of years in *age?*
6. How many *Fighting* Men?
7. How much *London* is, and by what steps it hath increased?
8. In what time the housing is replenished after a *Plague*?
9. What proportion die of each general and perticular *Casualties*?
10. What years are Fruitfull, and Mortal, and in what Space, and Intervals, they follow each other?
11. In what proportion Men neglect the Orders of the *Church*, and *Sects* have increased?
12. The disproportion of Parishes?
13. Why the Burials in *London* exceed the Christnings, when the contrary is visible in the Country?

To this I might answer in general by saying, that those, who cannot apprehend the reason of these Enquiries, are unfit to trouble themselves to ask them.
—John Graunt, 1662, Conclusion to his observations upon the Bills of Mortality

Source: Graunt (1662), p. 71.

Third, with an increasing diversity of data sources, it becomes more challenging to differentiate credible from noncredible sources of health statistics and the resulting knowledge. This challenge has several elements, including the challenge of evaluating information quality, when it is often difficult to evaluate the methods used to collect information, and the need to assess the analytic integrity of purported "knowledge," where it is often difficult to separate underlying data from "spin" that is introduced when information is used in advocacy or for proprietary purposes. Although federal agencies seek to address this challenge through clear documentation and official commentary on the quality of public information (USDHHS [hp] Guidelines for ensuring the quality), in a diverse health statistics enterprise no obvious counterpart policy exists for other data sources.

Finally, there are imbalances in knowledge about population health and the influences on it resulting from gaps in coverage of these topics by health statistics systems (see Box 10.2). As discussed in Chapters 1 and 3, our knowledge is now limited by data gaps in content (e.g., failure to understand the contextual influences on population health and lack of broader measures that integrate multiple aspects of health), as well as by restricted scope and insufficient detail (e.g., understanding variations in health status by geography and sociodemographic attributes). Uses of nontraditional sources of information (as outlined in Chapter 7) would help to address these gaps but are comparatively infrequent.

NOTES

1. Nikhil Sharma presents a brief history of the origin of the history of the hierarchy of these three terms, to which *wisdom* is often added to produce what is known as the *DIKW* hierarchy (Sharma [mg] Origin of DIKW). The authors acknowledge Mr. Sharma as a source for the idea of this section of our chapter. A nice discussion of the difficulties of defining information can be found at McInerney C. Information science—an art and a science [monograph on the Internet]. New Brunswick, NJ: Rutgers, The State University of New Jersey, NJ; 1997 [cited 2004 Mar 31]. Available from: http://www.scils.rutgers.edu/~clairemc/infsci.html.
2. Related—but not identical—to the second definition of research is the definition of research used by the U.S. Department of Health and Human Services in its regulations for the protection of human subjects: "a systematic investigation, including research development, testing and evaluation, designed to develop or contribute to generalizable knowledge" (45 CFR part 46 sec. 46.102(d)). (See Chapter 14 for a thorough discussion of the issue of the protection of human subjects involved in research.)
3. In 1739, the philosopher David Hume published eight "rules by which to judge of causes and effects" (Hume 1739). Henle in 1840 and Koch in the 1880s developed criteria for establishing a specific organism as the cause of an infectious disease (Evans 1993). Many epidemiologists have also addressed the issue of causation (e.g., Abramson and Abramson 1999, 305–327; Morabia 1991; Rothman and Greenland 1997; Susser 1973).
4. See Gordis (1996, 169–170) or other textbooks on epidemiology for a more complete discussion of ecological analyses and their potential for identifying spurious associations.
5. The 709 articles met the following criteria: publication date between 1 January 1990 and 8 April 2004; smoking included as a Medical Subject Heading (MeSH) term or as a text word in the abstract; and *infant, low birth weight* (MeSH), or *low birth weight* as a text phrase.
6. The additional criteria were articles in English, with abstracts, and with human subjects.

REFERENCES

Abramson JH, Abramson ZH. Survey Methods in Community Medicine: Epidemiological Research, Programme Evaluation, Clinical Trials, 5th ed. Edinburgh: Churchill Livingstone; 1999.

AcademyHealth [meeting agenda on the Internet]. Washington, DC: AcademyHealth [cited 2004 May 1]. Annual research meeting session: communicating your research to the media [about 1 screen]. Available from: http://www.academyhealth.org/arm/agenda/glance.pdf.

Ackoff RL [serial on the Internet]. On learning and systems that facilitate it. Center Qual Manag J 1996;5(2):27–35 [cited 2004 Mar 31]. Available from: http://cqmextra.cqm.org/cqmjournal.nsf/reprints/rp07300.

Aftab M, Kolben D, Lurie P. International cigarette labeling practices. Tob Control 1999; 8:368–372.

American Heritage Dictionary of the English Language, 4th ed. Boston MA: Houghton Mifflin; 2000.

American Legacy Foundation [homepage on the Internet]. Washington, DC: American Legacy Foundation; c. 2003 [cited 2004 Jun 9]. Truth campaign. Available from: http://www.protectthetruth.org/truthcampaign.htm.

American Statistical Association [homepage on the Internet]. Alexandria, VA: American Statistical Association; c. 2004 [cited 2004 May 1]. Statistics you can count on, information you can trust [about 5 screens]. Available from: http://www.amstat.org/pressroom/index.cfm?fuseaction=mediakit.

Arias E, Anderson RN, Kung HC, Murphy SL, Kochanek KD. Deaths: final data for 2001. Natl Vital Stat Rep 2003;52(3):1–115.

Aronson RA, Uttech S, Soref M. The effect of maternal cigarette smoking on low birth weight and preterm birth in Wisconsin, 1991. Wis Med J 1993;92(11):613–617.

Bell R, Lumley J. Low birthweight and socioeconomic status, Victoria 1982 to 1986. Aust J Public Health 1992;16(1):15–19.

Bellinger G, Castro D, Mills A. Data, Information, Knowledge, and Wisdom [monograph on the Internet]. OutSight, Inc; c. 2004 [cited 2004 Mar 30]. Available from: http://www.systems-thinking.org/dikw/dikw.htm.

Berry M, Bove F. Birth weight reduction associated with residence near a hazardous waste landfill. Environ Health Perspect 1997;105(8):856–861.

Beyer JM, Trice HM. The utilization process: a conceptual framework and synthesis of empirical findings. Adm Sci Q 1982;27:591–622.

Black N. Evidence based policy: proceed with care. Br Med J 2001;323:275–279.

Bonati M, Fellin G. Changes in smoking and drinking behaviour before and during pregnancy in Italian mothers: implications for public health intervention. Int J Epidmiol 1991;20(4):927–932.

Borland R. Tobacco health warnings and smoking-related cognitions and behaviours. Addiction 1997;92(11):1427–1435.

Brown D. Medical care often not optimal, study finds; failure to treat patients fully spans range of what is expected of physicians and nurses. Washington Post 2003 June 26; Sect. A:2.

Bulmer M. Governments and social science: patterns of mutual influence. In: Bulmer M, ed. Social Science Research and Government: Comparative Essays on Britain and the United States. Cambridge: Cambridge University Press; 1987, pp. 1–23.

Buxton M, Hanney S. How can payback from health services research be assessed? J Health Serv Res Policy 1996;1(1):35–43.

Canadian Research Transfer Network. Knowledge Transfer in Health: A Report on the second Annual Canadian Research Transfer Network Conference, Oct 24–25; 2002, Calgary, AL. Ottawa: Canadian Research Transfer Network.

CBSNews.com [homepage on the Internet]. New York: CBS Broadcasting Inc; c. 2004 [updated 2003 Jun 27; cited 2004 May 10]. Blunt warnings for French smokers. Available from: http://cbsnews.com/stories/2003/06/27/health/main560769.shtml.

Cecil H, Evans RI, Stanley MA. Perceived believability among adolescents of health warning labels on cigarette packs. J Appl Soc Psychol 1996;26(6):502–519.

Centers for Disease Control. Kaposi's sarcoma and pneumocystis pneumonia among homosexual men—New York City and California. MMWR 1981;30(25);305–308.

Centers for Disease Control and Prevention, National Center for Chronic Disease Prevention and Health Promotion, Tobacco Information and Prevention Service [homepage on the Internet]. Atlanta: Centers for Disease Control and Prevention [updated 2003

Mar 20; cited 2004 May 10]. Warning label fact sheet. Available from: http://www.cdc.gov/tobacco/sgr/sgr_2000/factsheets/factsheet_labels.htm.

Central West Health Planning Information Network. A Framework for Evaluating the Utilization of Health Information Products. Hamilton, Ontario: Central West Health Planning Information Network; 2000.

Chen LH, Petitti DB. Case-control study of passive smoking and the risk of small-for-gestational-age at term. Am J Epidemiol 1995;142(2):158–165.

Chong JR. California: smoking rates hit record lows in state, officials say. Los Angeles Times 2003 Apr 5; Sect. B:10.

Cohen BB, Friedman DJ, Mahan CM, Lederman R, Munoz D. Ethnicity, maternal risk, and birth weight among Hispanics in Massachusetts, 1987–89. Public Health Rep 1993;108(3): 363–371.

Cohen MD, March JG, Olsen JP. A garbage can model of organizational choice. Adm Sci Q 1972;17(1):1–25.

Cohen RA, Coriaty-Nelson Z, Ni H. Health Insurance Coverage: Estimates from the National Health Interview Survey, January–September 2003. Hyattsville, MD: National Center for Health Statistics; March 2004 [cited 2004 May 13]. Available from: http://www.cdc.gov/nchs/nhis.htm.

Crawford MA, Balch GI, Mermelstein R, Tobacco Control Network Writing Group. Responses to tobacco control policies among youth. Tob Control 2002;11:14–19.

Davis P, Howden-Chapman P. Translating research findings into health policy. Soc Sci Med 1996;43(5):865–872.

Day P. The media and the scientific message. J Health Serv Res Policy 1997;2(2):65–66.

deSemir V, Ribas C, Revuelta G. Press releases of science journal articles and subsequent newspaper stories on the same topic. JAMA 1998; 280(3):294–295.

Dietz PM, Adams MM, Kendrick JS, Mathis MP. Completeness of ascertainment of prenatal smoking using birth certificates and confidential questionnaires: variations by maternal attributes and infant birth weight. Am J Epidemiol 1998;148(11):1048–1054.

Entwistle V. Reporting research in medical journals and newspapers. BMJ 1995;310 (6984): 920–923.

Ericson A, Eriksson M, Kallen B, Zetterstrom R. Secular trends in the effect of socio-economic factors on birth weight and infant survival in Sweden. Scand J Soc Med 1993; 21(1):10–16.

Evans AS. Causation and Disease: A Chronological Journal. New York: Plenum; 1993, pp. 13–39.

Faden VB, Graubard BI. Alcohol consumption during pregnancy and infant birth weight. Ann Epidemiol 1994;4(4):279–284.

Fortier I, Marcoux S, Brisson J. Passive smoking during pregnancy and the risk of delivering a small-for-gestational-age infant. Am J Epidemiol 1994;139(3):294–301.

Fox SH, Koepsell TD, Daling JR. Birth weight and smoking during pregnancy—effect modification by maternal age. Am J Epidemiol 1994;139(10):1008–1015.

Gissler M, Merilainen J, Vuori E, Hemminki E. Register based monitoring shows decreasing socioeconomic differences in Finnish perinatal health. J Epidemiol Commun Health 2003a;57(6):433–439.

Gissler M, Pakkanen M, Olausson PO. Fertility and perinatal health among Finnish immigrants in Sweden. Soc Sci Med 2003b;57(8):1443–1454.

Google directory [database on the Internet]. Mountain View, CA: Google; c. 2004 [cited 2004 Apr 1]. Knowledge creation. Available from: http://directory.google.com/Top/Reference/Knowledge_Management/Knowledge_Creation.

Gordis L. Epidemiology. Philadelphia: W.B. Saunders; 1996.

Graunt J. Natural and Political Observations Mentioned in a Following Index, and Made upon the Bills of Mortality. London: John Martin; 1662 [cited 2004 Apr 4]. Available from: http://www.ac.wwu.edu/~stephan/Graunt/bills.html.

Haeckel SH, Nolan RL. The role of technology in an information age: transforming symbols into action. In: The Institute for Information Studies, The Knowledge Economy: The Nature of Information in the 21st Century. Queenstown, MD: The Aspen Institute; 1993, pp. 1–24.

Hammond D, Fong GT, McDonald PW, Cameron R, Brown KS. Impact of the graphic Canadian warning labels on adult smoking behaviour. Tob Control 2003;12:391–395.

Hanney SR, Gonzalez-Block MA, Buxton MJ, Kogan M [serial on the Internet]. The utilization of health research in policy-making: concepts, examples and methods of assessment. Health Res Policy Syst 2003;1(1):2 [cited 2004 Apr 8]. Available from: http://www.health-policy-systems.com/content/pdf/1478-4505-1-2.pdf.

Hill AB. The environment and disease: association or causation? Proc R Soc Med 1965; 58:295–300.

Hough R. Captain James Cook. New York: W.W. Norton; 1994.

Hueston WJ, Mainous AG III, Farrell JB. A cost-benefit analysis of smoking cessation programs during the first trimester of pregnancy for the prevention of low birthweight. J Fam Pract 1994;39(4):353–357.

Hume D. A Treatise on Human Nature, Book I, Sect. XV. London: Printed for John Noon, at the White Hart, near Mercer's-Chapel, in Cheapside; 1739, pp. 223–224.

Innvaer S, Vist G, Trommald M, Oxman A. Health policy-makers' perceptions of their use of evidence: a systematic review. J Health Serv Res Policy 2002;7(4):239–244.

Kaiserman MJ. The effectiveness of health warning messages. Tob Control 1993;2:267–269.

Kingdon JW. Agendas, Alternatives, and Public Policies, 2nd ed. New York: Longman; 2003.

Klein R. Research, policy, and the National Health Service. J Health Polit Policy Law 1990; 15(3):501–523.

Kluger R. Ashes to Ashes: America's Hundred-Year Cigarette War, the Public Health, and the Unabashed Triumph of Philip Morris. New York: Alfred A. Knopf; 1996.

Land GH, Stockhauser JW. Smoking and pregnancy outcome: trends among black teenage mothers in Missouri. Am J Public Health 1993;83(8):1121–1124.

Landry R, Amara N, Lamari M. Utilization of social science research knowledge in Canada. Res Policy 2001;30:333–349.

Lester JP. The utilization of policy analysis by state agency officials. Knowledge: Creation, Diffusion, Utilization 1993;14(3):267–290.

Lewis K. Evolution of Australia's health warning labels. World Smoking Health 1993;18(2):7–9.

Li DK, Daling JR. Maternal smoking, low birth weight, and ethnicity in relation to sudden infant death syndrome. Am J Epidemiol 1991;134(9):958–964.

Lindblom CE. The science of "muddling through." Public Adm Rev 1959;19:79–88.

Lindblom CE, Cohen DK. Alternatives to authoritativeness. In: Lindblom CE, Cohen DK. Usable Knowledge: Social Science and Social Problem Solving. New Haven, CT: Yale University Press; 1979, pp. 72–85.

Lipsky M. Street-Level Bureaucracy: The Dilemmas of the Individual in Public Service. New York: Russell Sage Foundation; 1983.

Lomas J. Finding audiences, changing beliefs: the structure of research use in Canadian health policy. J Health Polit Policy Law 1990;15(3):525–542.

Lomas J. Words without action? The production, dissemination, and impact of consensus recommendations. Annu Rev Public Health 1991;12:41–65.

Lomas J. Connecting research and policy. Isuma 2000;1(1):140–144.

Mahood G. Warnings that tell the truth: breaking new ground in Canada. Tob Control 1999;8:356–362.

Mainous AG III, Hueston WJ. The effect of smoking cessation during pregnancy on preterm delivery and low birthweight. J Fam Pract 1994;38(3):262–266.

Mathews TJ. Smoking during pregnancy in the 1990s. Natl Vital Stat Rep 2001;49(7):1–14.

McGlynn EA, Asch SM, Adams J, Kessey J, Hicks J, DeCristofaro A, et al. The quality of health care delivered to adults in the United States. N Engl J Med 2003;348(26):2635–2645.

Merriam-Webster Online Dictionary, 10th ed. [homepage on the Internet]. Springfield, MA: Merriam-Webster; c. 2004 [cited 2004 Apr 12]. Available from: http://www.m-w.com.
Millar WJ, Chen J. Maternal education and risk factors for small-for-gestational-age births. Health Rep 1998;10(2):43–51.
Miller DP, Villa KF, Hogue SL, Sivapathasundaram D. Birth and first-year costs for mothers and infants attributable to maternal smoking. Nicotine Tob Res 2001;3(1):25–35.
Morabia A. On the origin of Hill's causal criteria. Epidemiology 1991;2(5):367–369.
Mosteller F. Innovation and evaluation. Science 1981;211:881–886.
Nonaka I, Takeuchi H. The Knowledge-Creating Company. New York: Oxford University Press; 1995.
Okosun IS, Halbach SM, Dent MM, Cooper RS. Ethnic differences in the rates of low birth weight attributable to differences in early motherhood: a study from the Third National Health and Nutrition Examination Survey. J Perinatol 2000;20(2):105–109.
Olausson PM, Cnattingius S, Goldenberg RL. Determinants of poor pregnancy outcomes among teenagers in Sweden. Obstet Gynecol 1997;89(3):451–457.
Olsen J, Frische G. Social differences in reproductive health. A study of birth weight, still-births and congential malformations in Denmark. Scand J Soc Med 1993;21(2):90–97.
Pestiueau C. Evaluating policy research. Ottawa: Canadian Policy Research Networks; 2003.
Phillips D, Kawachi I, Tilyard M. The costs of smoking revisited. NZ Med J 1992;105(936): 240–242.
Ramsey AM, Blose D, Lorenz D, Thomas W, DePersio SR, Bruce FC. Cigarette smoking among women in Oklahoma: before, during, and after pregnancy. J Okla State Med Assoc 1993;86(5):231–236.
Reichman NE, Pagnini DL. Maternal age and birth outcomes: data from New Jersey. Fam Plann Perspect 1997;29(6):268–272, 295.
Rothman KJ, Greenland S. Causation and causal inference. In: Detels R, Holland WW, McEwen J, Omenn GS, eds. Oxford Textbook of Public Health, Vol. 2, The Methods of Public Health, 3rd ed. New York: Oxford University Press; 1997, pp. 617–629.
Schwartz L. Media coverage of scientific meetings: too much, too soon? JAMA 2002; 287(21): 2859–2863.
Sharma N [monograph on the Internet]. The Origin of the Data Information Knowledge Wisdom Hierarchy. [cited 2004 Mar 30]. Available from: http://www-personal.si.umich.edu/~nsharma/dikw_origin.htm.
Shimkhada R, Peabody JW. Tobacco control in India. Bull World Health Org 2003;81(1):48–52.
Singer E, Endreny P. Reporting on Risk: How the Mass Media Portray Accidents, Diseases, Disasters, and Other Hazards. New York: Russell Sage Foundation; 1993.
Singer E, Endreny P. Reporting on risk: how the mass media portray accidents, diseases, disasters and other hazards. Risk: Health, Safety Environ 1994;5:261 [cited 2004 Nov 12]. Available from: http://www.piercelaw.edu/risk/vol5/summer/singer.htm.
Stone D. Using knowledge: the dilemmas of "bridging research and policy." Compare 2002; 32(3):285–296.
Strahan EJ, White K, Fong GT, Fabrigar LR, Zanna MP, Cameron R. Enhancing the effectiveness of tobacco package warning labels: a social psychological perspective. Tob Control 2002;11:183–190.
Stratton K, Shetty P, Wallace R, Bondurant S, eds. Clearing the Smoke: Assessing the Science Base for Tobacco Harm Reduction. Washington, DC: National Academy Press; 2001.
Susser M. Causal Thinking in the Health Sciences. New York: Oxford University Press; 1973.
Taubes G. What if it's all been a big fat lie? New York Times Sunday Magazine 2002 July 7; Sect. 6:22 (col. 1).
Thomas HC [monograph on the Internet]. Fostering the Collaborative Creation of Knowledge: A White Paper. White Plains, NY: IBM [cited 2004 Apr 1]. Available from: http://www.research.ibm.com/knowsoc/project_paper.html.

Thomas P. The use of social research: myths and models. In: Bulmer M, ed. Social Science Research and Government: Comparative Essays on Britain and the United States. Cambridge: Cambridge University Press; 1987, pp. 51–60.

Thompson JM, Clark PM, Robinson E, Becroft DM, Pattison NS, Glavish N, Pryor JE, Wild CJ, Rees K, Mitchell EA. Risk factors for small-for-gestational-age babies: The Auckland Birthweight Collaborative Study. J Paediatr Child Health 2001;37(4):369–375.

Tighe RJ, Biersdorff KK. Setting agendas for relevant research: a participatory approach. Can J Rehabil 1993;7(2):127–132.

Tobacco Manufacturers' Association. History of warnings on packs in the UK [fact sheet on the Internet]. London: Tobacco Manufacturers' Association; 2003 Sep 26 [cited 2004 May 10]. Available from: http://tma.pr24x7.com/index.php?MRM_pmid=248.

U.S. Department of Health, Education, and Welfare, Public Health Service. Smoking and Health: Report of the Advisory Committee to the Surgeon General. Washington, DC: U.S. Public Health Service; 1964.

U.S. Department of Health and Human Services. Reducing Tobacco Use: A Report of the Surgeon General. Atlanta: U.S. Department of Health and Human Services, Centers for Disease Control and Prevention, National Center for Chronic Disease Prevention and Health Promotion, Office on Smoking and Health; 2000 [cited 2004 Jun 9]. Available from: http://www.cdc.gov/tobacco/sgr/index.htm.

U.S. Department of Health and Human Services [homepage on the Internet]. Washington, DC: U.S. Department of Health and Human Services [updated 2003 Nov 13; cited 2004 May 1]. Guidelines for ensuring the quality of information disseminated by HHS agencies. Available from: http://www.hhs.gov/infoquality.

USA Today [homepage on the Internet]. McLean, VA: USA Today; c. 2002 [cited 2004 May 20]. USA Today snapshot. Available from: http://www.usatoday.com/snapshot/news/nsnap085.htm.

Ventura SJ, Hamilton BE, Mathews TJ, Chandra A. Trends and variations in smoking during pregnancy and low birth weight: evidence from the birth certificate, 1990–2000. Pediatrics 2003;111(5 part 2):1176–1180.

Visscher WA, Feder M, Burns AM, Brady TM, Bray RM. The impact of smoking and other substance use by urban women on the birthweight of their infants. Subst Use Misuse 2003;38(8):1063–1093.

Von Krogh G, Ichijo K, Nonaka I. Enabling Knowledge Creation: How to Unlock the Mystery of Tacit Knowledge and Release the Power of Innovation. Oxford and New York: Oxford University Press; 2000.

Webb A, Wistow G. Whither State Welfare: Policy and Implementation in the Personal Social Services, 1979–80. London: Royal Institute of Public Administration; 1982.

Webb A, Wistow G. Planning, Need and Scarcity. London: Allen and Unwin; 1986.

Weiss CH. Introduction. In: Weiss CH, ed. Using Social Research in Public Policy Making. Lexington, MA: Lexington Books, pp. 1–22.

Weiss CH. The many meanings of research utilization. Public Adm Rev 1979;39(5):426–431.

Weiss CH. Knowledge creep and decision accretion. Knowledge: Creation, Diffusion, Utilization 1980;1(3):381–404.

Wikipedia: The Free Encyclopedia [encyclopedia on the Internet]. St. Petersburg, FL: Wikipedia Foundation; copyleft [updated 2004 Feb 19; cited 2004 Mar 31]. Knowledge. Available from: http://en.wikipedia.org/wiki/Knowledge.

Wikipedia: The Free Encyclopedia [encyclopedia on the Internet]. St. Petersburg, FL: Wikipedia Foundation; copyleft [updated 2003 Oct. 3; cited 2004 Apr 1]. Knowledge creation. Available from: http://en.wikipedia.org/wiki/Knowledge_creation.

Windham GC, Hopkins B, Fenster L, Swan SH. Prenatal active or passive tobacco smoke exposure and the risk of preterm delivery or low birth weight. Epidemiology 2000;11(4):427–433.

Wolff CB, Portis M, Wolff H. Birth weight and smoking practices during pregnancy among Mexican-American women. Health Care Women Int 1993;14(3):271–279.

Wolff CB, Portis M. Smoking, acculturation, and pregnancy outcome among Mexican Americans. Health Care Women Int 1996;17(6):563–573.

Wolfson MC. Social proprioception: measurement, data, and information from a population health perspective. In: Evans RG, Barer ML, Marmor TR, eds. Why Are Some People Healthy and Others Not? New York: Aldine de Gruyter; 1994, p. 314.

World Bank. Curbing the Epidemic: Governments and the Economics of Tobacco Control. Washington, DC: World Bank; 1999.

Wu T, Buck G, Mendola P. Can regular multivitamin/mineral supplementation modify the relation between maternal smoking and select adverse birth outcomes? Ann Epidemiol 1998;8(3):175–183.

CHAPTER 11

Why Truth Matters: The Role of Health Statistics in Health Policy

Judith Feder and Larry Levitt

Social organizations—whether they are businesses, nonprofits, or communities —rely on policies that define relationships, allocate resources, and determine the rules by which they operate. A hospital has policies for admitting patients, awarding privileges to physicians, and allocating resources across departments and roles across professions. A health plan has policies for paying claims, setting payments to providers, setting its premiums, and (in most cases) rewarding its stockholders. And a community—including the nation—has policies, implicit or explicit, on who has what kind of health insurance coverage, at what price, with what claims on physicians, hospitals, and other providers for the delivery of care.

Within an organization or a nation, policies have significant consequences. How a health plan selects or pays providers, for example, will determine the quality of care it provides, the patients it will attract, and its ability to stay in business. How the nation organizes its health insurance will determine who gets what kind of health care at what cost. Understanding the impact of policies and the factors that influence impacts is therefore critical to the formation of policies that promote organizational or community goals.

That statistics—or quantitative data—and their analysis are invaluable to understanding and therefore shaping policies should go without saying. How can an organization distinguish what works from what does not work without statistics on its revenues and costs and analysis of the factors that shape them? How can a community distinguish what works from what does not work without statistics and analysis? The answer is obvious: it cannot. But it is equally obvious that in organizations and communities, policies are not the simple outcomes of statistical analysis pursuant to the achievement of clearly articulated organizational goals. Organizations and communities have multiple goals (implicit and explicit). They also have entrenched bureaucracies and operating procedures alongside an array of competing interests and complex incentives. Policies will often be shaped at least as much by interests, incentives, and their interactions within institutions as by a rational, statistically based decision process. In other words, statistics will play a role in the policy process, but exactly what role will depend on the myriad other forces that determine how organizations and communities work.

The purpose of this chapter is to examine the role of statistical analysis in a very big and sometimes very visible policy process—health reform, or the making of the nation's policies on health insurance coverage. To observers of that process, relative to politics, statistics may appear to have had little if any role. But a closer look will reveal that statistical analysis is part of the political and policy process, even if it does not drive the debate or determine its outcome.

Our plan is as follows: We begin with an overview of the policy process in general, describing three critical stages—identifying the policy problem, analyzing possible solutions, and debating and deciding on political action. Then, after a brief discussion of what we mean by *health reform* and the policy and political process affecting it in the past decade, we describe the role of data and statistics in each phase of the process. Finally, we conclude with lessons from that experience for collection and analysis of statistics and the scholars and analysts who undertake it.

BACKGROUND: THE POLICY PROCESS AND HEALTH REFORM

John Kingdon's (1995) analysis of the factors shaping how issues emerge and fare on the political agenda provides a useful framework for examining the role of statistics in health policy. Kingdon's premise is that there are three *streams*, operating simultaneously and independently, that shape a policy agenda. First is the stream that identifies an issue as a *policy problem*—moves it from simply an unsatisfactory condition to a condition worthy of political attention. Kingdon argues that statistics can trigger such a move. Our first task is to demonstrate how.

The second stream of activity Kingdon identifies is that of policy solutions—use of the various tools government has at its disposal to resolve or mitigate the identified problem. In health reform, as in other policy areas, statistical analysis is key to the development and assessment of solutions that provide the focal point of policy action. Our second task is to describe the contributions and challenges statistical analysis makes to policy development.

The third stream from which political action items emerge is the political stream. It is in the political arena—the world of electoral, ideological, and interest group politics—that observers are most skeptical about the role of statistics. But, as we will describe, statistical analysis of policy impacts—for example, who wins and who loses from specific policy action—play a considerable role in policy debates. Although researchers may sometimes be horrified by the role statistics play, they are major contributors to the political process. Our third task is to illustrate that contribution.

Our intent is to examine the role of statistical analysis in the problem, policy, and political streams in the health reform debate of the 1990s. Our primary focus will be on health reform defined as coverage expansion, especially on the debate surrounding President Bill Clinton's proposal for universal health insurance in 1993–1994.

LACK OF HEALTH INSURANCE AS A POLICY PROBLEM

Clearly, lack of health insurance did not emerge as a problem for those affected by it just at the time of the 1992 election. Millions of Americans have always been without health insurance. And, after decades of expansion of coverage from the 1950s, private health insurance coverage began to decline in the late 1970s and early 1980s (Mishel 1997, 159). But the 1980s brought little political discussion of health insurance. How and why did lack of coverage move from an issue, recognized by experts and the people directly affected, to a policy problem in the 1990s? Did statistical analysis play a role?

Analyses of the 1990s debate tend to tie its emergence on the national scene with the 1991 special Senate election in Pennsylvania, when Harris Wofford made lack of health insurance an issue in his successful bid for the seat made vacant by the death of Senator John Heinz (Kingdon 1995, 218). Building on Wofford's success, 1992 presidential candidates—including, but not limited to, Bill Clinton—put health insurance high on the political agenda.

Statistics, then, did not place health insurance on the agenda. But a review of the early 1990s debate and of more current experience illustrates three ways in which statistical analysis established coverage as a problem requiring policy intervention: (*1*) by demonstrating that lack of health insurance matters, (*2*) by documenting the substantial and increasing number of people without insurance, and (*3*) by characterizing the uninsured population as worthy of support.

Evidence That Health Insurance Matters

From an equity perspective, it may be obvious that exclusion from the nation's health insurance system of tens of millions of people is problematic. But equity is unlikely to stimulate political action—and investment of resources—without evidence that lack of health insurance affects people's access to health care. Indeed, public opinion surveys fairly regularly indicate that the American public believes that most people get the care they need, whether or not they have health insurance (Institute of Medicine 2001, 2). Evidence aimed at refuting that point of view comes from statistics and their analysis.

This statistical evidence dates back to the New Deal debate on national health insurance (Anderson and Anderson 1999), became a national responsibility in the 1960s (Anderson and Anderson 1999, 19–20), and by the 1990s had become a fixture in health reform debates (Congressional Research Service 1988; U.S. Bipartisan Commission 1990).

The arguments used in the early 1990s debate relied heavily on surveys to make the case for universal health insurance. Along with the National Health Interview Survey, which documented that differences in service use were associated with differences in insurance status, analysis relied on a series of *access surveys* initiated in the1970s by The Robert Wood Johnson Foundation (RWJ)—surveys conducted to address the gap RWJ's leadership perceived in documentation of the access problem and support for measures to address it (Andersen and Anderson 1999, 25–27). Those surveys served to illustrate both that coverage expansion improved access, particularly among disadvantaged populations, and that lack of coverage posed barriers to access. Over time, the surveys moved from pure academic research to uses in policy advocacy, seeking more and more powerful ways to impress the public and the policy community (Anderson and Anderson 1999, 27). The 1986 RWJ survey, used by the Pepper Commission in 1990, demonstrated that people without insurance reported an inability to receive care for financial reasons, actual denial of care, based on ability to pay, and, for people with "serious symptoms," receipt of substantially less care for the uninsured than for the insured (U.S. Bipartisan Commission 1990, 34). In 1996 then-RWJ president Steve Schroeder used this survey evidence in *The New England Journal of Medicine* explicitly to challenge the myth that people without health insurance nevertheless receive health care when they need it (Schroeder 1996).

Today's arguments for health insurance continue to rely on survey data and continue to challenge myths (Institute of Medicine 2001, 2). And surveys by RWJ's Center for the Study of Health Systems Change, the Kaiser Family Foundation, and the Commonwealth Fund continue the earlier RWJ efforts to document access problems.

In contrast to the early 1990s, when only a handful of statistical analyses had provided detailed assessments of the impact of insurance, today's literature includes an abundance of analyses of the relationship between insurance and specific health conditions, as well as general access to and outcomes of care. Two recent reviews conclude that the preponderance of the evidence supports an argument that people who lack health insurance, compared to people who have it, get care later, get less care, and, as a result are likely to suffer poorer health—including a substantially higher probability of death (Hadley 2002; Institute of Medicine 2002). In his most powerful summary statistic, Hadley draws the conclusion that universal health insurance would reduce mortality rates among the uninsured population by 5% to 50%. However, no research is definitive. As Hadley notes, although the preponderance of evidence connects lack of insurance to poor health, studies use a wide range of imperfect methodologies, leading different studies to produce different results and some researchers to question strong inferences from any results (Levy and Meltzer 2001). Controversy as well as statistical analysis will undoubtedly continue, as will policy advocates' efforts to use statistical analysis to make their best case for policy interventions to expand insurance coverage.

Evidence on the Number of Uninsured

Although evidence on the importance of insurance is critical to any case for its expansion, evidence on the number of people without insurance is far more likely to be a motivator for action to achieve that result. The ability to count the uninsured—specifically, to demonstrate that the number is sizable and growing—provides the kind of indicator that Kingdon observes can transform an undesirable condition into a political problem.

Statistics from surveys are critical indicators in highlighting the health insurance problem. Most important as a regular source of indicators is the U.S. Census Bureau's Current Population Survey (CPS). Every year in September, Census reports on changes in the number of uninsured Americans during the previous year and over the past 20 years. Analysts and advocates have paid careful attention to its regular increases and—for the first time, recently—occasional decreases to inform and encourage policy action.

In the period leading up to the 1990s health reform debate, analysis of statistics from the CPS called attention to the negative trend in insurance coverage and, in conjunction with analysis of other surveys' statistics (Survey of Income and Program Participation [SIPP], National Medical Expenditure Survey [NMES]), illustrated the tie between unemployment and uninsurance—specifically, the loss of insurance associated with loss of jobs and the failure of insurance rates to climb at the recession's end (Congressional Research Service 1988; U.S. Bipartisan Commission 1990, 22). The recession at the beginning of the decade brought a dramatic drop in insurance coverage—by 4 million people between 1989 and 1992 (Cutler and Gruber 2002)—or, in campaign language, an increase in the uninsured of "a million a year." For most of the 1990s, the increases in the number of people without health insurance were regularly reported by the CPS and contrasted to historically high economic growth rates. The recession beginning in 2002 has again raised concerns that coverage will decline (Gruber and Levitt 2002). The policy/political conclusion: economic growth cannot be counted on to resolve the lack of health insurance, and economic decline can be counted on to exacerbate it.

For the first time since the Census Bureau began collecting comparable data, the March 2000 CPS showed a decline in the number of uninsured from 1998 to

1999 (U.S. Census Bureau [pr] Chances of having health insurance). Analysts' primary explanations were that enhancements in wealth and improvements in employer insurance offerings (at least for the better off) had finally improved insurance coverage for the employed. This good news for individuals, however, could have been bad news for policy activists—since it is declines, not improvements, in coverage that provide support for policy action. Hence the effort to tie improvements, at least in part, to a public policy initiative—the 1997 expansion of public coverage for children (Cunningham et al. 2002).

The ability of statistical analysis to highlight health insurance as a policy problem is sometimes clouded by problems in the surveys that generate the statistics. Uncertainty about respondents' understanding of some survey questions has called into question counts of the uninsured population. Changes in questions have created gaps in trends. And use of private insurance plans in public programs (Medicaid) makes it hard to interpret some survey responses (Lewis et al. 1998, 8). Such problems may be intrinsic to an ever-improving survey process. But efforts to minimize them are essential to maximize confidence in the power of statistics in the policy process.

Evidence on Characteristics of the Uninsured

Alongside information on the number of people with health insurance, analysts and advocates typically provide—and track—information on their characteristics. Survey statistics regularly provide evidence to challenge myths that associate lack of insurance with lack of personal responsibility.

The story of the uninsured that the data tell has been quite constant over the past decade or more. Reports leading to the reform debate characterized the uninsured as overwhelmingly in working families (only about a quarter unemployed), disproportionately low income (about 60% in families with incomes below twice the federal poverty level), and disproportionately tied to small businesses (about 60% in firms with fewer than 100 employees) (Congressional Research Service 1988; U.S. Bipartisan Commission 1990, 22). These characteristics highlight the challenges faced by hard-working people who lack insurance—the mismatch between their resources and affordable insurance policies. The tie to small business emphasizes problems small employers (who lack large employers' ability to pool risks and to self-insure) face in obtaining affordable, dependable coverage for their employees—identifying not only a policy problem but also a potential constituency for policy action. In the heat of the reform debate in the early 1990s, data were used to emphasize the risk of being uninsured across the full population—loss of affordable insurance with loss of a job and the probability of at least some period without insurance over a 2- or 3-year period.

Today's story looks quite similar, with only slight changes in proportions (Hoffmann and Pohl 2002). As a sign of the immigrant politics of the 1990s, analysts have emphasized that most of the uninsured are not immigrants (though immigrants are likely to be uninsured) (Institute of Medicine 2001, 5). In addition, surveys have been used to document that most of the uninsured are not offered insurance by their employers (O'Brien and Feder 1999)—a sign of dependence on the increasingly criticized individual market for insurance.

In addition to telling the story of the uninsured, survey statistics support analysis of specific segments of the uninsured population—particularly in today's environment, in which promoting new coverage for some has become more politically palatable than promoting coverage for all. For example, statistical analysis of the income distribution of the uninsured has led some to focus on the lowest-income uninsured, some to focus on the moderate-income population, and some to focus on different strategies for different income groups (Covering America 2001; Expanding health coverage 2001). Statistical analyses of the uninsured by age, access to employer coverage, and duration without insurance coverage have also been used to justify targeted policy interventions. The statistics can be used to justify different actions, reflecting the values, priorities, and political judgments of the analysts or advocates who use them. Whatever problem is selected, however, statistical analysis will be critical to putting it on the map.

Summary

Over the past decade, statistical analysis has been essential to defining lack of health insurance as a problem that requires political action—by demonstrating the human consequences of lack of insurance and the number and characteristics of people affected by it. However, statistical analysis by itself has not moved lack of insurance from a matter of concern to a matter of action. Today, as in the late 1980s, job loss causes concern about the loss of health insurance; rising health costs increase workers' burdens; and the number of uninsured appears to be on the rise. In the 1990s, politicians used statistical analyses of these problems to argue for political action. Today, similar conditions attract only modest political attention, despite even more extensive and sophisticated statistical support. Statistics do not force a political debate. Rather, they provide the raw material for that debate when it is, once again, ready to happen.

DEVELOPING POLICY SOLUTIONS

If events likely transcend data in the definition phase of the policy process, statistics and their analysis are a sine qua non in policy development. They are essential to crafting policy proposals that have the potential to produce the results policymakers intend. Given concern about the use of taxpayer resources and the politics of the budget process, it is impossible to imagine the development of a proposal to expand insurance coverage without analysis of its effects. Indeed, within government, institutions are dedicated to the use of statistics to evaluate policy impacts; witness the critical roles played by the President's Office of Management and Budget and the Congressional Budget Office. In health reform, these organizations' activities were supplemented by extensive analysis within the Departments of Health and Human Services, Treasury, and Labor. And, outside government, think tanks, interest groups, and academics are heavily engaged in similar tasks. Indeed, as others have observed (Bilheimer and Reischauer 1995; Congressional Budget Office 1994; Health Affairs 1994; Kronick 1999), it is hard to overstate the scope and intensity of the health policy community's investment in statistical analysis of the Clinton health reform proposal in the 1993–1994 period. That activity is the subject of this section.

Cost Estimates of the Clinton Health Reform Proposal

The primary task facing estimators was to determine how much health care its coverage would finance and how much taxpayers, businesses, and individuals would pay for it—both in total and relative to what they currently paid. That meant agreement on the current or *baseline* spending and distribution and an assessment of the changes that would result from the proposal's benefit requirements, insurance market changes, and cost containment provisions. The nation's health-care survey apparatus provided the statistics that facilitated and frustrated that task.

As estimators themselves described in looking back on the Clinton health reform debate, in 1993–1994 it was "impossible" to "construct a comprehensive picture" of the existing health care system. What was possible was to build a story from the mix of survey data they had available: census data on the number of insured and the uninsured, their characteristics, and the source of their health insurance coverage; the 1987 National Medical Expenditures Survey (statistically updated) for patterns of service use and—along with the Health Care Financing Adminstration's (HCFA's) National Health Accounts—for health care spending; the National Health Interview Survey to link health insurance coverage, health status, use of health services, and socioeconomic characteristics; and employer surveys to identify patterns of employment and health insurance offerings (Bilheimer and Reischauer 1995).

Then the task was to estimate what the proposal would do to that picture in terms of service use and spending, premiums charged, and distribution of who paid them. This task involved not only statistics but assumptions—in some cases heroic—about the behavior of individuals, businesses, providers, insurance plans, and governments in response to the rules and provisions of the reform proposal. Analyses were typically based on micro-simulation models, which rely on survey data and economic evidence of how individuals and employers behave under different circumstances, to simulate the effects of alternative policy proposals. Across the health policy community, premium estimates under the new proposal were generated by HCFA's Office of the Actuary (relying on data from Medicare,

Medicaid, and the National Health Accounts); by the Agency for Health Care Policy and Research (AHCPR) (relying on NMES and the agency's own simulation model); by private actuaries (ARC and Hewitt Associates); and by consulting firms (from the Health Insurance Association of America's employer surveys). Analysis of who faced what premium relied on survey and program statistics on the health status and service use patterns of different segments of the population (with employer-sponsored insurance, Medicaid, or no insurance). Analysts then made a variety of assumptions about how individuals with varying health status and likely health-care costs were distributed across the various insurance arrangements the proposal established. The resulting premium estimates were then combined—in various ways—with CPS and other data on employer plans and employer and employee characteristics to determine eligibility for taxpayer-financed subsidies that the Clinton health reform proposal made available to firms and individuals based on their respective incomes. And the combination of resulting expenditures by various parties was compared to the existing statistics on employer, individual, and government spending to determine the likely impact on each group's expenditures under the proposed reform—by income, by industry, by firm size, by previous insurance status, and so on.

The overall product—in combination with other analyses about the impact of market forces and regulatory arrangements on payments to providers, on service delivery in response to those payments, on overall health-care costs, on federal revenues, on economic growth—produced the postreform picture that allowed the Clinton administration, the Congressional Budget Office, and a host of outside analysts to report to the public on the impact of the Clinton health reform proposal on national health expenditures, individuals' and businesses' health expenditures, the government's health expenditures, and the state of the federal budget.

Generation of these estimates was viewed by participants and observers as a herculean effort, going well beyond what statistical analysis would comfortably support. In their retrospective, estimators bemoaned not only the need to piece together data from so many different sources, but also the inadequacy of the surveys they had and enormous gaps in information and understanding on which to base assumptions about behavior, both at the moment and into the future. Of particular concern were the lack of current data, the absence of data on the characteristics of workers and wage distribution within firms, limited understanding of the insurance market and of choices made by individuals and employers, and limited understanding of providers' responses to market and regulatory cost containment strategies (Bilheimer and Reischauer 1995; Nichols 1995; Sheils 1995; Thorpe 1995). The result was considerable uncertainty regarding the estimates.

Since the health reform debate, there has been substantial investment in data collection and statistical analysis aimed at reducing uncertainty. In particular, the federal government's Medical Expenditure Panel Survey (MEPS)—which has replaced the once-a-decade NMES—includes substantial improvements in information about insurance arrangements and now provides information about employers. Foundation-supported surveys of individuals and employers fill in some additional details. However, we still know little about the distribution of employee characteristics within firms, and about the health insurance purchasing behavior of individuals and employers in response to various financial subsidies.

Further improvement in statistics cannot address another factor creating uncertainty—disagreement among analysts about what the statistics mean. In the 1993–1994 effort, different analyses produced different premium estimates, different cost estimates, and different estimates of cost distribution that played a key role in the health reform debate. Most visible and probably influential were the disagreements between the Congressional Budget Office and the administration's Office of Management and Budget about how much the proposal would cost. But disagreements also occurred within the administration and, as discussed later, drove interest group and political challenges to administration claims.

Debate and dispute are intrinsic to the analytic process. But considerable disagreement on the interpretation of statistics clearly weakens the case for policy intervention.

Coverage Estimates During and After the Health Reform Debate

Although cost estimates predominated in the Clinton health reform debate, estimates of coverage impacts can be (and have been) equally important. Such estimates were briefly critical to coverage advocates aiming to hit the 95% target that had been deemed "good enough" at the end of the 1993–1994 debate;[1] were behind proponents' claims that the 1997 Children's Health Insurance Program would cover 5 million children; and are part of today's debate about tax credits versus public program expansions as an appropriate mechanism for achieving health reform. In the latter two debates, a new analytic challenge has arisen: determining the extent to which expansions in public programs or tax credits substitute for rather than add to existing sources of private coverage.

Estimating coverage in response to subsidies is no simpler than estimating costs. Although the nature of the estimates varies with the proposal, such estimates require assessing the impact of the subsidy on the price of insurance, the response by uninsured individuals to that price, and the response of insured individuals to that price (relative to the price they currently pay). Estimates of participation rely on price elasticities—measures of the sensitivity of consumers in differing circumstances to changes in price. But currently available statistics yield a tremendously broad range of possible results. Uncertainty in statistical analysis leads to debate among analysts on ideological as well as substantive grounds.

Summary

In his review of the Clinton health reform debate as of late 1993, Kingdon attributes its then-likely failure to produce action to conflict in the policy stream—disagreement in the policy community as well as the political community about which strategies would be most effective in expanding coverage (Kingdon 1995, 217–221). Although Kingdon was looking at disagreements on policy choices rather than disagreements on statistical analyses, the latter debate was also contentious. We believe the two debates had similar roots—not in analytic disputes but in the different values and political points of view held by policy analysts.

Statistical analysis is essential to policy design. But its inevitable uncertainty creates opportunities to politicize the analytic process. Challenges to cost and coverage estimates undermine confidence in proposed solutions and facilitate challenges that have nothing to do with analysis and everything to do with ideology. The more uncertain the analysis, the easier it is to mount those challenges and to disguise a political debate as an analytic one. Efforts to achieve that disguise are probably inevitable. The better the statistical data and the better grounded its analysis, the harder it becomes to disguise the real political choices.

DEBATING POLICY ACTION

When it comes to debating a policy proposal in the political arena, statistical analysis becomes more than a source of knowledge or even argument. It is better understood as ammunition—a weapon in a political battle. Advocates marshal analysis in support of their causes—or, often even more effectively, in opposition to the causes of others—to sway the public and legislators and the media that influence them. This section illustrates the power of analysis.

The Clinton health reform debate generated a mini-industry of consultants analyzing the Clinton proposal for various interest groups. That analysis profoundly affected the political debate by identifying "winners" and "losers"—describing the distributional impact of the proposal on specific groups and populations.

The Clinton administration sold its Health Security Act as a strategy that would simultaneously guarantee health coverage and slow the growth of health-care costs. It had something for everyone: insurance for those who did not have it; financial relief and "security" for those who did; subsidies to make insurance more affordable for small businesses, many of which do not sponsor coverage for their workers; and cost savings for larger companies that already offered coverage to workers and retirees. The goal of its design was to attract the broadest possible support for its enactment.

However, these specific promises—combined with the reality that the Clinton plan created new mandates for the purchase of coverage by employers and individuals and new sources of revenue—invited opponents to produce analyses showing that not everyone was, in fact, a winner. The result was a multitude of reports describing how much more small businesses not now providing coverage would have to pay; how much more consumers currently insured might pay; and how some employers currently offering coverage might have to pay more to upgrade that coverage to the minimums specified in the legislation. Just as the administration incorporated analysis in its efforts to mobilize support for legislation, critics used analysis to mobilize opposition. Analysis of health reform's losers fed naturally into the efforts of the Health Insurance Association of America to generate public skepticism through their Harry and Louise television ads: "There's got to be a better way." Public opinion polls at the end of the debate showed a far larger proportion of Americans believing they would be worse off, compared to better off, from the proposed Clinton reforms.[2]

The purpose of *dueling analyses* in the health reform debate was not to reveal truth and, from a research perspective, analyses on both sides varied considerably in quality. But, in the heat of battle, truth and accuracy were not the point. Statistical attacks on the Clinton administration's promise to benefit everyone undermined the potential for building the broad constituency necessary to pass legislation. To be sure, the proposal faced a multitude of challenges that have been well documented elsewhere. But the massive lobbying campaign by interest groups—fueled with analysis by consulting firms—played no small part in its defeat. And, the focus on potential losers from comprehensive health reform helped shift the political debate toward incremental—and less disruptive—change.

The Clinton reform debate is by no means the only example of the use of statistical analysis to reveal the losers from a political initiative. In 1995, Democrats successfully challenged a Republican effort to change the Medicaid program for low-income families, the elderly, and the disabled from a joint federal-state entitlement program to a block grant to states (Rosenbaum and Darnell 1996). Proponents of block grants claimed that they would increase states' flexibility to promote efficiency in the program and moderate cost growth (though costs would nevertheless continue to grow over time).

Opponents had an array of reasons for opposing block grants—including the threat to coverage from spending caps that failed to grow with inflation, and to reflect a growth in need that would come with an economic downturn. They relied on statistical analysis to make their case—in this instance, relying on program data rather than the survey-based statistics we have so far discussed. Statistical analysis documented the consequences of funding caps, probably proving most effective when estimating the number of frail elderly likely to lose Medicaid support for nursing home care (Holahan et al. 1995). Negative reactions to coverage loss helped add Medicaid to Medicare, education, and the environment in the Clinton administration's resistance to the budget proposals of the Republican Congress.

Also effective was the statistical analysis showing that some states would receive less federal assistance under the block grant proposal over time than they were getting in federal matching payments under the status quo. Drawing attention to the losers called into question proponents' claims that the block grant proposal would benefit states and undermined the governors' support for the proposal.

Summary

Political debate is rarely the finest hour in terms of research quality. But it is probably the time when data have their greatest impact. Policy advocacy requires claims as to the benefits of policy action. But claims are inevitably skewed: winners are emphasized, losers disguised. Using statistical analysis to identify who is disadvantaged by a policy proposal helps mobilize the opposition. And tapping into fears or concerns that resonate with the public (and, in turn, their representatives) helps undermine support.

CONCLUSION: LESSONS FOR ANALYSIS AND ANALYSTS

Although complicated and sometimes convoluted, the politics and policy of health reform have involved—even depended on—statistics in a variety of ways. Reviewing this experience reveals the potential for and limits to the use of statistics in policymaking. Understanding both suggests lessons for analysts and policymakers who want to make the most of statistical analysis in the policy process.

Potential and Limits of Statistical Analysis

Statistics Steer but Do Not Drive the Policy Process

Statistics are integral to all three stages of the policy process—defining a problem, developing a solution, and debating political action. In defining the problem, statistical analysis has framed lack of insurance as a problem that attracts political attention. Statistics have made development of solutions manageable—providing the means to assess how well alternative approaches work to achieve policy or political goals and to measure impacts on significant political stakeholders. And statistics have provided the tools and weapons these stakeholders use to promote their own policy and political objectives.

But it was politics, not statistics, that put health reform on the political agenda in the early 1990s; it is politics that keeps it off the agenda today; and it is politics—even among analysts—that has made agreement and action on solutions so difficult to achieve. Statistics cannot trump politics, but they provide the raw material for policy and political arguments, shape the form these arguments take, and significantly influence their ultimate impact.

Statistics Build Confidence, Not Certainty

Politicians who want to make a case on a controversial issue require some confidence that they are promoting the right thing, that is, that the battle is worth fighting. And, in the battle itself, they must instill confidence in order to mobilize the political will that action requires. Statistical analysis is the source of that confidence, providing the means to understand problems and to develop and contrast solutions.

But when policy and politics depend on analysis of potentially enormous behavioral changes projected well into the future, uncertainty is inevitable. Although they may lose perspective in the heat of battle, analysts are painfully aware of the limited data and the leaps of faith that underlie what appear as definitive or point estimates of policy impacts. The greater the uncertainty surrounding the consequences of action, the harder it is to accomplish. Alternatively stated, the better the data and the analysis, the greater the confidence and the potential to act.

Statistics Have More Power to Prevent than Promote Action

Statistics have perhaps demonstrated their greatest power in taking policy ideas off the political agenda rather than moving ideas into action. The Clinton administration had a wealth of statistical analysis to support its claims for the costs and benefits of health reform. However, statistical challenges to those claims fortified the already powerful opposition—severely damaging the Clinton administration's credibility. Statistical challenges similarly undermined the claims from Republicans in Congress regarding the proposed restructuring of Medicare and Medicaid. In neither case were statistics decisive, but their power as weapons proved far greater in preventing than promoting action.

The imbalance derives in part from the inevitable uncertainty about policy outcomes. Statistics cannot create certainty, but challenges to others' statistics can create a great deal of uncertainty. And—especially where powerful interests are at stake—uncertainty about the consequences of change can provide a major boost for those resisting it.

Good Analysis Is Essential to Effective Policy but Not to Effective Politics

The ability to distinguish policy interventions that will work from those that will not depends on the quality and comprehensiveness of the data, the knowledge behind behavioral assumptions, and the appropriateness and power of analytic methods. In other words, good analysis is essential to good policy.

As described above, good analysis also makes good politics—or, more precisely, builds confidence for political action. Unfortunately, however, bad analysis performs almost as well. In the heat of political battle, any analysis can be used to rationalize a political position or, in political terms, to provide cover to politicians. Sadly, neither the media nor the public seem able to distinguish good from bad analysis. Indeed, multiple analyses presenting conflicting conclusions tend to muddy the political debate—neutralizing the capacity of analysis to educate effectively.

Although we applaud the power of statistics as a tool, the contribution that tool will make will always depend on the objectives of its users. Statistics are at least as powerful a weapon to impede good policy as they are a tool to promote it.

Strengthening the Contribution of Statistical Analysis

Despite their limitations, statistics make an enormous contribution to policymaking. The health reform experience—and the conclusions we have just derived from it—provides some specific lessons to maximize that contribution.

The first lessons apply to the overall statistical enterprise. It is clearly in the public interest to have the statistics and analysis that are essential for making effective policy. It is therefore just as clearly a public responsibility to ensure the availability of the statistics and analysis needed to track and understand experience, define policy problems, and develop and evaluate solutions. To be helpful in the policy process, it is important that data collection be guided by policy questions; in that sense, it is a part of the policy process. But to be credible in the policy process, it is equally important that the accuracy and quality of the data be free from political oversight or manipulation. No one has impugned the health data that exist, but it is noteworthy that the statistical enterprise in health lacks the stature, the independence, and the focus of other significant statistical enterprises in the government (like those tracking unemployment, inflation, or gross domestic product). Greater attention to the way we conduct our data collection and analysis in health may enhance not only its quality but also the fiscal and political support it attracts.

The second set of lessons is for analysts both inside and outside government. In presenting these lessons, it is important to note that there are several stages of analysis and many kinds of analysts. Not all analysts put contributions to policy and policymaking at the top of their list of priorities. But to support analysts who want to make the most constructive contributions and to protect other analysts from being destructive, we offer the following suggestions:

- *Focus research on narrowing uncertainties in the policy debate.* Analysts know better than anyone else where the weaknesses are in our ability to evaluate possible solutions to the coverage problem—weaknesses not only in the availability of statistics but also in the adequacy of the analysis that underlies the behavioral assumptions so critical to the policy debate. More and better statistics and analysis—reinforced by debate and review in the field—can strengthen the foundation for the policy analysis that occurs in the political debate. Analysis central to the political process will always be subject to challenge. But the firmer its foundation, the greater will be its power in the political debate.

- *Produce timely data and research.* Political debates are unpredictable. Conflicts surrounding health reform are so substantial that action almost always seems unlikely. But moments—or, as Kingdon calls them, policy *windows*—occur. Timely research and analysis can take advantage of and sometimes even help create these windows. Presenting new statistical analysis helps attract attention and beats the challenge that "times have changed." Although researchers may feel they are rehashing old news, policymakers operate in the moment. To fill their needs, statistics must keep coming and analysis must keep improving, to update as well as enhance existing knowledge.
- *Treat all policy research as if it will make a difference.* As noted above, not every analyst wants to participate in the policy process. But regardless of the analyst's preferences, every analysis can become a part of that process. Participants engaged in political battle will take advantage of whatever analysis suits their needs and will present it as favorably as possible to support their position. Recognition of that likelihood has important implications for all analysts. If they want the analysis used accurately, it is their job to frame it—that is, use it to tell an easily accessible story, answer the "so what?" question, and spell out the inferences they believe can be drawn for policy, with any caveats they deem appropriate. Although analysts cannot control all uses of their research, they are better protected if they make this effort than if they do not.
- *Watch the line between research and propaganda.* Just as there are researchers who do not want to play the policy game, there are researchers who thrive on it. That is a boon to the policy process, for it generates the statistical analysis the process requires. But in the heat of political debate, the pressure to deviate from what the analysis says to what the policymakers or advocates want to hear can be powerful. Research is uncertain; policymakers want certainty. Research is ambiguous; policymakers want clarity. And research may not support the argument policymakers want to make. At their best, researchers involved in the policy process use analysis to, in Aaron Wildavsky's (1987) words, "speak truth to power." Any researcher working on social policy issues brings values to his or her work. But researchers who want to maintain their integrity must always be mindful of crossing the line that separates analysis from propaganda.

As stated at the beginning of this chapter, statistical analysis is only part of the policy process. And no matter how well the above lessons are followed, it will always take a back seat to politics as policy is made. Speaking the truth cannot guarantee that truth will triumph. But statistical analysis gives us the chance to find what the truth is and to make sure that, regardless of the political outcome, truth is at least on the table.

NOTES

1. In their retrospective on the debate, Congressional Budget Office analysts described the "programmatic contortions" pursued by various proposal sponsors to hit the desired target that their estimates would produce.

2. See, for example, Time/CNN/Yankelovich Partners Polls: July 1994 (31% worse off, 15% better off, 50% about the same) and August 1994 (31% worse off, 20% better off, 45% about the same). Both polls were conducted by Yankelovich Partners for Time and Cable News Network, and data were provided by The Roper Center for Public Opinion Research at the University of Connecticut. The first poll was conducted July 13–14, 1994, and was based on telephone interviews with a national adult sample of 600, which included an over-sampling of blacks to bring their total number to 250 (Catalog of Holdings [db] Health care). The second poll was conducted August 17–18, 1994, and was based on telephone interviews with a national adult sample of 1000 (Catalog of Holdings [db] Clinton).

REFERENCES

Andersen R, Anderson OW. National medical expenditures surveys: Genesis and Rationale. In: Informing American Health Care Policy: The Dynamics of Medical Expenditure and Insurance Surveys, 1977–1996. Monheit AC, Wilson R, Arnett RH, eds. San Francisco: Jossey-Bass; 1999, pp. 11–30.

Bilheimer L, Reischauer RD. Confessions of the estimators: numbers and health reform. Health Affairs 1995;14(1):39–40.

Catalog of Holdings [database on the Internet]. Storrs, CT: The Roper Center for Public Opinion Research; c. 2004 [cited 2004 May 24]. Time/CNN Poll: Clinton, the Clinton administration and Congress [Study# USYANK1994-94014]. Available from: http://roperweb.ropercenter.uconn.edu/cgi-bin/hsrun.exe/roperweb/Catalog40/stateid/CUWp3m8DqaG1smoocqo3AS5pYPZr—36HB/HAHTpage/summary_link?archno=USYANK1994-94014.

Catalog of Holdings [database on the Internet]. Storrs, CT: The Roper Center for Public Opinion Research; c. 2004 [cited 2004 May 24]. Time/CNN Poll: Health care, Haiti and the space program [Study# USYANK1994-94012]. Available from: http://roperweb.ropercenter.uconn.edu/cgi-bin/hsrun.exe/roperweb/Catalog40/stateidCUWp3m8DqaG1smoocqo3AS5pYPZr—36HB/HAHTpage/summary_link?archno= USYANK1994-94012.

Congressional Budget Office. An Analysis of the Administration's Health Proposal. Washington, DC: GPO; 1994.

Congressional Research Service, Library of Congress. Health Insurance and the Uninsured: Background Data and Analysis. Washington, DC: GPO; 1988.

Cunningham PJ, Hadley J, Reschovsky JD. The Effects of SCHIP on Children's Health Insurance Coverage. Research Report No. 7. Washington, DC: Center for Studying Health System Change; 2002.

Cutler D, Gruber J. Health policy in the Clinton era: once bitten, twice shy. In: Frankel JA, Orszag PR, eds. American Economic Policy in the 1990s. Cambridge, MA: MIT Press; 2002, pp. 825–899, which cites Employee Benefits Research Institute. Sources of Health Insurance and Characteristics of the Uninsured. Washington, DC: Employee Benefits Research Institute; 2000, p. 5.

Expanding health coverage. Health Affairs 2001;20(1):6–309.

Gruber J, Levitt L. Rising Unemployment and the Uninsured. Washington, DC: Kaiser Family Foundation; 2002.

Hadley J. Sicker and Poorer: The Consequences of Being Uninsured. Washington, DC: The Kaiser Commission on Medicaid and the Uninsured; 2002.

Health Affairs 1994;13(1):4–351.

Hoffmann C, Pohl MB. Heath Insurance Coverage in America, 2000 Data Update. Washington, DC: Kaiser Commission on Medicaid and the Uninsured; 2002.

Holahan J, Coughlin T, Liu T, Ku L, Kuntz C, Wade M, et al. Cutting Medicaid Spending in Response to Budget Caps. Washington, DC: Kaiser Commission on the Future of Medicaid; 1995 [cited 2004 May 24]. Available from: http://www.kff.org/medicaid/2056-index.cfm.

Institute of Medicine, Board on Health Care Services, Committee on the Consequences of Uninsurance. Coverage Matters: Insurance and Health Care. Washington, DC: National Academy Press; 2001.

Institute of Medicine, Board on Health Care Services, Committee on the Consequences of Uninsurance. Care without Coverage: Too Little, Too Late. Washington, DC: National Academy Press; 2002.

Kingdon JW. Agendas, Alternatives, and Public Policies, 2nd ed. New York: HarperCollins College; 1995.

Kronick R. Numbers We Need: Health Statistics and Health Policy. Washington, DC: National Committee for Vital and Health Statistics; 1999.

Levy H, Meltzer D. What do we really know about whether health insurance affects health? Unpublished paper presented at the Agenda Setting Meeting of the Coverage Research Institute. Ann Arbor, MI; 2001.

Lewis K, Ellwood MR, Czajka JL. Counting the Uninsured: A Review of the Literature. Occasional Paper No. 8 of Assessing the New Federalism. Washington, DC: Urban Institute; 1998, p. 8.

Meyer J, Wicks E, eds. Covering America: Real Remedies for the Uninsured. Washington, DC: Economic and Social Research Institute; 2001.

Mishel L, Bernstein J, Schmitt J. The State of Working America, 1996–1997. Armonk, NY: M.E. Sharpe; 1997, p. 159.

Nichols LM, Numerical estimates and the policy debate. Health Affairs 1995;14(1):56–59.

O'Brien E, Feder J. Employment-Based Health Insurance Coverage and Its Decline: The Growing Plight of Low-Wage Workers. Washington, DC: Kaiser Commission on Medicaid and the Uninsured; 1999.

Rosenbaum S, Darnell J. A Comparison of Medicaid Provisions under Current Law, the President's Balanced Budget Proposal, the Medigrant Provisions of H.R. 2491, and the Medicaid Restructuring Act of 1996 (Contained in S. 1795 and H.R. 3507). Washington, DC: Kaiser Commission on the Future of Medicaid; 1996.

Schroeder SA. The medically uninsured—will they always be with us? N Engl J Med 1996;334(17):1130–1133.

Sheils JF. Need for continued refinement in cost estimations. Health Aff (Millwood) 1995 Spring;14(1):60–62.

Thorpe KE. A Call for health services researchers. Health Aff 1995;14(1):63–65.

U.S. Bipartisan Commission on Comprehensive Health Care (Pepper Commission). A Call for Action: Final Report. Washington, DC: U.S. Government Printing Office; 1990.

U.S. Census Bureau [press release on the Internet]. Washington, DC: U.S. Census Bureau [updated 2001 Mar 14; cited 2004 May 24]. Chances of having health insurance increase, reversing 12-year trend, Census Bureau says. Available from: http://www.census.gov/Press-Release/www/2000/cb00-160.html.

Wildavsky, Aaron B. Speaking Truth to Power: The Art and Craft of Policy Analysis. Boston: Little, Brown; 1979.

CHAPTER 12

Health Statistics in Public Health Practice

John W. Oswald, Daniel J. Friedman, and Margaret Hargreaves

This chapter describes key uses of health statistics in public health practice, with an emphasis on state and local practice. Models of public health practice are presented as a framework for discussing these uses, which include monitoring community health status and outcomes, assessing community health, designing public health programs and targeting interventions, evaluating public health programs and policies, and informing the public. Emerging issues in the use of health statistics are then discussed. The chapter concludes with case studies of the successful application of health statistics in public health practice.

For public health practitioners, the use of health statistics is fundamental in assessing health trends and setting priorities for programs. The user at state and local levels must strike a balance between scientific rigor and practical considerations. The capacity to develop and appropriately use health statistics is an essential component of the public health infrastructure.

This chapter demonstrates the need for state-, county-, city-, and community-level health statistics to support public health practice in addition to national statistics. State and especially local-level data are often lacking in important areas for public health practice. Needed state and local public health statistics must continue to be developed, consistent with national health statistics, along such key dimensions as data content and format standards, statistical standards, and population health indicators.

MODELS FOR PUBLIC HEALTH PRACTICE

Within the past two decades, several influential models of public health practice have been developed. These models are useful for understanding the role of health statistics, for identifying gaps in health statistics that need to be filled in order to better support public health practice, and for improving the quality of health statistics.

The seminal 1988 Institute of Medicine (IOM) report, the *Future of Public Health*, presents three core functions of public health practice: assessment, policy development, and assurance (Institute of Medicine 1988). The assessment function is defined in the *Future of Public Health* as the "systematic collection, assembly, analysis, and dissemination of information about the health of a community." As illustrated later in this chapter, health statistics provide much of the core information utilized for the assessment function.

Ten Essential Public Health Services, developed by a task force convened by the U.S. Department of Health and Human Services in 1994, built on the core public health functions described in the1988 IOM report (U.S. Department of Health and Human Services 1994). The report described 10 services that constitute public health practice:

1. Monitor health status to identify community health problems.
2. Diagnose and investigate health problems and health hazards in the community.
3. Inform, educate, and empower people about health issues.
4. Mobilize community partnerships at the state and local levels to identify and solve health problems.
5. Develop policies and practices that support individual and community health efforts.
6. Enforce laws and regulations that protect health and ensure safety.
7. Link people to health services and ensure the provision of health care when it is otherwise unavailable.
8. Ensure the existence of a public health and personal health care workforce.
9. Evaluate the effectiveness, accessibility, and quality of personal and population-based health services.
10. Conduct research to develop new insights and innovative solutions to health problems.

Health statistics are needed for adequate performance of each of *The Ten Essential Public Health Services.* The use of health statistics can and should be embedded in all of the essential services, rather than being confined to monitoring health status (essential service 1). Table 12.1 provides illustrations of how health statistics are used in conducting the essential public health services in states, counties, and other local areas.

TABLE 12.1

Use of Health Statistics in Conducting Essential Public Health Services in States, Counties, and Other Local Areas

Essential Service	*Example of Use*
Monitor health status to identify community health problems	Ongoing collection, analysis, and dissemination of key population health indicators, such as infant mortality rates, adequacy of prenatal care, and smoking prevalence
Diagnose and investigate health problems	Identification of specific communities, population subgroups, and census tracts with higher than average infant mortality rates or lower than average adequacy of prenatal care percentages, followed by more detailed analyses to identify area-specific and group-specific factors requiring further investigation
Inform people about health issues	Well-publicized release of annual data on infant mortality to local media, accompanied by local public meetings to present these data to citizen advocacy groups
Mobilize community partnerships	Use of detailed analyses of local area birth and death data, development of: • Fetal and infant mortality review teams consisting of local public health practitioners and local health-care providers to identify specific correlates of infant mortality in the local area • Coalitions of health-care providers, local government officials, community groups, and state officials to design public health interventions and advocate for sufficient funding
Support individual and community health efforts	Use of over-time trend data in order to track progress on key indicators.
Enforce laws and regulations	• Use of hospital-level analyses of birth data, fulfilling state legislative mandates to inform public of primary and repeat cesarean section rates at birth hospitals • Fulfillment of state legislative mandates to monitor health status and outcomes among patients enrolled in managed care organizations through using managed care organization use data, birth data, death data, hospital discharge data, and other state data
Link people to health services	Identification of specific service needs at the census tract and neighborhood levels
Ensure an adequate health-care workforce	Use of data on distribution of physicians and nurses to designate and monitor medically underserved areas
Evaluate effectiveness of health services	Use of publicly available data to evaluate performance of individual health-care institutions on key performance indicators with population-based comparison data
Research for new insights	Investigation of key findings, such as over-time increases in low birth weight rates, using multivariate statistical measures to formulate etiologic hypotheses

USES OF HEALTH STATISTICS FOR STATE AND LOCAL PUBLIC HEALTH PRACTICE

Types of Public Health Practice Data

Virtually all of *The Ten Essential Public Health Services* entail data collection. Core data sets contributing to health statistics at state and local levels are varied and typically include (adapted from Centers for Disease Control and Prevention 1999a, 7):

Health Status and Outcome Data

- Birth and death registries
- Communicable disease registries
- Cancer registry
- Birth defects registry

Risk Factor Data

- Behavioral risk factor surveys
- Prenatal risk assessment surveys
- Tobacco use surveys

Health Services Data

- Immunization program registry
- Program use data sets, such as breast and cervical cancer screening registries, Early Intervention services use, and Women, Infants, and Children services use
- Hospital discharge and emergency department data sets

Demographic Data

- Census data on trends in age, geographic distribution, race, and other characteristics of the population
- Health insurance coverage survey

These and other health statistics data sets are used by state and local public health agencies on a daily basis for public health practice in five ways: monitoring health status and outcomes; assessing community health; designing public health programs and targeting interventions; evaluating programs; and informing the public.

Monitoring Health Status and Outcomes

Chapter 2 makes it clear that the initial rationale for the government-sponsored development of health statistics capacities in the United Kingdom, other European nations, and the United States in the eighteenth and nineteenth centuries was to monitor the health status and health outcomes of the population. Typical examples of the use of health statistics for monitoring health status and outcomes can be found in ongoing national and subnational publications. In the United States, *Health, United States* has been published annually since 1975. *Health, United States* contains point-in-time and trend data on multiple topics, such as demographics, health risks and health risk behaviors, preventive health care, mortality, fertility, and natality, health services use, health-care resources, and health-care expenditures (National Center for Health Statistics 2003). Similar publications are regularly released in other countries as well. Excellent examples include *Australia's Health*, Canada's *Toward a Healthy Future* and *Statistical Report on the Health of Canadians*, Singapore's *State of Health: the Report of the Director of Medical Services*, Sweden's *Yearbook of Health and Medical Care*, and *United Kingdom Health Statistics* (Australian Institute of Health and Welfare 2002; Federal, Provincial, and Territorial Advisory Committee on Population Health 1999a, 1999b; Ministry of Health 2001; National Board of Health and Welfare 2002; Pearce and Goldblatt 2001). Health statistics enabling comparative monitoring of multiple nations are available in the World Health Organization's annual *World Health Report.*

In the United States, virtually every state publishes annual vital statistics reports, containing statewide and generally county or even city- and town-level data on births, deaths, fetal deaths, and key natality and mortality indicators. Some of these reports have been published on an uninterrupted basis for many years; for example, the *Annual Report of Vital Statistics of Massachusetts* (*Public Document #1*) has been published annually since 1841.

The World Wide Web has revolutionized the use of health statistics for monitoring health status and outcomes by providing broad, immediate, and generally free, flexible access to multiple population health indicators at multiple geographic levels. Such Web sites are now maintained by individual subnational areas, by individual nations, and by international agencies and private firms. In the United States, many states maintain interactive Web sites that provide on-line, flexible access to a variety of population health data sets (Friedman et al. 2001). Similar subnational Web sites are maintained in other countries, such as Canada. Many nations also provide a wealth of health statistics data on the Web, sometimes also available for subnational areas and with customizable demographic parameters (CDC [db] CDC Wonder). Finally, the World Health Organization's Statistical Information System (WHOSIS) and several private organizations also provide health statistics that can be used for the comparative monitoring of health status and outcomes for multiple nations (Nationmaster.com [hp]; WHO [hp] WHOSIS).

Health status and outcomes are typically monitored in three ways: tracking over-time trends; comparing geographic areas and population groups; and "drilling down" from larger to smaller geographic areas or from broader populations to specific subpopulations, defined demographically or geographically.

A classic example of the use of health statistics to monitor over-time trends is presented in Figure 12.1, which shows the percentage of deaths due to communicable diseases, chronic diseases, infant mortality, and injuries from 1842 to 2002 for Massachusetts. A contemporary example of the use of health statistics to monitor over-time trends is the longitudinal analysis of low birth weight trends, both in individual states as well as internationally (Blondel et al. 2002; Cohen et al. 1999). For example, although the low birth weight rate in Massachusetts increased from 1989 to 1996, over-time monitoring revealed that "the increase in the proportion of multiple births is directly responsible for the increase in crude LBW rates in Massachusetts" (Cohen et al. 1999).

Table 2.1 illustrates the use of health statistics to compare geographic areas. Developed by William Farr and published in 1865 in the *Supplement to the 25th Annual Report of the Registrar-General of Births Deaths, and Marriages in England*, this table shows the number of deaths by age group in 30 large town districts for 1851–1860, what the number of deaths for those town districts would have been if they had the same death rates as 63 healthy town districts, and what the excess

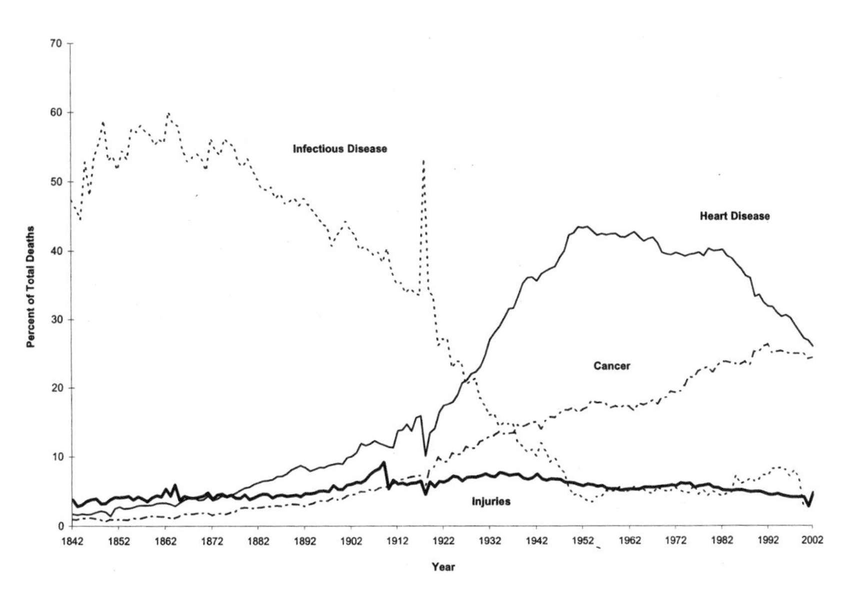

FIGURE 12.1
Percentage of deaths due to communicable diseases, chronic diseases, infant mortality, and injuries from 1842 to 2002, Massachusetts. (Source: Massachusetts Department of Public Health, personal communication, March 8, 2004.)

number of deaths were for the 30 town districts based upon the prevailing rates in the 63 healthy town districts.

Current examples of the use of health statistics to compare geographic areas and population groups abound. A typical example is the Australian Institute of Health and Welfare's *The Health and Welfare of Australia's Aboriginal and Torres Strait Islander Peoples*, which compares indigenous to other Australians on multiple indicators in each of eight Australian and Torres Strait Islander Commission regions; indicators range from health services access and use, to perinatal and maternal health, to dental health, to diabetes and obesity (Edwards and Madden 2001). Another example of the use of health statistics to compare geographic areas and populations is the U.S. Department of Health and Human Services' Indian Health Service report on *Regional Differences in Indian Health, 1997*, which compares the health of Native Americans in the 12 Indian Health Service regions on such indicators as years of potential life lost, infant mortality, and so forth (Indian Health Service 1997).

Most ongoing health statistics publications include examples of drilling down from larger to smaller geographic areas or from broader populations to specific subpopulations. For example, the Manitoba Centre for Health Policy's 2003 report *The Manitoba RHA Indicators Atlas: Population-Based Comparisons of Health and Health Care Use* provides over-time data for 3 major geographic regions in Manitoba, 11 Regional Health Authorities, and Manitoba as a whole on multiple population health indicators, organized around Premature Mortality Rates for each geographic region (Martens et al. 2003). The report drills down from the province of Manitoba as a whole, to the 3 major geographic areas, to the 11 Regional Health Authorities within those larger areas. Interactive health statistics Web sites also often provide a drilling-down capacity.

Assessing Community Health

A cornerstone of health statistics in public health practice has been its use in community health assessment, which is the first function described in *The Ten Essential Public Health Services.* As Keppel and Freedman (1995) indicate, assessment is an ongoing effort that includes three facets, all of which involve health statistics: first, identifying health needs by monitoring community health status and risks; second, ascertaining the community's ability to respond to needs by identifying and evaluating the effectiveness of available health resources; and third, presenting to the public and community leaders the results of the initial two facets so that actions can be chosen. A leading tool for conducting community health assessment and planning is the Assessment Protocol for Excellence in Public Health (APEXPH), developed by the National Association of City and County Health Officials (1991; [hp] APEXPH). The Centers for Disease Control and Prevention (CDC) Planned Approach to Community Health (PATCH) process builds on APEXPH, and emphasizes the use of health statistics to select program priorities and evaluation strategies, and to evaluate public health programs (U. S. Department of Health and Human Services no date).

Another example of the use of health statistics in community assessment is the World Health Organization's (WHO) Healthy Cities initiative, which was "founded on the moral and political beliefs that inequalities in social conditions (and therefore health) are unjustified and that their reduction should be an overriding public health objective" (Awofeso 2003). Since its inception in 1987, the WHO Healthy Cities effort has involved over 120 cities in its network (WHO Regional Office for Europe [hp] Healthy cities and urban governance). Participants in the Healthy City Network develop city health profiles that are intended to "help the city introduce programmes that will reduce the differences in health that can be changed [and can serve as] an important lever for change" (World Health Organization, Regional Office for Europe 1998). The WHO has developed a set of 53 indicators to aid in Healthy Cities community assessments and to compare Healthy Cities in widely different national settings (Doyle et al. 1997). The Healthy Cities indicators include health, health services, environmental, and socioeconomic measures. Especially prominent among the Healthy Cities indicators are a wide variety of pollution and waste, green and living spaces, transport, and broadly conceived socioeconomic indicators. The breadth of the Healthy Cities indicators reflects the WHO framework, which emphasizes nonmedical determinants of population health. In the United States, the Healthy Communities movement has built on the basic Healthy Cities concepts and has contributed to the development of broad-based community indicator data sets (Kingsley 1998; National Civic League [hp] Healthy Communities Initiatives; Tyler Norris Associates 1997; Urban Institute [hp] NNIP).

The growth of public health observatories is another major international development in community assessment. Public health observatories "serve to combine the qualities of academic and state based public health by providing high quality, relevant regional health intelligence for those who need it. They provide reliable intelligence on a shorter timescale, enabling rapid responses to regional foci" (Hemmings and Wilkinson 2003, 325). *Saving Lives: Our Healthier Nation*, the 1999 report from the Secretary of State for Health of the United Kingdom, calls for the establishment of public health observatories in each National Health Service region (Secretary of State for Health 1999). In France, the Observatoire Regional de la sante de'Ile-de-France was created in 1974. Since 2000, it has published a wide variety of regional health statistics data, including reports on urban pollution and health, the elderly and youth, attitudes toward tobacco and acquired immunodeficiency syndrome (AIDS), and addictions (Observatoire Regional de la sante de'Ile-de-France [hp]).

The common philosophy underlying community health assessments is the importance of bringing together community leaders, community-based organizations, and community members to develop agreement on specific health priorities based on data presented to them. In pursuing this agreement, the goal is for public health practitioners to gain the commitment of other community leaders to work together on commonly identified high-priority public health problems.

Regardless of the specific approach, informed use of health statistics is the basis of all community assessments. Traditional health statistics indicators are typically employed, such as infant mortality rates, cause-specific mortality rates, primary site-specific cancer incidence rates, percentages of cancers diagnosed at late stages, and so forth (e.g., see Coulton 1999). Health services data, to the extent that they are population-based, can be included as proxy measures of morbidity as well as indicators of the resource burden of illness. Community health assessments also employ a broad array of socioeconomic and environmental indicators reflecting the myriad influences on population health.

Less common but still important for community health assessments are local-level population health surveillance surveys. One example is the SHAPE (Survey of the Health of Adults, the Population, and Environment) survey, conducted in 1998 and 2002 in Minnesota by the Hennepin County Community Health Department in collaboration with the Minneapolis Department of Health and Family Support and the Bloomington Division of Health (Hennepin County Community Health Department, Bloomington Division of Health 2003a, 2003b, 2003c). The 2002 survey collected data on overall health, health-care access and use, lifestyles/behaviors, and social-environmental factors for six racial/ethnic groups (American Indians, Southeast Asians, U.S.-born blacks, African-born blacks, Hispanics/Latinos, and whites) and 20 geographic regions within the county. The information was used to identify local health disparities, determine progress on local health objectives, monitor the impact of policy changes and programmatic initiatives at the community level, and plan new local public health programs.

Designing Public Health Programs and Targeting Interventions

To be effective in reaching their target populations and efficient in using scarce public health resources to achieve public health goals, program design and intervention must be based on health statistics, typically used through analysis of data collected on an ongoing basis; analysis of data specifically collected for the purpose of designing a particular program; or review of multiple analyses of multiple data sets, combined in order to shed light on basic policy and programmatic choices.

New Jersey, North Carolina, and Manitoba offer excellent examples of the use of routinely collected data for developing and targeting programs. In New Jersey, routinely collected tuberculosis surveillance data were linked to zip code–based census data. This analysis revealed that "substantial numbers of employed foreign-born tuberculosis patients now reside in affluent New Jersey locations," indicating that tuberculosis control programs would need to re-examine traditional assumptions regarding the relationship between tuberculosis and poverty

(Davidow et al. 2003). North Carolina examined occupational mortality differences among working-age state residents for colorectal, prostate, female breast, and cervical cancers. Based on these death certificate analyses, worksite health promotion information and disease screening in North Carolina could be targeted to workers in specific occupational categories (Surles et al. 1999). In Manitoba, longitudinal analyses of hospital admissions and discharge data revealed that seasonal increased use and perceived overcrowding were due not to prior hospital bed closures but to seasonal influenza patterns; due to these analyses, the Winnipeg Regional Health Authority implemented a new influenza vaccine program rather than add new hospital beds (Menec et al. 2002; Roos et al. 2004).

Data are sometimes collected specifically for the purpose of designing programs and targeting interventions. Working with the National Opinion Research Center, the CDC's Racial and Ethnic Approaches to Community Health (REACH 2010) program has undertaken community surveys at 21 sites in order to obtain detailed information from adults about health services use, exercise, eating habits, height and weight, and screening for cardiovascular disease and breast and cervical cancers. Analyses of the survey data, together with information garnered from focus groups, helped the Nashville REACH 2010 program to discover that "'plump is considered good' by many of the African American women in this community" and helped in the design of cardiovascular and diabetes interventions specifically targeted to the views held by women in the specific site (National Center for Chronic Disease Prevention and Health Promotion 2002).

In addition to informing the design of public health programs and the targeting of interventions through analyses of data collected on an ongoing basis or through collection of new data, multiple analyses of multiple data sets can also be reviewed to build a cohesive argument for designing a related set of programmatic interventions. The Manitoba Centre for Health Policy (MCHP) has accomplished this through its ongoing analyses. Put simply, the MCHP has used health statistics to demonstrate that "more investment in health care does not translate into more health" and that "what is needed is better management of the health care sector, not more money." For the Province of Manitoba, one clear implication has been the need to shift physician expenditures from urban to rural areas (Roos and Shapiro 1999).

Evaluating Programs

Effective public health practice depends on evaluating whether implemented programs have their intended impacts. Multiple examples of the use of health statistics in program evaluation exist. Such evaluations typically use health statistics based on the full panoply of health statistics data collection methods and sources: population-based health surveys, administrative health data, data from registries, complementary data, and linkages of data sets from any of the previous data sources.

Ongoing state population-based surveys have proved to be a fruitful data source for evaluating state public health programs, both because such surveys provide an opportunity for longitudinal tracking of health status, behaviors, and outcomes and because the samples can be sufficiently large to enable analysis of longitudinal changes and subgroup differences. For example, the Behavioral Risk Factor Surveillance System, an ongoing CDC- and state-funded random digit dial survey of adults, has been fruitfully used to assess the impact of a comprehensive tobacco control program in Massachusetts from 1990 to 1999, as well as to study the program's impact on adults with disabilities ((Brawarsky et al. 2002; Weintraub and Hamilton 2002). When ongoing population-based surveys do not provide the needed topical detail or sample size, special-purpose surveys can be conducted. Examples of such surveys used for program evaluations include a random digit dial survey of California households to assess longitudinal changes in attitudes and patronage behaviors in response to a newly implemented smoke-free bar law, Massachusetts surveys of public school students to assess changes in youth tobacco use in response to a state tobacco control program, and a Massachusetts random digit dial telephone survey of teenagers to determine their receptivity to antitobacco television advertisements implemented through the state tobacco control program (Biener 2002; Soldz et al. 2002; Tang et al. 2003). Evaluation surveys can also use sample frames based on administrative health data, such as a survey of enrollees in a state-sponsored children's health insurance program to assess whether the program had a differential impact based on familial income (Feinberg et al. 2002).

Administrative health data and data from registries can be linked to evaluate the impact of public health programs on health status and outcomes. In evaluating the impact of participation in the U.S. Special Supplemental Nutrition Program for Women, Infants, and Children (WIC) and Medicaid on Medicaid costs and infant outcomes, North Carolina has linked Medicaid cost and health-care service use data, WIC enrollment data, and birth certificate data (Buescher and Horton 2000; Buescher et al. 2003).

An important new development in the use of health statistics in program evaluation is health impact assessment. In its 1999 Gothenburg consensus paper, WHO and the European Centre for Health Policy defined health impact assessment as "combination of procedures, methods and tools by which a policy, program or project may be judged as to its potential effects on the health of a population, and the distribution of those effects within the population" (Mindell et al. 2003; World Health Organization, European Centre of Health Policy 1999). Health impact assessment extends the concept of environmental impact assessment to the examination of the potential impact of new policies and programs on population health, using quantitative as well as qualitative data (Northern and Yorkshire Public Health Observatory 2001). Health impact assessment has been adopted as a key approach within the United Kingdom, where all "major new Government policies should be assessed for their impact on health" (Secretary of State for Health 1999). Methodologies for health impact assessments are being developed (Department of Health 1999). Although not without controversy, health impact assessment has been applied to evaluate a wide variety of potential policies and programs in the United Kingdom, Canada, and other countries (Krieger et al. 2003; Northern and Yorkshire Public Health Observatory 2001).

Informing the Public

The fifth and final use of health statistics in public health practice is to inform the public about population health issues. Health statistics serve this purpose through multiple mechanisms, including press releases, the increasing use of the World Wide Web to disseminate health statistics, and release of regularly scheduled and special reports. The popular media sometimes serve as intermediary distributors of health statistics, as with *Macleans'* annual issue on regional health care in Canada or *Boston Magazine*'s periodic issue on health status in Massachusetts' cities and towns (Blanding 2003; Hawaleshka 2002).

CASE STUDIES OF THE SUCCESSFUL APPLICATION OF HEALTH STATISTICS TO PUBLIC HEALTH PRACTICE

Two case studies that illustrate the application of health statistics to public health practice follow. The first addresses how health statistics in Minnesota and other states have helped to identify public health needs and then assisted in developing policies and programs to meet those needs. The second case study examines how Florida and other states have used health statistics to evaluate tobacco control programs.

Case Study: Minnesota and the Assessment of Racial and Ethnic Health Disparities

According to *America's Health: United Health Foundation State Health Rankings*, Minnesota was ranked as the healthiest state in the country in 2001 (Insure.com [hp] Lankarge; United Health Foundation 2001). In addition, the state has among the highest rates of public health spending and the highest percentage of population with health insurance coverage in the United States. However, Minnesota's periodic statewide health assessment, done in partnership with local public health agencies, revealed the poor health status of the state's racial and ethnic populations (Minnesota Department of Health 2000). In 1994, the Minnesota Department of Health (MDH) established an Office of Minority Health to assist in improving the health of people of color in the state. The Minnesota legislature subsequently commissioned the MDH Office of Minority Health to analyze and report on the health status of the state's four largest communities of color: African Americans, American Indians, Hispanics/Latinos, and Asians. Published in 1997, 1998, and 2002, the *Populations of Color in Minnesota: Health Status Report* highlighted significant health disparities between the health of these minorities and the health of whites (Minnesota Department of Health 2002). The report found differentials in rates of low-weight births and infant mortality and potential years of life lost, as well as gaps in other morbidity, behavioral risk, and health-care access measures. The report included policy recommendations that were developed in consultation with community groups serving the four identified populations.

At the national level, President Clinton announced in February 1998 an initiative to Eliminate Racial and Ethnic Disparities in Health as part of a broader White House Initiative on Race. A national report published at that time compared the health status of the 50 states and identified significant racial and ethnic health disparities within Minnesota, including teen birth rates by race/ethnicity (Centers for Disease Control and Prevention 2000). While Minnesota had the lowest teen birth rate for whites among the 50 states, it had the highest rate for African Americans. Additional support was provided for the development of this as a state priority when the U.S. Department of Health and Human Services (USDHHS) identified the elimination of health disparities as one of two primary public health goals in its *Healthy People 2010* initiative report (USDHHS 2000). In 1999, with funds from the USDHHS Office of Minority Health, the MDH Office of Minority Health issued grants to local public health agencies for local and regional minority health assessments. A number of local public health agencies throughout the state conducted assessments and published their findings in 2000 and 2001. One of the largest of these projects was a minority health assessment of the seven-county metropolitan area encompassing Minneapolis and St. Paul, which was conducted by a consortium of local health departments and was coordinated by the Minneapolis Department of Health and Family Support. Findings from these local, state, and federal disparity assessments were highlighted at area conferences, reported in the media, and shared in community meetings sponsored by the MDH and local public health agencies (Minnesota Department of Health 2003). During the 2000–2001 session, the Minnesota legislature passed an initiative to eliminate racial and ethnic health disparities within the state, with an appropriation of $12.6 million per year. The Eliminating Health Disparities Initiative (EHDI) is designed to close racial and ethnic health gaps in the following areas: infant mortality, breast and cervical cancer screening, cardiovascular disease, accidental injuries and violence, adult and child immunizations, HIV/AIDS and sexually transmitted infections, diabetes, and teen pregnancy (Minnesota Department of Health [hp] EHDI). As part of the Initiative, the MDH developed a community grants program. In February 2002, the MDH Office of Minority and Multicultural Health awarded 59 grants to tribes and community agencies throughout the state for the planning and implementation of disparity reduction services. The MDH Center for Health Statistics is responsible for the tracking and evaluation of these EHDI programs.

Case Study: Evaluation of Florida's Comprehensive Program to Prevent Tobacco Use by Youth

In the late 1990s, several states initiated litigation against the tobacco industry to recover health-care costs incurred for people with tobacco use–related diseases. Florida was the first state to agree to a settlement with the tobacco industry; the settlement created a $20 billion endowment for use by the state government. A comprehensive program to prevent adolescent tobacco use was launched that included both a major media campaign and community and school-based programs to counter marketing by the tobacco industry (Bauer et al. 2000).

State health officials developed a rigorous evaluation plan to counter anticipated scrutiny of the program's spending. This evaluation included a statewide survey with county-level estimates to track overall trends in the use of tobacco by youth on an annual basis. The evaluation included an impact assessment of the media campaign (Sly et al. 2000). In addition, evaluations of community programs were established to estimate the impact of such programs (Weatherby et al. 2000).

The evaluations documented a dramatic reduction in youth tobacco use in Florida within a year of the implementation of the media campaign (Centers for Disease Control and Prevention 1999b). These results were very timely in the spring of 1999, when the federal negotiations were taking place between 44 states and the tobacco industry for a national settlement of the tobacco litigation. The proven effectiveness of the Florida countermarketing campaign was such that the national settlement created the American Legacy Foundation, which implemented a comparable marketing campaign on a national basis (American Legacy Foundation 2002).

CONCLUSION

The major applications of health statistics in public health practice include monitoring community health status and outcomes, assessing community health, designing public health programs and interventions, evaluating public health programs and policies, and informing the public. Health statistics need to drive public health practice. The challenge for the field of health statistics has been and remains strengthening ongoing links between health statistics and program design, targeting, and evaluation.

REFERENCES

American Legacy Foundation. Building the Foundation: Progress Report 2000–2001. Washington, DC: American Legacy Foundation; 2002.

Australian Institute of Health and Welfare. Australia's Health, 2002. Canberra: Australian Institute of Health and Welfare; 2002.

Awofeso N. The Healthy Cities approach—reflections on a framework for improving global health. Bull World Health Org 2003;81(3):222.

Bauer U, Johnson T, Hopkins R, Brooks R. Changes in youth cigarette use and intentions following implementation of a tobacco control program: findings from the Florida Youth Tobacco Survey, 1998–2000. JAMA 2000;284(6):723–728.

Biener L. Anti-tobacco control advertisements by Massachusetts and Philip Morris: what teenagers think. Tob Control 2002;11(suppl II):ii43–ii46.

Blanding M. The healthiest towns. Boston Magazine 2003 Apr, pp. 78–85.

Blondel B, Kogan MD, Alexander GR, Dattani N, Kramer MS, Macfarlane A, et al. The impact of increasing number of multiple births on the rates of preterm birth and low birthweight: an international study. Am J Public Health 200;292(8):1323–1330.

Brawarsky P, Brooks DR, Wilber N, Gertz RE Jr, Walker DK. Tobacco use among adults with disabilities in Massachusetts. Tob Control 2002;11(suppl II):ii29–ii34.

Buescher PA, Horton SJ. Prenatal WIC participation in relation to low birth weight and Medicaid infant costs in North Carolina—a 1997 update. CHIS Studies 2000;122.

Buescher PA, Horton SJ, Devaney BL, Roholt SJ, Lenihan AJ, Whitmire JT, et al. Child participation in WIC: Medicaid costs and use of health care services. Am J Public Health 2003;93(1):145–150.

Centers for Disease Control and Prevention. Public Health Data: Our Silent Partner. Atlanta: Centers for Disease Control and Prevention; 1999a [cited 2004 Mar 3]. Available from: http://www.cdc.gov/nchs/products/training/phd-osp.htm.

Centers for Disease Control and Prevention. Tobacco use among middle and high school students—Florida, 1998 and 1999. MMWR 1999b;48(12):248.

Centers for Disease Control and Prevention. National and state-specific pregnancy rates among adolescents—United States, 1995–1997. MMWR 2000;49(27):605.

Centers for Disease Control and Prevention [database on the Internet]. Atlanta: CDC [updated 2003 Nov 14; cited 2004 Mar 7]. CDC Wonder [about 2 screens]. Available from: http://wonder.cdc.gov.

Cohen BB, Friedman DJ, Zhang Z, Trudeau EB, Walker DK, Anderka M, et al. Impact of multiple births on low birthweight—Massachusetts, 1989–1996. MMWR 1999;48(14): 289–292.

Coulton CJ. Vital Records: A Source for Neighborhood Indicators. Cleveland: Center on Urban Poverty and Social Change, Case Western University; 1999.

Davidow AL, Mangura BT, Napolitano EC, Reichman LB. Rethinking the socioeconomics and geography of tuberculosis among foreign-born residents of New Jersey, 1994–1999. Am J Public Health 2003;93(6):1007–1012.

Department of Health. Health Impact Assessment: Report of a Methodological Seminar. London: Department of Health; 1999.

Doyle Y, Brunning D, Cryer C, Hedley S, Hodgson CR. Healthy Cities Indicators: Analysis of Data from Cities Across Europe. Copenhagen: World Health Organization Regional Office for Europe; 1997.

Edwards RW, Madden R. The Health and Welfare of Australia's Aboriginal and Torres Strait Islander Peoples. Canberra: Australian Bureau of Statistics; 2001.

Farr W. Letter to the Registrar General. In: Supplement to the 25th Annual Report of the Registrar General for the Years 1851–1860. London: HMSO; 1864.

Federal, Provincial, and Territorial Advisory Committee on Population Health. Toward a Healthy Future: Second Report on the Health of Canadians. Ottawa: Health Canada; 1999a.
Federal, Provincial, and Territorial Advisory Committee on Population Health. Statistical Report on the Health of Canadians. Ottawa: Health Canada; 1999b.
Feinberg E, Swartz K, Zaslavsky A, Gardner J, Walker DK. Family income and the impact of a children's health insurance program on reported need for health services and unmet need. Pediatrics 2002;109(2):E29.
Friedman DJ, Anderka M, Krieger JW, Land GZ, Solet D. Accessing population health information through interactive systems: lessons learned and future directions. Public Health Rep 2001;116(2):132–147.
Hawaleshka D. Measuring health care. Macleans 2002 June 17;115(24) [cited 2004 Mar 7]. Available from: http://www.macleans.ca/topstories/article.jsp?content=967885.
Hemmings J, Wilkinson J. What is a public health observatory? J Epidemiol Commun Health 2003;57:325.
Hennepin County Community Health Department, Bloomington Division of Public Health. SHAPE 2002: A Preview, Survey of the Health of Adults, the Population and the Environment. Minneapolis: Hennepin County Community Health Department; 2003a.
Hennepin County Community Health Department and Bloomington Division of Public Health. SHAPE 2002: Geographic Data Book, Survey of the Health of Adults, the Population and the Environment. Minneapolis: Hennepin County Community Health Department; 2003b.
Hennepin County Community Health Department, Bloomington Division of Public Health. SHAPE 2002: Racial and Ethnic Data Book, Survey of the Health of Adults, the Population and the Environment. Minneapolis: Hennepin County Community Health Department; 2003c.
Indian Health Service. Regional Differences in Indian Health. Washington, DC: U.S. Department of Health and Human Services; 1997.
Institute of Medicine, Division of Health Care Services, Committee for the Study of the Future of Public Health. The Future of Public Health. Washington, DC: National Academy Press; 1988.
Insure.com [homepage on the Internet]. Darien, IL: Insure.com; c. 1995–2002 [updated 2001 Dec 13; cited 2004 Mar 7]. Lankarge V. The healthiest states in America [about 5 screens]. Available from: www.insure.com/health/healthystates1001.html.
Keppel KG, Freedman MA. What is assessment? J Public Health Manag Pract 1995;1(2):2.
Kingsley GT. The information revolution and community building. Community 1998;1(1): 20–25.
Krieger N, Northridge M, Gruskin S, Quinn M, Kriebel D, Davey-Smith G, et al. Assessing health impact assessment: multidisciplinary and international perspectives. J Epidemiol Commun Health 2003;57:659–662.
Martens PJ, Fransoo R, Burland E, Jebamani, Burchill C, Black C, et al. The Manitoba RHA Indicators Atlas: Population-Based Comparisons of Health and Health Care Use. Winnipeg: Manitoba Centre for Health Policy; 2003.
Menec VH, Roos NP, MacWilliam L. Seasonal pattern of hospital use in Winnipeg: implications for managing winter bed crises. Healthc Manag Forum 2002;Suppl:58–66.
Mindell J, Ison E, Joffe M. A glossary for health impact assessment. J Epidemiol Commun Health 2003;57:647–651.
Ministry of Health. State of Health 2001: The Report of the Director of Medical Services. Singapore: Ministry of Health; 2001.
Minnesota Department of Health. Populations of Color in Minnesota Health Status Report: Update Summary. St. Paul: Minnesota Department of Health; Fall 2002.
Minnesota Department of Health. Healthy Minnesotans: Special Report. 2000;1(4):

1–16 [cited 2004 Mar 7]. Available from: http://www.health.state.mn.us/divs/chs/healthmnvol1d.pdf.
Minnesota Department of Health. Eliminating Health Disparities Initiative: 2003 Report to the Legislature. St. Paul: Minnesota Department of Health; 2003 [cited 2004 Mar 7] Available from: www.health.state.mn.us/ommh/legrpt012103.pdf.
Minnesota Department of Health [homepage on the Internet]. St. Paul: The Department [updated 2003 Nov 25; cited 2004 Mar 7]. About eliminating health disparities initiative (EHDI) [about 2 screens]. Available from: http://www.health.state.mn.us/ommh/aboutehdi.html.
National Association of County and City Health Officials. APEXPH Workbook. Washington, DC: NACCHO; 1991.
National Association of County and City Health Officials [homepage on the Internet]. Washington, DC: NACCHO; [cited 2004 Mar 3]. Assessment protocol for excellence in public health. Available from: http://www.naccho.org/project47.cfm.
National Board of Health and Welfare. Yearbook of Health and Medical Care 2002. Stockholm: Statistics Sweden; 2002.
National Center for Chronic Disease Prevention and Health Promotion. We must identify the gaps before we can close them. Chronic Dis Notes Rep 2002;15(3):17–22 [cited 2004 Mar 8]. Available from: http://www.cdc.gov/nccdphp/cdnr/cdnr_fall0205.htm.
National Center for Health Statistics. Health, United States, 2003 with Chartbook on Trends in the Health of Americans. Hyattsville, MD: National Center for Health Statistics; 2003.
National Civic League [homepage on the Internet]. Denver: National Civic League; c. 2003 [cited 2004 Mar 3]. Healthy Communities Initiatives [about 4 screens]. Available from: http://www.ncl.org/cs/services/healthycommunities.html.
Nationmaster.com [homepage on the Internet]. Sydney: Nationmaster.com; c. 2003–2004 [cited 2004 Mar 3]. Available at http://www.nationmaster.com.
Northern and Yorkshire Public Health Observatory. An Overview of Health Impact Assessment. Occasional Paper No. 1, May 2001. Stockton on Tees: Northern and Yorkshire Public Health Observatory; 2001.
Observatoire Regional de la sante d'Ile-de-France [homepage on the Internet]. Paris: O.R.S Ile-de-France [cited 2004 Mar 3]. Available from: http://www.ors-idf.org.
Pearce D, Goldblatt P, eds. United Kingdom Health Statistics. London: HMSO; 2001.
Roos LL, Menec V, Currie RJ. Policy analysis in an information-rich environment. Soc Sci Med 2004;59(7):1435–1447.
Roos NP, Shapiro E. From research to policy: what have we learned? Med Care 1999;37(6):6.
Secretary of State for Health. Saving Lives: Our Healthier Nation. London: HMSO; 1999.
Sly DF, Ray S, Heald G. Florida Anti-Tobacco Media Evaluation: 30th Month Report, December 2, 2000. Tallahassee: Florida State University; 2000 [cited 2004 Nov 3]. Available from: http://tobacco.med.miami.edu/reports/octreport.pdf.
Soldz S, Clark TW, Stewart E, Celebucki C, Walker DK. Decreased youth tobacco use in Massachusetts 1996 to 1999: evidence of tobacco control effectiveness. Tob Control 2002;11(suppl II):ii14–ii19.
Surles KB, Gizlice Z, Buescher PA. Using death certificates to target occupation groups for health promotion and disease screening in North Carolina. SCHS Studies 1999;117:1–11 [cited 2004 Mar 8]. Available from: http://www.schs.state.nc.us/SCHS/pdf/SCHS117.pdf.
Tang H, Cowling DW, Lloyd JC, Rogers T, Koumjian KL, Stevens CM, et al. Changes of attitudes and patronage behaviors in response to a smoke-free bar law. Am J Public Health 2003;93(4):611–617.
Tyler Norris Associates, Redefining Progress, Sustainable Seattle. The Community Indicators Handbook: Measuring Progress Toward Healthy and Sustainable Communities. Oakland, CA: Redefining Progress; 1997.

U.S. Department of Health and Human Services, Public Health Functions Steering Committee. Ten Essential Public Health Services. Washington, DC: USDHHS; 1994.
U.S. Department of Health and Human Services. Healthy People 2010, 2nd ed. Washington, DC: GPO; 2000.
U.S. Department of Health and Human Services. Planned Approach to Community Health: Guide for the Local Coordinator. Atlanta: National Center for Chronic Disease Prevention and Health Promotion; no date [cited 2003 Nov 3]. Available from: http://www.cdc.gov/nccdphp/patch/index.htm.
United Health Foundation. America's Health: United Health Foundation State Health Rankings, 2001 Edition. Minneapolis: United Health Foundation; 2001.
Urban Institute [homepage on the Internet]. Washington, DC: Urban Institute; c. 2004 [updated 2004 Feb 23; cited 2004 Mar 8]. National Neighborhood Indicators Partnership [about 2 screens]. Available from: http://www.urban.org/nnip.
Weatherby N, Bauer U, Klein S, et al. Impact of community anti-tobacco partnerships on youth tobacco us and committed non-smoking [abstract #10137]. In: American Public Health Association. Program Listing of the 128th Annual Meeting of the APHA, Nov. 12–16, 2000. Boston: Washington, DC: APHA; 2000 [cited 2004 Mar 8]. Available from: http://apha.confex.com/apha/128am/techprogram/paper_10137.htm.
Weintraub JM, Hamilton WL. Trends in prevalence of current smoking, Massachusetts and states without tobacco control programmes, 1990 to 1999. Tob Control 2002;11 (suppl II):ii8–ii13.
World Health Organization [homepage on the Internet]. Geneva: WHO; c. 2004 [cited 2004 Mar 8]. WHO Statistical Information System (WHOSIS): evidence and information for health policy [about 1 screen]. Available from: http://www3.who.int/whosis/menu/cfm.
World Health Organization, European Centre of Health Policy. Health Impact Assessment: Main Concepts and Suggested Approach. Copenhagen: WHO Regional Office for Europe; 1999.
World Health Organization, Regional Office for Europe. City Health Profiles: A Review of Progress. Copenhagen: World Health Organization Regional Office for Europe; 1998, p. 11.
World Health Organization, Regional Office for Europe [homepage on the Internet]. Copenhagen: WHO Regional Office for Europe; c. 2004 [updated 2004 Feb 27; cited 2004 Mar 8]. Healthy Cities and urban governance [about 2 screens]. Available from: http://www. who.dk/healthy-cities.

PART IV

Identifying Current and Forthcoming Issues in Health Statistics

This part focuses on current and forthcoming issues in health statistics. These issues cut across the major sources of health statistics discussed in Part II and the uses of health statistics delineated in Part III.

Two chapters in this part concentrate on current issues in health statistics. In Chapter 13, Stoto explores how health can be assessed at the community and population levels, using both summary and performance measures. Stoto presents criteria for performance measures used in community health profiles, and identifies statistical issues that must be addressed as community health profiles are developed in more communities and countries. Stoto explains a variety of summary measures of population health, including both frequently used mortality-based measures and population-based health indices that use more than mortality information. Although methodological challenges remain in the application of both performance and summary measures, both will be essential areas of emphasis in the continued evolution of health statistics in the twenty-first century.

In Chapter 14, Fanning defines basic but often poorly understood concepts and clarifies the role of laws in protecting privacy and safeguarding confidentiality. He discusses both practical and policy issues related to protecting privacy and maintaining confidentiality in the health statistics enterprise, such as national organizational structures to protect privacy and privacy review mechanisms; reducing identifiability of data; and special disclosure mechanisms to enable data access for qualified researchers. Rapid changes in data collection, in data set linkage, and in electronic availability of and access to data will continue to make these concepts, laws, and issues relevant throughout the twenty-first century.

Part IV also focuses on two issues that will develop and attract increasing attention in coming years. In Chapter 15, Detmer and Steen draw a vivid portrait of how technology will affect the collection and use of health statistics at the end of the twenty-first century, highlighting four areas of future technological development: information and communications technology, genomics, personal health technology, and nanotechnology. They predict that these technologies will converge around several trends, all of which will have the potential for creating dramatically new uses for and users of health statistics.

In Chapter 16, Wolfson argues for the expansion of the uses of health statistics to include construction of simulation models. Simulation models can help policymakers to address "what if" questions in the formulation of new health policies and to explore the causal relationships inherent in answers to those questions. To facilitate the increased use of health statistics for simulation modeling, Wolfson emphasizes the importance of fulfilling two needs: first, the need for coherent frameworks for collecting the data that become health statistics and, second, the need to use electronic health records for the generation of health statistics.

CHAPTER 13

Population Health Monitoring

Michael A. Stoto

Many of the challenging health problems facing the United States in the twenty-first century require an understanding of the health not just of individuals, but also of communities. Problems such as providing immunizations to all children, controlling epidemics and infectious diseases, addressing the causes and consequences of obesity, and dealing with environmental health risks all demand comprehensive rather than disease-specific solutions that take into account the needs of entire populations. While individual access to quality health care is a necessity, medical care alone is not sufficient to address problems related to personal behavior (e.g., diet, exercise, smoking, alcohol abuse) and social problems (e.g., violence, drugs) or caused by diffuse environmental threats. Moreover, while the control of emerging infections and the threat of bioterrorism require a substantial medical response, such problems also require population-based solutions such as risk assessment and risk communication, quarantine, and mass immunization. Due to the complexity of these multifaceted challenges, a community's health problems can be addressed most effectively through collaboration among health-care systems, community groups, government, and business.

The challenge of dealing with community health issues has led to the development of a *population health* perspective (Friedman and Starfield 2003). Population health can be defined as "the health outcomes of a group of individuals, including the distribution of such outcomes within the group" (Kindig and Stoddart 2003). A focus on population health implies a concern for the determinants of health for both individuals and communities. According to this perspective, health is a dynamic state that embraces well-being as well as the absence of disease. The health of a population grows out the community's social and economic conditions as well as the quality of its medical care. Thus, a community's health is determined by interactions among multiple factors, including the social environment, the physical environment, genetic endowment, an individual's behavioral and biological responses, disease, health care, health and function, and well-being (Evans and Stoddart 1990). The population health perspective also requires attention to resource allocation and accountability, implying the need for measures of health outcomes and evidence linking interventions to those outcomes (Kindig and Stoddart 2003).

This broader understanding of health and its determinants suggests that many public and private entities have a stake in or can affect the community's health. These stakeholders include health-care providers (clinicians, health plans, hospitals, and so on), public health agencies, and community organizations explicitly concerned with health. They can also include entities that may not see themselves as having an explicit health role, such as schools, sports clubs, employers, faith communities, and agencies providing social and housing services, transportation, education, and justice (Institute of Medicine 2003).

The increasingly common acceptance of this perspective by health professionals and community leaders has important implications and poses challenges for public health statistics. This chapter will address statistical issues that arise when implementing population health concepts in public health: the development and use of community health indicators and profiles, summary measures of population health, and community-based public health performance measures.

Because so many diverse entities can influence health, the public's health must be seen as a shared responsibility (Institute of Medicine 2003; Stoto et al. 1996). Managing a shared responsibility, however, is a major challenge, especially in an era that increasingly demands accountability in the public as well as the private sector, and has important implications for public health statistics. Toward this end, the Institute of Medicine (IOM) has developed a model Community Health Improvement Process (CHIP) as a tool to address a community's collective responsibility for its health (Durch et al. 1997). The CHIP perspective distinguishes between two kinds of population health measures—summary and performance—and this distinction will be used to organize this chapter.

Drawing on a variety of existing community health improvement processes, the CHIP includes two principal interacting cycles based on analysis, action, and measurement (Fig. 13.1). The health assessment activities that are part of a CHIP's problem identification and prioritization cycle should include production of a community health profile that can provide basic information to a community about its demographic and socioeconomic characteristics and its health status and health risks. This profile would provide background information that could help a community identify issues that need more focused attention and put other health data in context. Community health profiles and related issues are presented in the first section of this chapter. The second section discusses approaches to developing a single-measure community health summary.

Within the CHIP framework, a community may have a portfolio of health improvement activities, each progressing through its own analysis and imple-

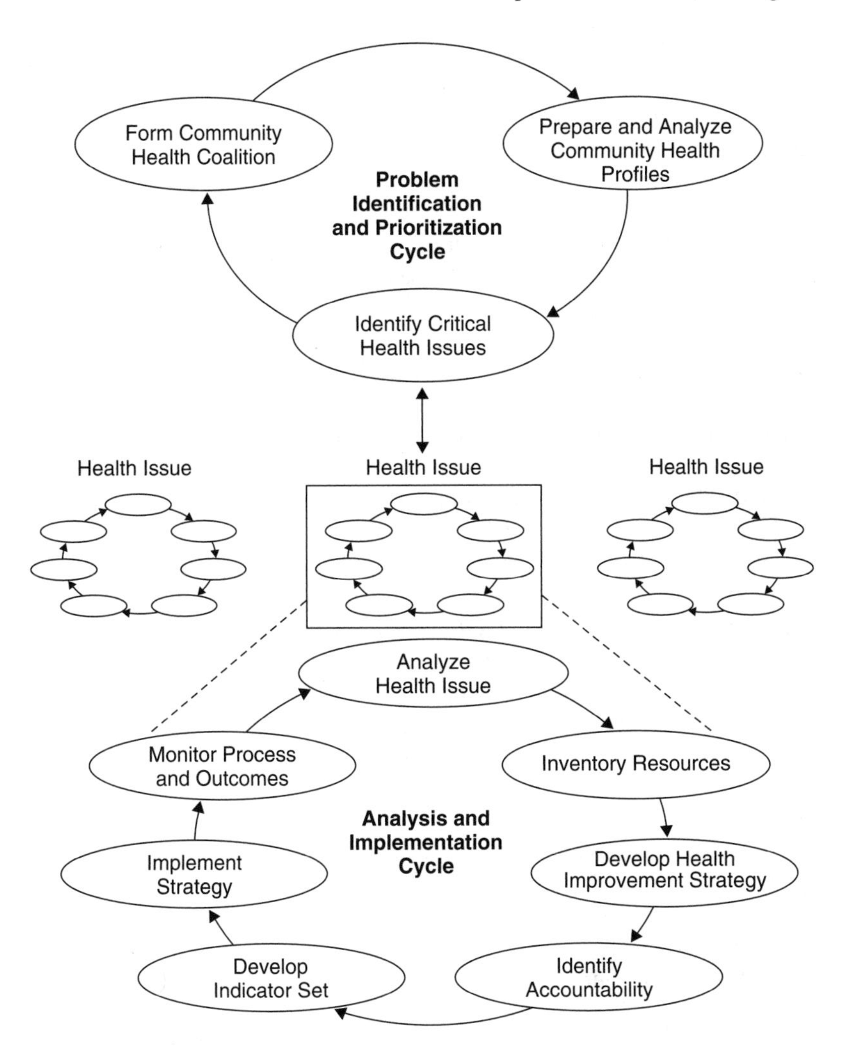

FIGURE 13.1
The Institute of Medicine's Community Health Improvement Process (CHIP).
(Source: Durch et al. 1997.)

mentation cycle at its own pace. To operationalize the concept of shared responsibility for community health, stakeholders need to know how the actions of each potentially accountable entity are contributing to the community's health. Thus, a CHIP includes the development of a set of specific, quantitative performance measures, linking accountable entities to the performance of specific activities expected to lead to the production of desired health outcomes in the community. The final section of the chapter, therefore, deals with statistical issues in performance monitoring in public health.

COMMUNITY HEALTH PROFILES

The population health perspective takes the community rather than an individual as the patient. To properly manage this patient's health, policymakers need regular measurement of the community's health status, as well as its determinants and consequences. In the IOM's CHIP process, community health profiles are the population-based health equivalent of regular medical checkups, helping to identify problems that need to be addressed and informing community priority setting activities (Stoto 1992).

Community health profiles include a set of measures that summarize the health of a community and facilitate comparisons over time and with other communities. Experience with social indicators suggests that a community health profile includes a set of indicators that is limited in number so that the story is not lost in the details and must be comprehensive so that all major issues are addressed. The indicators must be individually significant to keep the reader's attention and work together to tell a coherent story of the community's health. To be useful, the indicators must be capable of being monitored over time and disaggregated to subgroups of the population that might suffer from health disparities or be vulnerable in some other way. The indicators must also be valid and well conceptualized so that they can be clearly interpreted. They also must have sufficient reliability so that changes over time and among different groups in the population can be discerned.

For example, the set of indicators for a community health profile might include measures of:

- Sociodemographic characteristics, such as the high school graduation rate and median household income.
- Health risk factors, such as child immunization coverage, adult smoking rate, and obesity.
- Health care resource consumption, such as per capita health-care spending.
- Health status, such as the infant mortality rate by race/ethnicity, number of deaths due to preventable causes, and confirmed child abuse and neglect cases.
- Functional status, such as the proportion of adults in good to excellent health.
- Quality of life, such as the proportion of adults (in a population survey) satisfied with the quality of life in the community (Durch et al. 1997).

A variety of principles have been used to suggest appropriate measures for community health profiles (Fielding et al. 1997). To guide their proposed "California Health Report," Halfon et al. (2000) use a comprehensive and integrative model of community health that includes a range of health outcomes and determinants over the life course. The IOM suggested three different organizational principles in its suggestion for *Healthy People 2010's Leading Health Indicators: Understanding and Improving Health*: health determinants and health outcomes, life course determinants, and prevention (Chrvala and Bulger 1999; U.S. Department of Health and Human Services 2000).

Community health assessments are intended to help a community maintain a broad strategic view of its population's health status and factors that influence health in the community. They are not expected to be comprehensive surveys of all aspects of community health and well-being, but they should be able to help a community identify and focus attention on specific high-priority health issues. The background information provided by a health assessment can help a community interpret data on those issues (Durch et al. 1997).

Health assessments can help motivate communities to address health issues (Rhein et al. 2001). For example, evidence of low immunization rates among children or the elderly might encourage various sectors of the community to respond through official actions (e.g., more systematic provider assessments of patients' immunization status) and through community action (e.g., volunteer groups offering transportation to immunization clinics). Comparisons based on health assessment data may also motivate and help communities in assessing health priorities. These comparisons can be based on measurements over time within an individual community, comparisons with other communities or with state of national measures, or comparisons with a benchmark or target value such as those put forth in *Healthy People 2010* (Durch et al. 1997). Community health assessments can also help a community focus on reducing health disparities (Alameda County Public Health Department 2003).

More generally, community health assessments can provide the basis for all local public health planning, giving the local health department the opportunity to identify and interact with key community leaders, organizations, and interested residents about health priorities and concerns. New York State's Public Health Agenda Committee, for instance, has suggested that "a Community Health Assessment should be judged by how well it tells the story of the health of a particular community." The committee also recommended that the document should have multiple uses; relate to multiple local, state, and federal agencies, organizations, and audiences (grant makers, facilities, citizens); and meet the needs of both state and local governments for assessment (Public Health Agenda Committee 1998).

Experience in New York and elsewhere suggests that community health profiles should:

- be flexible,
- be less cumbersome to complete,
- be responsive to community needs,
- identify critical/core community health information,
- enable information sharing,
- facilitate review and timely feedback,

- recognize that community health assessment is an ongoing process that is open and collaborative, and
- demonstrate a link between community health assessment and the local health department's plans (Public Health Agenda Committee 1998).

Example: Community Health Indicators for the Washington Metropolitan Region

The Metropolitan Washington Public Health Assessment Center at the George Washington University School of Public Health and Health Services has recently developed a set of *Community Health Indicators for the Washington Metropolitan Region* (Metropolitan Washington Public Health Assessment Center 2001) that illustrates the challenges of assembling accurate, appropriate, and comparable demographic and other public health data for a community health profile.

To ensure its relevance to local public health officials and others in the community, the report was prepared under the guidance of an advisory committee that included representatives from area health departments. With a focus on health promotion and disease prevention efforts in the region and the *Healthy People 2010* leading health indicators as an organizing framework, 29 indicators were selected after several rounds of review (U.S. Department of Health and Human Services 2000). (See Box 13.1.) The choice of indicators was guided by several considerations:

- Presenting a mix of measures for health outcomes, such as death rates, and preventable health risks, such as smoking.

BOX 13.1
Healthy People 2010 Leading Health Indicators

1. Physical activity
2. Overweight and obesity
3. Tobacco use
4. Substance abuse
5. Responsible sexual behavior
6. Mental health
7. Injury and violence
8. Environmental quality
9. Immunization
10. Access to health care

Source: U.S. Department of Health and Human Services (2000).

- Focusing on health concerns for which effective preventive interventions are available (flu shots, for example, were chosen over Alzheimer's disease rates because we do not currently have ways to prevent or cure Alzheimer's disease).
- Having data available for each of the nine county-level jurisdictions in the region.

Nine of the indicators used data from vital statistics, and an additional 10 indicators were based on special county-level tabulations of the Centers for Disease Control and Prevention (CDC's) Behavioral Risk Factor Surveillance System (BRFSS) data (Centers for Disease Control and Prevention [hp]). The state health departments supplied data for five measures on reportable infectious diseases, and data for the other indicators were gathered from various state and local sources. However data for Washington-area jurisdictions were not available for most of the measures selected at the national level to track the *Healthy People* leading health indicators.

Based on these data, the report concluded that, overall, the adult population of the Washington metropolitan area is healthier than the nation as a whole. For 19 of 27 indicators, the Washington region is doing as well as or better than the national average. For instance, the region's coronary heart disease death rate and mammography rate already more than meet national targets for 2010, and the estimated rate of adult obesity in the region is almost at the national target. On some measures, however, the region appears less healthy than the nation. Particular problems are acquired immunodeficiency syndrome (AIDS), gonorrhea, and other sexually transmitted infections; binge drinking and firearm-related deaths; and infant mortality and low birth weight.

The data also show that the region is diverse, and that every jurisdiction shows some strengths and some weaknesses. Jurisdictions with higher average socioeconomic status still face challenges in promoting health and preventing disease in pockets of poverty and among growing immigrant communities with varying cultural and linguistic characteristics. Rates for whites were better than the national average for 17 of 19 indicators analyzed by race, but were better for blacks for only 5 of the 19 indicators (smoking, suicide, motor vehicle deaths, dental care, and mammography). The data available for 10 indicators also confirm that people with more education and higher household incomes tend to have more healthful behaviors.

Finally, the analysis highlighted some key regional health data needs. In particular, the region needs data comparable across jurisdictions on behavioral risk factors for adolescents and more data on risk factors for younger children. Also needed are data on the use of hospital and emergency department services, such as visits for asthma, injury, or mental health care, compiled in forms suitable for regional or jurisdiction-based analysis.

Furthermore, regional analysis often suggests that political boundaries of states or even counties do not adequately reflect geographical patterns of health determinants or health outcomes. A recent report from the Brookings Institution, *A Region Divided: The State of Growth in Greater Washington* (Center on Urban and Metropolitan Policy 1999), suggests that many socioeconomic indicators are substantially lower to the south and east of a line that roughly follows Interstate Highway 95 through Virginia, the District of Columbia, and Maryland. Some health indicators seem to follow this same pattern. For other indicators, the areas of Maryland and Virginia near the most disadvantaged parts of the District of Columbia have the worst health indicators. Patterns like these can be seen clearly, however, only if subcounty data are available.

Statistical Issues in the Development of Community Health Profiles

The development of community health profiles reminds us of the limitations of population-based data for *small areas*, which include most governmental units below the state level. Community-level data frequently suffer from large relative random variation due to rare outcomes in the numerator. The infant mortality rate, for instance, is a widely used public health measure, but in most communities the number of infant deaths is small and statistical fluctuations from year to year can be relatively large. This problem may be addressed in a variety of ways. Measures with problems of this sort, for instance, might be smoothed by averaging over time (using time series methods and weighted moving averages, for instance) and perhaps over space using spatial analogues of these methods. This solution, however, leads to problems with timeliness of the results and perhaps their understandability. Alternatively, proxy measures might be developed. In some circumstances, the proportion of children born with low birth weight (with a larger numerator) might be a more stable summary measure of infant health than the infant mortality rate (Stoto 1992, 2003). Empirical Bayes and mixed effects models can be very useful in this context (Devine and Louis 1994; Manton et al. 1989; Nandram et al. 2000; Pickle 2000; Shen and Louis 1999, 2000). One such model was used in the preparation of the *Atlas of United States Mortality* (Pickle et al. 1999).

Indicators based on survey data are also problematic. Most health surveys are designed to make estimates at the national or state level and incorporate a sample of thousands of respondents at these levels. The number of observations for substate areas, however, is substantially less and is often too small to provide reliable estimates. This problem might be approached through hierarchical Bayesian statistical models (Borgoni and Billari 2003) or through reweighting (Rao 2003). Alternatively, synthetic estimates or regression models might be developed to incorporate reliable local data based, say, on vital statistics or administrative records (Malec and Sedransk 1993).

Spatial models depend on the assumption that geographically proximate areas have similar health outcomes and, on this basis, "borrow strength" to overcome the limitations of small numbers. Alternatively, one could assume that nongeographic factors such as socioeconomic status are more appropriate and build regression models to estimate local area rates. These and other statistical techniques for model-based small area estimation (see, e.g., National Research Council 2000a, 2000b) are well developed but have rarely been used for public health data.

Statistical models of this sort, it must be acknowledged, are better for some purposes than for others. Depending on the variability in the data for the target area and the desired degree of smoothing, more or less weight is put on a community's own area data. Because of the assumptions that underlie them, these models are not good for looking for outliers or differences between adjacent or similar communities; depending on the degree of smoothing and the statistical model, differences of this sort will be minimized. These techniques can be very useful, however, in seeing the big picture in geographical and other patterns.

SUMMARY MEASURES OF HEALTH

Boston Magazine's annual "Healthiest Towns" report (Blanding 2003) and the United Health Foundation's *State Health Rankings* (United Health Foundation et al. 2003) illustrate a common type of community health summary. This type of summary is typically based on a variety of indicators of health outcomes, as well as environmental and socioeconomic indicators known to be related to health outcomes. A single score for each state or community is then computed, giving roughly equal weight to all of the indicators, and rankings are prepared based on the summary score. One problem with measures of this sort is that the choice of measures to be included and the weighting scheme are essentially arbitrary. Measures that have a lot of natural variability can inordinately influence the summary, and as a result, including different measures of similar concepts can sometimes lead to dramatically different rankings. Perhaps more troubling is that reports about such community summaries in the media tend to focus on the horserace aspect rather than suggesting what a community might do to improve its health.

Rather than monitoring and arbitrarily summarizing a large set of community health indicators, a number of authors have advocated the development and use of a theory-based summary measure of population health that could be expressed in a single number. Wolfson (1994, 296–299) offers a hypothetical example from a future national health status report:

> Average health status of Canadians was 82.7 percent [where 100 percent would indicate that all residents were in full health]. This is 0.3 percent higher than reported . . . in the last survey. For those over age sixty-five, average health status was 68.3 percent. . . . If the elderly had not suffered from mobility impairments, their health status would have averaged 79.1 percent. . . .

> Over two-thirds of these mobility impairments were associated with arthritis and other musculoskeletal diseases.

Wolfson also suggests that the results could be broken down by geographic region and compared, and as the example suggests, the summary measure should be disaggregated by age, by the causes of ill health, and other factors. Analyses of this sort, however, implicitly assume that the summary measure has the same meaning in every population compared.

Setting aside for a moment the challenges of developing and using such a single-number summary, one must first ask whether it is beneficial. For certain economic analyses, the answer to both questions is decidedly yes. If one is comparing the cost effectiveness of interventions that impact different dimensions of health, such as the potential benefits of vaccines for different diseases (Stratton et al. 2001), a common unit of health gains is essential. However, whether a single-number index effectively engages the public or serves as a useful guide for policymakers remains an open question. It seems likely that if overall health were 5 percentage points lower in community A than in community B, people would want to know what this statistic means, whether it is important, and what they can do about it.

Until recently, summary measures of population health have typically been based on mortality statistics, in part because vital statistics exist for countries, states, and smaller geographic areas. Perhaps the most common summary measure is life expectancy, which summarizes the age-specific mortality experience rates of the current population by calculating the average age of death if a cohort were to experience these rates throughout its life (Young 1998, 33–35). Although a cumbersome concept, life expectancy can be explained simply: "In 2002, the life expectancy for women in the United States was 80 years" (National Center for Health Statistics 2003a). By virtue of its definition, life expectancy does not depend on the age distribution of the population, so it is a pure summary of the age-specific mortality rates and can be used to compare different populations.

Despite its limitations, life expectancy can be a powerful tool in summarizing population health. Tobias and Cheung (2003), for instance, estimated the life expectancy for New Zealanders categorized by ethnicity (European, Maori, and Pacific) and by a small-area deprivation index, calculated using socioeconomic and demographic census data using the smallest possible geographic units. They found a strong negative relationship between small area deprivation and life expectancy.

Life expectancy values each year of life equally, but for some purposes one might want to give more weight to *premature mortality* or lives lost among younger people. One measure of this concept is called *years of potential life lost* (YPLL). It sums the average number of years "lost" by individuals, assuming that all who die younger than some arbitrary age, such as 65 or 75 years, would have lived until that age. The YPLL is typically calculated for particular causes of death.

Young, for instance, shows that although there were 25,687 cancer deaths and 10,286 injury deaths in Canada in 1993, the YPLL for injuries surpassed that for cancer: 336,593 versus 302,585 (Young 1998, 35–36). As this illustration suggests, YPLL gives more weight to causes of death that tend to occur at younger ages. The difficulty with this measure is that the cutoff age is arbitrary, and changes in mortality above that age, or of quality of life at any age, do not enter into the calculation.

Life expectancy, YPLL, and similar calculations, such as premature mortality rates, summarize only a population's mortality experience, not the health conditions with which they live. As chronic diseases and other conditions became more prominent through the twentieth century, an increasing proportion of individuals' lives was lived with health conditions that reduced their level of functioning and quality of life. To address these conditions, a number of indices that incorporate both mortality and health-related quality of life have been developed and used at the population level.

The development and use of a population-based health index that incorporates more than mortality information consists of two steps, both of which involve statistical and ethical challenges. First, a one-dimensional scale must be developed to represent the *health utility*—*H*—of every conceivable combination of health states that an individual could experience. How, for instance, does diabetes with blindness due to diabetic retinopathy and the risk of other complications compare to having a bad case of the flu? Second, the *H*'s must be combined across everyone in the population into a summary measure (Field and Gold 1998; Murray and Frenk 2002; Murray et al. 2002a, 2002b). As will be seen, neither of the two steps in the process is currently developed well enough to provide valid and reliable single-number summaries of population health in the United States.

Estimation of *H* at the Individual Level

The assignment of a single number, *H*, in a reliable and consistent way requires many theoretical and practical choices that can greatly influence the results. For instance, if blindness is 0.5 on a scale of 0 to 1, what is a bad case of the flu that requires 3 days of bed rest and time away from work? Does it matter that the blindness is a lifelong condition, whereas the flu lasts only a few days? How should past and future health states be factored in? Should a 50-year-old smoker's health index reflect the likelihood of future cancer and heart disease? Should *H* for a 70-year-old man be measured relative to the typical health status of 70-year-old men or should it be independent of age and sex? Should distinctions be based on social role or function, or on some more intrinsic valuation of the health states? Should the valuation be based on the opinions of people who have the condition in question, a random sample of the population looking across all conditions, or a group of physician judges who are familiar with all of the conditions?

Substantial progress has been made in the past two decades on the development of survey methods to assess health utilities across many diseases and conditions. The Health Utility Index (HUI), for instance, focuses on an individual's assessment of his or her functional capacity in eight dimensions of health (vision, hearing, speech, ambulation, dexterity, emotion, cognition, and pain) (Grootendorst et al. 2000; McDowell and Newell 1996). Then, using preference weights developed in a separate study in which participants were asked to compare pairs of combinations of health states, a single numerical summary measure of health-related quality of life is computed. The use of preference weights based on a single survey in one country (Canada), however, limits the usefulness of this scale in other countries.

The Short Form 36 (SF-36), now translated into many languages and dialects for international use (McDowell and Newell 1996; Ware and Sherbourne 1992), represents another approach. This self-administered instrument includes 36 items and produces results in eight dimensions of health: physical functioning, social functioning, role limitations (physical), role limitations (emotional), well-being (mental health), vitality, pain, and overall evaluation of health. The SF-36 has been carefully tested and validated, but does not include any means to combine the results across the eight component dimensions into a single numerical score. Rather, the SF-36 is commonly used to compare both individuals and population profiles, that is, changes and differences in the pattern of scores in the eight dimensions.

A far simpler approach is to simply ask survey respondents about their general health. The Health Survey for England, for instance, asks, "How is your health in general? Would you say it was (*1*) very good, (*2*) good, (*3*) fair, (*4*) bad, or (*5*) very bad?" Similarly, the U.S. National Health Interview Survey (National Center for Health Statistics 2003b) asks, "Would you say [subject name's] health is excellent, very good, good, fair, or poor?" Sturgis and colleagues (no date) conclude that single-item questions such as those pertaining to self-assessed general health are simple to ask and answer, and extensive use of such questions allows for comparisons over time and place. They are valid in the sense that they are a good predictor of mortality. Measures of this sort, however, do not provide for a single numerical value for H.

In summary, the only currently available and validated instrument that provides for single-value estimates of H is the HUI. The calculation of this index, however, relies on a survey of the preference of one group of Canadians, and its validity for other populations is not known.

Calculation of H at the Population Level

To calculate a community-level health summary, individual-level estimates of H must be combined over the entire population. This can be done in a number of ways. Conceptually simplest, H might be determined for everyone in a survey of a representative sample of the population and then simply averaged. A simple summary of this sort, however, would reflect the age distribution of the population, so it would have to be standardized or adjusted in some way for meaningful comparisons.

Another approach is to build on the framework used for mortality statistics. Age-specific estimates of *H* might be combined with mortality rates into a *health expectancy*. Continuing with Wolfson's example, the future health report might say (Wolfson 1994, 297):

> Life expectancy for women is currently 82.2 years. However, adjusting for average observed deviations from full health at each age reduces this to 74.4 years of *healthy* life expectancy. Most of the 7.8 year difference occurs after age 65. . . . A more detailed analysis reveals that limb and joint disorders have three times as great an impact on this healthy life expectancy as all cancers combined.

To calculate healthy life expectancy, one can apply the current age-specific average *H* to the proportion surviving to each age in the population's life table and then sum over the life span, as in the standard calculation of life expectancies. The problem with this *prevalence-based* approach is that it combines summaries of *H* in the current population with survival fractions that would be experienced in a hypothetical population that experienced all of the current-period age-specific mortality rates. Another problem is that this formulation does not allow for calculations of the impact of changes in specific health problems or the disaggregation of the overall summary health measure by specific conditions, as in Wolfson's example.

An *incidence-based* approach is more theoretically appropriate but also more difficult to implement. If estimates were available on the age-specific rates of transition between every possible health state, they could be combined in a multistate life table approach and values of *H* for each state factored into the calculation of health life expectancy. Lack of data on the transition rates prohibits the general use of this approach.

Other measures are reported with some number of years (less than the population life expectancy) as the unit but are conceptually different. Disability-free life expectancy (DFLE), for instance, essentially assumes that *H*—freedom from disability in this case—is a dichotomous value; people are either disability free or not (Crimmins et al. 1997). The DFLE is calculated by multiplying the age-specific life table survivorship rates by the proportion disability free by age and then summing across the life span. Some variants of disability-adjusted life years (DALY), commonly used in international comparisons, weight the value of health at different ages differently—for example, applying lower weights for the very young and the very old to reflect economic productivity (Murray and Lopez 1996).

Every method for calculating population health summaries by building on individual-level measures of *H* embodies a number of ethical choices (Field and Gold 1998). Should everyone's *H* count equally or should some count more, depending on their social role? Distinctions of this sort are typically not made, except for age. It is appropriate to discriminate by age, some argue, because everyone eventually passes through all ages. The standard practice in economic analyses is to discount future costs and benefits, including expected future changes in health expectancy. This is necessary to avoid economic paradoxes, but might it be better to address intergenerational issues more directly in ethical terms?

Conclusions on Summary Health Measures

Despite substantial advances in theory and methods, many issues remain to be resolved before summary health measures can be implemented on a regular basis, and the data needed to calculate a single-number population-level summary health measure are generally not available. Thus, while single-number health summaries are necessary for economic analyses, the jury remains out on whether they would be useful for monitoring the community's health. Moreover, while a single-number summary may gain the public's attention, questions such as "Is this important?," "What does it mean?," and "What should we do about it?" will soon arise. If the summary must be disaggregated to be useful, would it not be preferable to simply monitor a well-chosen set of individually meaningful indicators? Continuing with the population as patient metaphor, could a single summary number (even if exceptionally well developed) ever be enough to guide medical choices?

PERFORMANCE MEASUREMENT

In recent years, public health and health-care policymakers have come to realize the importance of population-based data on health status and the determinants of health for improving the accountability of managed care organizations, public health agencies, and other entities that can contribute to the public's health. Part of this realization is due to the nature of public health and the emerging importance of preventive medicine: their impact can only be seen in statistical terms such as declining rates of lung cancer attributed to smoking reduction many years earlier. There are no grateful patients or families who know that they have been saved by the intervention of a particular physician or hospital.

Personal health services providers have increasingly embraced performance measurement as a way to improve health care. Governmental agencies, private quasi-regulatory bodies, and professional associations have all promulgated measures, increasingly with a focus on quality of care. Examples include the Center for Medicare and Medicaid Services (Jencks et al. 2000), the Joint Commission on Accreditation of Healthcare Organizations (2003), the National Committee for Quality Assurance (2003), and physician professional groups (Kania et al. 1996) that have developed a variety of performance measures for hospitals, providers, health plans, and managed care organizations. In 1999 Congress mandated two new annual reports to be prepared by the Agency for Healthcare Research and Quality (AHRQ): the *National Healthcare Quality Report* and the *National Healthcare Disparities Report* (AHRQ 2003a, 2003b).

Though it has a long history (APHA 1934), performance measurement is less common in public health, although it is becoming more widespread (Derose et al. 2002, 2003; Perrin and Koshel 1997; Perrin et al. 1999). *Healthy People 2010* (U.S. Department of Health and Human Services 2000) and its predecessors have clarified the importance of specific, quantitative, population-based health measures for setting public health policy. Other examples include the Model Standards (American Public Health Association et al. 1991), the Assessment Protocol for Excellence in Public Health (APEX/PH) (National Association of County Health Officials 1991), and the Mobilizing for Action through Planning and Partnerships (MAPP) program (National Association of County and City Health Officials 2001). Taking this approach further, and consistent with the Government Performance and Results Act (GPRA), the Health Resources and Services Administration's (HRSA) Maternal and Child Health Block Grants, for instance, now require annual performance measures at the state level (Maternal and Child Health Bureau [hp]).

As noted above, the IOM's CHIP includes the development of a set of specific quantitative performance measures, linking accountable entities to the performance of specific activities expected to lead to the production of desired health outcomes in the community. Selecting these indicators requires careful consideration of how progress is achieved in health. A set of indicators should balance population-based measures of risk factors and health outcomes and health systems–based measures of services performed. Capacity (sometimes known as *structure*, e.g., the availability of trained staff) and process measures (such as availability of insurance coverage for immunizations) might be included, but only to the extent that there is evidence that links them to health outcomes. To encourage full participation in the health improvement process, the selected performance measures should also be balanced across the interests and contributions of the various accountable entities in the community, including those whose primary mission is not health specific. It has also been suggested that the set of performance measures should include some for which progress may be seen in the short run in order to maintain a sense of momentum for the participants (Durch et al. 1997). In the population-as-patient metaphor, once a disease or health problem has been diagnosed, numerous clinical indicators are needed to assess treatment progress.

Example: Performance Measurement for Tobacco Control

If a community chooses to target tobacco-related issues as part of its community health improvement plan, Box 13.2 illustrates the types of performance measures it might monitor. Deaths from tobacco-related conditions would be included because reducing this is the ultimate goal, but it is recognized that even effective actions taken today will not result in a reduction of mortality for many years. Tobacco-related mortality can be estimated as a proportion of deaths due to heart disease, stroke, various cancers, and other conditions (Shultz et al. 1991), so this measure is available even for small communities. Smoking-related residential fires is included as a more immediate outcome measure.

The sample indicator set includes two smoking behavior indicators. Smoking prevalence in adults can be measured in a population survey, and reflects cumulative efforts to promote smoking cessation as well as reduce initiation. Smoking initiation is more difficult to measure in a population, but it is included as a more immediate measure of a key component of a communitywide tobacco control effort. The proportion of high school seniors who smoke is a reasonable proxy.

Two of the indicators reflect legal efforts to address smoking. First, the existence of environmental tobacco ordinances such as indoor smoking laws reflects the commitment of the community as a whole to tobacco control. Laws on tobacco sales to youth are normally determined at the state level, but the community's efforts in this regard can be measured in terms of enforcement of these and federal regulations. Enforcement can be measured through sting operations, and reflects the contributions of both the police and the business community to tobacco control.

Box 13.2

Sample Performance Indicator Set for Tobacco Use and Health

- Deaths from tobacco-related conditions
- Smoking-related residential fires
- Prevalence of smoking in adults
- Initiation of smoking among youth
- Ordinances to control environmental tobacco smoke
- Local enforcement of laws on tobacco sales to youth
- Tobacco use prevention in school curricula
- Counseling by health-care providers
- Availability of cessation programs
- Health plan coverage for cessation programs

Source: Durch et al. (1997).

Tobacco control also requires educational efforts, which are reflected in the next two indicators. An indicator reflecting the amount of tobacco prevention material in the curriculum measures the schools' contribution. Physicians and other health-care providers have a role to play as well, and an indicator on smoking counseling summarizes their contribution. The extent to which they ask their patients whether they smoke and counsel them to quit if they do, for instance, can be measured in population surveys.

The final two indicators relate to the accessibility of smoking cessation programs. Whether and to what extent they exist in the community is a measure of the effectiveness of voluntary health associations such as the local chapters of the American Cancer Society or the American Lung Association, which typically run such programs. The proportion of health plans that cover the costs of such programs is a measure of the contribution of the plans as well as the employers who purchase them.

Statistical Issues in Performance Measurement

The development of appropriate performance indicators in public health must consider validity, reliability, and trade-offs between them. Reliability assesses whether the indicator consistently measures the concept. The primary issues relate to the small number of events and sample sizes for small areas, as discussed above. Because performance measures are typically followed over time to assess progress, *sensitivity to change*—an indicator's ability to measure change—is particularly important. Some changes simply reflect chance fluctuations in epidemiologic rates. For most communities, for instance, infant mortality rates fluctuate substantially from year to year simply because the numerator, the number of infant deaths, is small. Statistical tests can be used to assess the degree to which the indicator changes if and only if the concept being measured also changes.

Validity, on the other hand, is an indicator's capacity to measure the intended concept. One must ask whether the measure is really within the control of the entity whose performance is being assessed, and consider risk adjustment to control for differences in the populations being served. Changes in the social process of measuring health, and the distinction between real and artifactual changes in mortality statistics and self-reported health conditions, are also important. A common problem, for instance, occurs when health service records are used to assess changing disease burdens. Does a decrease in emergency department visits for asthma indicate the success of a prevention program or measures to restrict access to individuals without insurance?

Compromises must generally be made among validity, reliability, data availability, and sensitivity to change. In the area of prenatal care, for instance, evaluators often use the receipt of prenatal care in the first trimester, rather than more complex measures based on official recommendations of the U.S. Public Health Service for the frequency and content of prenatal care, because the former measure is available on birth certificates and the latter is not. This is a case of trading validity for increased data availability. In many communities, annual infant morality rates are not reliable due to the small number of infant deaths. Instead of annual rates, therefore, epidemiologists commonly calculate running averages by the average infant mortality rate over 3 or 5 years. This is a case in which reliability is gained at the expense of timeliness and responsiveness to change. Another approach frequently used to deal with sparse data is to use proxy measures that reflect trends and differences. The percentage of infants born with a low birth weight, for example, is used rather than infant mortality because low birth weight has been shown to be strongly associated with infant morality. This is a case of trading validity for reliability.

Example: Promoting Successful Birth Outcomes

Access to Health Care in America, a 1993 IOM report, suggests a number of measures of access to health care, and one group of these measures illustrates the statistical issues in the development of performance measures in public health (Milman 1993). The measures below address only one of five access objectives: promoting successful birth outcomes. Although each of the proposed indicators has limitations as well as strengths, it is thought that the combination of these four should provide a reasonably complete and accurate set of performance measures for this objective.

The first indicator is based on the use of health care, specifically prenatal care. Using information on birth certificates, one can calculate the percentage of pregnant women obtaining adequate prenatal care. The strength of this indicator is that it is a direct measure of health-care access. There are, however, a number of weaknesses. First, "adequate" prenatal care is measured only by what is available on the birth certificate, which is usually limited to the time of initiation and the frequency of care. There is no information on the distribution of visits over time or their content. Indeed, a large number of visits could represent a problem pregnancy. More complex indices of the adequacy of care are available, but their calculation can be confounded by missing or incomplete data, and there might be problems in recalling the number or timing of visits when the birth certificate is being filled out.

The second indicator proposed by the IOM is an outcome measure: the infant mortality rate. This is a commonly used measure of access and is available even for small communities from vital statistics. The infant mortality rate, however, provides little information about access barriers and includes causes of death that cannot be affected by the health-care system. Moreover, because infant deaths are now uncommon, there is high chance variability in infant deaths in many areas.

As an alternative, the third indicator proposed is the low birth weight rate, the proportion of infants weighing less than 2500 g at birth. The strengths of this indicator are that it is known to be specific to adequate prenatal care and access to nutrition services and is an important predictor of infant survival. Moreover, since the numerator is not as rare as infant deaths, the rate is more stable. Like the infant mortality rate, however, the low birth weight rate provides little information about access barriers.

The final indicator is the rate of congenital syphilis. This is a reportable condition in most states, so the data are available, and the condition is very specific to lack of or inadequate prenatal care. The weaknesses are that reporting may be incomplete, and since syphilis is rare in most states, the measure often lacks reliability.

CONCLUSIONS

The population health perspective that is becoming increasingly common in medicine and public health has important implications for public health statistics. Treating the population as the patient means that new and better statistical tools are needed to monitor the community's overall health (including the social, environmental, and behavioral factors that determine health) on a regular basis in order to set priorities for improving it. Performance measures are also needed to manage population-based interventions, including those based in managed care organizations, to address specific population health issues.

The development of statistical measures to meet the needs of population health is difficult for a number of reasons, including the relatively small size of the populations in question, which are often communities smaller than states. There is also the challenge of developing valid and reliable measures using existing data. New statistical methods exist and are being developed, and the acceptance of the population health perspective will likely advance their development and use.

Acknowledgments

Preparation of this chapter was supported by the RAND Corporation.

REFERENCES

Agency for Healthcare Research and Quality. National Healthcare Quality Report. AHRQ Publication No. 04-RG003. Rockville, MD: Agency for Healthcare Research and Quality; 2003a [cited 2003 Dec 29]. Available from: qualitytools.ahrq.gov/qualityreport/download_report.aspx.

Agency for Healthcare Research and Quality [monograph on the Internet]. National Healthcare Disparities Report AHRQ Publication No. 04-RG004. Rockville, MD: Agency for Healthcare Research and Quality; 2003b [cited 2003 Dec 29]. Available from: qualitytools.ahrq.gov/disparitiesreport/download_report.aspx.

Alameda County Public Health Department [monograph on the Internet]. Alameda County Health Status Report 2003. Oakland, CA: Alameda County Public Health Department; 2003 [cited 2003 Dec 21]. Available from: http://www.co.alameda.ca.us/publichealth/information/info.htm.

American Public Health Association. Appraisal Form for City Health Work, 4th ed. New York: American Public Health Association; 1934.

American Public Health Association et al. Healthy Communities 2000: Model Standards. Washington, DC: American Public Health Association; 1991.

Blanding M. The healthiest towns. Boston Magazine 2003 Apr, pp. 78–85.

Borgoni R, Billari FC [article on the Internet]. Bayesian spatial analysis of demographic survey data: an application to contraceptive use at first sexual intercourse. Demogr Res 2003;8, Article 3 [cited 2003 Dec 21]. Available from: http://www.demographic-research.org.

Center on Urban and Metropolitan Policy [monograph on the Internet]. A Region Divided: the State of Growth in Greater Washington, D.C. Washington, DC: The Brookings Institution; 1999 [cited 2003 Dec 21]. Available from: http://www.brookings.edu/es/urban/dc/regiondividedexsum.htm.

Centers for Disease Control and Prevention [homepage on the Internet]. Atlanta: Centers for Disease Control and Prevention [cited 2003 Dec 21]. About the BRFSS. Available from: http://www.cdc.gov/brfss/about.htm.

Chrvala CA, Bulger RJ, eds. Leading Health Indicators for Healthy People 2010: Final Report. Washington, DC: National Academy Press; 1999.

Crimmins EM, Saito Y, Ingeneri D. Trends in disability-free life expectancy in the United States, 1970–90. Pop Dev Rev 1997;23:555–572.

Derose SF, Asch SM, Fielding JE, Schuster MA. Developing quality indicators for local health departments: experience in Los Angeles County. Am J Prev Med 2003;25:347–357.

Derose SF, Schuster MA, Fielding JE, Asch SM. Public health quality measurement: concepts and challenges. Annu Rev Public Health 2002;23:1–21.

Devine OJ, Louis TA. A constrained empirical Bayes estimator for incidence rates in areas with small populations. Stat Med 1994;13:1119–1133.

Durch JS, Bailey LA, Stoto MA, eds. Improving Health in the Community: A Role for Performance Monitoring. Washington, DC: National Academy Press; 1997.

Evans RG, Stoddart GL. Producing health, consuming health care. Soc Sci Med 1990;31: 1347–1363.

Field MJ, Gold MR, eds. Summarizing Population Health: Directions for the Development and Application of Population Metrics. Washington, DC: National Academy Press; 1998.

Fielding JE, Halfon N, Sutherland C. Characteristics of community report cards—United States, 1996. MMWR 1997;46:647–649.

Friedman DJ, Starfield B. Models of population health: their value for U.S. public health practice, policy, and research. Am J Public Health 2003;93:366–369.

Grootendorst P, Feeny D, Furlong W. Health Utilities Index Mark 3: evidence of construct validity for stroke and arthritis in a population health survey. Med Care 2000;38:290–299.

Halfon N, Ebener PA, Sastry N, Ahn P, Cherman L, Hernandez J, et al. [monograph on the Internet]. California Health Report (MR-1205-TCWF). Santa Monica, CA: RAND Corp.; 2000 [cited 2003 Dec 21]. Available from: www.rand.org/publications/MR/MR1205.

Institute of Medicine, Board on Health Promotion and Disease Prevention, Committee on Assuring the Health of the Public in the 21st Century. The Future of the Public's Health in the 21st Century. Washington, DC: National Academy Press; 2003.

Jencks SF, Cuerdon T, Burwen DR, Fleming B, Houck PM, Kussmaul AE, Nilasena DS, et al. Quality of medical care delivered to Medicare beneficiaries: a profile at state and national levels. JAMA 2000;284:1670–1676.

Joint Commission on Accreditation of Healthcare Organizations [monograph on the

Internet]. Oryx Performance Measurement. Oakbrook Terrace, IL: JCAHO; 2003 [cited 2003 Dec 21]. Available from: http://hcpc.uth.tmc.edu/pihome/oryx/oryx.html.

Kania C, Richards R, Sanderson-Austin J, Wagner J, Wetzler H. Using clinical and functional data for quality improvement in outcomes measurement consortia. Jt Comm J Qual Improv 1996;22:492–504.

Kindig DA, Stoddart G. What is population health? Am J Public Health 2003;93:380–383.

Malec D, Sedransk J. Bayesian predictive inference for units with small sample sizes. The case of binary random variables. Med Care 1993;31(suppl):YS66–YS70.

Manton KG, Woodbury MA, Stallard E, Riggan WB, Creason JP, Pellom AC. Empirical Bayes procedures for stabilizing maps of U.S. cancer mortality rates. J Am Stat Assoc 1989;84: 637–650.

Maternal and Child Health Bureau [homepage on the Internet]. Rockville, MD: Health Resources and Services Administration [cited 2003 Dec 21]. Guidance and forms for the Title V application/annual report. Available from: http://ftp.hrsa.gov/mchb/blockgrant/bgguideforms.pdf.

McDowell I, Newell C. Measuring Health: A Guide to Rating Scales and Questionnaires, 2nd ed. New York: Oxford University Press; 1996.

Metropolitan Washington Public Health Assessment Center [monograph on the Internet]. Community Health Indicators for the Washington Metropolitan Region. Washington, DC: Metropolitan Washington Council of Governments; 2001 [cited 2003 Dec 21]. Available from: www.mwphac.org.

Milman M, ed. Access to Health Care in America. Washington, DC: National Academy Press; 1993.

Murray CJL, Frenk J. Summary measures of population health in the context of the WHO framework for health system performance assessment. In: Murray CJL, Salomon JA, Mathers CD, Lopez AD, eds. Summary Measures of Population Health: Concepts, Ethics, Measurement and Applications. Geneva: World Health Organization; 2002.

Murray CJL, Lopez AD, eds. The Global Burden of Disease: A Comprehensive Assessment of Mortality and Disability from Diseases, Injuries, and Risk Factors in 1990 and Projected to 2020. Cambridge, MA: Harvard School of Public Health on behalf of the World Health Organization and the World Bank; distributed by Harvard University Press; 1996.

Murray CJL, Salomon JA, Mathers CD. A critical examination of summary measures of population health. In: Murray CJL, Salomon JA, Mathers CD, Lopez AD, eds. Summary Measures of Population Health: Concepts, Ethics, Measurement and Applications. Geneva: World Health Organization; 2002a.

Murray CJL, Salomon JA, Mathers CD. The individual basis for summary measures of population health. In: Murray CJL, Salomon JA, Mathers CD, Lopez AD, eds. Summary Measures of Population Health: Concepts, Ethics, Measurement and Applications. Geneva: World Health Organization; 2002b.

Nandram B, Sedransk J, Pickle LW. Bayesian analysis and mapping of mortality rates for chronic obstructive pulmonary disease. J Am Stat Assoc 2000;95:1110–1118.

National Association of County Health Officials. APEX/PH: Assessment Protocol for Excellence in Public Health. Washington, DC: National Association of County Health Officials; 1991.

National Association of County and City Health Officials [monograph on the Internet]. MAPP—Mobilizing for Action through Planning and Partnerships. Washington, DC: National Association of County and City Health Officials; 2001 [cited 2003 Dec 21]. Available from: http://www.naccho.org/project77.cfm.

National Center for Health Statistics [monograph on the Internet]. Health United States 2003. Hyattsville, MD: National Center for Health Statistics; 2003a [cited 2003 Dec 21]. Available from: http://www.cdc.gov/nchs/hus.htm.

National Center for Health Statistics [questionnaire on the Internet]. Hyattsville, MD:

National Center for Health Statistics; 2003b [cited 2003 Dec 21]. 2003 National Health Interview Survey questionnaire, family core. Available from: http://ftp.cdc.gov/pub/Health_Statistics/NCHS/Survey_Questionnaires/NHIS/2003/Family.pdf.

National Committee for Quality Assurance [monograph on the Internet]. The State of Managed Care Quality 2003. Washington, DC: National Committee for Quality Assurance; 2003 [cited 2003 Dec 21]. Available from: www.ncqa.org/Communications/State%20Of%20Managed%20Care/SOHCREPORT2003.pdf.

National Research Council. Small-Area Estimates of School-Age Children in Poverty: Evaluation of Current Methodology. Washington, DC: National Academy Press; 2000a.

National Research Council. Small-Area Income and Poverty Estimates: Priorities for 2000 and Beyond. Washington, DC: National Academy Press; 2000b.

Perrin EB, Durch JS, Skillman SM, eds. Health Performance Measurement in the Public Health Sector: Principles and Policies for Implementing and Information Network. Washington, DC: National Academy Press; 1999.

Perrin EB, Koshel JJ, eds. Assessment of Performance Measures for Public Health, Substance Abuse, and Mental Health. Washington, DC: National Academy Press; 1997.

Pickle LW. Exploring the spatio-temporal patterns of mortality using mixed effects models. Stat Med 2000;19:2251–2263.

Pickle LW, Mungiole M, Jones GK, White AA. Exploring the spatial patterns of mortality: the new atlas of United States mortality. Stat Med 1999;18:3211–3220.

Public Health Agenda Committee [monograph on the Internet]. Planning and Funding Local Public Health Services in New York State: The New Public Health Agenda. Albany: New York State Department of Health; 1998 [cited 2003 Dec 21]. Available from: http://www.health.state.ny.us/nysdoh/chac/pdf/phagenda.pdf.

Rao JNK. Small Area Estimation. New York: Wiley; 2003.

Rhein M, Lafronza V, Bhandari E, Hawes J, Hofrichter R [monograph on the Internet]. Advancing Community Public Health Systems in the 21st Century: Emerging Strategies and Innovations from the Turning Point Experience. Washington, DC: National Association of County and City Health Officials; 2001 [cited 2003 Dec 21]. Available from: http://www.naccho.org/GENERAL322.cfm.

Shen W, Louis TA. Empirical Bayes estimation via the smoothing by roughening approach. J Comput Graph Stat 1999;8:800–823.

Shen W, Louis TA. Triple-goal estimates for disease mapping. Stat Med 2000;19:2295–2308.

Shultz JM, Novotny TE, Rice DP. Quantifying the disease impact of cigarette smoking with SAMMEC II software. Public Health Rep 1991;106:326–333.

Stoto MA. Public health assessment in the 1990s. Annu Rev Public Health 1992;13:59–78.

Stoto MA [monograph on the Internet]. Statistical Issues in Interactive Web-Based Public Health Data Dissemination Systems (WR-106). Santa Monica, CA: RAND Corp; 2003 [cited 2003 Dec 21]. Available from: http://www.rand.org/publications/WR/WR106.

Stoto MA, Abel CA, Dievler A, eds. Healthy Communities: New Partnerships for the Future of Public Health. Washington, DC: National Academy Press; 1996.

Stratton KR, Durch JS, Lawrence RS, eds. Vaccines for the 21st Century: A Tool for Decisionmaking. Washington, DC: National Academy Press; 2001.

Sturgis P, Thomas R, Purdon S, Bridgwood A, Dodd T [monograph on the Internet]. Comparative Review and Assessment of Key Health State Measures of the General Population. London: Department of Health, United Kingdom; no date [cited 2003 Dec 21]. Available from: http:// www.doh.gov.uk/public/healthreport.htm.

Tobias MI, Cheung J [article on the Internet]. Monitoring health inequalities: life expectancy and small area deprivation in New Zealand. Pop Health Metr 2003;1:2 [cited 2003 Dec 21]. Available from: http://www.pophealthmetrics.com/content/1/1/2.

United Health Foundation, American Public Health Association, Partnership for Prevention [monograph on the Internet]. America's Health: State Health Rankings—2003 Edition. Minnetonka, IL: United Health Foundation; 2003 [cited 2003 Dec 21]. Available from: www.unitedhealthfoundation.org/download/UHC_037304_book.pdf.

U.S. Department of Health and Human Services. Healthy People 2010: Understanding and Improving Health. Washington, DC: GPO; 2000.

Ware JE, Sherbourne CD. The MOS 36-item short-form health survey (SF-36®): I. conceptual framework and item selection. Med Care 1992;30:473–483.

Wolfson MC. Social proprioception: measurement, data, and information from a population health perspective. In: Evans RG, Barer ML, Marmor TL, eds. Why Are Some People Healthy and Others Not? The Determinants of Health of Populations. New York: Aldine de Gruyter; 1994. pp. 287–316.

Young TK. Population Health: Concepts and Methods. New York: Oxford University Press; 1998.

CHAPTER 14

Privacy, Confidentiality, and Health Statistics

John P. Fanning

THE IMPORTANCE OF PROTECTING PERSONAL INFORMATION

The public is entitled to fair, respectful treatment of personal information that is used in health statistical activities. Both the ethical principle of respect for persons and the practical necessity of securing cooperation of the public require that health statistics practitioners collect, hold, and disclose individually identifiable personal information, with attention to the privacy interests of the subjects.

The information about individuals that health statistical activities use is often sensitive. It may include information about diseases commonly recognized as creating social stigma (like sexually transmitted diseases), as well as information less widely recognized that, because of the particular circumstances of an individual, could be harmful if disclosed.

Collection of information could be an intrusion on the individual, and its use or disclosure beyond the purposes for which it was collected risks harm to the individuals concerned. Improper disclosure breaks faith with the individuals and is disrespectful of their dignity. And, as a simple pragmatic matter, if people are concerned that information about them will be improperly used or disclosed, they will be reluctant to provide information for these activities, institutions will be reluctant to provide information they hold, and there will be less public support for statistical activities.

This chapter discusses privacy principles that are valuable in making judgments about the use and disclosure of personal information, the legal requirements governing health statistical information, and some policy and practical problems encountered in managing this information.

SCOPE AND COVERAGE

The privacy protections for information in health statistical activities depend on the nature and purpose of the statistical activity. This volume addresses the wide range of activities that might be encompassed within the term *health statistics*:

- Collection of information by government statistical agencies like the National Center for Health Statistics.
- Individual research projects, including hypothesis-based research.
- Ongoing surveillance systems for health services research purposes, such as the Healthcare Cost and Utilization Project of the Agency for Healthcare Research and Quality.
- State and local public health activities such as surveillance for communicable diseases, which may include interventional components.
- Long-term surveillance for conditions and chronic diseases, such as birth defects registries.
- Activities with a civil administrative purpose as well as a statistical purpose, such as vital events registration.
- Activities with both health-care delivery and statistical components, such as immunization registries.

The basic principles for protecting information are applicable in all these settings, but the specifics of allowable uses and disclosures of information differ.

Institutions

This chapter does not address directly the protection of information about institutions or about individuals in their business or professional roles. It is often necessary to protect this information for some of the same reasons that are relevant to information about individuals, particularly as an encouragement to disclose information. Facts about institutions, such as hospitals, are gathered in the course of health statistical activities, and aggregate information about individuals will often communicate something about an institution. While this chapter does not address these issues specifically, a few points are important to note:

- Information about individuals collected from institutions may produce aggregate results revealing something about the institutions; this possibility may influence institutions' choices about providing this information.
- Individual health-care practitioners in their professional capacity are, by virtue of their professional status, licensure, and responsibility to the

public, not entitled to the same protections against use and disclosure of information about them as are individuals such as patients. But they do have the right to fair and respectful treatment in essentially the same way, and the principles applicable to protecting private individuals that we discuss here are relevant to protecting individuals in their professional roles.

- Legal protections for health statistical information about individuals sometimes apply equally to information about institutions.

Group Interests

Nor does this chapter deal directly with the rights of groups with respect to their information. However, information about groups—in particular culturally or ethnically related people—can have relevance for individual privacy, and some scholars argue that groups as such have rights with respect to information about them. One effect of producing data showing that a named group shares a particular characteristic to a higher degree than the population generally is the possibility that all members of the group will be perceived as having that characteristic. The stated purpose of the inquiry may not be to identify the characteristics of a particular group, but the result may be such an identification. This can have implications for others' views of the group and for treatment by others of individuals in the group. These considerations have produced suggestions to take account of group interests when designing data collection and to consult representatives of the group (Alpert 2000).

There is now little formal obligation to do this, and doing it could present serious practical difficulties: for example, how to identify a group, how to identify representatives who might be consulted, and how to take account of conflicting views within a group. In data collection for general-purpose health statistics, for example, a particular result about a group might be seen by some in the group as demeaning and disadvantaging them, and by others as benefiting them by identifying a health or social problem and leading to its correction. The regulation for protection of research subjects (discussed below in section on "Protection of Research Subjects Regulation") does not address this topic, although it does explicitly exclude from consideration by an institutional review board the "possible long-range effects of applying knowledge gained in the research (for example, the possible effects of the research on public policy)" (45 CFR sec. 46.111(a)(2)).

TERMINOLOGY AND DEFINITIONS

Effective discussion of the protection of personal information requires a vocabulary. Initially, it should be noted that this discussion is about informational privacy; it is not about other dimensions of privacy, such as the right to be free from government intrusion into one's home or the right to make decisions about personal matters.

Definitions in this area are somewhat subjective, but for operational purposes some terms are quite clear, and in many instances a precise term and its meaning are not important in making sound decisions about use and disclosure of personal information. It is more important to protect privacy than to be able to define it.

A definition commonly used comes from the work of Alan Westin (1967), who conceives of privacy as "an instrument for achieving individual goals of self realization," and defines it as "the claim of individuals, groups, or institutions to determine for themselves when, how, and to what extent information about them is communicated to others." Privacy conceived of in this way serves important human interests: it has been described as "an interest of the human personality that protects the inviolate personality, the individual's independence, dignity, and integrity" (Bloustein 1964).

For ease of discussion, we define the term *privacy* here as the claim of individuals, and the societal value representing that claim, to control the use and disclosure of information about them.

The "societal value" part of this definition presents privacy not only as a purely individual claim, somehow in opposition to, and to be balanced against, broader societal interests. It characterizes it as a value in which society generally has an interest, in the sense that an invasion of an individual's privacy is not simply a harm to the individual but also a diminution of a broader good. It is that broader good that must be compared to other broad goods, like public health and national security. The distinction has been formulated this way: "Instead of a conflict between an individual interest and a societal interest, the policy problem in fact involves a conflict between two societal interests—privacy and effective law enforcement, for example" (Regan 1995).

Formulas of the issue in terms of balance also emphasize that the simple invocation of a wider public interest does not itself answer the question of whether a particular disclosure is warranted (Gostin and Hodge 2002).

The term *confidentiality* refers to the status of information—a status intended to protect privacy. We define it here as a status accorded to information that means that it must be protected, and used or released only in a controlled manner. It does not imply absolute secrecy; information is gathered for a purpose, and the people who need it for that purpose have access to it within a confidentiality regimen.

The terms *privacy* and *confidentiality* are often used interchangeably or to mean the same thing; in most instances, the term chosen does not affect any actual decisions about the use of information. In some analyses, the term *privacy* is seen as encompassing as well "an individual's freedom from excessive intrusion in the quest for information" (Panel on Confidentiality and Data Access 1993).

There is more agreement on the term *security*. It refers to measures used to protect information and can be defined as the administrative, technical, and physical safeguards in an information system that protect it and its information against unauthorized disclosure (as well as ensure its availability and maintain its integrity) and limit access to authorized users in accordance with an established policy. Thus, it includes a wide range of features such as controls within computer systems to prevent hackers from breaking in remotely, training and management direction prohibiting leaving computers and paper records exposed to unauthorized persons, locks on doors and file cabinets, password controls to regulate access, and systems to record who has had access to a particular individual's record, permitting auditing of that access (National Research Council 1997).

To put them all in a sentence: "If the **security** safeguards in an automated system fail or are penetrated, a breach of **confidentiality** can occur and the **privacy** of data subjects invaded" (Ware 1993).

The term *data protection* is used in Europe, referring broadly to the legal, policy, and other arrangements to protect personal information. The European Union has a data protection directive, not a privacy directive (Directive 95/46/EC of the European Parliament and of the Council of 24 October 1995 on the protection of individuals with regard to the processing of personal data and on the free movement of such data [Eur. O.J. 95/L281]).

The term *fair information practice* refers to principles and practices found in codes governing the use of personal information, discussed below.

The varying definitions and understandings of these terms mean that, in practice, a simple statement that information will be held confidential is rarely useful or informative, or even honest.

Ownership, in the traditional property sense, is not generally used as an organizing concept for defining and protecting individual rights in information, but it may be an important issue in the use, sale, or other transfer of databases. Whatever the ownership of information en masse, the power to use or disclose it in identifiable form is constrained by subject privacy rights reflected in ethical principles and legal controls.

BASIC PRINCIPLES

Government agencies, international organizations, study commissions, and advocacy groups have developed principles for the protection of personal information. In practice, these principles are reflected in individual ethical and professional responsibilities, the codes of ethics of professions and professional organizations, the practices and policies of government agencies and private organizations, and legal controls.

In the United States, the efforts of the federal government to ensure protection of research subjects produced ethical principles as a basis for policymaking for such protection. *The Belmont Report* of the National Commission for the Protection of Human Subjects of Biomedical and Behavioral Research, a major foundational document springing from those government efforts, identified respect for persons, beneficence, and justice as such ethical principles (National

Commission for the Protection of Human Subjects of Biomedical and Behavioral Research 1978). When applied to protection of personal information, respect for persons means that individuals should be treated as autonomous agents, and thus be given the opportunity to choose what shall or shall not be done with personal information about them.

At about the same time as this professional and governmental attention to protecting research subjects, policymakers began to address informational privacy as they perceived the effects of new information and communications technologies on personal privacy. This attention produced a certain degree of consensus on principles to ensure the respectful treatment of personal information, called *fair information practice principles.* These principles are mainly formulated as procedural rights rather than as more basic human rights. They do not typically provide the basis for determining a priori which data should or may be recorded or used, or why, or when (U.S. Department of Health, Education and Welfare 1973). But their philosophical foundations are similar to those underlying the protection of research subjects. These principles were developed to apply to personal information of all kinds. The tradition of confidentiality in research and statistics, where respectful treatment of information was a longstanding ethical and often legal obligation, was an instructive model. The new principles also found ready applicability in these fields.

Principles of fair information practice, and the term *fair information practice,* were originally formulated in 1973 in a report of the Secretary's Advisory Committee on Automated Personal Data Systems, an advisory committee to the U.S. Department of Health, Education, and Welfare (Regan 1995; U.S. Department of Health, Education, and Welfare 1973; Westin 2003).

Another significant formulation of principles was the work of the Organisation for Economic Co-operation and Development (OECD), motivated by concern about the effect on human rights of increasing use and transfer of personal data, and by concern that individual countries' laws would interfere with desirable data flow. In 1980 the OECD developed a document with principles to guide nations in their development of data protection law to protect privacy in the context of transborder data flows (Organisation for Economic Co-operation and Development 1980). This document set forth eight basic principles that the member states agreed should guide choices about collection, use, and disclosure of personal information. They have become the basis for much of the thinking about privacy. Statutes in Canada (The Personal Information Protection and Electronic Documents Act [S.C. 2000]), Australia (Privacy Act 1988 [Act No. 119 of 1988 as amended]), and New Zealand (Privacy Act 1993) formulate obligations of record holders in terms of similar principles.

In summary, the principles are:

- Collection limitation: There should be limits to the collection of personal data; data should be obtained by lawful and fair means and, where appropriate, with the knowledge or consent of the data subject.

- Data quality: Personal data should be relevant to the purposes for which they are to be used and, to the extent necessary for those purposes, should be accurate, complete, and kept up-to-date.
- Purpose specification: The purposes for which personal data are collected should be specified not later than at the time of data collection and the subsequent use limited to the fulfillment of those purposes or such others as are not incompatible with those purposes and as are specified on each occasion of change of purpose.
- Use limitation: Personal data should not be disclosed, made available, or otherwise used for purposes other than those specified at the time of data collection except with the consent of the data subject or by the authority of law.
- Security safeguards: Personal data should be protected by reasonable security safeguards against such risks as loss or unauthorized access, destruction, use, modification, or disclosure of data.
- Openness: There should be a general policy of openness about developments, practices, and policies with respect to personal data. Means should be readily available of establishing the existence and nature of personal data and the main purposes of their use, as well as the identity and usual residence of the data controller.
- Individual participation: An individual should have the right to see any data about himself or herself and to correct or remove any data that are not timely, accurate, relevant, or complete.
- Accountability: Those holding data should be accountable for complying with measures that give effect to the principles stated above.

STATISTICAL PURPOSES AND ADMINISTRATIVE PURPOSES

For privacy analysis, there are two general types of use of personal information: administrative, and research or statistical.

- An *administrative* use is one that involves a decision affecting the rights, benefits, or privileges of a specific individual. In such a use, the individual's identity is essential to the outcome. A clinical medical record is developed for such a use.
- A *research or statistical* use does not involve a decision affecting an individual. Here the identity is irrelevant to the outcome (even if identity is necessary within a research or statistical activity, e.g., to link records held in several places under an individual's name). The result is a statistic, and it makes no difference who the subjects were individually. A cancer registry is established for such a use.

There are data systems that serve both functions, as, for example, the vital registration system, and systems for surveillance and case identification and intervention, with intervention being a clear administrative use.

But the distinction is a useful one for privacy analyses of collection, use, and disclosure of personal information in the research and statistical context. The Privacy Protection Study Commission, created by Congress in the Privacy Act of 1974, used the distinction in its analysis of the privacy issues in research and statistical record keeping in its 1977 report. It proposed as a standard the principle of *functional separation*, which has served since as a starting point for much policymaking in this area. It can be formulated this way: "Information collected or maintained for a research or statistical purpose may not be used in individually identifiable form to make any decision or take any action directly affecting the individual to whom the record pertains, except within the context of the research plan or protocol" (Privacy Protection Study Commission 1977).

Based on this principle, the Commission recommended establishment by law of essentially absolute protection for individual research and statistical information from use and disclosure for any other purpose. The exceptions are disclosures to prevent grave danger to life (supporting what would normally be the ethical choice in such a situation) and research-related uses such as auditing of the research. The principle received support in a study sponsored by the Committee on National Statistics, and conducted by the Panel on Confidentiality and Data Access, which recommended consistent legislation to protect statistical records across all federal agencies (Panel on Confidentiality and Data Access 1993).

The professional communities that use personal information in research and statistical activities have codes of practice and ethics that reflect this principle as well. Among them are the American Statistical Association (1999), the International Statistical Institute (1985), and the American College of Epidemiology (2000).

Mixed Activities

As indicated above, there are data systems that serve both administrative and research or statistical functions. Health statistics may appear in administrative activities, in research and statistical activities, or in mixed activities. The functional separation principle is applicable to research and statistical activities and to the research and statistical portion of mixed activities.

One significant such activity, where the principle is applicable to only one of its purposes, is the vital registration system, which at once has administrative purposes (civil registration for establishing identity, legal rights, etc.), health intervention purposes (as in newborn screening), and broader statistical purposes (for research and ongoing monitoring of the health of the population).

The state laws that establish the vital registration system sort among these purposes, and often allow different uses and disclosures based on the purpose of particular items of information in the record. Most states restrict the use of some information in their birth and death registration systems to statistical and public health purposes.

The model certificate of live birth promulgated by the National Center for Health Statistics and recommended for adoption by the states identifies certain items of information as "information for medical and health purposes only" (National Center for Health Statistics [hp] 2003 Revisions).

State and local health departments also collect other information, such as that relating to immunization and the prevalence and incidence of communicable diseases, that serves principally to provide information about the health of the populace generally—a classic statistical activity. But its public health purpose includes the possibility of intervention: use of information about a specific individual for finding that individual and, for example, recommending treatment and taking other actions to interrupt the transmission of disease.

A precise taxonomy of systems by purpose is not necessary here. What is most important is that, in establishing a data system, there should be great clarity as to the purposes of the system, transparency to those immediately concerned and to the public about the purposes, and clear policies (including, as appropriate, laws), based on the stated purposes, governing the use and disclosure of personal information in the system.

THE PLACE OF INDIVIDUAL AWARENESS AND CONSENT

The obligation to get the individual's consent to the collection, use, and disclosure of personal information appears significantly in research ethics and privacy policy thinking. Commonly accepted principles of fair information practice, such as those in the OECD guidelines mentioned above, envision that individuals will play a distinct and active role in decisions about their personal information.

Those principles, as well as formulations like the regulation for protection of research subjects (discussed below), suggest that, ideally, the individual should know about his or her inclusion in a health data system, and should have a choice about being included and about disclosures of identifiable information from the system.

But in practice, the details of individual involvement are complex, and range from distinct informed consent to a specified research or statistical use of information, through presumption of implied consent, to statutory authority for research or statistical use of information with no individual involvement (Lowrance 2002).

In practice, and under many laws governing use of information, the individual does not get the degree of control envisioned in the ideal. Even the OECD principle that information will be collected with the knowledge or consent of the data subject is qualified by a "where appropriate" condition. In many instances, a public health statistical system could not operate if it needed approval, either for initial inclusion or for subsequent disclosures, of all individuals identified within it.

Further, true informed consent for use and disclosure of a record would require that the individual know what is in the record, and know to whom and for what purpose it is being disclosed, before signing a paper permitting its disclosure. Even in situations where there is individual involvement, the individual will often not know the content of the record.

Many confidentiality enactments permit disclosure for public health and research and statistical activities without authorization or other direct involvement by the individual. Some, like the Federal Privacy Act and the Health Insurance Portability and Accountability Act (HIPAA) Privacy Rule, discussed below, require entities subject to them to involve the public by publishing notices of their information practices, including possible disclosures. But they do not generally require that individuals be offered an opportunity to object to disclosures.

The use of existing administrative records for research and statistical purposes without direct contact with the individual is discussed in more detail below in the section on "Availability of Information for Public Health and Research."

Those developing or using data systems must make choices about the need for and the form of individual consent. Involving the individual directly remains the approach most respectful of individual autonomy, despite the many instances in which there is ethical or legal support for using records without individual involvement.

THE ROLE OF LAW

Understanding the Role of Law

Societal choices about how to use personal information are, in the case of health statistics, often expressed in legal enactments. A legislative body (like Congress or a state legislature) or an executive agency with legal authority to do so (like the U.S. Department of Health and Human Services or a state health department) determines how personal information may be used or disclosed and formulates it in a statute or regulation binding, often with penalties for disobedience, on those who hold the information. In many instances, legal confidentiality obligations coincide with the ethical obligations of practitioners and the needs of the programs collecting data.

This section identifies and discusses some of those enactments. They are important both for operational reasons (i.e., officials, researchers, and statisticians must heed them) and, from a broader perspective, in order to understand

and appreciate the privacy-based societal choices about how this information may be used.

It is essential that all who work with individually identifiable health information in a statistical activity be knowledgeable about the laws applicable to the information. In particular, frank, detailed communication between an agency's or organization's legal counsel and its health and statistical professionals is important. The operator of a health statistics system must understand the laws (and the principles and policies behind them) that govern the information. Legal counsel must understand the public health and scientific goals to be served by the activity. It is also important that the health statistical community play a role in policymaking to ensure that the policy process is informed by accurate scientific information about how it conducts its business.

Protective Laws for Federal Statistical Programs

The federal statistical agencies have strong legal protection for their information, generally restricting its use to the statistical purposes for which it was collected. While many federal agencies compile some health statistics—often program-specific and derived from operational program data—this section will focus on federal entities whose principal mission is statistical.

The National Center for Health Statistics (NCHS), in the Centers for Disease Control and Prevention in the Department of Health and Human Services, is one of the U.S. government's major statistical agencies, and is responsible for the collection, analysis, and dissemination of statistics on the nature and extent of the health, illness, and disability of the U.S. population; the impact of illness and disability on the economy; the effects of environmental, social, and other health hazards; the use of health-care services; health resources; family formation, growth, and dissolution; and vital events (i.e., births and deaths).

Identifiable information (about both individuals and entities, like businesses) collected or obtained by the NCHS and its agents is protected by a confidentiality provision in the statute that authorizes the NCHS's activities. Under this provision the purposes of any data collection, as specified to the source of the information, define the allowable uses of the data. It commands NCHS to maintain and use the information solely for the purposes for which it was collected and prohibits unauthorized disclosures. Thus, it protects against compulsory legal processes, such as court orders or subpoenas, that would seek information for purposes other than those specified (Public Health Service Act sec. 308(d), 42 U.S.C. 242m(d)). The basic elements of this protection date from 1970. It resembles and was derived from the Bureau of the Census's confidentiality statute that applied to the predecessor federal organization that collected health statistical data as part of the U.S. Department of Commerce. The firm assurance of confidentiality that can be offered under this protection has been the basis for effective data collection in the many activities of the NCHS, including the National Health and Nutrition Examination Survey, the National Health Interview Survey, and the National Survey of Family Growth.

Other health statistical activities of the U.S. Department of Health and Human Services that enjoy similar protection are those of the Agency for Healthcare Research and Quality (AHRQ) and certain public health surveillance activities of the Substance Abuse and Mental Health Services Administration (SAMHSA) (Public Health Service Act secs. 924(c) and (d), 42 U.S.C. 299c-3(c) and (d), and Public Health Service Act sec. 501(n), 42 U.S.C. 290aa(n)).

In many instances, the prohibitions on disclosure of these statutes apply as well to nonfederal entities that receive grant or contract funds under the legal authorities under which the federal agencies operate.

For research activities, the Secretary of Health and Human Services has statutory authority to grant a protection (typically in the form of a certificate of confidentiality for a particular research project) so that the researcher cannot be compelled by legal process (e.g., a subpoena or a court order) to disclose the identity of research subjects (Public Health Service Act sec. 301(d), 42 U.S.C. 241(d)).

Other Federal Laws

A few words are in order about other laws that address information disclosure and use at the federal level. The Privacy Act of 1974 applies to record systems operated by federal agencies and their contractors in which information is retrieved by personal identifier. It controls the use and disclosure of that information, establishes requirements for transparency in collecting and maintaining it, and permits individuals to see their own records. It states a general rule that information may not be disclosed unless the individual consents, but it identifies many disclosures that agencies can make without consent, and also gives agencies administrative power to make other disclosures, called *routine uses*, as long as they are compatible with the purpose for which the information was collected, by announcing them in the *Federal Register* (5 U.S.C. 552a).

Federal statistical agencies are subject to the Privacy Act but are also constrained by their own confidentiality statutes, as described above, which are more restrictive, and thus are not free to make all of the disclosures that the Privacy Act permits. An agency may exempt itself from the Privacy Act's requirement that individuals have access to their own records with respect to records that are "required by statute to be maintained and used solely as statistical records" (5 U.S.C. 552a(d) and (k)(4)).

Under the Confidential Information Protection and Statistical Efficiency Act of 2002 (CIPSEA) (Pub. L. No. 107–347, tit. V, 44 U.S.C. 3501 note), if a federal agency collects identifiable information (about individuals or entities, like businesses) and promises to use it purely for statistical purposes, it may not use or disclose it for any nonstatistical purpose. There are criminal penalties for violation. The act provides federal agencies that do not have confidentiality statutes of their own a protection for their information.

The Freedom of Information Act is an open government statute that makes government records available to any inquirer, but it has several exceptions to its general rule of full disclosure. The exceptions for disclosures that would invade privacy and for disclosures forbidden by other statutes effectively shield individually identifiable statistical information from release (5 U.S.C. 552(b)(3) and (6)).

Protection of Research Subjects Regulation

Some statistical activities are subject to the regulation promulgated by federal agencies for protection of research subjects. This regulation imposes requirements on the agencies and their grantees and contractors to ensure that the subjects of their research are treated with respect and dignity. For the U.S. Department of Health and Human Services it is codified at 45 CFR part 46.

The regulation requires review of research projects by an institutional review board (IRB) and specifies some factors that the board must consider. It does not have substantive rules for keeping personal information confidential, but it requires that IRBs, in their review of projects, consider the provisions for protecting the subjects' privacy, and it requires that research subjects be told the extent to which confidentiality will be maintained (secs. 46.111(a)(7) and 46.116(a)(5)).

The regulation applies to *research*, which it defines as "a systematic investigation, including research development, testing and evaluation, designed to develop or contribute to generalizable knowledge" (sec. 46.102(d)). Some health statistical activities fall under this definition. Other activities, such as surveillance, are more properly public health practice activities, not research, and do not fall under the regulation. The distinction in any particular case is not always fully clear, and there are competing views of how an activity might be categorized and the extent to which traditional public health activities need, as an ethical matter, the review required for research (Elster et al. 2002; Mariner 1997; Snider and Stroup 1997).

Guidelines developed by the Centers for Disease Control and Prevention (1999) distinguish research (with its goal of "generalizable knowledge," as defined in the regulation) from public health practice activities, where the primary intention of the endeavor is to benefit clients participating in a public health program or to benefit a population by controlling a health problem in the population from which the information is gathered.

A possible new approach to this issue may be to apply to public health activities ethical requirements that parallel those for research but that are tailored to the special situation of public health practice (Burris et al. 2003). Such an approach can move beyond vocabulary discussions to direct ethical analysis (Fairchild 2003; Fairchild and Bayer 2004).

The regulation for protection of human subjects, while applicable to all research, was conceptualized around biomedical and clinical research, and was not formulated with detailed attention to the special issues in collecting, analyzing, and using personally identifiable information—activities of which health statistical activities are a significant example. Statistical agencies often struggle with IRBs on how to use this framework to provide the appropriate ethical review for nonclinical research. Recent policy consideration of this issue offers the hope of more fine-grained approaches. A panel convened by the National Research Council has made recommendations in this area. They include a call for more attention to the conditions under which the general rule of informed consent might be waived in such research, guidance on what activities fit under the protection of research subjects regulation's definition of research, and more explicit attention to protecting confidentiality (Panel on Institutional Review Boards, Surveys, and Social Science Research 2003).

Whatever the technical applicability of the protection of human subjects regulation, the mechanisms of that protective system may be helpful in evaluating data use and collection in nonresearch activities. The IRB, for example, can ensure full consideration of a proposed collection, use, or disclosure of information from a variety of perspectives, including those of the professional community that conducts the inquiries and those of the community from which the information will be collected. The National Center for Health Statistics regards its activities as subject to the regulation and, for example, advises the public specifically that the protocol for the National Health and Nutrition Examination Survey of the National Center for Health Statistics has been reviewed by an IRB.

The HIPAA Privacy Rule

The Secretary of Health and Human Services has promulgated a health information privacy regulation in accord with the requirements of the Health Insurance Portability and Accountability Act of 1996 (HIPAA)(Pub. L. No. 104–191, amending Social Security Act to create new Title XI, part C, 42 U.S.C. 1320d to 1320d-8)(Regulation at 45 CFR parts 160 and 164 (2003)).

It sets out a comprehensive scheme of protection, controlling uses and disclosures of personal health information, providing patients with access to their records, and imposing requirements on record holders for careful treatment of the information, including security requirements. It applies to health-care providers who use electronic administrative transactions established under other provisions of the HIPAA law; to health plans (insurers, health maintenance organizations, and certain named government health programs); and to clearinghouses (which perform certain functions in electronic transactions). The widespread use of electronic administrative transactions means that the vast majority of health-care providers will be subject to it.

It does not apply to health statistical activities as such, but can be significant because some health department activities involving health care may be covered by it, and because it regulates disclosure of information by health-care providers for public health and research purposes. Its provisions governing these disclosures are discussed below in the section on "Availability of Information for Public Health and Research."

State Law

The federal legal enactments discussed above often have counterparts in state law. A review of them in substantive detail is not warranted here in light of their number and scope, but some examples illustrate the context. The wide variety of state laws and practices means that there are considerable variations in the protection of health statistical information and in the requirements for access to data for research and statistical purposes.

All states have laws governing health information, but their coverage, scope, and protective power vary greatly. There are several states with comprehensive statutes for the confidentiality of health information held by health-care providers. Virtually all states have statutes protecting specialized classes of information considered sensitive, such as information about human immunodeficiency virus (HIV) infection and mental health treatment (Gellman 1984; Institute for Health Care Research and Policy 2002).

Some states have privacy statutes governing information held by state and local government agencies analogous to the Federal Privacy Act. All have freedom of information acts, but not all provide explicit exceptions for privacy, as does the federal law (Schwartz et al. 1996).

All states have statutes explicitly protecting some classes of individually identifiable information obtained by government agencies and virtually all states protect information obtained in public health activities. Not all states restrict use of the information in individual form solely to public health purposes; some, for example, permit disclosure pursuant to subpoena or court order (Gostin et al. 1996, 1999a).

The Model State Public Health Privacy Project at Georgetown University has produced a model law for adoption by states to address "privacy and security issues arising from the acquisition, use, disclosure, and storage of identifiable health information by public health agencies at the state and local levels." It specifies what the drafters believe are appropriate protections, and allowable disclosures, of personal information in the public health system (Gostin et al. 1999b).

In many instances, laws establishing particular collections of identifiable data by state agencies include confidentiality provisions. Reports to the California cancer registry, for example, are declared confidential except for enumerated purposes, all of which are for the purposes of research and related activities. The statute is detailed in permitting disclosure for research only after review by an

IRB constituted in accord with the federal regulation for protection of research subjects, and receipt of assurances by recipients as to their ability to maintain the information confidentially and to limit disclosure to "the information necessary for the stated purpose of the requested disclosure" (California Health and Safety Code sec. 103885 [West 1996 and Supp. 2002]). The state's freedom of information act explicitly mentions cancer registry information as not disclosable under it (California Government Code secs. 6276 and 6276.10)[West Supp. 2002]; von Tigerstrom et al. 2002).

There are some research and statistical confidentiality statutes analogous to the federal ones mentioned above. Minnesota, for example, protects information obtained by the Commissioner of Health, or by others "for the purpose of reducing the morbidity or mortality from any cause or condition of health," by commanding that it "be used solely for the purposes of medical or scientific research" (Minn. Stat. Ann. sec. 144.053 [1998]).

New Hampshire similarly protects personal medical data obtained for medical or scientific research by the commissioner of health, or by any person, organization, or agency authorized by the commissioner to obtain such data, by limiting its use "solely for medical or scientific purposes" (N.H. Rev. Stat. Ann. sec. 126–A:11 [1996]).

The laws establishing the vital events registration system in each state address what information from these records is disclosable and to whom. The National Center for Health Statistics recommends, in conjunction with the National Association for Public Health Statistics and Information Systems (representing the state officials who operate the system), a model act for adoption by states. States are not obliged to adopt it; many have adopted it, but with varying degrees of congruence (National Center for Health Statistics 1995). Related are model certificates of birth, death, and fetal death (National Center for Health Statistics [hp] 2003 Revisions).

PRACTICAL AND POLICY ISSUES

Organizational Structures to Protect Privacy

The infrastructure for protection of personal information, including health statistical information, includes government regulatory and consumer protection agencies, but there is little in the way of a general-purpose privacy regulatory apparatus in the United States. Government enforcement agencies are typically devoted to enforcing privacy laws governing particular sectors (such as the Office for Civil Rights of the U.S. Department of Health and Human Services, which administers the HIPAA Privacy Rule). Two states (Hawaii and California) have privacy offices, with mainly educational and advocacy functions. General-purpose privacy regulatory laws are better developed outside the United States than within it (Bennett and Raab 2003).

The Canadian federal government has a Privacy Commissioner, and each province has an official with privacy oversight responsibilities. Canada and its provinces have privacy laws applicable to personal information held both by government agencies and by private entities. The legal structure permits the provinces to have their own laws, including sector-specific ones, and some provinces have laws specific to health information.

At least as significant as their regulatory activity is those offices' analytic capacity to do research on privacy issues, develop best practice guidelines, comment on proposals, and otherwise contribute to policies for protecting information. The Ontario Information and Privacy Commissioner has, for example, produced a document setting out best practices in survey research (Information and Privacy Commissioner [Ontario] 1999).

Likewise, all European Union (EU) countries have general data protection laws and regulatory bodies to enforce them, in accord with requirements of the EU data protection directive. Australia and New Zealand have laws of general applicability and agencies to enforce them.

Health and other statistical activities fall within the purview of these general regulators, and they have had occasion to comment on such activities. In some instances, these agencies or other government or private entities have developed privacy codes, based on their statutes, specific to the health sector.

Privacy Review Mechanisms

Those designing data systems have to give the fair information practice principles and legal controls discussed above careful consideration at every stage of development, and apply them as they design a new system or consider possible uses and disclosures for existing ones. One technique for ensuring such consideration is the privacy impact assessment (PIA). It is described as "a systematic process that evaluates a proposal in terms of its impact upon privacy" (Privacy Commissioner of New Zealand 2002).

In the United States, the E-Government Act of 2002 requires a privacy impact assessment when the federal government develops information technology for processing personal information or initiates a new collection of personal information that will be maintained using information technology (Pub. L. No. 107-347, sec. 208). The Canadian government requires such assessments for Canadian federal government data systems (Treasury Board of Canada Secretariat [mg] Privacy Impact Assessment Policy). The Canadian Institute for Health Information (CIHI), a private entity that assembles health information for research and statistical purposes, identifies the privacy impact assessment as a key element of its privacy program and has developed a template for the necessary analysis (Canadian Institute for Health Information 2002).

Whether formally required or not, such an analysis can weigh, in a focused, systematic way, the effects on individual privacy of a new data system or a change in a system such as a new category of disclosure, and can force conscious policy decisions about the privacy questions it raises. The designers of any system must address the purposes of the collection, the information to be collected and the population about whom it is collected, policies for its use and disclosure, the applicable legal controls, and the administrative, technical, and physical measures used to safeguard it. Thoughtful system designers have always taken these into account; the formal mechanism assists the process, ensures attention and deliberate choices by policy officials, and makes the choices apparent to others.

The analysis can address such issues as:

- whether the intended purpose can be accomplished without personally identifiable information
- if personally identifiable information is needed, what is the minimum necessary to accomplish the purpose
- what the information is to be used for, who can get the information, for what purposes, pursuant to what showing, and upon whose authority
- what legal controls apply to the system, and the implications of those controls both for the initial assemblage of information and for its use and disclosure (accompanied by a recognition that legal obligations alone do not define the policies for collecting, using, and disclosing personal information)
- what the general public and sources of the information (either individuals or entities providing data about individuals) will be told about the uses and disclosures
- whether the method of collecting the information is appropriate

Availability of Information for Public Health and Research

Privacy controls on use and disclosure of personal information affect the availability of information in administrative files (like clinical records) for public health and research purposes. In general, policy thinking and legal enactments have supported the use and disclosure of personally identifiable information for public health and research purposes, with identifiers and without explicit individual consent, under certain conditions.

It is essential that health statistics practitioners understand the controls on such information, and the steps needed to obtain it in accord with the law that covers the information and in accord with ethical considerations and respect for the individuals. The policy justification and legal basis differ somewhat, depending on whether the purpose is public health or research.

Public Health

The theoretical justification for the collection of personal information for public health purposes is found in the police power of the state to protect its citizens (Gostin et al. 2002).

On this basis, there have been long-standing requirements for reporting certain diseases, and related power to compel disclosure of additional information as needed by public health authorities. The traditional thinking in this regard has been in the context of communicable disease and protective interventions. But the underlying public good principle is also a basis for collection of individually identifiable information in longer-range, nonemergency inquiries, such as cancer registries and occupational health inquiries, both on a voluntary basis and as required by statute. The Occupational Safety and Health Act of 1970, for example, provides authority to require employers to maintain and disclose information for occupational health inquiries (Occupational Safety and Health Act of 1970 secs. 8 and 20, 29 U.S.C. 657 and 669).

The most recent significant health information privacy enactment, the HIPAA Privacy Rule, reflects this policy. It explicitly permits the use and disclosure of patient information for public health purposes under specified conditions. This provision is broad in that it permits disclosure to a "public health authority that is authorized by law to collect or receive such information for the purpose of preventing or controlling disease, injury, or disability, including, but not limited to, the reporting of disease, injury, vital events such as birth or death, and the conduct of public health surveillance, public health investigations, and public health interventions" (45 CFR sec. 164.512(b)).

This permission to disclose is not predicated on a specific legal obligation to report. If the activity is an authorized public health activity, the rule permits an entity holding the information to disclose it to the public health authority voluntarily or pursuant to a simple request. The regulation also permits disclosure to nongovernment entities operating at the direction of a public health agency. Information once disclosed to a public health agency is not covered by the HIPAA Privacy Rule unless the agency is otherwise covered by the Rule in its public health activities (Centers for Disease Control and Prevention 2003).

Research

The use of information for research generally does not share the same foundation in legal compulsion, but policy studies and inquiries in recent years have supported the use of individually identifiable information, without individual consent, for research under specified conditions for protecting the individuals. These conditions typically set out the determinations that the record holder must make before disclosing the information and the requirements the recipient must meet.

The studies have included those of the Department of Health, Education, and Welfare Secretary's Advisory Committee on Automated Personal Data Systems, the Privacy Protection Study Commission, and the Privacy Working Group of the President's Information Infrastructure Task Force (Information Infrastructure Task Force 1995; Privacy Protection Study Commission 1977; and U.S. Department of Health, Education, Welfare 1973).

Studies prepared within a more distinct advocacy context, such as by the Health Privacy Working Group, under the auspices of the Georgetown Health Privacy Project, have also supported these uses under careful controls, such as "an objective and balanced process to review the use and disclosure of personally identifiable information for research" (Institute for Health Care Research and Policy 1999).

Legal controls have often followed the same course, and many health information confidentiality statutes permit disclosure for research. For example, the federal substance abuse confidentiality statute, an early and significant protection, permits disclosure for scientific research, with a prohibition on further disclosure (Public Health Service Act sec. 543(b)(2)(B), 42 U.S.C. 290dd-2(b)(2)(B), regulation at 42 CFR sec. 2.52).

The protection of research subjects regulation permits waiver of its usual requirement for informed consent under certain conditions. That provision has been the basis for use of existing records for research without individual consent (45 CFR sec. 46.116(c)).

Similar approaches appear in state law. The Maryland health information privacy law, for example, permits disclosure of information from clinical records for "educational or research purposes, subject to the applicable requirements of an institutional review board" on the condition that the recipient sign an acknowledgment of the duty under this act not to redisclose any patient identifying information (Maryland Code-Health General sec. 4-305(b)(2) [2000]).

The HIPAA Privacy Rule permits use or disclosure for research if the project is approved either by an IRB constituted under the regulation for protection of research subjects or by a privacy board meeting conditions set out in the Privacy Rule. The Privacy Rule sets out conditions that the project must meet to warrant approval; they are similar to those required for waiver of informed consent under the protection of research subjects regulation, but are more specifically focused on privacy in the required findings and the assurances restricting further use and disclosure of the information (45 CFR sec. 164.512(i)).

The EU data protection directive takes a similar approach. While it regards heath data as sensitive and generally forbids processing sensitive categories of data without consent, individual nations may establish exceptions with "suitable safeguards," and scientific research is mentioned as a basis for the exception (Directive 95/46/EC of the European Parliament and of the Council of 24 Oct 1995 on the protection of individuals with regard to the processing of personal data and on the free movement of such data, art. 8.4 and recital 34 [Eur. O.J. 95/L281]). The EU press release about the directive noted that sensitive information like health information could be disclosed without consent "where there is an important public interest (e.g., for medical or scientific research) where alternative safeguards have to be established" (Delegation of the European Commission to the United States 1998).

Ethical Foundations

The philosophical or ethical foundations for research disclosure can be found in arguments for the common good, including the theme that since patients benefit from the experience of the medical care system with past patients, there is some obligation to contribute to the good of patients in the future by the use of one's experience (Etzioni 1999). In this regard, the propriety of this use of personal information may be examined by asking whether it is selfish to deny future patients the benefit of one's experience (Lowrance 1997). Gostin (1995) notes that "a complex modern society cannot elevate each person's interest in privacy above other important societal interests" and that "higher quality, better research" is one such interest.

Public Opinion

Despite the strong support in the professional and analytic communities that have produced the reports mentioned above, it is important to recognize that the public may not be as positive about the use of records for research. One commentator has analogized the use of records for research to the actions of a trespasser who enters a home, looks around, reads letters and personal papers, and leaves without stealing or harming anything (Woodward 1997).

There are some survey data showing that a substantial portion of the population would not want its records used for research or would want to be asked specifically about particular uses. In one survey, 58% of respondents thought it was "not very acceptable" or "not at all acceptable" for their records to be used for research without contacting them in response to a question that made it clear that the research would be reviewed by a board, and that no identifiable information about them would be published (Louis Harris and Associates, Inc. 1994). In a survey of patients already being treated for serious or chronic illnesses, when asked whether medical researchers should be able to get their medical records without their permission "if it will help them to do research that will advance medical knowledge in the future," 55% of them did not agree (Kass et al. 2003).

While, as indicated above, many health confidentiality laws do permit disclosure of health information for research, there has been some movement toward restrictions, including a Minnesota law that requires patient permission for use of records for research, although with some provisions that simplify the obtaining of permission and permit disclosure in some instances based on absence of affirmative objection (Melton 1997; Minn. Stat. Ann. sec.144.335, subd. 3a.(d) [West Supp. 2001]; Yawn et al. 1998).

These public concerns should be instructive with regard to the need to communicate with the public effectively. It is important that the health statistical community inform the public about statistical and research activities, and about their value and use in improving the health of the nation. Respect for the value of privacy demands that activities that may be seen as violating it—such as use of records for research and statistical activities without individual consent—be explained and justified, with enough information so that the merits of the use are apparent.

Identifiability

This chapter focuses on information described as *identified* or *identifiable*. These familiar terms conceal serious issues, since whether information about a person fits into those categories is not always easy to determine. The framework for determining that is changing. There is no privacy interest unless there is a named person to whom the information can be connected. In turn, the ethical and legal controls are formulated to apply to identified or identifiable information. The definition of these terms thus determines whether the ethical and legal controls are applicable.

There is a strong imperative to make the aggregate information in health statistics systems available for use for policymaking, design of health interventions, and other planning purposes. Aggregate information sufficiently detailed to be useful risks disclosing information about an individual. The statistical community has always recognized that identifiers much less precise than overt identifiers such as name, Social Security number, or street address have the potential to render information identified or identifiable.

This issue was brought into focus for people beyond the statistical community when Latanya Sweeney, then at the Massachusetts Institute of Technology, identified the records of Massachusetts Governor William Weld and his family from a public use data tape—presumably with anonymous data—of state employee health insurance claims by matching data from the tape against the voter list of the city of Cambridge (Lynne 2001; National Committee on Vital and Health Statistics 1998).

There is a substantial literature on statistical disclosure avoidance, originally focused on the possibility that a published statistical table would permit identification of an individual because small numbers of persons share a particular characteristic. Similar issues exist more vividly with microdata—person-specific information but without overt identifiers, as shown by the preceding example. The literature includes techniques for estimating the risk of statistical disclosure, and for disclosing information in a fashion that makes it usable without disclosing any identity (Doyle et al. 2001; Federal Committee on Statistical Methodology 1994).

But legal definitions of what information must be kept confidential are typically general. They use the simple term *identifiable* (Public Health Service Act sec. 308(d) 42 U.S.C. 242m(d)) or rely on a concept of reasonableness, such as "that permits the identity of the respondent to whom the information applies to be reasonably inferred by either direct or indirect means" (Confidential Information Protection and Statistical Efficiency Act of 2002, sec. 502(4), 44 U.S.C. 3501 note); or use an *effort* test—for example, "An individual shall not be regarded as 'identifiable' if identification requires an unreasonable amount of time and manpower" (Appendix to Recommendation No. R (97) 5 and Explanatory Memorandum of the Council of Europe on the protection of medical data). As this shows, the content of the concept of reasonableness has been left to technical determination by the statistical community.

However, the recent HIPAA Privacy Rule has moved the process forward by formulating a distinct legal standard for identifiability. It specifies that information may be considered deidentified either when determined so by qualified personnel applying scientific standards (the traditional approach), or by removal of all of a list of 18 items of identification set out in the regulation (45 CFR sec. 164.514(a)).

Policy in this area continues to evolve. The new standard in the HIPAA Privacy Rule categorizes as identifiable, and thus subject to the regulation's requirements governing use and disclosure, much information that previously was considered nonidentifiable and was handled as such. While the rule did not preclude the use of such information for research or public health purposes, it did add additional steps. Questions from the health-care community about the burden of the additional steps induced a change in the regulation by creating an intermediate category of identifiable information, the *limited data set*, which can be used and disclosed without complying with all of the regulation's requirements for, for example, research disclosure. The limited data set lacks overt identifiers but includes some items useful in analysis (particularly patient age and hospital dates of service and discharge) that would have to be removed to attain full deidentification. Limited data set information may be disclosed for research or public health purposes pursuant to an agreement by the recipient that it will be used only for such purposes and that there will be no effort to identify any individual (45 CFR sec. 164.514(e), and 67 Fed. Reg. 53,181, at 53,217 [Aug.14, 2002]).

Policymaking in this area will require continued attention not only from state and federal executive branch officials and legislatures, but also from the health statistical community and from persons familiar with information technology.

Special Disclosure Mechanisms

The full value of health statistical information is best achieved if it is available for use beyond its original purpose and if raw data can be made available for further analysis. But this goal of making data available and useful conflicts somewhat with the privacy needs of the individuals identified in those data. There are mechanisms to make data available with different degrees of identifiability, to permit further analysis, with safeguards to ensure its respectful use (Panel on Confidentiality and Data Access 1993).

Public use data, sometimes in microdata form, are available to anyone, and are prepared with care to ensure that no identifiable information is in them or able to be derived from them (Federal Committee on Statistical Methodology 2002). For analyses that require access to data that are identifiable or, if not overtly identifiable, at risk of ready identifiability, other techniques and mechanisms are available. They make data available under carefully controlled conditions, permitting the necessary analysis while reducing the possibility of inappropriate disclosure.

One approach used in federal statistical agencies is the temporary incorporation of an outside researcher into an agency, under an oath or similar commitment that binds the researcher to the same confidentiality obligations as employees of the agency (13 U.S.C. 9 and 23(c)). The Confidential Information Protection and Statistical Efficiency Act of 2002 provides for this (secs. 502(2) and 512(a), 44 U.S.C. 3501 note).

A related approach is a licensing program, in which the holding agency licenses a researcher to use the identified or identifiable information under a data use agreement or similar commitment, including, inter alia, promises not to use the identifiable information for anything but the stated project (Seastrom 2001). Another is the data center, where a researcher from outside the agency goes to a location with computer access to the data, but can access them only in the limited fashion necessary for a research project, which will have been approved by the holding agency. The computer available to the researcher is not connected to the outside of the agency, and will reach only the limited data within the agency needed by the researcher (National Center for Health Statistics [hp] Research data center).

In addition, there are methods of coding identifiable information in such a way that it is not overtly identifiable, but can be matched for research purposes with other bodies of information in a way that ensures effective matches without transmitting names (Pommerening et al. 1996). To the extent that such mechanisms can reduce the sharing of identifiable information, they serve to protect privacy.

Security

The protection of identifiable information from unauthorized disclosure is an essential element of the ethical responsibility to subjects and a requirement of fair information practice principles. It is achieved through administrative, technical, and physical safeguards to protect against deliberate or inadvertent disclosure of information to persons not permitted to receive it. Confidentiality enactments often impose an explicit obligation to establish appropriate administrative, technical, and physical safeguards to ensure the security of personal information; the specifics are left up to the organization.

While security is often seen as a technical matter, with little resonance in policy circles, it is essential. Much public concern over privacy is related to the possibilities of inappropriate disclosure, and many of the horror stories and cautionary examples spring from essentially inadvertent security breaches, not from considered judgments to disclose information.

CONCLUSION

Public health practitioners need an ethical and conceptual framework for making decisions about the use and disclosure of identifiable information about individuals. Tradition and ethical commitment, often supported by legal protections, have provided that framework and resulted in careful stewardship of personal health information (Bayer 1992).

Current developments in information and communications technology present new problems for that stewardship. They call for continuing attention to ensure that policy, legal, and technical measures to protect sensitive information keep pace with those developments.

The fair information practice principles discussed above provide a framework for that attention. They are sufficiently general to permit application to a variety of activities, including health statistical activities, and reflect a wide, indeed international, consensus about how individual rights in this area should be protected. Legal controls are important to the management of the data in health statistical systems. The broader framework of the fair information practice principles can help health statistics practitioners apply the law, address new issues, and provide the public with the respectful treatment of the data that it deserves.

REFERENCES

Alpert S. Privacy and the Analysis of Stored Tissues. Research Involving Human Biological Materials: Ethical Issues and Policy Guidance. Commissioned Papers. Rockville, MD: National Bioethics Advisory Commission; 2000.

American College of Epidemiology. Ethics Guidelines. Raleigh, NC: American College of Epidemiology; 2000 [cited 2004 Mar 7]. Available from: http://www.acepidemiology.org/policystmts/EthicsGuide.htm.

American Statistical Association. Ethical Guidelines for Statistical Practice [guidelines on the Internet]. Alexandria, VA: American Statistical Association; 1999 [cited 2004 Mar 7]. Available from: http://www.amstat.org/profession/ethicalstatistics.html.

Bayer R, Toomey KE. HIV prevention and the two faces of partner notification. Am J Public Health 1992;82:1158–1164.

Bennett CJ, Raab CD. The Governance of Privacy: Policy Instruments in Global Perspective. Aldershot, UK: Ashgate; 2003.

Bloustein EJ. Privacy as an aspect of human dignity: an answer to Dean Prosser. NYU Law Rev 1964;39:962–1007.

Burris S, Buehler J, Lazzarini Z. Applying the common rule to public health agencies: questions and tentative answers about a separate regulatory regime. J Law Med Ethics 2003;31: 638–653.

Canadian Institute for Health information. Privacy and Confidentiality of Health Information at CIHI: Principles and Policies for the Protection of Personal Health Information, 3rd ed. Ottawa: Canadian Institute for Health information; 2002 [cited 2004 Mar 15]. Available from: http://secure.cihi.ca/cihiweb/en/downloads/privacy_policy_priv2002_e.pdf.

Centers for Disease Control and Prevention [guidelines on the Internet]. Guidelines for Defining Public Health Research and Public Health Non-Research. Atlanta: Centers for Disease Control and Prevention; 1999 [cited 2004 Mar 7]. Available from: http://www.cdc.gov/od/ads/opspoll1.htm.

Centers for Disease Control and Prevention. HIPAA Privacy Rule and public health: guidance from CDC and the U.S. Department of Health and Human Services. MMWR 2003;52(suppl):1–20 [cited 2004 Mar 16]. Available from: http://www.cdc.gov/mmwr/pdf/wk/mmsu5201.pdf.

Delegation of the European Commission to the United States [press release no. 89/98]. EU directive on personal data protection enters into effect. Washington, DC: European Union, Delegation of the European Commission to the United States; Oct. 23, 1998.

Doyle P, Lane JA, Theeuwes JJM, Zayatz LV, eds. Confidentiality, Disclosure, and Data Access. Amsterdam: Elsevier; 2001.

Elster NR, Hoffman RE, Livengood JR. Public health research and health information. In: Goodman RA, Rothstein MA, Hoffman RE, Lopez W, Mathews G, eds. Law in Public Health Practice. New York: Oxford University Press; 2002.

Etzioni A. The Limits of Privacy. New York: Basic Books; 1999.

Fairchild A. Dealing with humpty dumpty: research, practice, and the ethics of public health surveillance. J Law Med Ethics 2003;31:615–623.

Fairchild A, Bayer R. Ethics and the conduct of public health surveillance. Science 2004;303: 631–632.

Federal Committee on Statistical Methodology, Confidentiality and Data Access Committee [monograph on the Internet]. Identifiability in Microdata Files. Washington, DC: Office of Management and Budget; 2002 July 5 [cited 2004 Mar 7]. Available from: http://www.fcsm.gov/committees/cdac/resources.html.

Federal Committee on Statistical Methodology, Subcommittee on Disclosure Limitation Methodology. Report on statistical disclosure limitation methodology (Statistical Policy Working Paper 22). Washington, DC: Office of Management and Budget; 1994 [cited 2004 Mar 15]. Available from: http://www.fcsm.gov/working-papers/spwp22.html.

Gellman R. Prescribing privacy: the uncertain role of the physician in the protection of patient privacy. North Carolina Law Rev 1984;62:255–294.

Gostin LO. Health information privacy. Cornell Law Rev 1995;80:451–528.

Gostin LO, Burris S, Lazzarini Z. The law and the public's health: a study of infectious disease law in the United States. Columbia Law Rev 1999a;99:59–126.

Gostin LO, Hodge JG. Modern studies in privacy law: national health information privacy regulations under HIPAA: personal privacy and common goods: a framework for balancing under the national health information privacy rule. Minn Law Rev 2002;46:1439–1479.

Gostin LO, Hodge JG, Members of the Privacy Law Advisory Committee [monograph on the Internet]. Model State Public Health Privacy Act as of October 1, 1999. Washington, DC: Model State Public Health Privacy Project, Georgetown University Law Center; 1999b [cited 2004 Mar 9]. Available from: http://www.publichealthlaw.net/Resources/ResourcesPDFs/modelprivact.pdf.

Gostin LO, Koplan JP, Grad FR. The law and the public's health: the foundations. In:

Goodman RA, Rothstein MA, Hoffman RE, Lopez W, Mathews G, eds. Law in Public Health Practice. New York: Oxford University Press; 2002.
Gostin LO, Lazzarini Z, Neslund VS, Osterholm MT. The public health information infrastructure: a national review of the law on health information privacy. JAMA 1996;275: 1921–1927.
Information and Privacy Commissioner (Ontario). Best Practices for Protecting Individual Privacy in Conducting Survey Research. Toronto: Information and Privacy Commissioner; 1999 [cited 2004 Nov 3]. Available from: http://www.ipc.on.ca/docs/bestpr-f.pdf.
Information Infrastructure Task Force, Information Policy Committee, Privacy Working Group [monograph on the Internet]. Privacy and the National Information Infrastructure: Principles for Providing and Using Personal Information. Washington, DC: Information Infrastructure Task Force; 1995 June 6 [cited 2004 Mar 7]. Available from: http://aspe.hhs.gov/datacncl/niiprivp.htm.
Institute for Health Care Research and Policy, Health Privacy Project, Georgetown University. Best Principles for Health Privacy. Washington, DC: Health Privacy Project; 1999 [cited 2004 Mar 7]. Available from: http://www.healthprivacy.org/usr_doc/33807.pdf.
Institute for Health Care Research and Policy, Health Privacy Project, Georgetown University. The State of Health Privacy, 2nd ed. Washington, DC: Health Privacy Project; 2002 [cited 2004 Mar 8] Available from: http://www.healthprivacy.org/info-url_nocat2304/info-url_nocat.htm.
International Statistical Institute. Declaration on Professional Ethics. Voorburg, the Netherlands: International Statistical Institute; 1985 [cited 2004 Mar 7]. Available from: http://www.cbs.nl/isi/ethics.htm.
Kass N, Natowicz MR, Hull SC, Faden RR, Plantinga L, Gostin LO, Slutsman J. The use of medical records in research: what do patients want? J Law Med Ethics 2003;31(3):429–433.
Louis Harris and Associates, Inc. Equifax-Harris Consumer Privacy Survey 1994. New York: Louis Harris and Associates; 1994.
Lowrance WW. Privacy and Health Research: A Report to the U.S. Secretary of Health and Human Services. Washington, DC: U.S. Department of Health and Human Services; 1997 [cited 2004 Mar 15]. Available from: http://www.aspe.hhs.gov/admnsimp/PHR.htm#Contents.
Lowrance WW. Learning from Experience: Privacy and the Secondary Use of Data in Health Research. London: The Nuffield Trust; 2002.
Lynne L. Confidentiality and privacy of electronic medical records. JAMA 2001;285:3075.
Mariner WK. Public confidence in public health research ethics. Public Health Rep 1997; 112(1):33–36.
Melton LJ III. The threat to medical-records research. N Engl J Med 1997;337:1466–1469.
National Center for Health Statistics. Model State Vital Statistics act and Regulations. 1992 rev. DHHS publication no. (PHS) 95–1115). Hyattsville, MD: National Center for Health Statistics; 1995.
National Center for Health Statistics [homepage on the Internet]. Hyattsville, MD: National Center for Health Statistics [updated 2004 Mar 11; cited 2004 Mar 16]. 2003 Revisions of the U.S. Standard Certificates of Live Birth and Death and the Fetal Death Report [about 7 screens]. Available from: http://www.cdc.gov/nchs/vital_certs_rev.htm.
National Center for Health Statistics [homepage on the Internet]. Hyattsville. MD: National Center for Health Statistics [updated 2003 Mar 3; cited 2004 Mar 8]. Research data center [about 5 screens]. Available from: http://www.cdc.gov/nchs/r&d/rdc.htm.
National Commission for the Protection of Human Subjects of Biomedical and Behavioral Research. The Belmont Report: Ethical Principles and Guidelines for the Protection of Human Subjects of Research. Bethesda, MD: U.S. Department of Health, Education, and Welfare; 1978 [cited 2004 Mar 15]. Available from: http://ohrp.osophs.dhhs.gov/humansubjects/guidance/belmont.htm.
National Committee on Vital and Health Statistics, Subcommittee on Privacy and Confi-

dentiality [transcript on the Internet]. Roundtable discussion: identifiability of data. Testimony of Latanya Sweeney, Wednesday, Jan. 28, 1998. Washington, DC: U.S. Department of Health and Human Services; 1998 [cited 2004 Mar 8]. Available from: http://ncvhs.hhs.gov/980128tr.htm.

National Research Council, Computer Science and Telecommunications Board, Commission on Physical Sciences, Mathematics, and Applications, Committee on Maintaining Privacy and Security in Health Care Applications of the National Information Infrastructure. For the Record: Protecting Electronic Health Information. Washington, DC: National Academy Press; 1997.

Organisation for Economic Co-operation and Development. OECD Guidelines on the Protection of Privacy and Transborder Flows of Personal Data. Paris: OECD; 1980 [cited 2004 Mar 13]. Available from: http://www.oecd.org/document/20/0,2340,en_2649_33703_15589524_1_1_1_1,00.html.

Panel on Confidentiality and Data Access. Private Lives and Public Policies: Confidentiality and Accessibility of Government Statistics. Washington, DC: National Academy Press; 1993.

Panel on Institutional Review Boards, Surveys, and Social Science Research. Protecting participants and facilitating social and behavioral sciences research. Washington: National Academies Press; 2003.

Pommerening K, Miller M, Schmidtmann I, Michaelis J. Pseudonyms for cancer registries. Meth Inform Med 1996;35:112–121.

Privacy Commissioner of New Zealand. Privacy Impact Assessment Handbook. Aukland, NZ: Office of the Privacy Commissioner; 2002 [cited 2004 Mar 7]. Available from: http://www.privacy.org.nz/comply/pia.html.

Privacy Protection Study Commission. Personal Privacy in an Information Society. Washington, DC: GPO; 1977.

Regan PM. Legislating Privacy: Technology, Social Values, and Public Policy. Chapel Hill: University of North Carolina Press; 1995.

Schwartz PM, Reidenberg JR. Data Privacy Law: A Study of United States Data Protection. Charlottesville, VA: Michie; 1996.

Seastrom MM. Licensing. In: Doyle P, Lane JI, Theeuwes JJM, Zayatz L, eds. Confidentiality, Disclosure, and Data Acess. Amsterdam: Elsevier; 2001.

Snider DE, Stroup DF. Defining research when it comes to public health. Public Health Rep 1997;112 (1):29–32

Treasury Board of Canada Secretariat [monograph on the Internet] Privacy Impact Assessment Policy. Ottawa: Treasury Board of Canada; 2002 May 2 [cited 2004 Mar 8]. Available from: http://www.tbs-sct.gc.ca/pubs_pol/ciopubs/pia-pefr/paip-pefr-PR_e.asp?printable=True.

U.S. Department of Health, Education, and Welfare, Secretary's Advisory Committee on Automated Personal Data Systems. Records, Computers, and the Rights of Citizens. Washington, DC: Government Printing Office; 1973 [cited.2004 Mar 7]. Available from: http://aspe.os.dhhs.gov/datacncl/1973privacy/tocprefacemembers.htm

von Tigerstrom B, Deschenes M, Knoppers BM, Caulfield TA. Legal regulation of cancer surveillance: Canadian and international perspectives. Health Law J 2000;8:1–94.

Ware W. Lessons for the future: privacy dimensions of medical record keeping. In: Proceedings, Conference on Health Records: Social Needs and Personal Privacy, sponsored by the Department of Health and Human Services. Washington, DC: GPO; 1993, p. 44.

Westin AF. Privacy and Freedom. New York: Atheneum; 1967.

Westin AF. Social and political dimensions of privacy. J of Soc Issues 2003;59:431–453.

Woodward B. Medical record confidentiality and data collection: current dilemmas. J Law Med Ethics 1997;25(2–3):88–97.

Yawn BP, Yawn RA, Geier GR, Xia Z, Jacobsen SJ. The impact of requiring patient authorization for use of data in medical records research. J Fam Pract 1998;47(5):361–365.

CHAPTER 15

New Technologies and Health Statistics

Don E. Detmer and Elaine B. Steen

How will technology affect the generation and use of health statistics in the twenty-first century? To explore this question fully, we must live it. To speculate on it, we must first identify the technologies that are likely to shape the health sector as the century progresses. We must then consider how these technologies will be used and the kinds of data they will generate. Finally, we need to visualize how data and information will flow within the health system as it evolves.

This chapter reviews cutting-edge technologies that are likely to be pivotal to health system development and to influence the generation and use of health statistics as the twenty-first century unfolds. Some of these technologies are already widely diffused but continue to evolve; others are just nascent; and still others are theoretical. It is impossible to be certain if these technologies will develop as anticipated. It is certain, however, that at least some of them will transform both the nature of health-care delivery and the field of health statistics.

LOOKING AHEAD

It is 2090. As John Jones (JJ) shaves each morning, he can view as much or as little of his current health status as he chooses on a screen that is part of his bathroom mirror. He can, for example, see his temperature, blood pressure, cholesterol level, and key protein profiles. He can request that his personal readings be compared to age/sex-specific norms that have been developed from population-based aggregations of deidentified personal health data. If any of JJ's statistics show significant change or deviate significantly—actual statistical significance, as determined weekly by automatic calculations using standard statistical packages within the software itself—from population norms, he is automatically alerted to the trend, as is his personal health coach (see below). Given his phenotype, JJ pays particular attention to the reports from the nanobots that monitor his colon for polyps and sessile lesions, as well as his arteries for intimal roughness and early atherosclerosis.

If he chooses to do so, JJ can view his total caloric intake for the past 24 hours or the past week. He can see how his nutritional intake compares to the plan recommended to him by his health coach based on his genetic map. He can see how many calories he expended in various activities for the same time periods and how frequently he raised and maintained his heart rate at the recommended target level. More important, he gets information on how often his resting blood pressure rises above 115/75.

JJ receives confirmation that his time-release medications are providing the appropriate dosage and reaching the correct locations. He is prompted to record any side effects that he may experience as a result of his drug regimen. JJ's pharmacist has sent a note to inquire whether his monthly medications should be forwarded to his home or office. While he is thinking of it, JJ requests a report that compares the current pollen profile and mold predictions to his own known allergies. This report recommends the specific aerosol that will be most effective for JJ this season.

JJ is pleased that his recent hip cartilage replacement treatment was successful and that his personal health coach recommends a return to his normal level of physical activity and regular exercise regime. He remembers that his grandfather actually had surgery to replace his hip for the same condition early in the century. JJ receives a survey regarding the process and effectiveness of the hip treatment and the accompanying physical therapy. The data he provides are forwarded to the group responsible for the treatment and, after being deidentified, are sent to the national database that tracks the effectiveness of treatments and therapies.

JJ's personal health data are coded and routinely forwarded to his personal health coach. JJ has authorized his personal health data to be made available for health research, so they are encoded to protect his privacy and then shared with the regional health database. JJ's family has agreed to share their personal data with a family health database that captures information on all of his blood relatives. JJ's parents are participants in the automatic health monitoring and notification program, so he receives an update if his parents experience any significant change in health status or personal behavior (e.g., sudden decrease in activity level).

Before JJ heads to breakfast, he requests that a list of suggested meals to fill nutritional gaps be forwarded to his quantum personal assistant (QPA), which can, in turn, check the inventory of JJs' kitchen and generate a shopping list that JJ can approve to be forwarded to his favorite grocery delivery service.

Mary Murphy is a licensed personal health coach. Her training included both primary care and infomediation. She relies heavily on smart software systems with embedded intelligence that provide links to the most current health knowledge and guide her decisions for her clients. She interacts regularly with her colleagues, who include an organizational knowledge broker and a population health manager.

Before Mary sees her first client of the day, she opens the report on the health status of her clients. Of the 2500 individuals she regularly coaches, 17 are flagged as having changes in health status that require follow-up; 2 of these appear to require immediate attention. After reviewing individual health records, she contacts their QPAs and requests that they contact her immediately. She sends a note to the remaining 15 and requests that they have their nanobots checked for accuracy; she then flags their files as needing ongoing review.

When Mary's first client arrives, she invites him into her comfortably furnished office. While Mary is chatting with Mr. Brown, she uses external sensors to confirm the readings of his nanobots. They review his health trends since his last visit, comparing them to age- and sex-adjusted population norms and giving attention to changes that both have noted in his automatically gathered data. As Mary reviews Mr. Brown's lifestyle data, she notes his new job and discusses whether this change may be responsible for the recent decline in the quality of his diet.

When Mary asks Mr. Brown if he has any concerns about his health, he mentions his family history of heart disease. Mary accesses the current protocols for screening young men for heart disease and looks to see how Mr. Brown's personal and family data relate to the protocols. She also glances at the output from a recently updated statistical package that uses deidentified patient data to compare local norms with national data to see if there are local variations that might alter her recommendations. Mary is able to show Mr. Brown how his profile compares to the protocol for further diagnostics. Mr. Brown does not meet the threshold criteria for further tests, but Mary adjusts his exercise program and offers suggestions for diet modifications. Before turning to his other questions, Mary links the heart disease screening protocols to Mr. Brown's database so that they are automatically reviewed each time his health data are updated.

THE TECHNOLOGIES: AN OVERVIEW

This futuristic but not implausible view of the late twenty-first century highlights four technological domains that will transform how we pursue health as individuals and as a society in the coming century.

- *Information and communications technology* (ICT) refers to both connective (e.g., Internet) and computing capabilities provided by information technology.

- *Genomics* refers to the study of the functions and interactions of all the genes in the genome and their contribution to health. Genomic medicine is the application of knowledge of the human genome to medical practice (Guttmacher and Collins 2002).
- *Personal health technology* encompasses the set of tools—both tests and equipment—that extend an individual's ability to manage his or her health care. This technology enables individuals to conduct diagnostic tests or monitor chronic conditions outside formal health-care settings. It also includes e-health technology (i.e., ICT that enables communications between an individual and health professionals or connects an individual to electronic health knowledge sources).
- *Nanotechnology* is focused on controlling matter at the atomic or molecular level to create and use "structures, devices, and systems that have novel properties because of their small or intermediate size," generally between 1 and 100 nanometers (one nanometer is a billionth of a meter or the width of 10 hydrogen atoms placed side by side) (National Nanotechnology Initiative [hp]; Fritz 2002).

Three of these domains—nanotechnology, genomics, and ICT—have been described as being "poised to spark a series of industrial revolutions in the next millennium" (Williams 1999). Varying admixtures of human and computer-based imagination and bioscience research will drive their remarkable advances. The fourth domain is actually the repackaging of other technology to make it widely accessible to the public. Personal health technology is already enabling a shift in the locus of control and responsibility from health professionals to patients, and its importance in the health sector is growing steadily.

There are areas of overlap among these fields. For instance, bioinformatics applies the "analytical theory and practical tools of computer science and mathematics" to biological data such as genomes (Lee and Mallick 1999). As we seek to apply the lessons of nanoscale science to all aspects of human endeavor, cross-fertilization and knowledge sharing among traditionally distinct fields such as physics and biology will become a hallmark of twenty-first-century science (Anderson 1996; Stix 2002; Williams 1999). For example, nano-engineered quantum dots are "minuscule, light-emitting particles" originally developed for electronics (Frantzell 2003). These dots are now being used to detect biological activity in cells. Human immunodeficiency virus (HIV) researchers are using quantum dots to determine the specific arrangement of proteins that maximize HIV binding to the host cell's fat molecules, with the ultimate goal of designing a way to prevent HIV from getting to the cell.

These technologies will influence the future of health statistics in two ways. First, the continuing evolution and diffusion of ICT will provide health statisticians with increasingly powerful tools for collecting and analyzing data and disseminating results to interested audiences. Second, by dramatically changing the nature of health-care delivery, the technologies will provide new kinds of data to be analyzed, new questions to be answered, and new users of health statistics.

Health statisticians will likely see five major trends in the coming decades as a result of emerging technologies. The first trend will be increased automation for both the creation and application of traditional health statistics. This will be accompanied by increased democratization of health statistics as they become more easily accessible to health professionals and the general public. These trends will be counterbalanced by increased demands for customization to address specific questions for a limited population and increased sophistication in the methodology employed by statisticians as they master increasingly complex tasks. Underpinning all of these activities will be increased collaboration as technology facilitates sharing of data and methodologies among disciplines and as patients and health professionals, enabled by technology and new knowledge, become stronger partners in the pursuit of health.

These technologies are at various stages of maturation, and it is impossible to predict how soon they will become routinely used. There are, however, exciting examples of how the technologies might work or are already working that provide a glimpse of what the future holds.

TECHNOLOGICAL POSSIBILITIES AND REALITIES

Information and Communications Technology

Information and communications technology contributes to the health system by providing connectivity among the multitude of players in the health sector, storage for the ever-growing health data and knowledge, the means of analyzing the expanding volume of increasingly sophisticated health data, and mechanisms for accessing and disseminating health data, information, and knowledge. These functions—connectivity, storage, processing, and access—are essential to sound decision making at all levels of the health sector and to the continued generation and application of new knowledge to advance health. They are also foundational elements of the envisioned National Health Information Infrastructure (NHII) (Detmer 2003; National Committee on Vital and Health Statistics 2001). The NHII will enable more efficient sharing of data, higher quality of data captured for clinical use and subsequent reference and analysis, easier access for authorized users to health data, and direct links between needed and available knowledge. It will eventually encompass a wide range of applications to meet the diverse needs of the various domains of the health sector.

Computer-based patient record systems, computer-based physician order entry systems, and computer-assisted decision support systems already contribute to improved quality of care and decreased costs associated with adverse events (Bates et al. 2001; Dexter et al. 2001; Pestonik et al. 1996). These systems are a critical element of the NHII, and their diffusion throughout the health system would constitute a huge step toward strengthening the health-care delivery capabilities in this nation. Work is underway to expand the functionality and scope of clinical information and decision support systems. For example, dynamic prognostic models could use pathologic and histologic data to provide clinicians and patients with more sophisticated calculations of prognosis for certain conditions (e.g., breast cancer) at the point of care (van Houwelingen 1997).

Public health surveillance systems that instantaneously generate health statistics using data gathered during normal clinical workflow are already emerging (Lober et al. 2002). Although still in active development with a limited number of actual deployments, these systems mark a significant achievement in the transformation of clinical data into useful health statistics by minimizing the demands placed on health-care professionals, improving data capture, rapidly analyzing data, and enabling overlay of other relevant data (Lober et al. 2002; RODS Laboratory [mg] 2003). The Center for Biomedical Informatics at the University of Pittsburgh first deployed the Real-time Outbreak and Disease Surveillance system (RODS) in 1999. By 2002, RODS encompassed a 13-county region of western Pennsylvania and covered 56% of the central urban region emergency department (ED) visits and 37% of urban and suburban ED visits. In addition, RODS was deployed in Utah for the 2002 Olympic Games and has become a permanent system for collecting data on more than 70% of the health-care visits in the State of Utah. This surveillance system uses only data collected routinely for other purposes—ED registration data, microbiology culture results, reports of radiographs, dictations of ED clinicians, test orders, and results of laboratory tests. The RODS database receives new data in real time from other computer systems (e.g., registration or laboratory systems) in the form of Health Level 7 (HL7) messages.

The RODS system provides analytic tools to detect the presence of a disease outbreak. Daily registrations with viral, respiratory, diarrheal, rash, and encephalitic chief complaints are plotted. Graphs and analyses are updated every 5 minutes to reflect real-time data. The system allows inspection of frequency of respiratory, diarrheal, or other cases by zip code. When the frequency of the predefined prodromes exceeds expectations for normal ED rates of occurrence, RODS notifies ED staff by electronic mail and pager. The RODS system also can overlay in real time health-care data and environmental data (e.g., ozone levels obtained in real time over the Internet and clinical data about the incidence of respiratory illness).

The successful, focused model of collaboration and technology could be extended in several ways. It has strong potential as a tool to detect intentional outbreaks of disease. Primary care offices could be added as a source of clinical data and included in notification of suspected disease outbreaks. The concept of tracking diagnoses over geographic areas could be applied to those diseases that are linked to environmental factors (e.g., cancer) to help identify more quickly when toxic conditions may be putting the public at risk. Finally, in light of the outbreak of severe acute respiratory syndrome (SARS) in 2003, the model may well have global applications.

A specialty area of ICT, bioinformatics, has been an important enabler of basic science and a major contributor to the success of the Human Genome Project. Further, researchers are increasingly turning to computational analysis and computer simulations to support basic and clinical research. For example, vascular researchers are using computational analysis to explore how and why blood components adhere to arterial walls, to study carotid endarterectomy reconstruction, and to create a virtual vascular laboratory (Archie 2001). Researchers can simulate clinical trials to estimate the impact of alternate drug therapies to determine if the risks to patients and the expense of the trial are merited, thereby streamlining clinical drug development. For example, pharmacokinetic and pharmacodynamic models were used to evaluate docetaxel to determine if patients would benefit from dose intensification. The simulated trial showed only a slight improvement in efficacy over the standard regimen and thus supported the decision not to perform a full clinical trial (Veyrat-Follet et al. 2000). Other simulations have evaluated the cost effectiveness of different strategies for treating patients with coronary disease, the cost effectiveness of combination antiretroviral therapy for HIV, and the impact of delays in discharge from the postanesthesia care unit (Dexter et al. 2001; Freedberg et al. 2001; Gaspoz et al. 2002).

An important computer research area—grid computing—may eventually play a pivotal role in health care and health statistics, as it provides even greater connectivity, storage, and processing capabilities for the health sector (Butler 2003; Foster 2003). *Grid computing* refers "to the large-scale integration of computer systems (via high-speed networks) to provide on-demand access to data crunching capabilities and networks not available to one individual or group of machines" (Foster 2003). As with the Internet, the early focus of the grid is on meeting research needs. For example, the European DataGrid testbed will support the Large Hadron Collidor (LHC) scheduled to come online in 2007. This grid includes 1000 networked machines in 15 countries with 5 terabytes (5×10^{12} bytes) of disk space and 350 test users. Eventually this network will serve 8000 physicists across the globe, provide the equivalent of 200,000 of today's fastest personal computers, and store up to 8 petabytes of data annually (Butler 2003).

Grid technology is already being used to manage the estimated 28 terabytes of image data generated in the United States each day by digital imaging and to facilitate comparison of mammograms and other body scans across time for individual patients and across case populations. Digital image libraries are now being created in the United States and the United Kingdom to address problems arising from the inability to locate previously prepared images (which occurs an estimated 20% of the time). The grid systems link physicians with advanced analytic tools for automated diagnosis (which offsets the misdiagnosis rate of 20%) and support real-time expert consultation (Foster 2003).

Eventually, computers will become so powerful that they will be capable of doing their own thinking and will reopen the field of artificial intelligence

(Kurzweil 1999). Well before such levels of complexity are achieved, people will be able to converse in natural language with a "virtual" colleague that is capable of providing cognitive psychological support for the management of simple depression, phobias, and panic disorders. These developments will expand the functionality of ICT to include computer-based knowledge generation and individualized knowledge application.

Genomics

The genome—the complete set of human genes that resides within each cell of the human body—has been described as a book or, more precisely, an autobiography that captures the history of the human species (Ridley 2000). Genomics seeks to decipher that book, to articulate how healthy and diseased cells function, and to develop tools that will enable prediction, prevention, interruption, or elimination of disease. Genomics encompasses several broad categories of activity that will have clinical applications—diagnosis of genetic diseases and conditions; manipulation of genes to treat genetic diseases; and drugs, vaccines, and enzyme replacement therapies made possible by genomic research. Genomics has already begun to transform the drug discovery process, is refining our understanding of what determines the effectiveness of drugs, and will likely shift the focus of therapies from treating the symptoms of disease to eliminating the root cause of disease (Ginsburg and McCarthy 2001; Reiss 2001). Further, the understanding of the molecular nature of disease may profoundly change clinical care by eventually enabling the practice of personalized and predictive medicine (Ginsburg and McCarthy 2001; Khoury et al. 2003).

Genomics has opened two new exciting areas of focus within pharmaceutical research. Pharmacogenomics applies genomic knowledge to the discovery of new drugs and enables researchers to identify drugs that can disable the proteins that cause disease. For example, molecular targeting led to the discovery of imatinib mesylate (Gleevec). This drug blocks the rapid growth of white blood cells and has received approval for treatment of chronic myeloid leukemia (Food and Drug Administration 2001, 2003). Pharmacogenetics uses genetic testing to guide drug treatment choices for individuals because genetic factors can influence the efficacy of a drug and the likelihood of an adverse reaction (Weinshilboum 2003). Gene expression profiling has been used to determine which breast cancer patients will respond well to particular drugs (Gorman 2002). Limited pharmacogenetics tests are currently available, but eventually a pharmacogenetics test that predicts the therapy response based on a patient's genomic profile will accompany many drugs. Further, research is underway to use molecular profiles to predict adverse drug reactions for new drugs.

Researchers now understand that lymphomas that look identical under the microscope can differ in terms of the genes involved in cell proliferation and immune-cell response (Lemonick 2000). This difference explains why only some patients respond to current treatments. Some researchers predict that eventually we will be able to read the entire genome of an individual human in the time it takes to do a routine medical diagnosis using magnetic resonance imaging (MRI) and, based on that reading, clinicians will be able to diagnose an illness and prescribe specifically tailored treatments that best suit the individual. Among those treatments for some conditions may be the actual manipulation of defective genes to eliminate disease. Gene therapy is, however, still nascent, and its safety and effectiveness are under close scrutiny.

Other researchers are focusing on the possibility of preventing disease by screening populations for genetic information to "target interventions to individual patients that will improve their health and prevent disease" (Khoury et al. 2003). Such screening will be able to identify individuals at risk for common conditions such as heart disease, diabetes, or cancer so that appropriate prevention efforts (e.g., diet, exercise, pharmacologic interventions) can be implemented (Ginsburg and McCarthy 2001). This practice will allow physicians "to move from intense, crisis-driven intervention to predictive medicine" (Khoury et al. 2003).

Many researchers and the media have widely heralded the promise of genomic medicine, but other researchers have cautioned that translating this genomic research into clinical applications will be "intellectually challenging, time-consuming, and expensive" (Goldstein 2003). A major challenge to be managed will be the increasing complexity of science and the huge number of tests—and accompanying costs—that could become part of routine clinical care (Varmus 2002). Thus, clinical genomic applications may emerge slowly, and the broad impact of genomics is not likely to be evident for at least another 15 years (Melzer et al. 2003).

Personal Health Technology

Personal health management refers to the deliberate effort by individuals to prevent disease through lifestyle choices, to participate actively in decisions about clinical care, and to assume greater responsibility for self-care. Today personal health technology allows patients to be better informed about treatment options, monitor their health status, and integrate their care over time. In the future, personal health technology will increasingly enable patients to manage their own therapies from home with the guidance of their health professionals.

Although far from a fully mature domain of the health sector, personal health management constitutes an important element of the evolving health system. Consumers accounted for approximately one-third of the 250 million MEDLINE searches conducted in 2000. To meet consumer needs, in 1998 the National Library of Medicine launched MEDLINEplus, a service that provides selective MEDLINE results along with Web links to "authoritative, full-text health information written for the general public" (Lindberg 2000). Some patients are using electronic support groups to share concerns and information (Benton Foundation 1999). Growing numbers of patients are maintaining contact with their primary (or multiple) health care professional(s) via e-mail at mutual convenience, thereby reducing the number of telephone calls and office visits (Borowitz and Wyatt 1998).

Personal health records enable patients or citizens to manage their health by maintaining a complete record of all previous health-care providers, significant health events, and medications. Families can develop intergenerational health records so that knowledge about family disease experiences is not lost. On-line personal health risk assessments can be performed in the comfort and privacy of one's home. The results of these assessments can link citizens to health promotion resources or flag the need to contact a health-care professional.

The home diagnostics industry is booming, with $2.6 billion in sales in 2002 (Powell 2003). Glucose testing and monitoring accounted for $2.1 billion in sales. Most home tests involve looking for signs of a disease or monitoring a condition—such as colon cancer, sperm count, blood glucose level, urinary tract infection, onset of menopause, pregnancy tests, or human immunodeficiency virus. Some health insurers have begun to pay for home tests and equipment used by patients to manage chronic conditions.

More comprehensive approaches are being developed. For example, Columbia University is conducting a 4-year demonstration project with 1500 participants to assess the feasibility, acceptability, effectiveness, and cost effectiveness of telemedicine in the management of older patients with diabetes (Shea et al. 2002). Intervention participants receive a home telemedicine unit that provides synchronous videoconferencing with a project-based nurse, electronic transmission of home finger stick glucose and blood pressure data, and access to a project Web site. The project will be evaluated on the basis of clinical measures, patient satisfaction, health-care service use, and costs.

Nanotechnology

The term *nanotechnology* is often applied imprecisely to nanoscience (i.e., basic research) and to microtechnology (i.e., structures and devices on the scale of microns or millionths of a meter). Some scientists caution that nanotechnology is "an enterprise of the future" because they are just beginning to decipher the properties that govern the nanoworld. Others warn that some visionaries have gone too far in their promises of what nanotechnology will be able to do (e.g., predictions that nanoscopic machines can help revive frozen brains from suspended animation) (Stix 2002). Nonetheless, the possibilities of nanotechnology are far-ranging—from fashion to sports to manufacturing to electronics to computing to biomedical applications—and quite intriguing even if the field is still emerging. Despite the hyperbole of some prognosticators, the field is being taken very seriously and is expected to become very big business. The National Science

Foundation estimates that the nanotechnology industry could grow to $1 trillion worldwide in 15 years (Ratner and Ratner 2003).

Nanotechnology may ultimately become the foundation for the next industrial era. A complete review of all the aspects of nanoscale discovery and application that lie before us is beyond the scope of this chapter. Highlights of applications in use or under development will, however, provide a sense of how different the future will be.

Nanotechnology has been in limited use for some years. For example, zeolites, also known as *molecular sieves* because their physical shapes allow them to sift materials, are used as domestic water softeners and can be used to produce petroleum more efficiently. They enable up to 40% more gasoline to be extracted from a barrel of crude oil and account for an estimated 400 million barrels of oil saved per year in the United States (Ratner and Ratner 2003). The first generation of consumer products based on nanotechnology has begun to appear in the market. These products include skin creams and suntan lotions, fabrics that are resistant to stains or incorporate biocidal agents intended to prevent the spread of pathogens, and a plethora of sports equipment such as lightweight bikes and sailboats, improved hockey pads, and tennis balls that bounce longer.

The impact of nanoscience and nanotechnology will be visible throughout the health-care sector from research to diagnosis to therapy. Scanning tunneling microscopes provide topographic maps of material surfaces in which it is possible to see individual atoms. These technologies enable biologists to look into the nucleus of a living cell and observe the interaction of proteins, watch neurons grow inside a living brain, or make movies of proteins shuttling cargo into and out of the nucleus of a cell through miniature doughnut-shaped pores (Boyd 2003). Nanotechnology can enhance biomedical research by revealing which sets of genes are active in cells under various conditions. Nanoscale models are helping to make the drug discovery process less happenstance and more a matter of design. Since many proposed nanodrugs work by well-understood and very specific mechanisms, there should be fewer side effects and more beneficial behavior. For example, intelligent nanoscale development of antidepressants is focused on restoring the concentration of neurotransmitter molecules to normal levels by blocking their destruction through modification of their binding properties (Ratner and Ratner 2003).

In the diagnostic realm, the introduction of nanoparticles into home pregnancy tests has made them easier to use, faster, and more accurate (Ratner and Ratner 2003). Miniaturization is improving diagnostic capabilities in novel ways. For example, Given Imaging has developed "an ingestible grape-sized capsule that transmits direct images of the entire GI tract—including for the first time the small bowel—as the device travels through and is eventually expelled from the body" (Levin 2002). Capsule enteroscopy dramatically improves the ability to diagnose problems in the small intestines, and is much less invasive and more comfortable for patients. Other anticipated diagnostic applications of nanotechnology include implants to monitor blood chemistry, improved contrast agents for noninvasive imaging, detection of cancerous tumors that are only a few cells in size, and diagnostic screens to determine an individual's susceptibility to different disorders or to reveal which genes are mutated in a person's cancer.

On the therapeutic front, nanotechnology is very useful in developing new schemes for increasing bioavailablity and improving drug delivery. Scientists are combining "advances in nanotechnology and microfabrication to make implantable microchips that can deliver drugs precisely and on schedule" (Langer 2003). The successful development of implants that release drugs on demand would benefit diabetics and cancer patients, as well as offer better forms of birth control. The ability to get drugs through cell walls and into cells is important in many diseases. Nanopharmaceutical drug-binding molecules tiny enough to travel through the body's smallest capillaries may provide a way to spare the heart and other organs from the toxic effects of drug overdoses.

Beyond drug delivery, nanoshells are envisioned as a potential tool against cancer (Altivisatos 2002). Nanoshells that bind specifically to tumor cells would be administered and then heated. Heating the nanoshells would in theory destroy the cancerous cells but not harm nearby tissue. In addition, nanoscale building blocks may one day mimic the processes of biology by repairing damaged tissues and regenerating bone, cartilage, and skin. Researchers at Northwestern University reported that they have designed molecules that "self-assemble into a three-dimensional structure that mimics the key features of human bone at the nanoscale level" (UniSci 2001). These designer molecules provide the starting point for the development of "bonelike material to be used for bone fractures or in the treatment of bone cancer patients" and may have implications for the regeneration of other kinds of cells such as neurons, cartilage, muscle, liver, and pancreas (UniSci 2001).

Meanwhile, the success achieved by microelectronics and anticipated in nanoelectronics in extreme miniaturization of computing power and storage has given rise to predictions that by the end of the century, people will unobtrusively wear computer power that is more powerful than the supercomputers of the early twenty-first century—as a watch-like appliance, inside the frame of glasses, or woven inside clothing (Williams 1999). It is conceivable that a personal health record will include a lifetime of experiences captured with sensors that are worn on or in the body.

Work currently underway will provide the foundation for such possibilities to become realities. For example, consumers can now purchase microdrives that function exactly like traditional computer hard drives but store four gigabytes on disks roughly the size of quarters. IBM's Millipede storage system is even smaller. By using thousands of levers that are about 10 micrometers wide, Millipede can store roughly 1 trillion bits of data per square inch of media, 20 times more than is possible with magnetic storage devices. Even more ambitious chips are in the works. IBM plans to test a chip that uses 4000 levers in a 7 square millimeter area of plastic and expects the chip to handle several gigabytes of data. The Millipede-based memory device could be available by the end of 2005 (Eng 2002).

The relatively young field of quantum information science combines computer science and nanoscience. It expands our understanding of information to include its physical attributes (Nielson 2003; Zeilinger 1998). Thus, while classical information science expresses information in terms of bits, which can be either 0 or 1, quantum information science expresses information as quantum bits (or qubits), which can be in both the 0 and the 1 state at the same time (i.e., superposition). This superposition gives rise to parallelism that would allow a quantum computer to perform traditional computing tasks faster than classical computers (e.g., calculate the prime factors of a 300-digit number). Although quantum computers are a distant proposition, quantum information scientists have begun to decipher the basic laws of quantum information and have made inroads on specific applications such as cryptography (which should aid computer security) and quantum teleportation.

Consider the potential of quantum computing as described by George Johnson in *A Shortcut Through Time* (2003). In 2003, one of the most powerful computers in the world—called Blue Mountain—occupies approximately one-quarter of an acre and has 6144 processors that can work jointly to perform 3 trillion mathematical operations per second (i.e., 3 teraops). Its successor—known as Q—will have twice as many processors, each running five times faster, resulting in a 30 teraops machine and requiring about an acre of space. A quantum computer made with 13 atoms could outperform Blue Mountain. A quantum computer with 14 atoms could match Q's performance. A quantum computer with 64 atoms could perform 2^{64}—18 quintillion—simultaneous calculations. For a traditional supercomputer to achieve that level of performance, it would have to occupy 750 trillion acres—or the surface of 5000 Earths (including the oceans).

Even more thought-provoking to contemplate is the possibility that neuroelectronic interfaces could eventually enable computers to be linked to the human nervous system. Neural implants are already being used to suppress tremors associated with cerebral palsy and multiple sclerosis; cochlear implants combined with electronic speech processors perform the job of the inner ear by analyzing the frequency of sounds waves (Kurzweil 1999). Nanoscale neuro-devices will require "the building of a molecular structure that will permit control and detection of nerve impulses" (Ratner and Ratner 2003). This constitutes a challenge for both computational nanotechnology and bionanotechnology. Research is underway on this topic, but little practical progress has been reported.

IMPLICATIONS FOR HEALTH STATISTICS

The technologies of the twenty-first century have the potential to transform health statistics from static snapshots of distant events into dynamic contributors to decision making at a wide range of levels in the health sector. These technologies will create new uses for and users of health statistics and allow faster production of and access to health statistics. The twenty-first-century technologies will create new modes of data collection, more sources of data, a growing volume of data, and more complex data to be managed as part of the process of creating health statistics. These technologies will also require increasingly sophisticated capabilities to analyze new kinds of data.

One of the most critical determinants of the future of health statistics is the level of success achieved in building a NHII that includes widespread availability of emerging ICT capabilities to manage health data. If the United States builds a robust NHII, we can expect improved depth, breadth, and quality of health data available to generate statistics, reduced costs of gathering and maintaining traditional health statistics, and better linkages across data and health statistics systems (Friedman et al. 2002; Woodward 2001). A robust health information infrastructure and the accompanying development of electronic health data sets will provide multidimensional information for analysis. Data standards and research to improve methods of managing deidentified data will be essential for progress on this front. For example, the movement toward functional requirements for computer-based health records will have important implications for the creation of health statistics (Institute of Medicine [mg] 2003).

The NHII will provide improved access and ability to format health statistics to support immediate decision making. Physicians or other health providers will be able to call on applications that gather relevant population data and apply appropriate analytic models to provide more precise analysis of treatment options for individual patients. Perhaps most important, the NHII will enable the creation of a continuous feedback loop that captures data on the actions of the health system and accompanying outcomes, analyzes those data, disseminates new information and knowledge arising from the data to inform future decisions, and repeats the loop to refine the knowledge base that supports health-care decisions at the individual, organizational, and system levels.

As individuals increasingly begin to maintain personal health records for themselves and family members, a new source of data is being established. While under the control of individual citizens, many are created through access to systems provided by health-care provider organizations, such as PatientSite (Caregroup Health-Care System [hp]), or on-line health management companies, such as Personal Path (PersonalPath Systems, Inc. [hp]), and patients may be willing to authorize access to their data if their identity can be protected. An important development that will be made possible by the NHII is the collection of follow-up data for patients outside the hospital setting. Through personal health records, patients can record their outcomes for given treatments and forward them to databases maintained by their health-care providers. In this way, clinicians and researchers will be better able to assess the effectiveness of various treatments.

Further, health-care organizations can track the kinds of knowledge sought by patients and the frequency of hits as a means of assessing health concerns in the population. *Clicks and mortar* e-health programs that allow patients to contact health sites on the Internet, as well as link to their regular sources of health care, show that clicks precede clinic appointments and visits. That is, many people search the Web for information before they make appointments for new symptoms. These searchers may constitute the earliest evidence available on emerging threats from either infectious disease or bioterrorism.

Information and communications technology has the potential to change time and space for health statistics. With data and greater computing capacity more readily available, we can anticipate increased speed of analysis and faster production of health statistics. Information and communications technology can shorten the time it takes to convert raw data into health statistics and put health statistics into use, thereby placing real-time statistical systems on the horizon. With resources like grid computing available, statisticians and researchers will be able to share computing and data resources across distances and not be limited by computing power and data storage at one institution. Such capabilities will facilitate the linkage environmental and health data (Thomas 2002).

Genomic, personal diagnostic, and nanotechnologies broaden the sources of data available to generate health statistics and contribute to the growing amounts of and complexity of data to be analyzed. Pharmaceutical companies and academic medical centers are already collecting biological specimens along with traditional clinical data (Ginsburg and McCarthy 2001; Hartge 2001). It is conceivable that eventually a genomic profile will be a standard component of health records for individuals. Thus, a preliminary bioinformatics challenge created by these technologies is the need to manage the massive flow of clinical, genetic, and personal behavior data from a multitude of sources on many patients and "to effectively store and integrate extremely large and diverse datasets and to support sophisticated querying of these data in a multitude of ways in reasonable time frames" (Brookes 2001). Genomic and other complicated data will require new analytical models and methods (van Houwelingen 1997). The major biostatistics challenge will be to discriminate between "marginal signals and background noise in extremely large, diverse and complex data sets" (Brookes 2001).

Along with technological advances, other developments are shaping the health sector and will influence the demand for and use of health statistics. Safety, quality, evidence-based medicine, population health management, personal health management, public health including bioterrorism preparedness, and more selective contracting with health-care providers by purchasers all depend on timely (in some cases immediate) access to current information and knowledge. Easier access to and faster generation of health statistics will strengthen these efforts. These initiatives will also likely raise new questions to be answered by health statistics and introduce new users to health statistics.

CONCLUSION

To date, health statistics have been overwhelmingly retrospective analyses with varying degrees of continuity. The technologies of the twenty-first century have the potential to transform health statistics into an increasingly continuous, prompt, and ubiquitous reflection of experiences in personal and population health care and health status. Future health data analysis may become so timely that all users—individuals, communities, or governments—will give health statistics much greater attention.

The ultimate impact of emerging and maturing technologies on health statistics will be determined by the system within which those technologies are applied. Will the health system have the mechanisms and processes in place to capture and analyze the data that are produced by new technologies to create useful statistics, information, and knowledge? Will it have the personnel who are capable of applying that information to advance the health of individuals, populations, and the nation? Will it encourage patients and citizens to adopt available technologies and to assume a more active role in managing their health?

The health system is a function of policies, funding, and incentives created for the multitude of actors in the health sector. The key question facing the health sector is whether it will take advantage of the capabilities offered by technology—particularly ICT—to create a true system of health for the nation (Detmer 2001). Such a system will require investment in the NHII, continued support for basic research that is the foundation of the future technologies, and prudent decisions to strengthen the nontechnological infrastructure components of the health system—including universal health insurance coverage, incentives that are aligned with desired behaviors by patients and health-care professionals, support of ongoing knowledge generation (i.e., clinical and basic research) to support evidence-based medicine, and a workforce that is equipped to fulfill the changing role of health professionals.

REFERENCES

Alivisatos, AP. Less is more in medicine. In: Fritz, S, ed. Understanding Nanotechnology. New York: Warner Books; 2002, pp. 56–69.

Anderson, WT. Evolution Isn't What It Used to Be. New York: W.H. Freeman; 1996.

Archie JP. Presidential address: a brief history of arterial blood flow from Harvey and Newton to computational analysis. J Vasc Surg 2001;34:398–404.

Bates DW, Cohen M, Leape LL, Overhage JM, Shabot MM, Sheridan T. Reducing the frequency of errors in medicine using information technology. J Am Med Inform Assoc 2001;8:299–308.

Benton Foundation [monograph on the Internet]. Networking for Better Care: Health Care in the Information Age. Washington, DC: Benton Foundation; 1999 [cited 2002 Mar]. Available from: http://www.benton.org/publibrary/health/home.html.

Borowitz SM, Wyatt JC. The origin, content, and workload of e-mail consultations. JAMA 1998;280:1321–24.

Boyd RS. Devices watch time (almost) stand still. Charlotte Observer 2003 Apr 11;Sect. A:2 (col. 1).

Brookes AJ. Rethinking genetic strategies to study complex diseases. Trends Mol Med 2001; 7:512–516.

Butler D. [article on the Internet]. The grid: tomorrow's computing today. Nature 2003;422: 799–800 [cited 2003 Apr]. Available from: http://www.nature.com.

CareGroup Healthcare System [homepage on the Internet]. Boston: Caregroup Healthcare System; [cited 2004 Mar 9]. PatientSite. Available from: http://www.caregroup.org/patientsite.asp.

Detmer DE. A new health system and its quality agenda. Front Health Serv Manag 2001; 18(1):3–30.

Detmer DE. Building the national health information infrastructure for personal health, health care services, public health, and research. BMC Med Inform Decis Mak 2003;3:1.

Dexter F, Penning DH, Traub RD. Statistical analysis by monte-carlo simulation of the impact of administrative and medical delays in discharge from the postanesthesia care unit on total patient care hours. Anesth Analg 2001;92:1222–1225.

Dexter PR, Perkins S, Overhage JM, Maharry K, Kohler RB, McDonald CJ. A computerized reminder system to increase the use of preventive care for hospitalized patients. N Engl J Med 2001;13:965–970.

Eng P. [article on the Internet]. Mega-data stored in mini-spaces: nanotechnology will cram more data in tiny storage devices. New York: ABC News; 2001 [cited 2003 Apr]. Available from: http://abcnews.go.com/sections/scitech/FutureTech/futuretech030110.html.

Food and Drug Administration [article on the Internet]. FDA Approves Gleevec for Leukemia Treatment. Rockville, MD: Food and Drug Administration; 2001 May 10 [cited 2003 Jun]. Available from: http://www.fda.gov/bbs/topics/NEWS/2001/NEW00759.html.

Food and Drug Administration [article on the Internet]. FDA News: FDA converts Gleevec in second line setting to regular approval. Rockville, MD: Food and Drug Administration; 2003 Dec 8 [cited 2004 Feb]. Available from: http://www.fda.gov/bbs/topics/NEWS/2003/NEW00990.html.

Foster I. The grid: computing without bounds. Sci Am 2003;288:78–85.

Frantzell A. Small-scale warfare: researchers at UCD are using the tiniest tools of the trade to fight HIV. The California Aggie 2003 Apr 14.

Freedberg KA, Losina E, Weinstein MC, Paltiel AD, Cohen CJ, Seage GR, et al. The cost effectiveness of combination antiretroviral therapy for HIV disease. N Engl J Med 2001; 344:824–831.

Friedman DJ, Hunter EL, Parrish RG, eds. Shaping a Health Statistics Vision for the 21st century. Final Report, November 2002. Hyattsville, MD: Centers for Disease Control and Prevention, National Center for Health Statistics; Washington, DC: U.S. Department of Health and Human Services Data Council, National Committee on Vital and Health Statistics; 2002.

Fritz S, ed. Understanding Nanotechnology. New York: Warner Books; 2002.

Gaspoz JM, Coxson PG, Goldman, PA, Williams LW, Kuntz KM, Hunink MGM, et al. Cost effectiveness of aspirin, clopidogrel, or both for secondary prevention of coronary heart disease. N Engl J Med 2002;346:1800–1806.

Ginsburg GS, McCarthy JJ. Personalized medicine: revolutionized discovery and patient care. Trends Biotechnol 2001;19:491–496.

Goldstein DB. Pharmacogenetics in the laboratory and the clinic. N Engl J Med 2003;6:553–556.

Gorman C. Rethinking breast cancer. Time 2002 Feb 18, [cited 2004 Nov 11]. Available from http://www.time.com/time/archive.

Guttmacher AE, Collins FS. Genomic medicine—a primer. N Engl J Med 2002;347:1512–1520.

Hartge P. Epidemiologic tools for today and tomorrow. Ann NY Acad Sci 2001;954:295–310.

Institute of Medicine [monograph on the Internet]. Key Capabilities of an Electronic Health Record System: Letter Report. Washington, DC: National Academy Press; 2003 [cited 2003 Aug]. Available from: http://www.nap.edu/books/NI000427/html.

Johnson G. A Shortcut Through Time: The Path to the Quantum Computer. New York: Alfred A. Knopf; 2003.

Kallioniemi, A. Molecular signatures of breast cancer—predicting the future. N Engl J Med 2002;347:2067–2068.

Khoury MJ, McCabe LL, McCabe ERB. Population screening in the age of genomic medicine. N Engl J Med 2003;348:50–58.

Kurzweil R. The Age of Spiritual Machines. New York: Viking; 1999.

Langer R. Where a pill won't reach. Sci Am 2003;288:50–57.

Lee C, Mallick P [monograph on the Internet]. The UCLA Bioinformatics Interdepartmental Program. Los Angeles: University of California at Los Angeles; 1999 [cited 2002 Jan]. Available from: http://www.bioinformatics.ucla.edu/leelab/outlineRFCv8.pdf.

Lemonick MD [article on the Internet]. The genome is mapped. Now what? Time 2000 Jul 3; [cited 2002 Jan]. Available from: http://www.time.com/time/archive/preview/from_search/0,10987,1101000703–48105,00.html 1;http://time.qpass.com/time/magazine/article.

Levin A [article on the Internet]. Given imaging: a capsule view of GI diagnostics' future. IN VIVO: The Business and Medicine Report; 2002 May 1 [cited 2003 May]. Available from: http://sis.windhover.com/windbuy/lpext.dll/windbuy/iv/2002/2002800102.htm.

Lindberg DAB. Internet access to the National Library of Medicine. Eff Clin Pract 2000; 3:256–260.

Lober WB, Karras BT, Wagner MW, Overhage M, Davidson MJ, Fraser H, et al. Roundtable on bioterrorism detection: information system-based surveillance. J Am Med Inform Assoc 2002;9:105–115.

Melzer D, Simmern RL, Detmer DE, Ling T. Regulatory options for pharmacogenetics [editorial]. Pharmagenomics 2003;4(5):1–4.

National Committee on Vital and Health Statistics. Information for health: a strategy for building the National Health Information Infrastructure, report and recommendations from the National Committee on Vital and Health Statistics [monograph on the Internet]. Washington: U.S. Department of Health and Human Services; 2001 Nov 15 [cited 2004 Mar 15]. Available from: http://aspe.hhs.gov/sp/nhii/Documents /NHIIReport2001/default.htm.

National Nanotechnology Initiative [homepage on the Internet]. What is nanotechnology?; [cited 2003 Apr] Available from: http://www.nano.gov/html/facts/whatIsNano.html.

Nielsen MA. Simple rules for a complex quantum world. Sci Am, special ed 2003;13(1):24–33.

PersonalPath Systems, Inc. [homepage on the Internet]. Upper Saddle River, NJ: PersonalPath Systems, Inc.; [cited 2004 Mar 9]. PersonalPath.com. Available from: http://www.personalpathsystems.com/pself.html.

Pestonik SL, Classen DC, Evans RS, Burke JP. Implementing antiobiotic practice guidelines through computer-assisted decision support: clinical and financial outcomes. Ann Intern Med 1996;124:884–890.

Powell C. Medical tests are making some house calls these days. Charlotte Observer 2003 Apr 28;Sect. E:1 (col. 2).

Ratner M, Ratner D. Nanotechnology: A Gentle Introduction to the Next Big Idea. Upper Saddle River, NJ: Prentice Hall; 2003.

Reiss T. Drug discovery of the future: implications of the Human Genome Project. Trends Biotechnol 2001;19:496–499.

Ridley M. Genome: The Autobiography of a Species in 23 Chapters. New York: Perennial; 2000.

RODS Laboratory [monograph on the Internet]. Demonstration Systems in Public Health Surveillance. Pittsburgh: RODS Laboratory [updated 2003 April 28; cited 2004 Mar 9]. Available from: http://www.health.pitt.edu/rods/RODS%20Demonstration% 20Systems6.pdf.

Shea S, Starren J, Weinstock RW, Knudson PE, Teresi J, Holmes D, et al. Columbia University's Informatics for Diabetes and Telemedicine (IDEATel) Project. J Am Med Inform Assoc 2002;9:49–55.

Stix G. Little big science. In: Fritz S, ed. Understanding Nanotechnology. New York: Warner Books; 2002, pp. 6–16.

Thomas DC. Some contributions of statistics to environmental epidemiology. In: Raftery AE, Tanner MA, Wells MT, eds. Statistics in the 21st Century. Alexandria, VA: American Statistical Association; 2002, pp. 75–83.

UniSci. Nanoscale designer molecules recreate bone structure. Daily University Science News, 27 Nov 2001 [cited 2003 Apr]. Available from: http://unisci.com/stories/20014/1127012.htm.

Varmus H. Getting ready for gene-based medicine. N Engl J Med 2002;347:1526–1527.

van Houwelingen HC. The future of biostatistics: expecting the unexpected. Stat Med 1997; 16:2773–2784.

Veyrat-Follet C, Bruno R, Olivares R, Rhodes GR, Chaikin P. Clinical trial simulation of docetaxel in patients with cancer as a tool for dosage optimization. Clin Pharmacol Ther 2000;68:677–687.

Weinshilboum R. Inheritance and drug response. N Engl J Med 2003;348:529–537.

Williams RS [article on the Internet]. Industrial revolutions in the 21st century. Physicsweb; 1999 Dec [cited 2003 Apr]. Available from: http://physicsweb.org/article/world/12/12/31/1.

Woodward PR. Measuring patient reported data and outcomes. Health Manag Technol 2001;2:28–30, 32.

Zeilinger, A [article on the Internet]. Fundamentals of quantum information. Physicsweb 1998 Mar [cited 2003 Apr]. Available from: http://physicsweb.org/article/world/11/3/9.

CHAPTER 16

Modeling Health: The Role of Simulation Models in Health Information Systems

Michael C. Wolfson

The health sector in any society is largely about information. Everyone who has seen a doctor or had a one-on-one encounter with another health provider will likely have experienced from the receiving end the process of diagnosing an ailment, prescribing a course of action, and monitoring the results. All of these tasks involve information flows; the action itself is often the lesser part of health-care encounters.

Many roles, of course, are played by information in the health sector and by the main precursors of information—data and health statistics.[1] Not least is assembling and analyzing the data to produce the evidence needed to underpin the processes of diagnosis and prescription. This entails collecting data from representative samples of health-care encounters. Often the data are collected as part of controlled experiments, notably randomized clinical trials of drugs. But these collections may also involve routine administrative data on all health-care encounters of a population, such as the members of a health plan (e.g., see Chapters 6 and 18). These kinds of data help us decide if a given drug or surgical procedure is efficacious and what proportion of the population is being treated in this way.

In addition, a major use of health information is to describe trends and patterns. Among the most widely used indicators for these purposes is life expectancy. Other widely used measures are based on self-reported health status and related measures from population health surveys, such as the proportion of the population reporting themselves to be in excellent or very good health or to be current smokers.

But descriptive statistics are not sufficient for managing countries' health systems or for informing many of the policy choices faced by those responsible, typically ministries of health, or for individuals trying to make the best choices for their own health. Policymakers, health system managers, and citizens need the best possible answers to "what if" questions—which of these new interventions is most deserving of new health care resources?; or what if I made a particular change in my health-related behavior (e.g., losing weight, increasing physical activity)?; or what if the government required employers to provide a minimum of health insurance?

For one group of relatively simple questions, the results of experiments such as randomized clinical trials may be sufficient: Would it help me or not if I took drug X to cure my ailment? However, many important questions are not in this simple class since the necessary experiments, even if we could imagine how to set them up, could never be done because they would be infeasible, unethical, or just too costly. For example, imagine a randomized trial to determine which offers a greater public health benefit per dollar—a regulatory initiative for the food industry to reduce dietary fat intake or a series of municipal zoning and transportation policies designed to increase physical activity?

In most cases, adequate answers to such "what if" questions require a carefully articulated causal chain, based on a series of detailed empirical results, quantified statistically, brought together in a coherent manner, and expressed as a computer simulation model. This chapter focuses on simulation models as critical components of health information systems. It includes several examples of simulations used in health analysis, an overview of simulation methods, particularly *micro*simulation, and a discussion of the implications of supporting simulation modeling for health information systems in general.

Simulation models are not new, even in the health sector. They are taken for granted in many other domains. For example, in ministries of finance, policy-oriented computer simulation models as a basis for personal income tax policy have been in regular use in a number of Organisation for Economic Co-operation and Development (OECD) countries since the 1960s. And in many facets of astrophysics research, computer simulation models play an increasingly central role in the interplay between observation and theory.

The parallels with tax policy and astronomy are notable. Astronomy is essentially an observational, not an experimental, science. It has long since moved beyond discovering single instances of a new kind of object (e.g., galaxy, supernova) to collecting data on populations of objects, and then exploring the distributional patterns of their characteristics in order to make inferences about their laws of motion or patterns of evolution (e.g., color and luminosity and the *main sequence* for stellar evolution leading to the Herzsprung-Russel diagram, red shifts, and expansion of the universe.). These inferences are increasingly based on computer simulations, since the theories that are coevolving with the observations are themselves too complex to be written as formulae and then solved with traditional pencil-and-paper (analytic) methods.

Tax policy simulation models also start with detailed observational data on a population, in this case individual taxpayers. The heterogeneity of taxpayers' circumstances is a critical factor, for example to predict who will gain and who will lose from a particular change in tax law. And even though it is obvious that changing some provision in the tax law will affect individuals' disposable incomes, it is equally obvious that there is a wide range of other factors that are at least as important (e.g., employment choices, investment portfolio choices). Thus, predicting the effects of a tax law change requires detailed microsimulation, which takes account of the unique circumstances of (at least a representative sample of) individual taxpayers.

The health domain shares a number of these attributes. Health policy, as well as decision aids designed to help individuals make health treatment choices where there are risks or difficult trade-offs, inevitably has to deal with data on populations, and should take account of their heterogeneity. While the results of randomized trials are regularly reported in the media, most empirical evidence is observational rather than experimental for the reasons just noted. And many questions involve singling out one factor in what is obviously a more complex causal web.

By comparison with domains like astronomy and tax policy, computer simulation models are seriously underdeveloped in the health sector. One major reason is that the information systems needed to support such models, the underlying efforts of developing and exploiting coherent data sets on myriad facets of the population's health and health care, are generally absent, though this situation is changing, as described below and in other chapters (see Chapter 17).

Another reason may be that the dominant activity in the health sector, one-on-one health-care interventions, often provided by solo or small groups of practitioners, entails a psychology that is antithetical to standing back and observing patterns or regularities at the population level. But again, with the rise of quantitative epidemiologic methods and the growth of concerns about effectiveness, appropriateness, and quality of care, the autonomy of individual practitioners has increasingly been overlaid by institutional structures designed to meet these concerns.

LIFE EXPECTANCY AND SIMULATION

The notion of computer simulation models in health may seem alien and may conjure up images of complex and impenetrable software systems. However, the single most widely used indicator of population health status, life expectancy, is not a datum that is measured directly; rather, it is the result of a simulation, albeit a very simple one.

Life expectancy (more specifically, *period*, as opposed to *cohort*, life expectancy) in year *t* (e.g., a few years ago, since it takes some time to assemble the mortality and population data) is the answer to the following hypothetical question: How long, on average, could a cohort of individuals expect to live if they were each exposed to the chance of dying at each year of age that we observed a few years ago in year t? No actual individual or cohort of individuals faces these mortality risks because mortality rates vary from year to year (most often declining), and at age $a + 1$, we face a mortality rate from a year later (i.e., $t + 1$, not t) than we did at age a.

The modeling method by which this synthetic indicator is constructed is straightforward, relying on the idea of a life table. At its simplest, this is a table with three columns: the first with simply the labels for single years of age ($a = 0, 1, 2, \ldots 100$), the second with the age-specific mortality rates all as observed in year t, and the third with the surviving population at each age, starting arbitrarily with a number like 100,000 at age 0. The surviving population at each subsequent age $a + 1$ is computed recursively by taking the population at age a and removing the proportion who die according to the mortality rate at age a. Life expectancy is then essentially the sum of all the numbers in the last column divided by the number we started with (i.e., 100,000).[2]

The "what if" character of life expectancy measures does not stop at positing a cohort "out of time," facing at each age the mortality rates observed in a single year, t. Several families of derived indicators are also fairly widely used, such as cause-deleted life expectancy and potential years of life lost (PYLL). If we replace the mortality rates in the second column of the life table just described with an alternative set based on all deaths *except* those from heart disease or lung cancer, say, but otherwise follow exactly the same procedures, we obtain *heart disease deleted* and *lung cancer deleted* life expectancies, respectively.

Alternatively, we could add up all the "missed" person-years of life (the count of deaths in each age interval multiplied by the number of years between the age at death and age 70, and then summed over ages at death up to 70) for the rows corresponding to ages 0 to 70; this is the definition of PYLL (though the choice of age 70 is arbitrary). We could do this calculation again but first exclude from the mortality rates all deaths from motor vehicle crashes. The difference between these two PYLL figures is often computed and in this specific case is called the PYLL *attributable* to motor vehicle injuries.

These are very simple simulation results. But they are by no means innocent. These kinds of figures have been used for decades to trace broad epidemiologic trends (reasonable) and to argue relative priorities (not so reasonable). For example, those interested in advocating a high priority for funding of heart disease research will tend to focus on cause-deleted life expectancy measures (as well as crude death rates by cause of death), since heart disease typically has the biggest impact of any disease in these kinds of calculations. On the other hand, those concerned about carnage on the nation's roads will focus on PYLL for motor vehicle injuries, since these deaths tend to occur at younger ages, and PYLL-type measures give more weight than cause-deleted life expectancy–type measures to deaths at earlier ages.

Moreover, it is a deeply embedded part of the underlying health information system that death certificates, the foundation of mortality rate data, after recording age at death and sex, focus on the cause of death defined in biomedical terms, using the International Classification of Disease (ICD). They do not, as a result, record "smoking tobacco" or "sedentary lifestyle," for example, as a cause of death. On the one hand, this is understandable, because there is only a statistical association between smoking and other lifestyle factors and many causes of death; we do not have the knowledge to ascribe this level of causality at the individual level.

Still, this is unfortunate. Most deaths from lung cancer are caused by smoking. As a result, any plausible scenario that would come close to achieving lung cancer deleted life expectancy, as mechanically calculated by the procedures just described, would require a radical reduction in the prevalence of smoking among the population. But in turn, such a reduction in smoking would also reduce deaths from a range of other tobacco-sensitive conditions, not least of them heart disease.

Thus, from the viewpoint of our understanding of the basic science of lung cancer and heart disease mortality, so-called cause-deleted life expectancy indicators are quite naive. Mechanically or algorithmically, it is straightforward to construct these "what if" simulation scenarios and compute the indicators. But the underlying causal stories are too simple for these kinds of measures to be used as anything more than broad indicators.

In addition, while mortality, ICD-defined causes of death, and derived indicators like life expectancy are obviously useful, they are seriously incomplete. They give us indications of how long we can expect to live but virtually nothing about the quality of life during those years. For this reason, there is a growing consensus for a generalization of life expectancy called *health-adjusted* life expectancy (HALE).

The usual method for estimating HALE is to combine a life table with age- and sex-specific data on average levels of health status in the population. In turn, these average health status levels usually come from a health interview survey. In Canada, HALE is estimated using national health interview survey data (from either the National Population Health Survey or the Canadian Community Health Survey) where the questions for the McMaster Health Utility Index have been included (Feeney et al. 2002).

In terms of the life table calculation sketched above, the basic addition to compute HALE is to add one more column—the average health status at each age (e.g., 0.99 at age 30, 0.75 at age 70)—and to multiply the person-years lived by the hypothetical cohort at each age by this fraction before adding up over the columns and dividing by the starting number of individuals. In other words, a year of life lived, but in less than perfect health, while given a weight of 1.0 in computing life expectancy, is given an "actual" weight of less than 1.0 in computing HALE.[3]

Just as life expectancy can be generalized to produce indicators like cause-deleted life expectancy and PYLLs by (biomedical) cause, HALE can also form the basis for an extended and coherent family of indicators. Such HALE-based indicators give a considerably modified view of the major sources of health problems. For example, depression and arthritis are nowhere near the top 10 of the league table of *burden of disease* if measured only in terms of mortality rates or cause-deleted life expectancy. However, they are much more significant health problems when assessed in terms of cause-deleted HALE (Manual et al. 2003; Mathers et al. 1999; World Health Organization 2000).

Since HALE indicators are based on the concept of life expectancy, they are really hypothetical measures derived from simulations. The most commonly used Sullivan method just sketched is a very naive simulation. For example, the use of cross-sectional health status data does not reflect the underlying disease dynamics. But as we shall see, the more sophisticated microsimulation approach can transform HALE into a very powerful set of health indicators.

MODELING HEALTH CARE

While the focus of this chapter is on simulation models of population health, simulation models can also play fundamental roles in understanding the implications of various health-care policy options. At the same time, for these benefits to be realized, the models must be based on appropriate health data and health statistics infrastructures.

Perhaps the most striking example of a *lack* of statistical preparedness for policy modeling was the Clinton health care reform debate in the United States in the early 1990s. The driving concern in this major policy initiative was the sizable "uninsured" population,[4] which is tracked annually by the Current Population Survey (CPS) conducted by the U.S. Census Bureau. The central policy proposal in the Clinton reform initiative was mandated minimum health insurance coverage to be paid for by employers with federal subsidies. Key policy questions in this context included the overall costs to employers of the additional health insurance premiums, and to the government for the subsidies, plus estimates of the distributions of these costs by geographic region, by the size of the employer, and by industry.

The appropriate methods for answering these fundamental questions include microsimulation modeling, and several models were developed specifically to inform the policy debate (reviewed in U.S. Congress 1994). Ideally, these models would have had as their foundation a data set for all employers, with a description of the kind of health insurance offered by each, including no plan at all. An appropriately designed microsimulation model would then step through each employer, check whether it already offered a package of health insurance above the mandated minimum, and if not, simulate the added employer costs of providing the minimum insurance, as well as the federal premium subsidy. Then, using the starting database on employers and their insurance plans, augmented by the simulated costs of the newly required minimum insurance, the proposed minus the current insurance costs could be summed across employers to get expected new costs to employers, total subsidy costs for the government, and cross-tabulated by geographic region, employer size, and industry to provide estimates of the distributional impacts of the reform.

Partial versions of this data set were available from the government's Health Insurance Plan Survey, as well as the Health Insurance Association of America's Health Insurance Survey. Unfortunately, the first survey was essentially useless because it was missing the most important part of the employer population in the context of the reforms—those employers who did *not* offer any health insurance to their employees. As a result, the Office of Technology Assessment (U.S. Congress 1994, 16) concluded, "These issues place a great demand on the data system, especially in the case of employer subsidies. There is, however, no consensus among analysts on the appropriate sources for firm-level data for the estimation of employer subsidies."

This is a simple, albeit major, example of the close relationships among a national health statistics program, fundamental policy questions, and simulation modeling. In this case, inadequate data severely limited the quality of information available to support the policy debate.

CAUSALITY AND "WHAT IF" QUESTIONS

Concerns about health care, for example the impacts of alternative payment organizations and the extent of the uninsured population, dominate health policy discourse in the United States. However, in most other OECD countries, there is much broader health-care coverage. As a result, policy issues more often focus on the effectiveness and quality of care and on the actual health of the population. In the United States, an increased focus on population health could well have salutary effects on policy discourse. The simple reason is that the health of the population is the proverbial bottom line for health policy, and health-*care* policy is an important, but by no means the only, or even necessarily the most important, determinant. As a result, we focus on population health in the balance of this chapter.

The preeminent summary measure of population health is the generalization of life expectancy to HALE. Coherent families of related HALE indicators, analogous to cause-deleted life expectancy, provide a framework within which trends and patterns in HALE can be understood. Regular production of HALE and related indicators by statistical agencies is therefore central for the ongoing monitoring of population health patterns and trends.

However, these kinds of monitoring indicators, while providing the basis, are insufficient as a guide to action. Decisions, whether for broad matters of health policy, more local issues faced by health system managers, or the daily decisions of individuals, need to be connected to likely health outcomes, including overall population health status as summarized by HALE. In turn, connecting potential changes in behavior or new policy or program initiatives to likely health outcomes should be informed by explicitly articulated causal stories. Ideally, the decision maker wants to know the likely effects of the change being considered. In turn, such projections require an understanding of the most relevant causal relationships.

For example, Figure 16.1 shows a simple diagram representing a *web of causality.* The various boxes represent states or characteristics of an individual, and the thin arrows indicate pathways of causal influence. The block arrows pointing from the "health and health care intervention" oval denote the fact that many interventions modify causal pathways at least as much as individual characteristics.

Some of the relationships shown in the diagram are very familiar, such as the influence of smoking on both coronary heart disease (CHD) and lung cancer. Others are obvious once you think of them but are not as widely appreciated, such as the connection between socioeconomic status (SES) markers like education and smoking. Still others represent areas of active research and debate, for example the idea that unobserved characteristics such as generalized immune resilience might be broadly protective for a wide range of clinical diseases. Finally, this diagram makes a clear distinction between biomedical concepts like clinical disease and vernacular aspects of health status such as pain, mobility, communicating, and remembering.

From the viewpoint of the information needed to support decision making, the causal stories implicit in this diagram, ideally, would be quantitative.

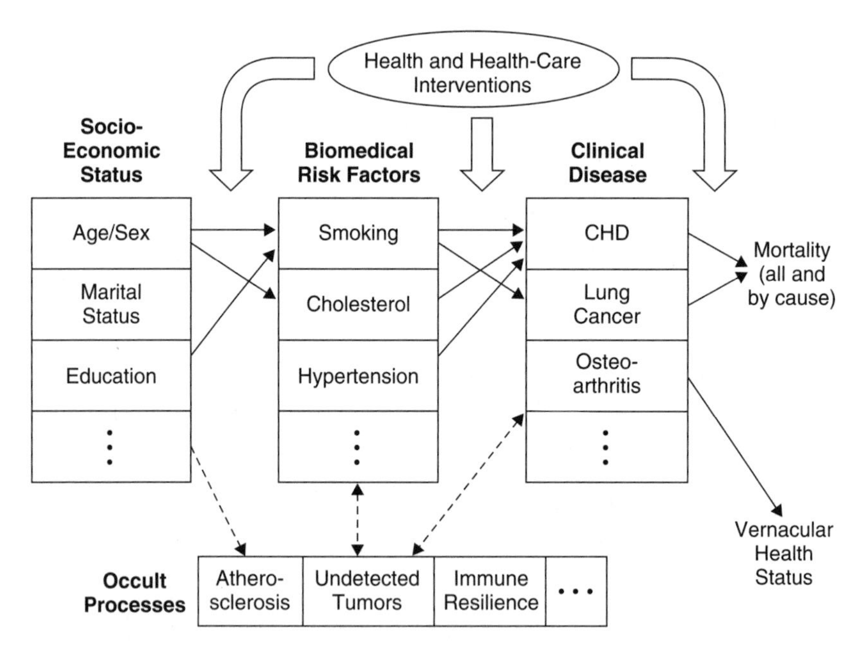

FIGURE 16.1
An illustrative web of causality for health. CHD = coronary heart disease.

They would be crystallized as statistical descriptions of disease processes. These process descriptions would include not only the progression of diseases in terms of severity, but also the multivariate risk functions or transition probability functions connecting diseases to their antecedent risk factors—both the more immediate and widely recognized biomedical factors and the further "upstream" socioeconomic ones. The process descriptions would also include disease sequelae, particularly fatality, and health status expressed vernacularly in terms of disability and functioning. And they would include points where health interventions could modify the way the various processes unfold—whether it is risk factor patterns (e.g., hypertension screening and treatment), disease progression (e.g., coronary bypass surgery), or the expression of vernacular health problems (e.g., pain management or wheelchairs).

Moreover, these statistical descriptions need to capture the heterogeneity of the population—the variety of risk factor profiles and the myriad ways disease processes unfold in actual cases. And finally, they need to be represented in a format that allows the rigorous posing and answering of "what if" questions—such as "What would happen to life expectancy and the (vernacular) burden of illness if we could lower the prevalence of hypertension in the population?" or "What would happen to health disparities if persons with lower education had the same lower smoking rates we observe among those with higher education?". In addition, there should be a "drill-down" capacity to answer questions at a finer level of detail; for example, what are the differences in population health impacts (and health system costs) between lowering cholesterol levels only for those with multiple heart disease risk factors compared to a more broadly targeted intervention?

Answering questions such as these requires not only the ability to estimate a measure like HALE for the population, but also the ability to estimate a hypothetical *counterfactual* HALE—the HALE we would observe if part of the data (e.g., hypertension prevalence) or part of the causal story (e.g., the arrow from education to smoking) were different from what is observed. Moreover, both the projected HALE and the counterfactual HALE need to be estimated jointly, with considerable underlying detail on the population. In other words, what is needed is a policy-oriented or decision support computer simulation model to evaluate prospectively the likely impacts of possible courses of action.

One fundamental challenge is describing the features of the health information system needed to support such modeling. However, before addressing this question, it is important to appreciate the challenges in explicitly and quantitatively modeling the kinds of health processes shown in Figure 16.1. The best-known effort in shifting the focus toward HALE-type measures in health policy discourse, while embedding the derivation of this summary measure of population health in a causal framework, is the WHO estimates of the global burden of disease (GBD), which, in turn, is based on disability-adjusted life years (DALYs) (World Bank 1993; World Health Organization 2000).[5]

The core of the World Health Organization's (WHO) GBD analysis is a series of quantitative descriptions of diseases. For each of over 100 ICD-defined diseases, rates of age- and sex-specific incidence are either observed directly or, much more often (given pervasive data limitations), inferred from corresponding data on the prevalence of each disease, combined with expert judgments on the time individuals can expect to live with the disease before dying of it or recovering. Total mortality (by age group and sex) is also exhaustively partitioned among each of these same 100 or so diseases. The (usually inferred from prevalence data) incidence and duration patterns of disease morbidity are combined with more conventional disease-specific mortality data. Then, in a large series of spreadsheets, all these data are put together in something roughly equivalent to a giant life table. Effectively, at each age and for each disease, the number of years of life individuals "lose," relative to some posited target life expectancy, due to the disease in question, and the number of years lived in a state of less than full health ascribed to the disease, scaled by a *disability weight*, are both estimated. The sum of years lost to premature mortality and the (weighted) years lost to living in less than full health are summed over ages and sex to produce the estimated burden of a given disease, and then summed over diseases to derive the overall burden of disease.[6]

The WHO 2000 GBD analysis was roundly criticized from many perspectives (see Health Systems Performance [hp] Debates by Topic). For the purposes of this chapter, we can note one group of criticisms: that the 2000 GBD exercise was at too high a level of generality. Policymakers reviewing the GBD statistical results could not determine what actions or initiatives they could take that would have the most beneficial impacts. In terms of Figure 16.1, it is as if the causal story included only the clinical disease and mortality boxes.

For example, a Pan American Health Organization (PAHO) meeting noted the idea of a series of *dashboard* health indicators like immunization rates that would be much closer to actions that health ministers could take and be held accountable (Murray and Evans 2003, chapter 3; World Health Organization, Pan American Health Organization 2001; World Health Organization, Regional Office for the Western Pacific 2001). The more recent GBD has taken steps in this direction by focusing on a set of the most important risk factors (e.g., hypertension, overweight, tobacco use, physical inactivity within developed countries) (World Health Organization 2002). The main features of this subsequent analysis that make it more relevant to health policy discussion are, first, the inclusion of this extra set of highly relevant boxes (in terms of Figure 16.1) and, second, a series of carefully constructed "what if" questions and answers. These "what if" questions were based on a series of counterfactual scenarios for potential changes in major risk factor prevalences and their distributions among the population.

These counterfactuals used a series of theoretical minima or targets for each risk factor, such as no smoking at all in the population or lowering a country's mean body mass index to 21. The 2002 GBD study also examined a range of more specific interventions. Rather than supposing that hypertension just disappeared entirely from the population, for example, the analysis looked at a legislated reduction in the salt content of processed foods. However, this part of the analysis was not directly connected to the theoretical counterfactuals and their associated DALY estimates; rather, these were derived from a series of separate simulation models, and the details underlying the results have not been provided.

There is an enormous advantage in having a common metric and a coherent framework for judging the relative importance of different kinds of health problems—the most basic accomplishment of the GBD studies. Showing, for example, the much larger magnitude than is generally perceived of mental health problems compared to, say, infectious diseases, in the overall league table of disease demonstrates a clear policy implication for the relative balance of efforts in these two broad areas of health. However, this is still a rather general kind of advice, one in which specific actions are not obvious without further work. The extension of the work to upstream (in the web of causal pathways) risk factors such as smoking and hypertension moves the analysis in a direction that is closer to the kinds of concrete policy interventions with which health ministries, for example, are familiar. Similarly, extending the framework to include the health-care system, for example surgical and pharmaceutical interventions, would also greatly enhance the salience of the framework for matters of typical health policy discourse.

Still, the causal stories underlying extensions of the GBD analysis, particularly to include risk factors, remain limited. Some of these limitations are inherent in the current state of knowledge, for example determining disease etiology and disentangling the relative importance of various risk factors when the etiology is clearly multifactorial. Our knowledge is seriously constrained by the available data.

On the other hand, there are other limitations inherent in the spreadsheet methods being used that can be overcome by using readily available computer microsimulation methods. These include:

- Explicitly representing the heterogeneity of individuals, not only to reflect more accurately major details of the causal pathways, but also to enable drill-down levels of detail to be viewed.
- Taking account of co-morbidity, both for disease progression and for disability weighting.
- Recognizing correlations in the population among risk factors (e.g., those who are obese are also more likely to be physically inactive).
- Accurately reflecting (nonlinear) interactions among risk factors (e.g., hypertension and cholesterol level, as in the Framingham logistic risk functions for cardiovascular disease).
- Representing dependent as well as independent competing risk factors (e.g., smoking and the risk of either a heart attack or incident lung cancer, or death from stroke or from an automobile injury, respectively).
- Allowing coherent comparisons of the impacts of health and health-care interventions anywhere in the web of causality (e.g., from hypertension screening to stroke rehabilitation).

- Enabling analysis of health inequalities.
- More integrated consideration of the range of elements involved in the web of causality, from upstream SES to biomedical risk factors to clinical diseases to functioning to health interventions.

Essentially, by using more flexible analytical methods than spreadsheets, much more of the detail available from already existing data and published studies can be used.

Key among these better methods is microsimulation modeling (to be defined below). As noted in Mathers et al. (1999, 140), "Data analysis requirements for a complex burden of disease study with many disease categories and population subgroups can rapidly exceed the capabilities of spreadsheet or database software. Microsimulation methods potentially allow a very flexible approach to dealing with many disease and population categories and with the interactions between them (e.g., differing incidence rates for different groups, and comorbidities and interactions between conditions)."

As will be evident, however, there are costs associated with microsimulation modeling, which is why it has not generally been adopted in health analysis (though, as noted earlier, it has been fundamental in tax policy analysis and astrophysics for decades). The main barriers are lack of familiarity, higher initial costs to start the analysis compared to spreadsheets, and perhaps a culture in epidemiology to focus on summary results like "the" relative risk of a given factor, rather than an interest in appreciating and exploring population heterogeneities.

SPREADSHEETS AND MICROSIMULATION COMPARED—THE GLOBAL BURDEN OF DISEASE AS AN EXAMPLE

The fundamental point of "what if" simulations is to inform decision making—both at the level of individual choices and collectively, for example in the design and prioritization of government programs and policies. Key to their usefulness is the plausibility and realism of the underlying distillations of evidence on causal pathways. This depends largely on the availability of data, as well as high-quality published analyses of the data. But the plausibility and realism of the underlying causal stories in a simulation model also depend critically on the way the model itself is constructed.

There are many trade-offs in the development of simulation models, and often it is beneficial to make a range of simplifying assumptions about the underlying patterns of causality in order to reduce the costs of model construction or to make what otherwise would appear a "black box" to prospective users more transparent. There are no right answers here; these trade-offs are matters of judgment. However, spreadsheet-type models, particularly in contrast to microsimulation models, are too simplified, given the dramatic (and continuing) improvements in readily available and inexpensive computing power.

What are the differences between spreadsheet methods and microsimulation? Spreadsheets are an instance of cell-based or *compartment* or semi-aggregated models. The fundamental unit of analysis is a *group* of individuals, characterized by only a handful of attributes—for example, a specific age range (e.g., 30 to 34 years), a given sex, and a specific set of health-related characteristics (e.g., does or does not have CHD, is or is not a current smoker). In the other main approach, microsimulation, the fundamental unit of analysis is an individual; indeed, this is the natural unit of analysis given the kinds of questions to be examined.

In a cell-based or spreadsheet model, the core data structure is a multidimensional array of cells, for example broken down by age group, sex, disease, and risk factor status. With a microsimulation model, in contrast, the core of the model is the set of characteristics of a representative sample of heterogeneous individuals from the population in question.

With population data such as those from a national health interview survey, a set of cross tabs is never as flexible as the microdata file itself, containing all the survey respondents' records. One can always produce a new cross tab if one has the survey microdata file. But producing a new cross tab if all one has is a predefined set of tables is generally impossible, unless the new table is merely a proper subset of the rows or columns of one of the preexisting tables.

Analogously, a microsimulation model is much more flexible than a cell-based model in terms of the potential outputs it can produce since it generates the equivalent of a microdata file. Cell-based models can produce no more detail, and have no more flexibility, than the a priori array of cells on which they are based. More important, a microsimulation model can "absorb" or make use of more complex data without having to make as many strong, simplifying assumptions.

To illustrate these points, recall the calculation of life expectancy sketched above. This is an example of a cell-based simulation model in which the array of cells is called a *life table.* The cells are defined in terms of age (usually single years but, in an abridged life table, 5-year groups), sex, and life status (alive or dead).

As already noted, the commonly used (period) life expectancy is, in a conceptual sense, *out of time.* Even though in reality the mortality rates an individual of age a in year t can expect to face at age $a + 1$ are those of year $t + 1$, period life tables use age- (and sex-) specific mortality rates all from the same calendar year. The alternative, using either or both historical and projected time-varying mortality rates, is called *cohort life expectancy.*

This difference can be illustrated using Figure 16.2. The horizontal axis is calendar time. At any moment in time, such as today, the living population is a mixture of ages, with each age corresponding to a date of birth. If we collect individuals into 1-year or one-decade groups by birth dates, they represent annual or decennial birth cohorts. These successive and overlapping birth cohorts are shown in Figure 16.2 as a sequence of survival curves (in this case for 20-year birth cohorts), starting at the upper left and descending diagonally to the lower right.[7]

Period life expectancy, by far the most widely used health status indicator, uses mortality rates all from the same date. For example, for period life expectancy in the year 2000, individuals born in 2000 are assumed to face the mortality rates of individuals aged 1, 10, 50, 60, and 100 years, all as observed in 2000. It is as if a birth cohort lived its life in the vertical rather than the horizontal dimension in Figure 16.2, hence the notation that this indicator is conceptually out of time. Cohort life expectancies, on the other hand, draw on the mortality rates at each age that actually obtain in that year and are embedded in calendar time. This measure of life expectancy is far less common because it requires historical mortality rates going back for up to a century, as well as mortality rates projected far into the future, in effect spanning all the years on the horizontal axis covered by the birth cohort(s) in question.

Even though the mortality rates that are the main inputs in computing *period* life expectancy are all from observations in the same year, there is a substantive time dimension to the implicit simulation model used to construct the indicator. Everything starts at age 0, and the modeling proceeds one year at a time with advancing age. Indeed, the only difference between the calculation of period (out of time) and cohort (embedded in calendar time) life expectancy is the dates to which the various age-specific mortality rates pertain.

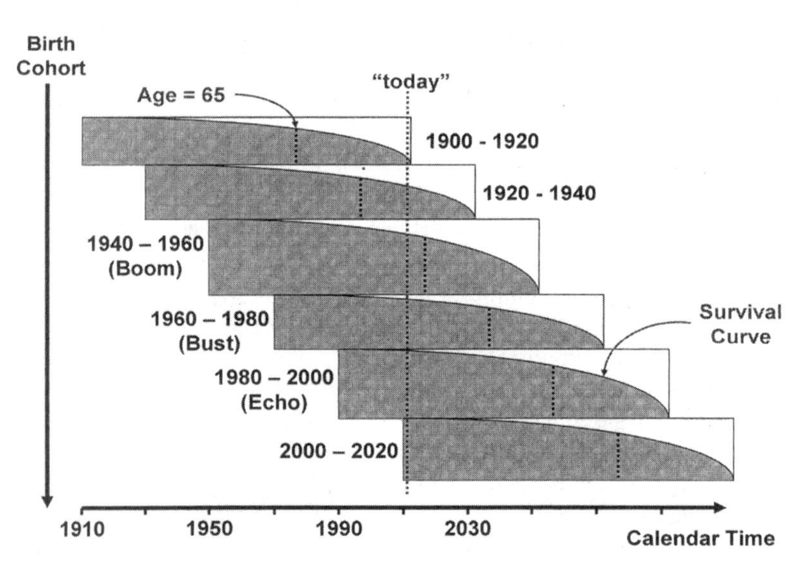

FIGURE 16.2
Overlapping birth cohort conceptual framework.

Turning to the GBD DALY analysis, several versions have been published. In the spreadsheets provided by WHO (Mathers et al. 2001), as well as those in Mathers et al. (1999), the calculation starts with the actual population in a given year and its distribution by age group and sex—equivalent to starting with the surviving populations from each birth cohort along the vertical line for "today" in Figure 16.2. Then, for each age (and sex) group, the burden of disease analysis proceeds in two parts. Years lived with disability (YLD) are estimated, disease by disease, with each disease considered separately. Based on extensive literature reviews and data analysis, YLD_i for disease i is entered into the spreadsheet either based on multiplying incident cases of disease by average duration in years or directly (deemed to be equivalent) as prevalent cases, then multiplied by a disease-specific disability weight for 1 year lived with the given disease.

Note that no explicit consideration is given to co-morbidity. For example, at age 73, some proportion of the individuals will be tagged as being alive with diabetes, and another proportion will be tagged with heart disease. The calculations take no account of, and indeed by construction are unable to represent, whether or not there are individuals alive and suffering from both diabetes and heart disease at the same time, though mathematically and in reality, there are certainly some such individuals. This entails two broad groups of simplification. First, in reality, disease progression and case fatality are influenced by co-morbid conditions. For example, the prospects for an individual who has just suffered a heart attack are quite different, depending on whether or not he is also diabetic. This is ignored in the GBD analysis. The other problem is what weight to assign to a person-year lived with both heart disease and diabetes or both blindness and deafness. The GBD analysis generally assumes (albeit implicitly) that it is simply the arithmetic sum of the disability weights of the co-morbid conditions, though this is unlikely to be an accurate reflection of disability weights elicited from a representative population sample.[8]

Years of life lost to mortality due to disease i (YLL_i) are imputed to the population, as part of a second completely separate and independent calculation, as the annual mortality rate from the given disease times the population at risk in the year times the average number of years between the actual age at death and a posited target age- and sex-specific life expectancy. In effect, cross-sectional incidences for both living with disease and "premature" mortality are imputed based on steady-state assumptions, and then using incidence (either for nonfatal disease or for mortality, all by disease) times expected duration.[9–11]

The "what if" counterfactuals in the GBD 2002 analysis go one step further. For each risk factor, the fraction of each disease that is "caused" by the given risk factor is determined. This *population attributable fraction* (PAF) is multiplied by the YLDs and YLLs for the given disease at each age and summed across ages to get the impact on DALY (i.e., YLD + YLL) of removing or changing the risk factor. One risk factor may have more than one PAF. For example, in the World Health Report for 2002, eliminating smoking in the population is estimated to avoid 90% of all lung cancers and 32% of all cases of cardiovascular disease among men in developed countries (WHO 2002, Annex Table 7). Other PAFs have been estimated for the remaining tobacco-sensitive diseases.

It should be evident from this explication of the underlying DALY algorithm and the counterfactual model that important simplifying assumptions have been made. In part, this is inevitable given data limitations. However, some of these simplifying assumptions derive from the use of a spreadsheet as the basic analytical tool.

One way to see this is to consider how DALYs or HALE would be computed in a more flexible microsimulation approach. This, in turn, is best illustrated by considering a population of individuals, each with a *health biography.* Figure 16.3 illustrates a set of these biographies for one birth cohort from a set of overlapping birth cohorts like that shown in Figure 16.2.

In real life, the population is made up of cohorts of heterogeneous individuals, each of whom can be characterized (for the purpose of health analysis here) by the various blocks of attributes shown down the rows of Figure 16.3. A key portion of these attributes is the disease history, which could be a block of 100 or more rows, one for each disease (as in the GBD analysis). For each disease row and age column, there would be an entry indicating whether or not the individual was suffering from the disease and, if so, its extent of progression or level of severity. In the last year of life, a special marker at the end of the appropriate row could indicate which disease was the cause of death. (Only one would be possible, as is standard on death certificates.)

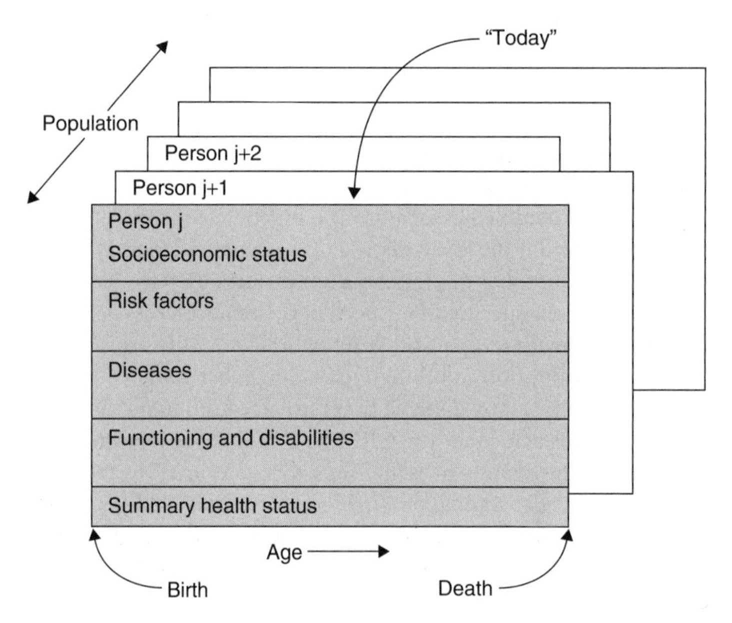

FIGURE 16.3
Illustrative population biographies for a birth cohort.

Each individual's biography could also contain a set of rows tracing his or her conventional biomedical risk factors (e.g., smoking, blood pressure, body mass index, physical activity). It could also track the individual's SES, including fertility and nuptiality, education and work activity, and income. Components of SES (e.g., age at first birth for women, marital status, income) are themselves risk factors for many diseases, often working indirectly through more proximal risk factors, such as the widely observed correlation of smoking with lower levels of income and education.

The most important sequelae of disease are reduced functioning, disability, and premature death. A set of rows is shown for characterizing functioning and disabilities (i.e., a systematic set of attributes characterizing, for example, the individual's ability to move around, communicate, and remember). While disabilities and diseases are related, there is generally no one-to-one relationship. Human immunodeficiency virus may be asymptomatic, for example, while mobility problems could derive from either heart disease or arthritis.

Finally, an algorithm embodying a health status preference function—*disability weights* in the terminology of WHO's GBD—would provide a mapping from the classifications entered into the set of functioning and disability rows to the proverbial bottom line, a row giving a summary health status index at each age—with values of 1 for full health and 0 for dead, with values usually in between for disabilities of various degrees of severity (though states worse than death, hence with values of less than 0, are observed).

Assuming we already had a set of filled-in health biographies like those shown in Figure 16.3 representative of a population, HALE is simply the sum over all ages from birth to death of the bottom row for each individual, then summed over individuals and divided by the number of individuals.

Note that this kind of HALE could be based on a set of biographies constructed analogously to period life expectancy, in which case all the underlying disease and mortality processes would be based on the transition dynamics observed "today," or more likely as estimated from recent data. Alternatively, the underlying transition dynamics could be based on actual historical and/or projected data, in which case the HALE estimate would be analogous to cohort life expectancy. The latter is obviously much more challenging from the viewpoint of data requirements but is also more realistic.

As another option, we could start with a cross-sectional description of the health of a representative sample of the population, for example using a microdata file for the U.S. National Health Interview Survey or the Canadian Community Health Survey. This would correspond to taking a slice down the vertical line for "today" in Figure 16.2 and starting the set of biographies in Figure 16.3 for a given cohort at the point marked "today" at some age $a > 0$ rather than at birth (for individuals of age a in the sample survey).[12]

Given this framework of a representative set of biographies, an alternative microanalytic (as opposed to a spreadsheet or cell-based) approach for calculating DALYs, in the contexts of Figures 16.2 and 16.3, is then straightforward.

Assume again that we have a very large number of Figure 16.3-style biographies already filled in for all birth cohorts (e.g., based on sampling with replacement from the starting representative population sample, and then filling out the biographies from "today" forward, based on methods to be described in a moment). The YLD is essentially the age at death minus HALE for whatever age the individual is at the end of the year considered "today"—in other words, the sum along the bottom row from age $a + 1$ to death of $(1 - \text{health status})$. In addition, for everyone who dies in the year considered "today," YLL is a posited or normative remaining life expectancy at the individual's actual age at death.[13]

A microanalytic reimplementation of the process for estimating DALYs such as this will give results identical to those of the cell-based spreadsheet approach, provided that the data inputs are the same and the number of biographies is large enough.

The process of filling in the biographies, either from birth to death or from age a until death, is what we call microsimulation. A set of these health biographies constitutes the core data structure of a microsimulation model. Ideally, it is based on a very rich set of data and analyses. Statistics Canada's POHEM (POpulation HEalth Model) and LifePaths are examples of this kind of microsimulation model.[14] Since these models are stochastic and follow individuals over their life cycles, they are generically called *longitudinal Monte Carlo microsimulation models.*

A microsimulation model essentially has two loops. The inner loop of the algorithm begins with a blank health biography, starts at the left side of the template, and recursively fills in all the cells, column by column, working from left to right, from age 0 to age at death. Alternatively, the model could start with an individual aged a "today," drawing data from a health survey, for example, and recursively filling out the biography from that age, moving to the right in terms of Figure 16.3.

The outer loop keeps generating new blank biographies (either blank from birth on or from age a on—depending on whether we are modeling a full birth cohort or starting with a representative cross-sectional population, respectively), hands them to the routines of the inner loop, and then accumulates the results. In effect, the model synthesizes one complete biography at a time, and keeps doing this until it has created a sample of millions of biographies.[15] The result of this simulation process is a synthetic data set that is akin to a microdata file from a complete ideal longitudinal panel survey of the population. This longitudinal file can then be cross-tabulated or manipulated to produce the desired indicators such as HALE and DALY, as just outlined. In addition, this microdata file for an idealized panel survey offers the ultimate flexibility for drilling down to obtain underlying detail on the results—such as distributional patterns for health disparities or inequality analysis—and identifying the groups that are better off.

The challenge is how to construct the modules of the inner loop that synthesize individual biographies. The methods for doing so are well developed in the social policy literature and date back to the seminal work of Guy Orcutt (e.g., Orcutt et al. 1978). One of the key challenges is data availability. Many diverse data sets have to be analyzed and assembled in combination with diverse results from the published literature.

To give an example, consider lung cancer and CHD. Both share one major risk factor, smoking, though the relationship is different. Lung cancer incidence depends on cumulative exposure, with a long lag, while CHD depends primarily on contemporaneous smoking rates. The most widely used CHD risk functions derive from the Framingham Study and are based on logistic regressions. As a result, there are interactions among risk factors; the quantitative importance of smoking one pack of cigarettes a day on an individual's risk of a heart attack depends on his or her body mass index, cholesterol level, and so on.

These pieces of data and evidence with regard to causal pathways can be embodied in the model by first including values in each biography for smoking, cholesterol, body mass index, and so on, at age a. These need not be assumed to be independent; data on the observed joint distribution can be directly used. Longitudinal data, to the extent available, can then be used to describe the multivariate risk factor dynamics in the population—for example, the chances of being a smoker and being obese, but not having elevated cholesterol (and so on) at age $a + 1$, given a set of values for these (and other) risk factors (and other attributes such as educational attainment) at age a. For any one biography in the process of being synthesized, random number generators are used to draw from the joint distribution of risk factors at age $a + 1$, conditional on the individual's risk factor (and other attribute) profile at age a.[16]

The risk factor trajectories in any one biography generated by this process will be completely "made up." However, over a sufficiently large sample of synthesized biographies, the joint distributions of risk factors at each age should reproduce those observed, as should the transition dynamics.

Given a profile of risk factors at age $a + 1$ for a biography in the course of being synthesized, the next step is to see if the individual becomes ill with one or another disease. Given the individual's cumulative lagged pack-year exposure to smoking (assuming that this is the relevant right-hand variable in the risk function), the individual's relative risk of developing (or, more accurately, being diagnosed with) lung cancer can be evaluated. Whether or not the individual actually will be tagged as an incident lung cancer case then depends on the draw from a random number generator (uniformly in the unit interval) and on whether this number is less than the observed age- (and sex-) specific baseline lung cancer incidence rate times the just calculated individual-specific relative risk.[17] If it is, the individual is tagged as having a newly diagnosed case of lung cancer, and the model proceeds to simulate further aspects of the disease, such as stage; otherwise, the individual lives another year free of lung cancer.

At the same time, the individual's risk factor profile is plugged into a CHD risk function, such as that from the Framingham Study. Again, a random number is generated and compared to the individual's baseline CHD risk multiplied by the relative risk derived from the risk factor profile. Depending on the comparison, the individual may be tagged as having a heart attack.

Note that effectively, this process, because it is operating at the individual level rather than at the level of some population subgroup, accurately (to the extent of the data) and naturally captures the competing risks of lung cancer incidence and heart attack. Furthermore, to the extent that there is evidence that the presence of one disease affects the incidence or progression of another, that can be readily incorporated—diabetes and CHD is a good example. Indeed, the risk of a heart attack, and the case fatality rate, could easily be made to depend not only on whether or not the individual had diabetes, but also on the severity of the diabetes. The main constraint is the richness of the available data.

Upstream from the risk factors, a range of data on schooling and from family history surveys (to pick two examples) can be drawn on to derive transition dynamics for education progression and attainment, and union formation and dissolution, respectively. Downstream from the diseases, population health surveys, ideally linked to clinical records from health-care administrative data, can be used to create cross-walks between ICD-defined diseases, and the vernacular health states shown at the lower right of Figure 16.1, and the penultimate rows of Figure 16.3. For example, as already noted, both arthritis and CHD cause pain and mobility limitations, though to varying degrees. Moreover, recent work at Statistics Canada (unpublished) shows that Canadians prefer to express their preference values across health states defined in vernacular rather than clinical terms. Additionally, defining health status in terms such as pain and mobility limitations allows the framework to assess interventions that not only reduce the incidence or severity of CHD but also address pain and mobility directly. The key here is the "Rosetta stone" data needed to produce the mapping between diseases (including co-morbid conditions) and vernacular health state descriptors.

Once this disease-to-vernacular health state mapping is available, the final step is the mapping from health states to the bottom line last row of Figure 16.3, a summary numerical index of health status. The sketches above have already shown how this bottom row can be used to compute either HALE or DALYs.

This is a very brief sketch of the microsimulation process.[18] In many ways, it is more general and richer than the risk factor, disease incidence and progression, and case fatality data embodied in the GBD analysis. Still, if the much simplified versions of these processes embodied in the GBD analysis were used in this microsimulation model approach, and if the number of simulated biographies were large enough, it would exactly reproduce the GBD spreadsheet-based results.

Of course, there is little point in replacing the GBD spreadsheets, let alone conventional life tables, with this more complex analytical machinery if that is all one wants to do. But now that we have briefly sketched the main steps in a microsimulation approach, it is immediately apparent where a number of the simplifying assumptions can be easily relaxed.

One is the modeling of risk factors—a key focus for policy interventions. With a microsimulation approach, it is not necessary to simplify the impact of a given risk factor to a single proportion (PAF), in effect assuming that the effects are identical irrespective of age, co-morbidity, and other risk factors. Indeed, the set of rows shown in Figure 16.3 for risk factors (and indeed SES) would be limited only by the availability of data. The values in these rows (e.g., systolic blood pressure, body mass index, smoking rate in packs per day) need not be based on a series of univariate independent distributions but can be drawn from observed multivariate joint distributions—further broken down by age, sex, and possibly other covariates such as marital status and income. For example, the observed correlations among obesity, physical inactivity, and lower SES could be readily incorporated. Moreover, if longitudinal data are available, the persistence of elevated risks revealed by these data could also be reflected in the biographies.

In turn, this would allow much more realistic and relevant counterfactual scenarios to be simulated and explored. For example, the effects on the distribution of hypertension would be far different if there were regulations on the amount of salt allowed in processed food, compared to increased screening followed by medical management of persons with hypertension, two of the scenarios examined in WHO 2002 (World Health Organization 2002, 115) but outside the GBD framework. The reason these scenarios were not integrated with the GBD analysis presumably is that the resulting spreadsheets would have become overwhelmingly complex; myriad added cells would be needed for risk factor levels to capture the differing impacts on the population distribution of hypertension. Indeed, alternatives for targeting risk factor interventions could be assessed from the viewpoint of health impacts.

Another major simplification in the spreadsheet-based models is the treatment of health status. Essentially, each person-year of a prevalent disease is treated as having one weight, independent of other prevalent disease.[19] Conceptually, a far better approach is to base disability or health status weights on a widely agreed-on and widely adopted generic health status measure, such as the McMaster Health Utility Index (Feeney et al. 2002), or the index implicit in the latest round of the WHO World Health Survey, or the new Classification and Measurement System of Functional Health (CLAMES) being developed at Statistics Canada. Doing so, however, would require explicit modeling not only of risk factor and disease dynamics, but also of the key attributes on which these generic health status measures are based—for example, mobility, and pain. Indeed, including these kinds of vernacular attributes in the chain risk factors → diseases → vernacular attributes of function → individual-level health status index would greatly increase the salience and face validity of the exercise. Moreover, it would have the very salutary effect of enlarging the universe of discourse to include interventions that directly target individuals' ability to function in society, thereby broadening the framework beyond biomedical interventions such as open heart surgery and antidepressant medications, and public health interventions such as smoking cessation programs, to include social environmental interventions such as wheelchair accessibility regulation.

A third area of major simplification in the GBD analysis is covariates. It is widely observed that mortality, health status, disease prevalence, and risk factors are all pervasively associated with nonhealth attributes, particularly SES—for example, race, ethnicity, income, and education. Mathers et al. (1999) extended the GBD framework to shed some light on these relationships. The method, however, was not integrated within the GBD analysis. Rather, separate and independent GBD analyses were done for each income quintile, to the extent that mortality and disease incidence rates were available by these quintiles, and the results were then juxtaposed. While this is an important first step, readily available data in many developed countries indicate that the picture is more complicated than this. At the same time that the incidence of disease varies by SES, so do the major risk factors such as smoking and obesity. Spreadsheet or cell-based model approaches to incorporating these data would quickly become intractable. Microsimulation approaches, on the other hand, can readily build in such relationships. For example Wolfson and Rispin (1996) showed that variations in smoking rates by education, working through the effects of smoking on lung cancer and heart disease incidence and mortality, could account for roughly one-fifth of the observed mortality gradient in Canada.

Another important simplification in GBD analyses is the treatment of competing and interacting risks, which are generally ignored. One response to this limitation is to increase the number of cells (or compartments) in cell-based models, so that instead of having either diabetes or CHD, the further possibility of having both is included as a distinct set of cells. However, this strategy requires an almost complete rewrite of the model each time the core structure (numbers, dimensions) of the cells is changed. It also leads quickly to a *combinatorial explosion* as ever more finely divided cells are created in the model. At some point, it becomes impractical to maintain and extend the model.[20]

In sum, then, microsimulation is a natural framework for the modeling of diseases, their upstream causal factors, the downstream sequelae of morbidity and mortality, and the potential impacts of health and health-care interventions. It is far more flexible than extant spreadsheet methods, such as those used in GBD analyses. However, the "costs of entry" to microsimulation are higher—the software and requisite data analysis are more complex. Still, given the great importance the public attaches to health matters and the large size of the health sector in most advanced countries' economies, it is difficult to understand why investments in this superior analytical technology have been lagging.

PREVENTIVE TAMOXIFEN—A MICROSIMULATION EXAMPLE

The discussion of microsimulation modeling so far started with a spreadsheet model and showed how it could be reimplemented using microsimulation. A key point is that microsimulation is *upwardly compatible* from spreadsheet or cell-based models. But the discussion, by focusing on WHO's GBD analysis, started from a point where a host of simplifying assumptions had already been made. Moreover, many of these assumptions were driven not by lack of data, but rather by the need to keep the spreadsheet model manageable.

In this section, we briefly summarize an analysis that was designed and developed with the power of microsimulation in mind from the start. It draws on the results from a major clinical drug trial, using the drug tamoxifen in a new way. Tamoxifen is already established as effective in preventing contralateral breast cancer in women who already have the disease. The question is whether tamoxifen is also beneficial in preventing breast cancer in women who are otherwise healthy but, according to specified criteria, such as having a close relative with breast cancer, are at higher risk.

Figure 16.4 displays the main results of the largest clinical trial designed to answer this question (Fisher et al. 1998). The horizontal axis shows relative risks based on almost 5 years of follow-up—1 is neutral; less than 1 means that the chances of the event happening were reduced. The horizontal bars show the 95% confidence intervals for the effects of this drug used in this preventive manner.

Breast cancer incidence, shown at the top of Figure 16.4, was cut in half, and the confidence interval is quite tight. The drug clearly has a beneficial impact on breast cancer incidence for the population targeted in the clinical trial. However, for other clinical endpoints examined in the trial, such as the incidence

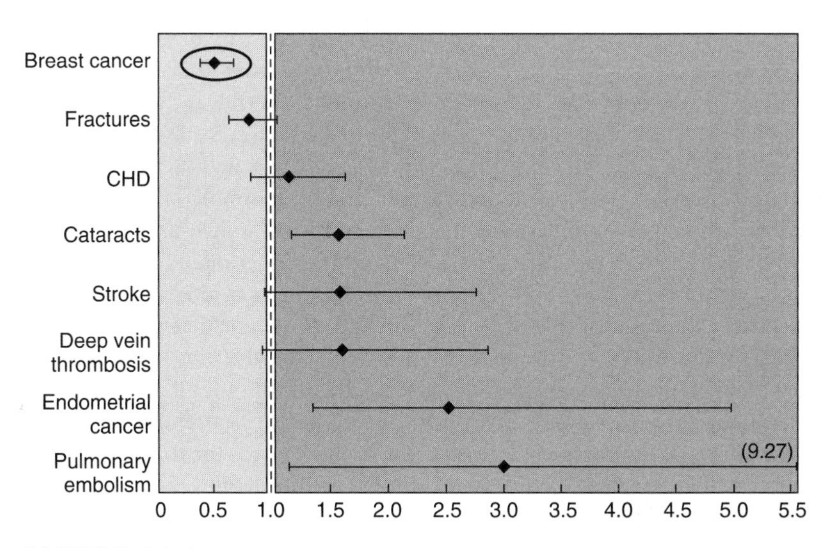

FIGURE 16.4
Relative risks of incident disease from taking preventive tamoxifen. CHD = coronary heart disease. (Source: Fisher et al. 1998.)

of CHD, stroke, deep vein thrombosis, and endometrial cancer, there are highly uncertain but often substantially adverse effects.

Given these ambivalent results, an informed judgment should be based on a careful assessment of the likely joint or overall impacts of all these effects on the population who would be the intended beneficiaries. Unfortunately, the Fisher et al. (1998) tamoxifen trial did not find any statistically significant differences in overall mortality rates between the tamoxifen and control groups, so the trial itself offers no guidance on this most basic question. When there are mixed results, as in the example just given, and population heterogeneities matter, differences between the trial population and the intended population of beneficiaries can be important.

To assess the potential effects of adopting preventive tamoxifen in the Canadian population, a detailed microsimulation analysis was undertaken (Will et al. 2001), building on ongoing work at Statistics Canada to develop a POHEM (Wolfson 1994). The POHEM already had many modules relevant to the task of assessing the tamoxifen clinical trial. The basic framework of demography and mortality was well developed, and a number of disease and risk factor modules had already been implemented (e.g., for breast cancer; Will et al. 2001). As a result, the marginal cost of extending the then current version of POHEM to undertake this analysis was modest. In fact, this illustrates well the point that the microsimulation architecture is open and readily extensible, a major advantage compared to cell-based or spreadsheet models. (Similarly, a recent analysis of colorectal cancer screening was completed using POHEM, where again, relatively modest extensions were required, given the existing investment in the basic model and modeling environment; see Flanagan et al. 2003.)

A central aspect of the trial was an algorithm to identify women at high risk of developing breast cancer. One basic question is, at what threshold of risk is the use of preventive tamoxifen optimal? Another concern was the uncertainty of the parameter estimates of the final published trial results, as illustrated in Figure 16.4. As a result, the model was first augmented by adding a third outermost loop. Recall that a longitudinal Monte Carlo microsimulation model typically has two loops—an inner loop that synthesizes one individual's biography at a time and an outer loop that generates millions of biographies. But the inner loop in this case generates a probability of breast cancer or other disease incidence based on a multivariate risk function with given coefficients. It is these coefficients that are part of the question in assessing the likely impact of preventive tamoxifen for Canadian women. As a result, a third outer loop was added that stepped through various draws from the joint distribution of coefficients for the effects of tamoxifen. To be efficient in this regard, the draws were not random; rather, they were based on a Latin hypercube design, so that 40 replicates of a single simulation were made, systematically sampling from the relative risk distributions illustrated above.[21]

The simulations were also run under a range of scenarios for the risk thresholds used to identify women who would be prescribed the drug. Other scenarios were explored to assess key assumptions where the published results were ambiguous, such as mortality rates for cancers and other disease endpoints not explicitly modeled in the published multivariate analysis, and for effects that might persist beyond the nearly 5-year time frame of the trial follow-up.

The results of this detailed microsimulation analysis were disturbing. At the risk threshold recommended in the trial, about 85% of otherwise healthy Canadian women would be eligible to take the drug at some point in their lives (Fisher et al. 1998). Even though the microsimulation analysis showed, not surprisingly, major reductions in breast cancer incidence, the overall results included a net *negative* effect on the longevity of Canadian women, depending on the assumptions in the sensitivity analysis. Nevertheless, the U.S. Food and Drug Administration has approved the use of tamoxifen as a primary preventive in high-risk women—accepting most of the algorithm for identifying high-risk women. (The main difference is not defining high risk as attaining age 65.)

This analysis of preventive tamoxifen illustrates the power and salience of microsimulation. It has enabled an extrapolation of the clinical trial to assess prospectively its potential impact in a general population. In this case, where the drug has both beneficial and adverse effects, all of which were determined only with a considerable range of uncertainty, the simulation analysis also enabled this uncertainty to be expressed in terms of the overall population health impact and in terms of much more relevant endpoints—all-cause mortality, for example, and not just the incidence of selected diseases.

As a final, more methodological point, this analysis points to a potential improvement in the management of large clinical trials. The tamoxifen trial was stopped early because of the obviously beneficial effects found for breast cancer incidence—notwithstanding Will et al.'s (2001) analysis suggesting the possibility of an opposite adverse result for overall life expectancy. However, if the stopping rule committee had had, at each of its successive meetings, not only access to the accrued data and the statistical results to that point in the trial, but also an updated projection based on a POHEM-style microsimulation analysis of the broader population health impacts, the trial might not have been stopped.

IMPLICATIONS FOR HEALTH INFORMATION SYSTEMS

These examples illustrate the potential of simulation models, especially microsimulation, in the health domain. In both cases, GBD-style analysis generally, and specific clinical analyses such as those concerning preventive tamoxifen use, the models sit on top of, and depend critically on, the infrastructure of routinely collected health data, regularly compiled health statistics, and a growing volume of health research producing multivariate analyses of these data.

However, the evolution of these data, statistics, and published analyses is not optimal from the viewpoint of simulation modeling and addressing important "what if" questions. In addition to analyses of a specific data set's data per se, the idea of meta-analysis, especially with clinical trials, has become widely accepted. When there are a number of trials or studies, all examining the same question but coming to different conclusions, it is sometimes beneficial to pool the results of the various trials and analyze them jointly. As an extension of this idea, simulation models are exercises in meta-synthesis. This involves pooling the results of many data sets and many studies, but not all pertaining to the same question; rather, they pertain to complementary questions.

But for meta-analysis to be practical, each study must include a minimum set of information about the study, as well as sufficient details on the findings, in order to facilitate pooling of results. Analogously, simulation modeling would be greatly facilitated if the underlying health data and statistical infrastructure had coherence and completeness of coverage. For example, it would help if a given concept was measured the same way in all relevant data sets (e.g., disability or vernacular health status) and key population subgroups were not always omitted (e.g., the institutionalized in health interview surveys).

At present, national health information systems development is generally fragmented. Comprehensive simulation models, like that implicit in GBD analyses, and Statistics Canada's POHEM, provide a coherent framework for guiding and prioritizing data development.

To return to some themes introduced at the beginning of the chapter, the idea of models driving (and then coevolving with) data development is by no means new and is well accepted in many fields. The design characteristics of the latest astronomic telescopes are deeply linked to the current state of theory and related observations that point to the next priority areas for new measurements. The characteristics of the System of National Accounts are closely tied to the evolution of the macroeconometric models used by central banks, finance ministries, and major private sector financial institutions.

The situation in health should be similarly guided. Of course, there are myriad specialized areas of research or policy questions where tailor-made data sets are required. There are two caveats, however. One is that there is an increasing appreciation of the need for an overview, a coherent integrated picture of the health of a population, its main determinants, and the most important areas where interventions will likely prove effective. The other is that the costs of collecting data with more than one use in mind are often only marginally higher than the costs of collecting data with only a single primary use. Thus, even specialized data development and collection efforts may be candidates for more generalized approaches. In other words, there are potentially major benefits if health information systems are designed with simulation modeling needs in mind.

This requirement is not as difficult as it might seem, given the current range of drivers for the development of twenty-first-century health information. In general, health information systems are moving in the direction of electronic patient or electronic health records (EHRs). The primary reason for EHRs is to improve the care of individual patients. Among the anticipated benefits are reductions in medical error, an improved continuum of care such as hand-off from one provider to the next, improved privacy protection compared to paper records, and a facility for building in real-time decision aids for clinicians, for example in prescribing drugs.

A secondary reason for EHRs is to provide the information base for better system management. This ranges from providing data to system managers so that they can better monitor the processes of care, such as risk-adjusted lengths of stay, to rates of compliance with appropriateness guidelines, managing waiting lists, monitoring procedure rates, and generating information on use patterns more generally. Even more important, these EHR data will provide a foundation for continuously generating information on the outcomes of interventions, which in turn can be analyzed to help assess what works.

Finally, and most important from the perspective of this chapter, population-level EHR (micro) data can provide many of the statistical foundations for the simulation models just described. These data, when appropriately analyzed (statistically and anonymously), not only provide basic descriptions of the nature and circumstances of the myriad treatment interventions of the health-care system, they also can provide the basis for statistical descriptions of change dynamics. For example, after a heart attack, how long do individuals spend in the hospital and then in postacute home care? What is the likelihood of a second heart attack (and its timing), conditional on the severity of the initial heart attack, the individual's risk factor profile (e.g., still smoking and obese), and the kind of treatment provided (e.g., aggressiveness of revascularization)?

These questions need not be answered only in terms of averages; it will also be possible to derive the distributions of these durations or intervals between events and probabilities of change expressed in terms of multivariate hazards using statistical analysis. Such information is central to the validity and quality of any simulation model results.

Beyond EHRs, another key element of twenty-first-century health information systems is a carefully designed and complementary program of population health surveys. The core already exists in most developed countries—a regular population health interview survey. But several features are fundamental if the health survey program is to attain its greatest usefulness. One is a core set of standard constructs used in all related surveys and operationalized in an equivalent manner. Age and sex are obvious. These constructs should also include at least a summary individual-level measure of health status and measures of key SES attributes such as income, education, and labor market experience.

It is also valuable to ask respondents for their permission to link their survey responses to their health-care administrative records, as has been done in Statistics Canada's health surveys since 1994, with over 90% agreement. The resulting linkages allow us to bring together the (up to now) two separate clinical and vernacular descriptions of health status: health status defined biomedically, in terms of disease from the administrative and clinical records, and health status defined vernacularly in terms of disabilities, activities, and participation (to draw on the main terms in the revised WHO International Classification of Functioning).

Finally, simulation models require more than descriptions of the state of the population and the many relevant attributes of health. They also require the best possible evidence on causal pathways. In turn, this means that our health information system will need to provide the foundations for causal analysis. This is a complex and challenging endeavor. It places a much higher premium on multivariate, multilevel microdata that are longitudinal—in a phrase, *multi, multi milo* data. For example, we need data to capture the evolution in the population not only of average levels of biomedical risk factors, but also how their joint distribution evolves—for example, how physical activity patterns are coevolving with indicators of obesity by age, sex, and SES, and, in turn, how these changes are affecting the incidence of clinical disease and the expression of vernacular health problems.

The vision, then, is for a coherent system of health information along the lines illustrated in Figure 16.5. At the apex of this figure (flattened slightly to indicate that there is no one overall summary indicator), the information system must offer a valid and salient but parsimonious set of top-level summary indicators for the health system as a whole, particularly a basic measure of population health, and its distribution, and the costs and resources used in the health system.

At the base of the pyramid, the foundation is a combination. One part is basic administrative data on the full range of individuals' health system encounters, preferably organized into EHRs for each individual; the other is a sample of responses from a systematic set of health surveys that go well beyond clinical disease to gather information on health, SES, and a range of risk factors, preferably with a core that is longitudinal.

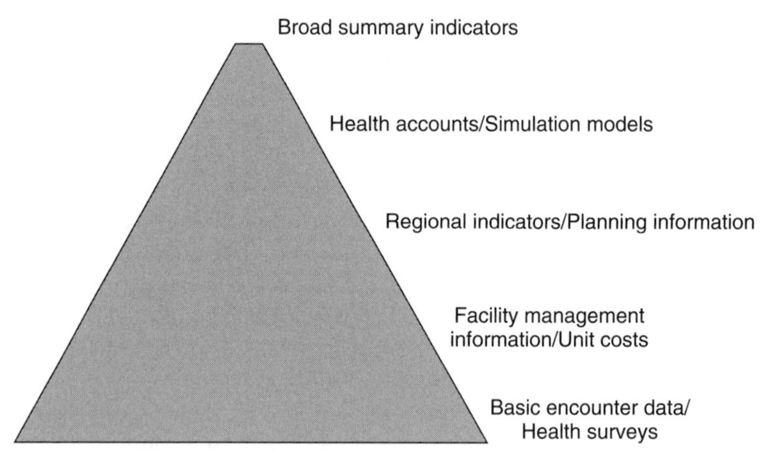

FIGURE 16.5
A vision for health information.

The foundational administrative data must be relevant to the myriad providers at ground level; otherwise, where is the incentive for them to generate high-quality data?

The system must have a bottom-up aspect so that data can be rolled up to local/regional/provincial or state and then national levels, for example to provide data to hospital managers and other health-care facility managers, and for region or province/state-level managers and responsible officials.

The information system must also have a top-down aspect. Overall or summary indicators cannot exist in splendid isolation; they cannot risk disconnection from practical policy choices. There must be a built-in drill-down capability.

There must also be a capacity, at various levels in the middle of the pyramid, to join the resources devoted to interventions with their outcomes. The information system has to support continuous monitoring and feedback on results achieved, as well as research and analysis to determine how well various activities are working.

And key among these mechanisms for integrating information, and providing the basis for planning for the future, is a coherent set of health accounts and (micro)simulation models

ACKNOWLEDGMENTS

I am indebted to editors, Jean-Marie Berthelot, Sally Thornton, and Colin Mathers, for helpful comments on earlier drafts. I remain responsible for any errors or infelicities.

NOTES

1. The focus in this chapter is more generally on health information, a broader notion than health statistics, which is the principal focus of this volume. A good definition of health statistics is "numerical data that characterize the health of a population and the influences that affect its health" (see Chapter 1). The main reason for our focus on information rather than statistics in this chapter on modeling is that the former builds on the latter by adding considerable processing, statistical inference, additional knowledge, and often assumptions. In particular, the outputs of computer simulation models are, in a fundamental sense, made up; they are not directly observed. Ideally, computer simulation model outputs are the same as the data and health statistics we would (eventually, in the case of projections) observe in a world where the assumptions posited in the simulation were true.

2. This description is likely very familiar to most readers; still, it provides the basis for more general ideas to be developed below. It is also simplified. For example, we actually want the numbers of years lived within each age interval, and a special assumption is required for the highest open-ended age interval.

3. This approach is known as the *Sullivan method* (Sullivan 1971). The derivation of the health status weights is a subject of considerable debate and development. Wolfson (1999) gives an overview of many of the issues. See also Murray et al. (2002).

4. The extent of an individual's insurance coverage in the United States is more complex than a simple dichotomy—insured or not. Uninsured individuals may get health care at public hospitals, while nominally insured individuals may find that substantial portions of their health-care costs are not fully covered by their insurance.

5. Even though the GBD analyses focus on DALYs, the HALE and DALY concepts are close enough that it does not matter for this part of the discussion.

6. Actual calculations are more complex than this. The DALYs (though not HALE) include the gap between observed ages at death and some posited target life expectancy. Also, DALYs may be age weighted and are typically discounted. (In principle, HALE could be either age-weighted or discounted, or both, though typically it is not.) Appendixes B and C of Mathers et al. (1999) give examples of spreadsheets for calculating DALYs for specific diseases, while the WHO Web site provides blank ready-made spreadsheets for general use. Both of these illustrate the actual calculations. Mathers et al. (2001) provide a detailed manual for these calculations.

7. The "boom," "bust," and "echo" labels reflect the title of a popular book on demography (Foot and Stouffman 2000) and refer to the sizes of the various birth cohorts in Canada and the United States, reflecting the post–World War II baby boom, the sharp decline in fertility rates in the 1960s, and then the increase in births, though not fertility rates, as baby boomers themselves entered their childbearing years.

8. For some disease pairs where comorbidity is common and the disability weight for individuals with both diseases is unlikely to be simply the arithmetic sum of the individual disease weights, a post hoc adjustment based on the judgment of the analyst using a kind of geometric mean is recommended by the GBD manual. In other cases, such as anxiety disorder and depression, the GBD manual (Mathers et al. 2001) suggests that they could be treated as one composite disease.

9. In algebra, $\text{YLD} = \Sigma_a \text{pop}_a \Sigma_i I_{ia} \text{L}_{ia} \text{D}_i$ or $\text{YLD} = \Sigma_a \text{pop}_a \Sigma_i \text{P}_{ia} \text{D}_i$ and $\text{YLL} = \Sigma_a \text{pop}_a m_a LE^*_a$, so that DALY = YLL + YLD, where a = age; i = disease; pop = population count; I = incidence rate; L = duration (years); P = prevalence (rate); D = disability weight; m = mortality rate; and LE^*_a = the standard or posited life expectancy at age a (based on a life table with LE^* = 80 males, 82.5 females).

10. Note that for conceptual convenience we are ignoring the discounting and age-weighting features of DALYs.

11. Interestingly, this approach to constructing the GBD entails possible inconsistencies. Consider case (a), where a person dies of a stroke at age 75, and therefore has a YLL equal to the posited life expectancy at age 75 and a YLD of 0; and then case (b), where a person suffers a stroke at age 75, lives for a decade, and then dies at age 85. In the latter case, the individual has a YLL equal to the posited life expectancy at age 85 and a YLD of 10 $\times$ the disability weight for stroke (e.g., 0.63 in Mathers et al. 1999). It is possible for case (b) to have a higher DALY than case (a), even though it is obvious that the individual in case (b) lives longer and has a higher health-adjusted life length than case (a). Such paradoxical assumptions are not obvious in the GBD spreadsheet approach. They are implicit, however, and their quantitative significance will depend on details of the estimated durations of various diseases and the choice of the standard life table. I am indebted to Dena Schantzer for pointing this out. Note that this example does not depend on discounting or age weighting.

12. For simplicity, we ignore the fact that the survey likely has a complex sample design, and hence not only has weights, but also has varying sample weights for different individuals.

13. Note that, without loss of generality, we continue to ignore discounting and age weighting.

14. See Wolfson (1994) for an early description of POHEM. Flanagan et al. (2003) and Will et al. (2001) are examples of recent applications of POHEM. Wolfson and Rowe (2004) provide an example of a LifePaths application.

15. This process is feasible on contemporary personal computers, based on experience with the LifePaths and POHEM models at Statistics Canada. See www.statcan.ca, and search on either model name for more information and to download a free copy of a simplified version of LifePaths.

16. Indeed, to the extent that richer data are available, there will likely be evidence that there is *duration dependence*, that is, that risk factors at age $a + 1$ are correlated not only with

risk factors at age a, but also at age $a-1$, $a-2$, and so on. Much of the data on obesity and the failure of weight loss programs suggest this kind of duration dependence. Such evidence can also be readily incorporated into the model.

17. Note that baseline risk is not the same as the observed incidence rate. Rather, it is the rate that would be observed if no one in the population had any elevated risks (or special protective factors). Deriving this baseline risk is challenging. It is estimated based on both the observed average incidence rate and the prevalence distribution in the population of relevant risk factors.

18. It should be noted that many details have still been omitted. For example, the description so far has been couched as if the simulation assumed discrete annual time steps. In fact, the Statistics Canada microsimulation models use continuous time and represent multivariate transitions in terms of waiting time functions. This enables the model, for example, to use hazard regression results directly rather than forcing them into discrete time approximations.

19. Mathers et al. (1999) is a partial counterexample; some of the more significant kinds of co-morbidity were explicitly taken into account and adjustments made, albeit in an ad hoc manner.

20. The original Dutch PREVENT model, while not as complex in terms of the number of diseases modeled, was more explicit about their relationships but only considered mortality and major risk factors (Gunning-Schepers 1989). Still, PREVENT did not allow an individual to have both lung cancer and heart disease at the same time. It was extended, in PREVENT Plus, to include morbidity, but this required a complete rewrite of the model.

21. Since the Will et al. (2001) analysis was constrained to the published data, and nothing was available on covariance, the coefficient distributions were assumed to be independent.

REFERENCES

Feeny D, Furlong W, Torrance GW, Goldsmith CH, Zhu Z, DePauw S, et al. Multiattribute and single-attribute utility functions for the health utilities index mark 3 system. Med Care 2002;40:113–128.

Fisher B, Costantino J, Wickerham DL, Redmond CK, Kavanah M, Cronin WM, Vogel V, Robidoux A, Dimitrov N, Atkins J, Daly M, Wieand S, Tn-Chiu E, Ford L, Wolmark N, other National Surgical Adjuvant Breast and Bowel Project Investigators. Tamoxifen for prevention of breast cancer: report of the national surgical adjuvant breast and bowel project P-1 study. J Natl Cancer Inst 1998;90(18):1371–1388.

Flanagan WM, Le Petit C, Berthelot J-M, White KJ, Coombs BA, Jones-McLean E. Potential impact of population-based colorectal cancer screening in Canada. Chronic Dis Can 2003;24(4):81–88 [cited 2004 Mar 22]. Available from: http://www.hc-sc.gc.ca/pphb-dgspsp/publicat/cdic-mcc/24–4/a_e.html.

Foot D, Stouffman D. Boom, Bust and Echo 2000: Profiting from the Demographic Shift in the new Millennium. Toronto: Stoddart; 2000.

Gunning-Schepers LJ. The health benefits of prevention, a simulation approach. Health Policy 1989;12(1–2):1–255.

Health Systems Performance [homepage on the Internet]. Geneva: World Health Organization; c. 2001 [cited 2004 Mar 22]. Debates by topic [about 1 screen]. Available from: http://www.who.int/health-systems-performance/docs/listofdebates.htm.

Manual DG, Luo W, Ugnat A-M, Mao Y. Cause-deleted health-adjusted life expectancy of Canadians with selected chronic conditions. Chronic Dis Can 2003;24(4):108–115 [cited 2004 Mar 22]. Available from: http://www.hc-sc.gc.ca/pphb-dgspsp/publicat/cdic-mcc/24–4/e_e.html.

Mathers CD, Vos T, Lopez AD, Salomon J, Ezzati M, eds. National Burden of Disease Studies:

A Practical Guide, ed. 2.0. Global Program on Evidence for Health Policy. Geneva: World Health Organization; 2001. The WHO spreadsheet "DALY template.xls" is available from: http://www3.who.int/whosis/menu.cfm?path=evidence,burden,burden_manual, burden_manual_other&language=english.

Mathers CD, Vos T, Stevenson C. The Burden of Disease and Injury in Australia. Canberra: Australian Institute of Health and Welfare; 1999 [cited 2004 Mar 22]. Available from: http://www.aihw.gov.au/publications/health/bdia/index.html#s01.

Murray CJL, Evans DB, eds. Health Systems Performance Assessment: Debates, Methods, and Empiricism. World Health Organization: Geneva; 2003. Available from: http://whqlibdoc.who.int/publications/2003/9241562455.pdf.

Murray CJL, Salomon JA, Mathers CD, Lopez AD, eds. Summary Measures of Population Health: Concepts, Ethics, Measurement and Applications. Geneva: World Health Organization; 2002 [cited 2004 Mar 22]. Available from: http://www.who.int/pub/smph/en.

Orcutt GH, Caldwell S, Wertheimer R, Franklin S, Hendricks G, Peabody G, Smith J, Zedlewski S. Policy Exploration Through Microanalytic Simulation. Washington, DC: Urban Institute; 1978.

Sullivan DF. A single index of mortality and morbidity. HSMHA Health Rep 1971;86(4):347–354.

U.S. Congress, Office of Technology Assessment. Understanding Estimates of the Impact of Health Reform on the Federal Budget. Publication No. BP-H-132. Washington, DC: U.S. GPO; July 1994 [cited 2004 Mar 22]. Available from: http://www.wws.princeton.edu/~ota/ns20/year_f.html.

Will BP, Nobrega KM, Berthelot J-M, Flanagan W, Wolfson MC, Logan DM, Evans WK. First do no harm: extending the debate on the provision of preventive tamoxifen. Br J Cancer 2001;85(9):1280–1288 [cited 2004 Mar 22]. Available from: http://www.bjcancer.com.

Wolfson MC. POHEM—a framework for understanding and modeling the health of human populations. World Health Stat Q 1994;47:157–176.

Wolfson MC. Health-adjusted life expectancy. Health Rep 1996;8(1):41–46.

Wolfson MC. Measuring health—visions and practicalities. Stat J UN Econ Commun Eur 1999;16:1–17.

Wolfson MC, Rispin P. Modeling health and socioeconomic status. Issues Lipidol 1996;5(1): 5–7, 15.

Wolfson MC, Rowe G. Disability and informal support: prospects for Canada. Presentation at the Eighth Conference on Health Survey Research Methods; 2004 Feb 20–23; Atlanta.

World Bank. World Development Report 1993: Investing in Health. New York: Oxford University Press; 1993.

World Health Organization. World Health Report 2000 Health Systems: Improving Performance. Geneva: World Health Organization; 2000 [cited 2004 Mar 22]. Available from: http://www.who.int/whr/previous/en.

World Health Organization, Pan American Health Organization [report]. Regional Consultation on Health System Performance Assessment; Washington, DC: World Health Organization; 2001 May 8–10.

World Health Organization. World Health Report 2002: Reducing Risks, Promoting Healthy Life. Geneva: World Health Organization; 2002 [cited 2004 Mar 22]. Available from: http://www.who.int/whr/previous/en.

World Health Organization, Regional Office for the Western Pacific. Regional Consultation on Health System Performance Assessment, Manila, Philippines; 3–5 July 2001. Manila (the Philippines): World Health Organization, Regional Office for the Western Pacific; 2001 [cited 2004 Mar 22]. Available from: http://www.who.int/health-systems-performance/regional_consultations/wpro_report.pdf.

PART V

Transforming Health Statistics Through New Conceptual Frameworks

In Chapter 1, Parrish, Friedman, and Hunter present a model of the influences on population health (Figure 1.3) that can be used to conceptualize the broad array of topics that need to be addressed by the health statistics enterprise. The four chapters in this part explicitly and implicitly build on Figure 1.3 and similar models of population health, and focus on new conceptual frameworks that can transform health statistics.

In Chapter 17, Zelmer, Virani, and Walker provide a global overview of new developments in health statistics and population health information systems. They argue that the evolving and expanding understanding of health, population health, and their determinants has led to increased demands for more and different data and information. In particular, these demands focus on the need for broader data on multiple determinants of health, as well as data capturing a broader concept of health. Different countries have responded to these new demands in different ways, but common themes are emerging in those national responses. Zelmer, Virani, and Walker, using a wealth of examples from countries throughout the world, explore these themes.

In Chapter 18, Black, Roos, and Roos also reflect on the need to adjust health statistics to a broader definition of population health. Stressing the importance of the use of models of the influences on population health, they emphasize that health care is only one of many factors that influence health. The recognition that multiple factors affect population health, including many factors outside of the health services sector, provides an important perspective necessary for developing enhanced and more useful health information systems. Black, Roos, and Roos go on to illustrate the possibilities of new health information systems through their discussion of POPULIS, a Manitoba Centre for Health Policy system that enables the study of many factors affecting population health.

In Chapter 19, Starfield expands on the evolving understanding of population health and its implications for health information systems. As she points out, diseases are becoming less important in managing population health and as a basis for allocating resources. Co-morbidities, rather than diseases, are emerging as a major challenge for health statistics, health information systems, and health policy. The recognition of the central role of co-morbidities, coupled with recognition that population health is not just the aggregation of the health states of individuals, is leading to new measurement issues that must be confronted by health statistics. Starfield illustrates these issues by discussing two promising new approaches for characterizing population health: Adjusted Clinical Groupings and mutually exclusive profiles of health.

In Chapter 20, Lumpkin and Deering show how the evolving definition of health is reflected in the need for the development of a National Health Information Infrastructure (NHII) in the United States. In terms of technology, the NHII will consist of an electronic web of computer and communications technologies. But, as represented by Lumpkin and Deering and as conceptualized by the National Committee on Vital and Health Statistics, the NHII will extend far beyond its technical infrastructure, and will include "values, practices, relationships, laws, standards, systems, [and] applications." The NHII will focus on finding the tools and structures, some technological and others not, to improve knowledge exchange and communication on a broad range of health issues, including health care, population health, and consumer health.

CHAPTER 17

Recent Developments in Health Information: An International Perspective

Jennifer Zelmer, Shazeen Virani, and Jennifer Walker

This chapter provides an overview of the status of recent developments in health information at a national level in selected developed countries, including common strategies, trends, and future directions. It draws primarily on the experience of countries other than the United States.

NATIONAL HEALTH INFORMATION STRATEGIES AND ORGANIZATION

Over the past decade, the organization and delivery of health services has changed significantly in many countries. At the same time, our understanding of health and its determinants is evolving, and there is greater demand for evidence on which to base health and health-care decisions. Every year there are also significant advances in information management and technology capabilities. As a result, expectations for health information are growing.

In response, many countries and jurisdictions within those countries have made major efforts to enhance their health information capacity. Typically, programs include enhancements to basic infrastructure, information systems and networks, standards, data collection and analysis, the capacity for timely access to relevant information, and much more. These coordinated programs represent significant multiyear investments. The ultimate goal, broadly, is to use information and information technology to improve health and health care.

As part of a health information strategy, some countries have created or enhanced their national data collection and analytic capacity, often within the ministry responsible for health. In France, for example, the Ministry of Employment and Solidarity houses the Directorate for Research, Analysis, Assessment, and Statistics (DREES). Established in 1998, DREES brings new analytic and assessment capacity to health information previously administered within the Ministry by the Office of Statistics, Research, and Information Systems and the Research Unit (National Institute for Statistics and Economic Studies [hp] The public statistical system). Another example is the New Zealand Health Information Service (NZHIS), set up by the Ministry of Health (New Zealand Health Information Service [hp] About NZHIS). The division collects and reports on data on health status, hospital use, health workforce, and mental health (New Zealand Health Information Service [hp] Data and services).

In addition, some countries have developed or used independent agencies responsible for coordinating health information and statistical activities at a national level, often in cooperation with the national statistical agency and/or ministry of health. Examples include the Australian Institute of Health and Welfare (AIHW) (Australian Institute of Health and Welfare [hp]), the Canadian Institute for Health Information (CIHI) (Canadian Institute for Health Information [hp]), the Korean Institute for Health and Social Affairs (Korean Institute for Health and Social Affairs [hp]), and the National Research and Development Centre for Welfare and Health (STAKES) in Finland (National Research and Development Centre for Welfare and Health [hp]).

In Australia, the AIHW was set up in 1987 to inform community discussion and decision making through national leadership in developing and providing health and welfare statistics and information (Australian Institute of Health and Welfare 1999). The AIHW is an integral player in carrying out Australia's National Health Information Agreement, which provides a framework for national health information activities and cooperation (Australian Institute of Health and Welfare [hp] National Health Information Management Group). It originally came into effect in 1993. The Commonwealth, State, and Territory health authorities, the Australian Bureau of Statistics, and the AIHW are signatories to the agreement (Australian Institute of Health and Welfare 2000). Within this broad context, a number of key activities have been undertaken, including the following:

1. *National Health Information Work Program*: annual programs outlining health information development projects to operationalize the rolling triennial AIHW Corporate Plans (Australian Institute of Health and Welfare 1999, 2003).
2. *National Health Information Development Plan*: a plan providing key stakeholders with a list of accepted priorities for national health information (Australian Institute of Health and Welfare, Australian Health Ministers' Advisory Council 1995).

3. *National Health Information Knowledgebase*: an Internet-based site covering national health metadata (data about data), integrating the National Health Information Model, the data dictionary, and other material (Australian Institute of Health and Welfare [hp] The Knowledgebase).
4. *National Aboriginal and Torres Strait Islander Health Information Plan*: a plan to improve the quality of indigenous health information (Aboriginal and Torres Strait Islander Health and Welfare Information Unit, Australian Health Ministers' Advisory Council 1998).

In Canada, the report of the National Task Force on Health Information in 1991 initiated a period of considerable national activity related to health information (National Health Information Council 1991). A key result of this report was the formation in 1993 of CIHI, an independent, not-for-profit organization mandated to coordinate the development and maintenance of a comprehensive and integrated health information system for Canada. Like Australia's AIHW, CIHI's plans are developed collaboratively with federal, provincial, and territorial governments, as well as a range of other stakeholders. Strong collaboration with Statistics Canada, the national statistical agency, is particularly important.

In 1999, pan-Canadian consultations on health information needs and the report of the Federal Minister of Health's Advisory Council on Health Info-Structure led to significant additional investments in health information (Advisory Council on Health Infostructure 1999). Funding was announced in the February 1999 federal budget to support enhancements to national surveillance activities; improved access to health information; the implementation of the Health Information Roadmap, a shared vision for modernizing Canada's health information systems; and other activities (Canadian Institute for Health Information 1999a, 1999b, 2001). The Roadmap initiative focuses on providing answers to two basic questions: "How healthy are Canadians?" and "How healthy is Canada's health care system?" Through this initiative, Statistics Canada, CIHI, and other agencies are collaborating to conduct special studies and produce regular reports, to address data gaps, to establish data standards, and to create a Canadian Population Health Initiative. In 2002, renewal of Roadmap funding for a second multiyear period was announced.

NATIONAL HEALTH DATA COLLECTIONS

Regardless of how a country has chosen to organize health information activities at a national level, most developed countries have implemented a common core set of data collections, including:

- Vital statistics (births, deaths, marriages, and divorces).
- National population-based health interview surveys.
- Statistics on key health risk factors, socioeconomic variables, and other

nonmedical determinants of health from surveys or other sources (e.g., unemployment, education, and income levels).
- Communicable disease statistics (e.g., tuberculosis, measles, and chlamydia).
- Hospital facility statistics (e.g., beds, services, and financial data).
- Hospital inpatient discharge statistics (e.g., length of stay, diagnoses, procedures, and patient demographics).
- Health human resources statistics for regulated health professions.
- Macro-level health expenditure data.

Beyond this core, data collections vary, depending on national priorities, progress of implementation efforts, and other factors. Particular countries have implemented a broad range of additional data collections, including:

- Immunization statistics.
- Expanded maternal and perinatal health data.
- Clinical registries for selected health conditions (e.g., cancer, diabetes, and end-stage renal disease).
- Facility statistics for health-care institutions other than hospitals (e.g., nursing homes and other residential care facilities).
- Data on outpatient hospital services, physician visits/payments, pharmaceutical use, mental health services, home care, oral health care, and other nonhospital services.
- Collection of physical measures (e.g., blood samples) as part of population health surveys.
- Surveys of patient and/or public satisfaction with health services.
- Waiting list and patient safety statistics.

The outcome is that the extent of countries' health data collections varies widely. Figure 17.1 compares the availability of health and health system indicators in 29 countries. The results are based on statistics reported in OECD Health Data 99 (Organisation for Economic Co-operation and Development 1999), the Organisation for Economic Co-operation and Development's (OECD's) annual set of health indicators for member states.[1]

The 1999 edition covers health status, health-care resources, health-care use, health expenditures, financing, and remuneration, social protection, the pharmaceutical market, nonmedical determinants of health, and contextual demographic and economic variables. Countries report national data for standardized indicators based on health surveys, administrative data, and other information sources.

COMMON TRENDS AND FUTURE DIRECTIONS

Fiscal, demographic, technological, and other factors are contributing to rapid change in the organization and delivery of health services in most developed

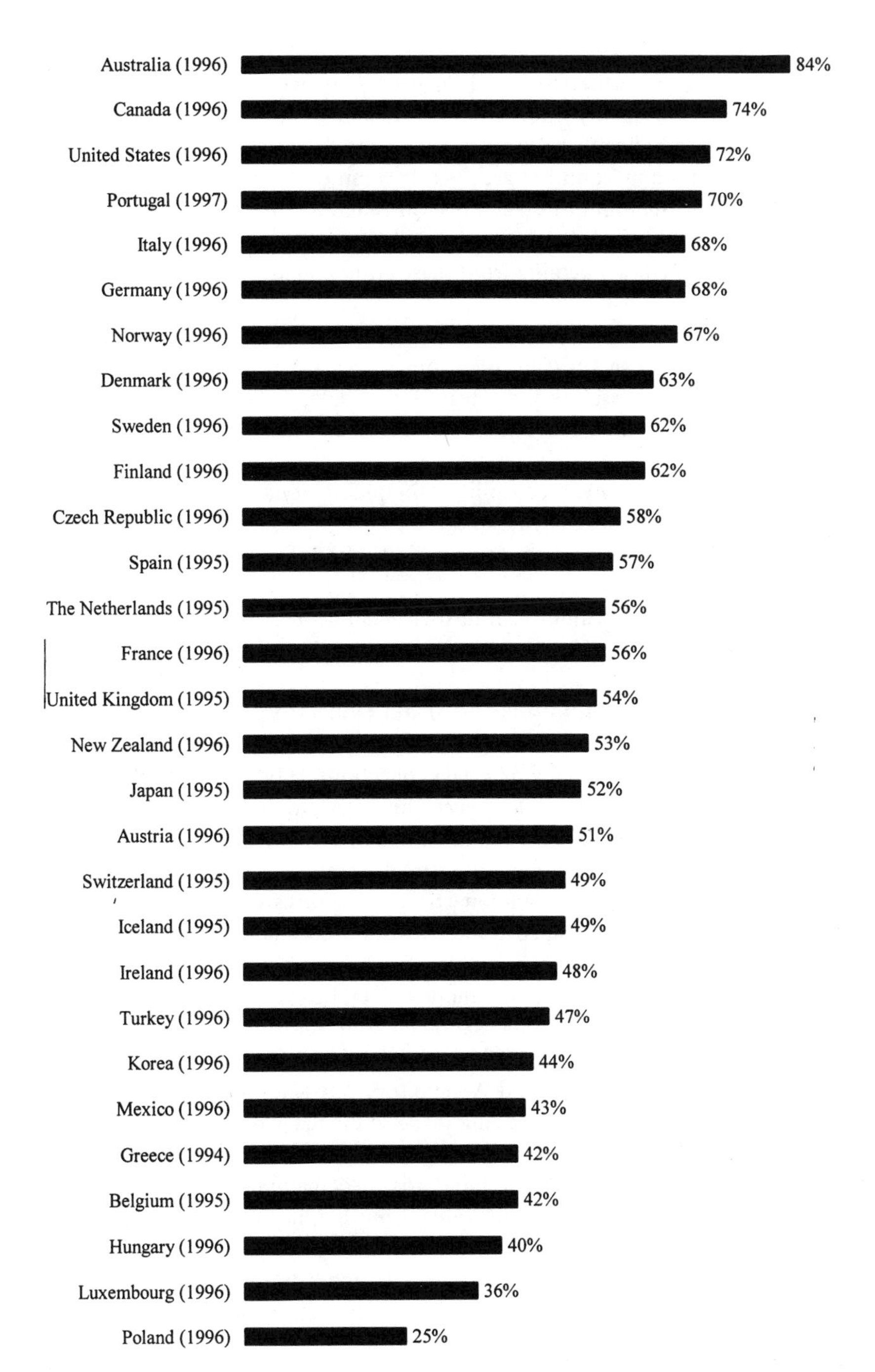

FIGURE 17.1
Coverage and timeliness (median year of most recent data) of health data in OECD countries. (Source: Organisation for Economic Co-operation and Development 1999.)

countries. Health information must keep pace. Enhancing the capture, dissemination, and use of quality information is often cited as one of the keys to improving health and health services.

As a result, many countries are making significant investments to enhance their health information infrastructures. Considerable effort is also being made to improve health information capacity at the national level.

Common themes emerging from these efforts include:

- Renewing traditional data collections and extending the content, coverage, and quality of key data collections.
- Increasing the flexibility and integration of data.
- Ensuring personal privacy and the confidentiality and security of personal health information.
- Improving the utility, accessibility, and quality of data through innovations in analysis and dissemination.
- Increasing international cooperation in health information.

These themes are examined in further detail below.

Renewing and Extending Health-Data Collections

Vital statistics were among the first data collections to be widely implemented in most countries. In the past 20–30 years, however, the emphasis has shifted to statistics related to population health, the health system, and the use of health services, particularly in the inpatient hospital sector.

In many countries, these traditional data collections are now being revised to reflect evolving patterns of practice and trends in information management. For example, in some countries, considerable effort has been invested in the development of national health information models, data dictionaries, and meta-data. A case in point is Australia, where the National Health Information Knowledgebase integrates a broad range of material in an accessible Internet-based application (Australian Institute of Health and Welfare [hp] The Knowledgebase).

Significant changes are also being made to the data collections themselves. Information systems are being upgraded; some minimum data sets are being revised; diagnosis and intervention standards are being updated worldwide; and options for reducing the survey respondent burden, facilitating the capture of administrative data, and improving data quality are being explored. New data collections, such as those used to monitor waiting lists and patient safety, are also being introduced to address emerging policy questions.

Other profound changes are also taking place. Several countries are designing and implementing an expanding range of data collections that will cover more of the continuum of care and track postcare outcomes. For instance, Australia,

Canada, New Zealand, and other countries are developing new minimum data sets in areas such as mental health and home care (Canadian Institute for Health Information [hp]; Grant and Petrie 2001; Ryan et al. 1999; New Zealand Health Information Service [hp] Mental Health Information National Collection). The number of clinical registries that follow individuals with particular health conditions (e.g., diabetes or end-stage renal disease) or interventions (e.g., transplants or joint replacements) longitudinally is also growing. In addition, there is increasing appreciation of the need to reorient health information activities to move beyond health services and focus on health and its broad determinants—from data on illness to data on health.

Increasing Data Integration

Addressing fundamental questions about health and health services requires data on factors that affect health, the health status of individuals and how it changes over time, and individuals' encounters with the health system. Historically, data have tended to be divided into silos—one for vital statistics, one for health surveys, one for hospitals, one for physician services, and one for financial data. Given that the determinants of health and illness are complex and that successfully addressing health issues frequently requires the collaboration of multiple institutions and professionals, this fragmented approach is no longer sufficient.

Many countries are recognizing that the ability to readily integrate different types of micro-level health data—within the context of stringent privacy, confidentiality, and security safeguards—is essential. Otherwise, systematic connections cannot be made between surgery in one hospital and complications treated in another. Likewise, the ability of an individual to return to his or her normal daily tasks after a knee or hip replacement and the amount of time spent in rehabilitation care in the interim are not routinely connected to the data on the surgery itself. These types of connections are necessary to assess the cost effectiveness and long-term outcomes of different health interventions and to disentangle the effects of a broad range of risk factors on health.

One new development in this area is the high level of investment in modernizing health information systems. A 2002 review of health information and technology activities underway in nine developed countries found many similarities in approaches being used (Table 17.1).

These activities, particularly the focus on developing electronic health record (EHR) systems, have the potential to significantly affect the health information capacity in the future. The EHR is visualized as an integrated health record that would follow individuals throughout their life span, capturing their experiences with the health system and other information, such as their health status and risk factors. Proponents argue that EHRs would enhance accessibility to a patient's complete health and health-care history within comprehensive privacy

TABLE 17.1

Health Information Activities Underway in Nine Developed Countries

	United Kingdom	*New Zealand*	*Australia*	*USA*	*Italy*	*France*	*Japan*	*Germany*
National Strategy	"Information for Health"	"Health Information Strategy for the Year 2000"	"Health Online"	"National Health Information Infrastructure"	Health Info. System	National Project	National Project	National Project
Standards*	Yes	Yes	Yes	Yes	Yes	Yes	Yes	Yes
Privacy and Security of Information†	Yes	Yes	Yes	Yes	Yes	Yes	Yes	Yes
Health Network‡	Yes	Yes	Yes		Yes	Yes	Limited	Limited
Digitization of Patient Information§	Yes	Yes	Yes	Yes		Yes	Yes	Yes
Telehealth//	Yes	Yes	Yes	Yes				Yes
Education and Training#	Yes	Yes	Yes	Yes	Yes			Yes
For further information	National Health Service (1998)	Ministry of Health (1996)	National Health Information Management Advisory Council (2001)	National Committee on Vital and Health Statistics (2001)	Rogers (1999)	Joch (1999)	Rogers (1999)	Nadarajah (1999)

*Standards: to allow seamless connectivity between systems and to improve the availability, quality, and reliability of health data and information.
†Privacy and Security: to ensure that personal health information, given in confidence, remains safe.
‡Health Network: a health system network through which information can flow securely between health service delivery locations.
§ Digitization: an electronic health record of comprehensive personal health information.
//Telehealth: the use of technology to enable remote diagnostic services and care.
#Education and Training: prerequisite education and training of service providers and managers.
Source: Adapted from Advisory Committee on Health Infostructure (2001).

and confidentiality protections. In addition, some suggest that one of the benefits of the proposed systems is the enhancement of clinical, epidemiologic, and health administration research.

Many countries have EHR initiatives underway. For example, Australia has tested the concept of a national health information network called HealthConnect (Australian Government Department of Health and Ageing [hp] Welcome to HealthConnect; HealthConnect Program Office 2001). In this project, electronic patient records (EPR) would be captured in a standardized format and networked for access by authorized health service providers. Patients would control access to their records and would have access themselves. Similarly, in England, the National Health Service plans to implement EPRs in all hospitals and Primary Care Trusts by 2006 (National Health 2002). A subset of the EPR will contribute to a lifelong EHR to improve the ability to assess the continuum of health status and health care over the life span. The vision is that all patients will have access to their EPR, health-care providers will have access to the patient's medical history, and health planners will have integrated aggregate information to support analysis and decision making (National Health Service Information Authority [hp] Information for health).

In addition, several countries have already made significant progress in building the infrastructure required to effectively integrate a wide range of health data. This includes establishing an appropriate policy and legislative framework and the professional and technical capacity to integrate existing data sets. Standards are also needed to reduce fragmentation and ensure comparable and integrable data. Examples include common geographic references, consistent data standards, and common identifiers. For instance, a uniform anonymous linkage code is created for each hospital patient in Switzerland. Other than a subset retained for epidemiologic purposes (children under 15 years of age, adults over 64 years of age, and a sample of the population between 15 and 64 years), these codes are destroyed after 10 years (Swiss Federal Statistical Office 1998).

Personal identifiers are generally developed for administrative rather than statistical purposes. Their sources and scope of use vary considerably from country to country. In some cases, civil registration numbers are used. In others, specific identifiers are created for use in the health system. The structure of identifiers also varies. For example, in the mid-1990s, Denmark, England, and Sweden had 10-digit numeric codes; New Zealand used a 7-digit alphanumeric National Health Index; and in Canada, 8- to 12-digit numeric or alphanumeric codes were assigned by the provinces/territories (Partnership for Health Informatics/Telematics 1996).

Many countries are regularly performing analyses that take advantage of those data that can already be integrated consistently. For example, expanding record linkage for research and statistical purposes was one of the priorities identified in Australia's National Health Information Development Plan in 1995. Substantial progress has been made in this area of the Plan (Australian Institute of Health and Welfare 2000). For example, the Australian Bureau of Statistics has announced that it will begin linking administrative data to household survey data with consent. Also, in 1998–1999, the AIHW approved 41 projects linking data from two large databases, the National Death Index and the National Cancer Statistics Clearinghouse. It reports that these studies have contributed to knowledge about the patterns of disease in specific populations and for specific diseases.

Canada has also made considerable progress in data integration. For some time, research institutes in several provinces have successfully brought together a wide range of data. These include administrative data on physician visits, hospitalizations, and pharmaceutical use; survey data from health interview surveys and the census; and a variety of other sources. Chapter 18 provides further information on the goals and results of these efforts in one province.

Similar initiatives are also underway at the national level. For instance, respondents to Canada's National Population Health Survey (NPHS) and the Canadian Community Health Survey (CCHS) are routinely asked for consent to link their survey responses with health services data from administrative data sets for statistical purposes (Statistics Canada 2000, 2001). The vast majority of respondents agree to this linkage. Over the coming years, Statistics Canada will be using the NPHS and other sources as part of its ongoing effort to develop person-oriented information, integrating individual-level microdata across time and data collections, to answer key health questions.

Similar programs also exist in several other nations. For example, Denmark regularly integrates a wide range of individual-level data using the Danish civil registration number. Data collected from services performed by general practitioners (generating approximately 72 million records per year), dispensed prescriptions, and hospitalizations are brought together in the Health Statistic System. Access rights depend on the user's professional affiliation (Ministry of Health, Denmark 1998).

Likewise, Finland's STAKES links its register-based data collections for statistical or, in special cases, scientific purposes. Identifiers are typically encrypted. In some cases, third parties perform the integration of data to ensure confidentiality (National Research and Development Centre for Welfare and Health [hp]).

Ensuring Privacy and Confidentiality

Privacy is a fundamental value that is widely recognized. In most developed countries, the collection, use, linkage, disclosure, and retention of health information take place within established privacy and confidentiality principles and policies. This framework builds on ancient professional pledges of confidentiality such as the Hippocratic Oath:

> Whatever, in connection with my professional service, or not in connection with it, I see or hear, in the life of men, which ought not to be spoken of abroad, I will not divulge, as reckoning that all such should be kept secret.
>
> (*Hippocrates, fifth century* B.C.)

Professional pledges of confidentiality remain a key component of the privacy protection landscape. However, today's multifaceted and increasingly computerized health systems also require a more complex set of legislative, policy, regulatory, and technical strategies to protect personal privacy and safeguard the confidentiality and security of health information.

Recent legislation is generally modeled on the core principles outlined in the OECD Guidelines on the Protection of Privacy and Transborder Flows of Personal Data (Organisation for Economic Co-operation and Development 1980):

- Data collection limitation
- Data quality
- Purpose specification
- Use limitation
- Security safeguards
- Openness
- Individual participation
- Accountability

For example, Australia and Canada have broad, cross-sector, federal privacy legislation covering the activities of associated government agencies. The Australian Privacy Commissioner recently augmented the existing legislation to cover health information in the private sector with the Privacy Amendment (Private Sector) Act 2000, including new Guidelines on Privacy in the Private Health Sector (Office of the Federal Privacy Commissioner [hp] Guidelines on privacy in the private health sector). Canada's federal legislation is also evolving to cover a broader scope of activities. As in most countries, this legislation is supplemented by state/provincial/territorial privacy laws and confidentiality clauses in health-related legislation. National guidelines and standards, such as Australia Standards' Personal Privacy Protection in Healthcare Information Systems (Australia Standards 1995) and the Canadian Standards Association's Privacy Code (Canadian Standards Association 1996), also play an important role.

Members of the European Union (EU) were required to implement the EU's Directive on Data Protection (Directive 95/46/CE) by October 1998 (European Commission, Legal Advisory Board 1995). Several European countries—Austria, Belgium, Finland, Italy, Portugal, Sweden, and the Netherlands—have revised their legislation as a result (European Commission [hp] Data Protection). For instance, an updated Data Protection Act received Royal Assent in England in July 1998 (provisions come into force over the following decade). Information related to an individual's health is categorized as *sensitive*, requiring special protection.

In addition to general legislation, New Zealand has a Health Information Privacy Code 1994 that specifically covers health information (Office of the

Privacy Commissioner 2000). It grants individuals the right of access to public health sector records and provides for the development of codes of conduct in liaison with the Privacy Commissioner, who is responsible for implementing access and other privacy policies in the private sector. The Code covers all health agencies and protects all personal information related to an identifiable individual. Health information protection legislation is also in place in several Canadian provinces (Privacy Commissioner of Canada [hp] Sector specific legislation dealing with privacy).

Technical security and other measures complement legislation and national standards/guidelines in most countries. The protection of privacy, confidentiality, and security is rapidly becoming a central design feature of health information systems in many countries. For example, some health authorities are investigating the use of innovative technological solutions to prevent unauthorized access to confidential data.

MAKING HEALTH INFORMATION MORE ACCESSIBLE

Data are useful only when they are analyzed and when the resulting information reaches its intended audience in a form that is accessible and easy to use. Many nations are taking advantage of advances in technology and improved health data to develop tools that make health information more accessible to a variety of audiences, including the general public. These tools are often supplemented with regular reports based on current statistics that present an overview of health and the health system in an understandable form.

In recent years, there has been increasing emphasis on the value and importance of reporting standardized comparative health data. Internationally, this has led to sustained efforts by the World Health Organization, OECD, and others to compile and disseminate consistent data for a range of indicators for member states. These data are also included in regular broad-based reports on health, such as the World Health Report (World Health Organization 2001).

A recent initiative by the International Organization for Standardization (ISO) focused on achieving an international consensus on a health indicator framework patterned after Canada's National Population Health Indicators Framework (International Organization for Standardization 2001). The framework would encompass indicators of health status, the determinants of health, health system performance, and community and health system characteristics. The belief is that adoption of a standard framework would foster cross-national comparisons and facilitate the setting of international benchmarks.

The World Health Organization's Regional Office for Europe has also called for countries to provide user-friendly access to an integrated set of national and subnational health statistics that would complement international efforts (World Health Organization, Regional Office for Europe 1998). Activities in many nations are already well advanced. For instance, according to a study in the late 1990s, 6 of 18 European countries surveyed had expanded national health information and monitoring systems to track progress against health targets (Van de Water and van Herten 1998). Another eight nations were expanding their systems or had plans to do so. The remainder were using existing information systems.

To meet the needs of a broad range of users, many countries are beginning to disseminate health statistics through flexible, user-friendly, Web-enabled applications and regular reports on the health of the population (often designed for the general public). In this way, data can be used for a wide range of purposes, including health surveillance, planning and management of the health system, and public reporting.

Achieving easy access to quality comparative information, however, is not a simple task. Building effective systems requires considerable financial and human resources. In addition, a number of complex issues must be addressed, such as:

- Preserving privacy, confidentiality, and security.
- Identifying, compiling, and integrating high-quality comparable data of different types from a wide range of sources.
- Achieving consistent and accurate statistical estimates for communities and regions, particularly if geographic boundaries change over time or if the population is highly mobile.
- Ensuring that nonspecialists can appropriately interpret the data, including on occasion making information available in multiple languages and formats.
- Preparing comprehensive, easy-to-understand reports for the public on health and the health system.

Nevertheless, a number of countries have made considerable progress in the development and dissemination of subnational comparative data. For example, Germany has developed a Health Information System (HIS) as part of the Setting up a Federal Health Monitoring System Research Project. The project's goal was to report comprehensively on the health status of the German population, as well as on factors affecting health (including health care). Topics covered include health status, behavioral and risk factors, diseases, health-care resources, production and consumption of health services, and health-care expenditures. The system brings together a range of national and subnational data, standard indicator definitions and associated metadata. The overall cost was close to 4.5 million DM and required approximately 10 person-years (Federal Statistical Office of Germany 1998).

France has also established an integrated set of data on demographics, causes of death, morbidity, hospital diagnoses, and a variety of other topics at a regional level (Direction Régionale des Affaires Sanitaires et Sociales [Stat] 2002). A similar concept, called Net-Hilmo, has been implemented in Finland (National Research and Development Centre for Welfare and Health [hp] STAKES statistical databases). In both cases, the initiatives include a set of health and health-care indicators that are available to the general public, with more sophisticated access for authorized users. Comparable projects are also underway or planned in several other countries, including Canada, Denmark, Japan, Lithuania, Norway, Sweden, the United Kingdom, and others.

Just as the World Health Organization publishes an annual World Health Report, individual countries are producing regular reports for public use on health and health care based on these types of statistics. These reports vary from vast compendiums of statistics to descriptive reports that draw on a range of data. Topics frequently covered include health status; the major determinants of health, including key risk factors; health expenditures; use and outcomes of health services, particularly acute care hospitals; and focused analysis related to special populations (e.g., children and the elderly).

Increased International Cooperation

While differences remain between the approaches taken and the degree of implementation in various countries, there is considerable convergence in national health information activities and strategies. In part, this may be the result of sustained international cooperation and information exchange.

For years, countries have collaborated in the compilation of mortality statistics and a limited range of other health statistics. Examples of efforts initiated more recently include:

- The acceleration of international health informatics standardization efforts, including the formation of the European Committee for Standardization (European) and ISO (international) standards committees (European Committee for Standardization [hp] CEN/TC 251; Inter-national Organization for Standardization [hp] TC 215 health informatics).
- The expansion of comparative health statistics reporting, including the World Health Organization's Health For All indicators (WHO 1981) and the OECD's indicators (Organisation for Economic Co-operation and Development [hp] OCED health data 2003).
- International surveys, such as the Commonwealth Fund International Health Policy Surveys (Commonwealth Fund [hp] International program in health care policy and practice).

- Joint ECE–WHO (United Nations Economic Commission for Europe—World Health Organization) meetings on health statistics to share information on issues such as the coordination of national and international health statistics, the role of information technology in the collection and dissemination of health data, the development and use of health output indicators, and the progress in implementation of health classification systems (United Nations Economic and Social Council 2001).
- An international conference on performance measurement, "Measuring Up: Improving Health Systems Performance in OECD countries," hosted by the OECD and Health Canada in November 2001 (Organisation for Economic Co-operation and Development [conference proceedings on the Internet]).
- The projects under the Global Healthcare Applications Project as part of the G7/G8 Information Society initiative (European Commission [hp] G8 global information society), including GLOPHIN, a Global Public Health Intelligence Network that uses the Internet to create an information base to detect worldwide communicable disease outbreaks, assess risks, manage responses, and implement control and prevention measures (Laaser et al. 1999).

In addition, the World Health Organization has developed an organization-wide strategy to build and enhance health information systems in member countries as a fundamental component of health systems development (World Health Organization [hp] EHSPI). In this way, developing countries are also improving their capabilities in routine collection of health information and in using information to guide decisions for health care.

CONCLUSION

As knowledge about health and the organization and delivery of health services evolves, so must health information. In most developed countries, significant activity is underway at a national level to meet changing health information needs. Focal points are developing to ensure national coordination; historical data collections are evolving and being extended; and there is increased emphasis on the dissemination and reporting of comparative information. At the same time, both awareness of the need to protect personal privacy and safeguard the confidentiality and security of health information and the demand for increased integration of health data for statistical purposes are growing. While the approaches taken by particular countries may differ, they share many opportunities and challenges. In general, they also share a common goal: using better health information for improved health and health care.

APPENDIX: LIST OF ORGANIZATIONS

Australia

Australian Bureau of Statistics http://www.abs.gov.au
Australian Institute of Health and Welfare (AIHW) http://www.aihw.gov.au
HealthConnect http://www.health.gov.au/healthconnect
National Centre for Classification in Health http://www2.fhs.usyd.edu.au/ncch
National Health Information Knowledgebase http://www.aihw.gov.au/knowledgebase/index.html
Office of the Federal Privacy Commissioner http://www.privacy.gov.au
Standards Australia http://www.standards.com.au

Canada

Canadian Institute for Health Information (CIHI) http://www.cihi.ca
Canadian Standards Association (CSA) http://www.csa.ca
Health Canada, Office of Health and the Information Highway http://www.hc-sc.gc.ca/ohih-bsi
Privacy Commissioner of Canada http://www.privcom.gc.ca
Statistics Canada http://www.statcan.ca

Europe

EUROSTAT Statistical Office of the European Communities http://europe.eu.int/en/comm/eurostat/serven/home.htm
European Committee for Standardization (CEN) http://www.cenorm.be/cenorm/index.htm

Finland

Net-Hilmo http://info.stakes.fi/nettihilmo/english/default.htm
National Research and Development Centre for Welfare and Health (STAKES, Finland) http://www.stakes.fi/english/index.html

France

Direction de la recherche, des études, de l'évaluation, et des statistiques (DREES) http://www.sante.gouv.fr/htm/publication/

Germany

German Institute for Medical Documentation and Information (DIMDI) http://www.dimdi.de/dynamic/en/

International

International Organization for Standardization (ISO) http://www.iso.ch
Organisation for Economic Co-operation and Development (OECD) http://www.oecd.org
World Health Organization http://www.who.int/en

Ireland

Department of Health and Children http://www.doh.ie/hstrat/nhis/index.html

Japan

MEDIS-DC: Medical Information Systems Development Centre http://www.medis.or.jp

Korea

Korean Institute for Health and Social Affairs, Information and Statistics Research http://www.kihasa.re.kr/english/info/info01.html

New Zealand

Privacy Commissioner http://www.privacy.org.nz/top.html
New Zealand Health Information Service (NZHIS) http://www.nzhis.govt.nz

Nordic

Medico-Statistics Committee http://www.nom-nos.dk/NOMESCO.HTM
Social Statistics Committee http://www.nom-nos.dk/nososco.htm

United Kingdom

Department of Health http://www.doh.gov.uk
National Audit Office for the United Kingdom http://www.nao.gov.uk
National Health Service Information Authority http://www.nhsia.nhs.uk
Office for National Statistics http://www.statistics.gov.uk
Statistics Division of the Department of Health http://www.doh.gov.uk/public/stats5.htm

United States

The Commonwealth Fund http://www.cmwf.org/

The Uniform Resource Locators for all of the organizations were checked and verified as functional on March 26, 2004.

NOTE

1. These results may partly reflect a country's commitment to international comparative reporting, as well as the availability of health data at a national level.

REFERENCES

Aboriginal and Torres Strait Islander Health and Welfare Information Unit, Australian Health Ministers' Advisory Council. Aboriginal and Torres Strait Islander Health Information Plan: This Time, Let's Make It Happen. Canberra: Australian Bureau of Statistics; 1998.

Advisory Committee on Health Infostructure. Tactical Plan for a Pan-Canadian health infostructure: 2001 Update. Ottawa: Office of Health and the Information Highway; 2001 [cited 2004 Feb 10]. Available from: http://www.hc-sc.gc.ca/ohih-bsi/pubs/2001_plan/plan_e.html.

Advisory Council on Health Infostructure. Canada Health Infoway: Paths to Better Health. Final Report. Ottawa: Advisory Council on Health Infostructure; 1999.

Australia Standards. AS 4400-1995: Personal Privacy Protection in Healthcare Information Systems. Sydney: Standards Australia; 1995. Available from: http://www.standards.com.au/catalogue/script/Details.asp?DocN=stds000013820.

Australian Government Department of Health and Ageing [homepage on the Internet]. Canberra: Australian Government Department of Health and Ageing [cited 2004 Mar 12]. Welcome to HealthConnect [about 2 screens]. Available from: http://www.health.gov.au/healthconnect.

Australian Institute of Health and Welfare, Australian Health Ministers' Advisory Council. National Health Information Development Plan. Canberra: Australian Government Publishing Service; 1995.

Australian Institute of Health and Welfare. Corporate Plan 1999–2000. Cat. No. AUS-18. Canberra: Australian Institute of Health and Welfare; 1999.

Australian Institute of Health and Welfare. Australia's Health 2000. Canberra: Australian Institute of Health and Welfare; 2000 [cited 2004 Mar 12]. Available from: www.aihw.gov.au/publications/health/ah00/index.html.

Australian Institute of Health and Welfare [monograph on the Internet]. Corporate Plan: 2003–2006. Canberra: Australian Institute of Health and Welfare; 2003 [cited 2004 Feb 29]. Available from: http://www.aihw.gov.au/publications/aus/cp03–06/cp03–06.pdf.

Australian Institute of Health and Welfare [homepage on the Internet]. Canberra: AIHW [updated 2004 Jan 5; cited 2004 Mar 12]. Available from: http://www.aihw.gov.au.

Australian Institute of Health and Welfare [homepage on the Internet]. Canberra: AIHW [updated 2002 Jun 20; cited 2002 May 23]. The Knowledgebase: Australia's health, community services and housing metadata registry [about 2 screens]. Available from: http://www.aihw.gov.au/knowledgebase/index.html.

Australian Institute of Health and Welfare [homepage on the Internet]. Canberra: Australian Institute of Health and Welfare [updated 2003 Sep 25; cited 2004 Mar 13]. National Health Information Management Group [about 1 screen]. Available from: http://www.aihw.gov.au/committees/health/nhimg/index.html.

Canadian Institute for Health Information. Health Information Roadmap: Launching the Process. Ottawa: Canadian Institute for Health Information; 1999a.

Canadian Institute for Health Information. Health Information Roadmap: Responding to Needs. Ottawa: Canadian Institute for Health Information; 1999b.

Canadian Institute for Health Information. Roadmap Initiative. Launching the Process: Two Years Later. Ottawa: Canadian Institute for Health Information; 2001 [cited 2004 Mar 12]. Available from: http://secure.cihi.ca/cihiweb/en/downloads/profile_roadmap_e_ProgReport2001.pdf.

Canadian Institute for Health Information [homepage on the Internet]. Ottawa: Canadian Institute for Health Information; c. 1996–2002 [cited 2004 Mar 12]. Available from: http://www.cihi.ca.

Canadian Standards Association. Privacy code [monograph on the Internet]. Mississauga, Ontario: Canadian Standards Association; 1996 [cited 2004 Mar 12]. Available from: http://www.csa.ca/standards/privacy/code/Default.asp?language=English.

Commonwealth Fund [homepage on the Internet]. New York: The Commonwealth Fund [cited 2002 May 27]. International program in health care policy and practice [about 8 screens]. Available from: http://www.cmwf.org/programs/policy.asp?link=2.

Direction Régionale des Affaires Sanitaires et Sociales, Direction de la recherche, des études, de l'évaluation, et des statistiques. Statistiques et Indicateurs de la Santé et du Social (STATISS) [statistics on the Internet]. Paris: DRASS, DREES [cited 2002 May 27]. Available from: http://www.sante.gouv.fr/drees/statiss/default.htm.

European Commission [homepage on the Internet]. Brussels: European Commission; c. 1995–2003 [cited 2004 Mar 12]. Data protection [about 2 screens]. Available from: http://europa.eu.int/comm/internal_market/privacy/index_en.htm.

European Commission [homepage on the Internet]. Brussels: European Commission; c. 1995–2000 [updated 2000 Nov 14; cited 2002 May 27]. G8 global information society pilot projects matrix [about 5 screens]. Available from: http://europa.eu.int/ISPO/intcoop/g8/i_g8pp_matrix.html

European Commission, Legal Advisory Board. Directive 95/46/EC of the European Parliament and of the Council of 24 October 1995 on the protection of individuals with regard to the processing of personal data and on the free movement of such data. Official Journal of the European Communities. 1995 Nov 23; No L. 281, p. 31. Also: European Commission, Legal Advisory Board [cited 2004 Mar 14]. Directive 95/46/EC [directive on the Internet]. Brussels: European Commission; 1995. Available from: http://europa.eu.int/ISPO/legal/en/dataprot/directiv/directiv.html.

European Committee for Standardization [homepage on the Internet]. Stockholm: Swedish Standards Institute [cited 2002 May 27]. CEN/TC 251: European Standardization of Health Informatics [about 1 screen]. Available from: http://www.centc251.org.

Federal Statistical Office of Germany. The German health information system. In: UN: Statistical Commission and Economic Commission for Europe, World Health Organization (WHO): Regional Office for Europe, and Conference of European Statisticians. Report on the Joint ECE-WHO Meeting on Health Statistics; 1998 Oct 14–16; Rome, Italy. Geneva: United Nations; 1998 [cited 2004 Mar 13]. Available from: http://www.unece.org/stats/documents/ces/ac.36/1998/14.e.html.

Grant B, Petrie M. Alcohol and Other Drug Treatment Services: Development of a National Minimum Data Set. Canberra: Australian Institute for Health and Welfare; 2001. Available from: http://www.aihw.gov.au/publications/hse/adts-dnmds/index.html [cited 2004 Mar 13].

HealthConnect Program Office. HealthConnect June 2001 update. Canberra: Australian Government Department of Health and Ageing; 2001 [cited 2004 Mar 16]. Available from: http://www.health.gov.au/healthconnect/pdf_docs/update0106.pdf.

International Organization for Standardization. Health Informatics: Health Indicators Conceptual Framework—Draft. ISO TC 215. Geneva: International Standards Organization; 2001.

International Organization for Standardization [homepage on the Internet]. Geneva: ISO; [cited 2002 May 27]. ISO technical programme: TC 215 health informatics [about 3 screens]. Available from: http://www.iso.ch/iso/en/stdsdevelopment/techprog/workprogTechnicalProgrammeTCDetailPage.TechnicalProgrammeTCDetail?COMMID=4720.

Joch A. Finland: centralised healthcare with a business bent. Healthc Inform 1999;16(8):61–64.

Korean Institute for Health and Social Affairs [homepage on the Internet]. Seoul: Korean Institute for Health and Social Affairs; c. 2002 [cited 2002 May 23]. Available from: http://www.kihasa.re.kr/english/info/info01.html.

Laaser U, Knogge T, Kugel T. Report on the G7–pilot towards a global public health information network. Int J Public Health Ed [serial on the Internet]. 1999 Jan 1 [cited 2004 Mar 13]; 1:C45–60. Available from: http://www.aspher.org/D_services/I-JPHE/Reports_Documents/Full%20text/report%20on%20the%20G7.pdf.

Ministry of Health. Health Information Strategy for the Year 2000. Wellington, NZ: Ministry of Health; 1996.

Ministry of Health, Denmark. The role of IT in providing ready access to statistics on health care in Denmark. In: UN: Statistical Commission and Economic Commission for Europe, World Health Organization (WHO): Regional Office for Europe, and Conference of European Statisticians. Report on the Joint ECE-WHO Meeting on Health Statistics; 1998 Oct 14–16; Rome, Italy [cited 2004 Mar 13]. Geneva: United Nations; 1998. Available from: http://www.unece.org/stats/documents/ces/ac.36/1998/12.e. html.

Nadarajah I. Looking for IT support from doctors. Healthc Inform 1999;16(8):61–64.

National Committee on Vital and Health Statistics. Information for Health: A Strategy for Building the National Health Information Infrastructure. Washington, DC: U.S. Department of Health and Human Services; 2001 [cited 2004 Mar 16]. Available from: http://www.ncvhs.hhs.gov/nhiilayo.pdf.

National Health Information Council. Health information for Canada: Report of the National Task Force on Health Information. Ottawa: National Health Information Council; 1991.

National Health Information Management Advisory Council. Health Online: A Health Information Action Plan for Australia, 2nd ed. Canberra: Commonwealth of Australia; 2001 [cited 2004 Mar 16]. Available from: http://www.health.gov.au/healthonline/docs/actplan2.pdf.

National Health Service. Delivering 21st Century IT Support for the NHS: National Strategic Programme. London: Department of Health; 2002.

National Health Service Information Authority [homepage on the Internet]. Birmingham: National Health Service Information Authority; c. 2004 [updated 2002 Jan 9; cited 2002 May 29]. Information for health: an information strategy for the modern NHS, 1998–2005 [about 2 screens]. Available from: http://www.nhsia.nhs.uk/def/pages/info4health/contents.asp.

National Institute for Statistics and Economic Studies [homepage on the Internet]. Paris: National Institute for Statistics and Economic Studies [cited 2002 May 23]. The public statistical system [about 1 screen]. Available from: http://www.insee.fr/en/a_propos/stat_pub/accueil_stat.htm.

National Research and Development Centre for Welfare and Health (STAKES) [statistics on the Internet]. Helsinki: STAKES; c. 1998 [updated 1998 June 6; cited 2002 May 27]). STAKES statistical databases. Available from: http://info.stakes.fi/nettihilmo/english/default.htm.

National Research and Development Centre for Welfare and Health (STAKES) [homepage on the Internet]. Helsinki: STAKES; c. 2004 [cited 2004 Mar 13]. Available from: http://www.stakes.fi/english/index.html.

New Zealand Health Information Service [homepage on the Internet]. Wellington, NZ: Ministry of Health [updated 2003 Sep 12; cited 2004 Mar 13]. About NZHIS [about 5 screens]. Available from: http://www.nzhis.govt.nz/aboutNZHIS.html.

New Zealand Health Information Service [homepage on the Internet]. Wellington, NZ: Ministry of Health [updated 2003 Oct 8; cited 2004 Mar 13]. Data and services [about 5 screens]. Available from: http://www.nzhis.govt.nz/Service_guide.html.

New Zealand Health Information Service [homepage on the Internet]. Wellington, NZ: Ministry of Health [updated 2003 Oct 21; cited 2004 Mar 13]. Guide to NZHIS National Collections: Mental Health Information National Collection [about 3 screens]. Available from: http://www.nzhis.govt.nz/collections/collections-mhinc.html.

Office of the Federal Privacy Commissioner [homepage on the Internet]. Sydney: Office of the Federal Privacy Commissioner; copyright [updated 2001 Nov 9; cited 2004 Mar 14]. Guidelines on privacy in the private health sector [about 90 screens]. Available from: http://www.privacy.gov.au/publications/hg_01.html.

Office of the Privacy Commissioner. Health Information Privacy Code 1994. Wellington, NZ: Privacy Commissioner; 2000 [cited 2004 Mar 13]. Available from: http://www.privacy.org.nz/comply/HIPCWWW.pdf.

Organisation for Economic Co-operation and Development. OECD Guidelines on the Protection of Privacy and Transborder Flows of Personal Data. Paris: OECD; 1980 [cited 2004 Mar 13]. Available from: http://www.oecd.org/document/20/0,2340,en_2649_33703_15589524_1_1_1_1,00.html.

Organisation for Economic Co-operation and Development. OECD Health Data '99. Paris: OECD; 1999.

Organisation for Economic Co-operation and Development [homepage on the Internet]. Paris: OECD [cited 2004 Mar 14]. OCED health data 2003 [about 3 screens]. Available from: http://www.oecd.org/document/30/0,2340,en_2649_34631_12968734_1_1_1_1,00.html.

Organisation for Economic Co-operation and Development [conference proceedings on the Internet]. Measuring Up: Improving Health Systems Performance in OECD Countries; OECD Health Conference on Performance Measurement and Reporting; 2001 Nov 5–7; Ottawa, Canada. Paris: OECD; c. 2001 [cited 2004 Mar 13]. Available from: http://www1.oecd.org/els/health/canconf/presentations.htm.

Partnership for Health Informatics/Telematics. Health Identification Systems: Background Document. Ottawa: Canadian Institute for Health Information; 1996.

Privacy Commissioner of Canada [homepage on the Internet]. Ottawa: Privacy Commissioner of Canada [updated 2002 Jan; cited 2001 Sep 19]. Sector specific legislation dealing with privacy [about 1 screen]. Available from: http://www.privcom.gc.ca/fs-fi/fs2001-02_e.asp.

Rogers R. Barriers to Global Information Society for Health: Recommendations for International Action. Final Report of the Project G8-ENABLE. Amsterdam: IOS Press; 1999.

Ryan T, Holmes B, Gibson D. A National Minimum Data Set for Home and Community Care. Canberra: Australian Institute for Health and Welfare; 1999 [cited 2004 Mar 13]. Available from: http://www.aihw.gov.au/publications/welfare/nmdshcc/index. html.

Statistics Canada. The Canadian Community Health Survey (Cycle 1.1): Content for September 2000. Ottawa: Statistics Canada; 2000 [cited 2002 May 27]. Available from: http://www.statcan.ca/english/concepts/health/pdf/cchs_quest.pdf.

Statistics Canada. 2000 National Population Health Survey (Cycle 4): Content for June 2000; Ottawa: Statistics Canada; 2001 [cited 2002 May 27]. Available from: http://www.statcan.ca/english/concepts/nphs/quest00e.pdf.

Swiss Federal Statistical Office. Data protection in relation to hospital medical statistics. In: UN: Statistical Commission and Economic Commission for Europe, World Health Organization (WHO): Regional Office for Europe, and Conference of European Statisticians. Report on the Joint ECE-WHO Meeting on Health Statistics; 1998 Oct 14–16; Rome, Italy. Geneva: United Nations; 1998 [cited 2004 Mar 13]. Available from: http://www.unece.org/stats/documents/ces/ac.36/1998/25.s.e.pdf.

United Nations Economic and Social Council. Report of the October 2000 Joint ECE/WHO Preparatory Meeting on Measuring Health Status. Geneva: United Nations; 2001 [cited 2004 Mar 13]. Available from: http://www.unece.org/stats/documents/ces/2001/28.e.pdf.

Van de Water HPA, van Herten LM. Health Policies on Target? Review of Health Target and Priority Setting in 18 European Countries. The Hague: TNO Prevention and Health, Public Health Division; 1998.

World Health Organization. Development of Indicators for Monitoring Progress Towards Health for All by the Year 2000. Geneva: World Health Organization; 1981.

World Health Organization. The World Health Report 2001. Geneva: World Health Organization; 2001 [cited 2004 Mar 13]. Available from: http://www.who.int/whr2001/2001/main/en/index.htm.

World Health Organization [homepage on the Internet]. Geneva: World Health Organization; c. 2001 [cited 2004 Feb 15]. Enhancing health systems performance initiative (EHSPI) [about 5 screens]. Available from: http://www.who.int/health-systems-performance/ehspi.htm.

World Health Organization, Regional Office for Europe, Unit of Epidemiology, Statistics and Health Information. Strengthening national health information systems: the concept of national integrated statistical health database. In: UN: Statistical Commission and Economic Commission for Europe, World Health Organization (WHO): Regional Office for Europe, and Conference of European Statisticians. Report on the Joint ECE-WHO Meeting on Health Statistics; 1998 Oct 14–16; Rome, Italy. Geneva: United Nations; 1998 [cited 2004 Nov 5]. Available from: http://www.unece.org/stats/documents/ces/ac.36/1998/5.e.html.

CHAPTER 18

From Health Statistics to Health Information Systems: A New Path for the Twenty-First Century

Charlyn Black, Leslie L. Roos, and Noralou P. Roos

Many countries are making significant investments to enhance their health statistics capabilities. These involve a range of activities, from renewing traditional data collections and extending their content and coverage, to increasing the flexibility and integration of data, to enhancing approaches to protecting privacy and confidentiality of data, and finally to improving the utility and accessibility of data (see Chapter 17).

As input into an initiative to develop a twenty-first-century vision for health statistics (Friedman et al. 2002), we have argued that a bold new vision is required to provide direction to these efforts. While enormous progress was made in developing health statistics systems during the twentieth century, current approaches fall short of providing a framework for moving into the future. Several major forces are moving us in a new direction: increased computerization, automation and computing power, improved ability to measure health, an increased appetite for evidence, a focus on accountability and outcomes, and an evolving conceptual understanding of health and the factors that contribute to health.

This chapter first outlines some of the forces that provide impetus for a new vision and, from this, identifies several characteristics that are critical to incorporate into future efforts. It then provides an update on experience gained in Manitoba, Canada, with development of a prototype health information system. The chapter concludes by considering opportunities for the future.

BACKGROUND

In the twenty-first century, a number of critical developments and perspectives are challenging us to rethink our approach to health statistics. Together, these factors support a more targeted and cohesive approach—one that focuses on health and the factors that influence health.

Evidence and the Outcomes Movement

In the 1970s and 1980s, research focusing on the health-care system revealed a surprising degree of variation in the way health-care services were delivered to populations. For a relatively small number of services, rates of intervention were quite similar across population groups. However, for the vast majority of services, profound variability in intervention rates was the norm. These patterns of variability in service delivery were found at many different levels, both across and within countries; and they were remarkably stable over time. Surprisingly, the variation often was most striking within—rather than across—countries and states.

These *small area variations* raised profound challenges for the health-care system. Subsequent research revealed that the variations are not clearly related to differences in population groups' underlying need for health care. Instead, they seem more likely to be driven by differences in providers' practice style. Most important, they raise the troubling question "Which rate is right?"—to which there is no simple answer. It became clear that there was very little evidence indicating that a higher level of intervention was more (or less) appropriate than a lower level of intervention. A quest to develop better evidence began, fueled by a new understanding of the importance of studying the impacts of health care in terms of the health outcomes it produced.[1]

In the 1990s, the United States embarked on a program of *outcomes* research that was designed to produce knowledge and evidence about the impact of the health-care system (Roper et al. 1988; U.S. Department of Health and Human Services 1990a, 1990b). Since then, the U.S. health agenda has been strongly influenced by the *outcomes* agenda. This massive effort has provided perspective on the relative risks and benefits of medical care and has led to a focus on clinical data sets and the development of detailed instruments for disease-based (as distinguished from health-based) research. Much has been learned, and much more remains to be learned, about the impact of specific medical interventions on the patients to whom they are applied.

The Population Health Agenda

Meanwhile, in Canada, a different conceptual and policy framework—one that encourages a focus on understanding factors that contribute to the health of populations—was gaining prominence in policy discourse. The framework underlying this perspective was most clearly articulated in an article by the Canadian health economists Robert Evans and Gregory Stoddart (Evans and Stoddart 1990). Of note in their model is the direct impact of *health care* on *disease*, but *not* on health and function or on well-being. The authors suggested that while tremendous value is ascribed to health, modern societies devote a very large proportion of their economic resources to the production and distribution of *health care*, reflecting a widespread belief that health care is central to the health of both individuals and populations. They argued that our understanding of the relationship between disease and health care that underpins our investments is simplistic. They developed a more complex model that incorporates factors *other* than health care that are known to influence health and well-being—factors such as the social and physical environments as well as the economic prosperity in which we live. They argued that ever-increasing investments in health care are unlikely to be the best way to improve the health of populations: "A society that spends so much on health care that it cannot or will not spend adequately on other health-enhancing activities may actually be reducing the health of its population." In other words, expansion of the health-care system consumes resources that would otherwise be available to address other factors that influence health.[2]

This *population health* framework, as it has come to be known, reorients us to consider health and the improvement of health (rather than a focus on disease) as fundamental goals of the health system. It builds on an earlier Canadian framework (Lalonde 1974) to encourage consideration of a broad range of factors that influence health, recognizing that both medical care and other determinants of health play important roles. It therefore supports a more explicit understanding of the contribution of medical care to the improvement of health. However, whereas the outcomes research agenda focuses on patients who receive specific interventions for identified diseases from the health-care system, the population health framework encourages conceptualization of populations defined by characteristics *other* than their interaction with the medical care system. More important, within the context of health reform, it challenges managers to understand how the health-care system, as currently structured, is responding to the goal of improving health, and how proposed changes may support or detract from that goal.[3]

The population health agenda, which has subsequently played a key role in the deliberations of the National Committee on Vital and Health Statistics (Friedman et al. 2002), provides a number of important perspectives that have important implications for the development of information systems. Most important, it has stressed the importance of health and underlined how little we really know about health and about what produces health. Second, it has provided conceptual models that challenge some of our central beliefs about what factors *do* contribute to health. This model suggests that factors outside of the health-care system may be as important as —or even more important than—the health-care system itself in producing health. Third, it has challenged us to think more broadly and more critically about the contribution of medical care to producing health in populations—beyond the perspective of the outcomes research agenda, which has focused specifically on patients rather than populations.

Expanding Data and Analytic Capabilities

A third major factor that provides important opportunities for rethinking our approach to health statistics in the twenty-first century relates to the remarkable improvements in our ability to routinely collect, store, and analyze data. We now have the potential to collect data about the environments in which people live and work, their social and economic status, educational experiences, states of health, contacts with the health-care system, involvement with various government programs, and health outcomes—all important aspects of understanding what contributes to health.

Whereas previously we had to rely on primary data collection activities that focused on answering specific questions with small samples on a one-time basis, we can now ponder the possibility of designing systems that will collect a rich set of data elements routinely. Whereas previously it was useful to think of developing statistics to address specific health issues (e.g., communicable disease control and surveillance, perinatal morbidity, hospital use), it is now possible to consider a set of data systems that provide a person-oriented, cradle-to-grave set of data records that provide the basic infrastructure to develop statistics and information to serve any number of purposes. Whereas previously compilation of statistics was laborious and resulted in outdated information, increased analytic power now provides us with opportunities to produce analyses that can be conducted in real time and are tailored to meet users' specific requirements.

Health Statistics or Health Information Systems?

Given the three major sets of influences outlined above—an increased emphasis on evidence and outcomes, a clearer recognition that producing health in the population requires attention to factors related to the health-care system as well as those external to it, and rapidly expanding opportunities to use data in powerful new ways—perhaps the real challenge before us is to think broadly and boldly enough as we develop health statistics systems for the twenty-first century. We argue that it may be time to shift our perspective from a focus on the production of health statistics to a focus on developing comprehensive and flexible health information systems that will be capable of producing statistics that can enhance decision making about programs and policies related to health and health care.

AN EARLY PROTOTYPE: THE POPULIS SYSTEM

Our experience in developing a unique database, created from the administrative data used to run a Canadian provincial health insurance system and now housed in a research data repository at the University of Manitoba, provides an important perspective for the development of a future system of health statistics. From this database, we have developed a population-based information system known as POPULIS. We believe that this system embodies a number of features that provide critical lessons for the development of health statistics and information systems of the future.

The Population-Based Information System

POPULIS is a system of data, an approach to analysis, a set of concepts and indicators, and a way of organizing these elements to produce information. It permits us to study, for a given population, the factors that influence health, the state of health, and the availability and use of health and other services. It uses a population-based approach to analysis whereby characteristics of defined groups of people are examined and compared. This concept is intuitive for studying health and social characteristics of populations, but is less so in the analysis of health services. Using this approach, all services, regardless of where they are provided, are attributed to the individual and the individual's region of residence. Population-based analysis therefore provides a perspective on how services *are used by population groups*, which is fundamentally different from understanding how services are delivered by providers. In so doing, it facilitates planning and evaluation from the viewpoint of the health needs of the population.

Information can be configured for many different population groups. For most of our applications, these groups are defined by geographic boundaries (and we have several different versions of these). However, we can also define populations by disease states, by social and economic circumstances, and by other characteristics. Another advantage of population-based analysis is that it makes it relatively easy to adjust for differences in the age and sex structure that may contribute to observed differences among populations. After adjustment, one can compare the use of health care across different regions, making it easy to compare indicators across population groups and across time.

The other important feature of POPULIS is that it enables the user to simultaneously relate characteristics that affect a population's *need* for health care to that population's *use* of health care, to that area's *supply* of health-care resources, and, finally, to the underlying *health status* of a population. The importance of this feature is that it permits the structuring of more complex and different questions (and answers) (Roos 1995). It allows us to ask, for instance: Does health status vary across regions? By how much? What factors are associated with poor health? Are high-risk populations poorly served by the health-care system or do they have poor health status despite being well served? What are we spending on acute hospital care per capita? How much does it vary across our health regions? Is reducing the investment in acute care compatible with good health? Where might cuts be made without jeopardizing at-risk populations? In short, we can focus on understanding the linkage between use of health-care resources and population health, instead of merely understanding how providers deliver care.

The Foundation: A Strong Underlying Data System

A recent initiative to make data available to Canadian researchers has stressed the central importance of data (Watkins 1994). The rationale for this project provides a perspective on the importance of constructing strong data systems to facilitate observational research:

> Data are unlike other tools of the research endeavor. They provide the raw material from which information can be created. . . . Unlike printed tables which, like a postcard, provide a larger view of a larger phenomenon, data can act as a camera, allowing the researcher to manipulate the foreground and more fully investigate the object under study.

The data system underlying the POPULIS system provides the critical foundation for its capabilities (see Fig. 18.1). The system relies on the unique Manitoba health research database, which comprises information produced in the administration of the provincial health insurance system. At the hub of this data system is a population-based research registry. This research registry, derived from a real-time provincial administrative system that provides insured benefits to

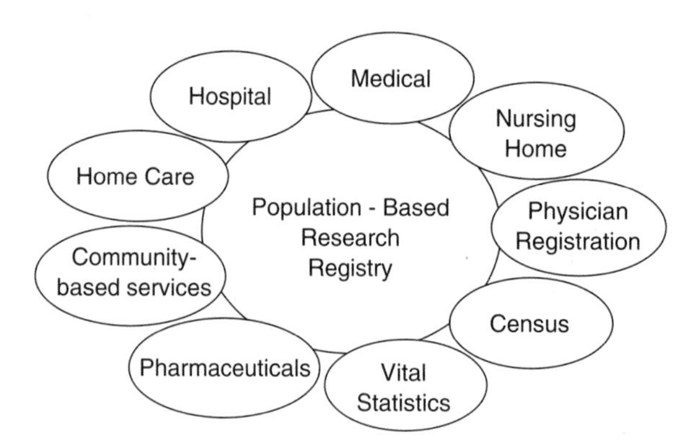

FIGURE 18.1
The data system underlying the population health information system.

provincial residents, contains a unique but nonidentifying research number that is assigned to each provincial resident, together with information about demographic characteristics, residence, and family composition. Other files within the data system use the same nonidentifying research number to track use of services, making it possible to compile comprehensive histories for individuals over time, as well as across types of services.

Administrative databases provide an information-rich environment for researchers; a system such as POPULIS fundamentally depends on the availability of such data. For billing and administrative purposes, every contact that the population has had with hospitals, nursing homes, and physicians over a 25-year period has been documented and is incorporated into the research database, even though, for some services, there are multiple payers. Recently, data on immunizations, pharmaceutical use, use of home care, and other community-based services have been added to the data holdings. Vital statistics data, documenting the date and cause of death, as well as public-use census information, have also been integrated into the database. More recently, data about educational attainment and use of social services have been added, making it possible to provide more comprehensive information—beyond the health-care system—about the population.

Population-based research registries, combined with administrative data files containing unique nonidentifying research numbers to indicate the service recipient, provide the ability to generate meaningful information on each individual's life course and multiply the types of studies that can be performed. Indicators focusing on quality of care (readmissions or emergency room visits within 30 days of discharge from a hospital) or indicators identifying disease cohorts (individuals with diabetes or hypertension whose outcomes can then be monitored across different delivery systems) are all enhanced if a population registry and cross-file linkages are possible.

The research database builds on currently available data, but can accommodate and potentially link other data, such as surveys, clinical data sets, electronic medical records, public health data sets, disease registries, and other data. Indeed, we have learned that when designing population-based health surveys, the possibilities of linking data and conducting validity studies using administrative data should be foreseen and incorporated into the study design (Muhajarine et al. 1997). Our data holdings include an important population-based panel survey of aging that has been linked to the administrative holdings (Havens 1996), as well as provincial samples of recent national surveys.

In the interests of protecting privacy, no identifying information is ever introduced into the research database. In addition, each of the individual data sets exists within the system in an unlinked format. Often, important data analyses can be conducted without the need for linkage. In fact, because of the focus on populations identified at the geographic level, most of the analyses undertaken for POPULIS projects require no linkage at the individual level. Linkages between the research registry and other data sets are undertaken only on a project-specific basis—once approvals from ethical review and data access review committees have been received. During the review process for each project, consideration is given to the importance of the research question and the offsetting potential risk of identification of individuals or violation of confidentiality. Strict protocols have been developed to reduce such risks during the research process, and security monitoring processes are in place and are continually upgraded.

An Approach to Analysis: Our Conceptual Model

Adoption of a conceptual model has been central to the progressive development of our POPULIS system (Roos et al. 1995). It has influenced many aspects: the data elements and files we have worked to add to our research database, the concepts and indicators we have developed, our approach to analysis, and the research questions we have pursued. Such a conceptual model has been critical in helping us move our research database from one that is focused on health care toward a resource that can begin to answer important questions about what produces health.

As presented in Figure 18.2, this model represents a modification of that proposed by Evans and Stoddart (1990). It recognizes a range of background factors that influence health status and well-being, including socioeconomic factors that characterize the economic, social, and physical environments in which individuals live and work, as well as demographic and genetic factors. Health states are influenced by these background factors, but are mediated by an individual's response to socioeconomic and biological circumstances. Health status reflects the absence or presence of disease and functional impairments. While it strongly influences a person's need for health-care interventions, the interplay between health status and health perception (which is shaped in part by other factors, such as practice patterns) influences an individual's sense of well-being and the resultant demand for health-care services. Need and demand influence the use of specific health-care services, but use is also affected by supply and practice pattern factors operating within the health-care system. Use of health-care services, mediated by individual responses, may affect the health status of individuals later at Time 2. Health states, as identified at Time 2, are influenced by socioeconomic factors, initial health status, and use of health-care services at an earlier time (Time 1). The model provides a framework for considering the relative contribution of each of these factors to health status and population health. Conversely, the model suggests that health status ultimately feeds back to influence the socioeconomic environment in which individuals operate and further influence use of health care.

This model recognizes that biological factors (including, but not limited to, the genetic predisposition to develop specific diseases), physical environmental factors (such as housing and pollution), social context (such as income inequality), and individual socioeconomic characteristics (poverty, lack of education, unemployment) have a strong impact on the health of a population. While we anticipate eventually incorporating several key environmental indicators into the

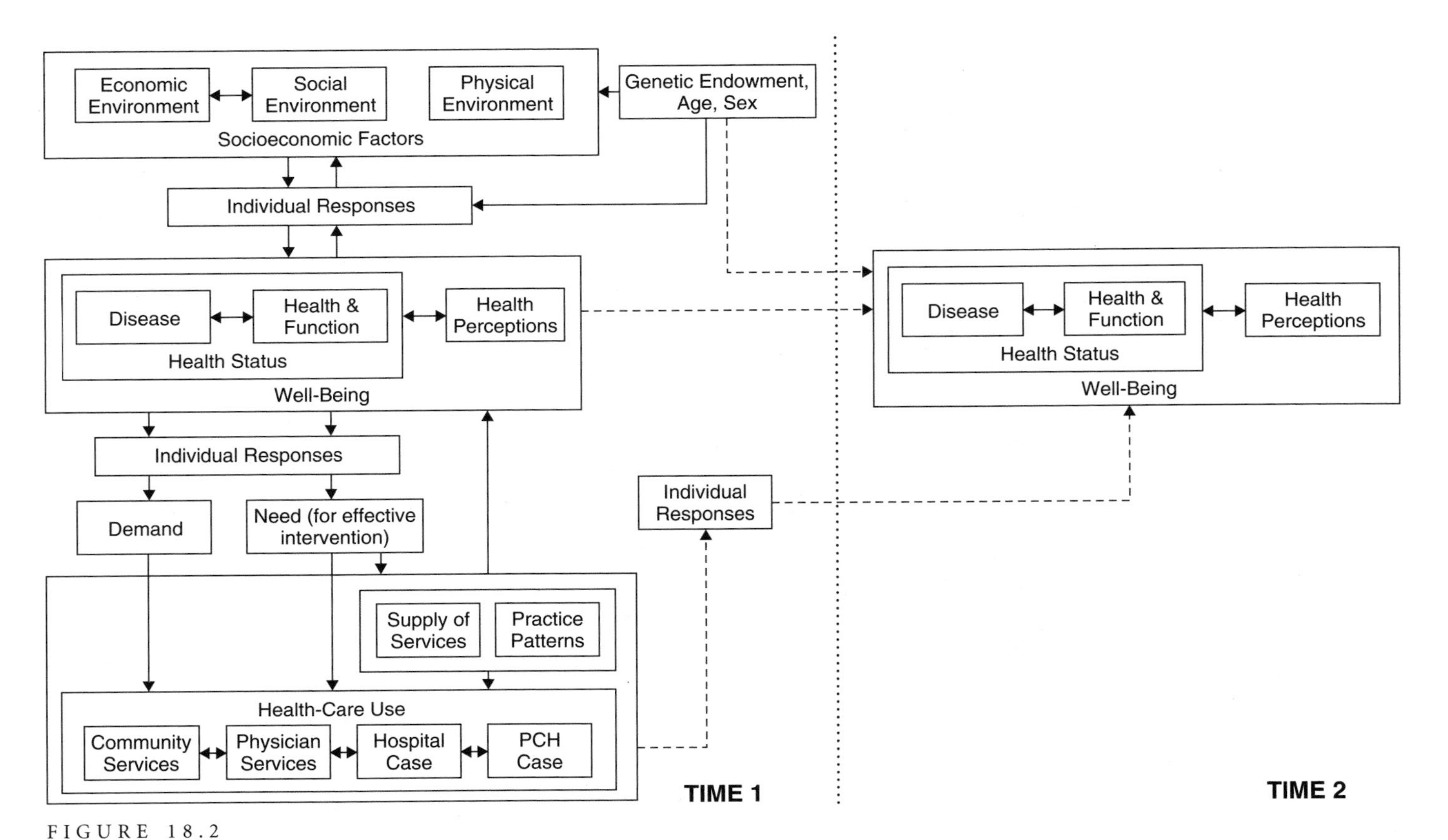

FIGURE 18.2
The conceptual model underlying the population health information system. PCH = personal care home.

information system, we have initially focused on the socioeconomic determinants of health and their relationship to use, supply, and health status indicators—and we have actively tried to increase our data and our analytic capabilities in this area.

Development of Key Concepts and Indicators

Another important principle in developing POPULIS has been the use of a consistent approach to operationalize key concepts and indicators—in other words, to develop a consistent and coherent set of statistics to underpin the system. Our approach builds on what is currently available—data created routinely as part of administering and paying for services delivered—and turns them into information about key concepts such as need, health status, use and supply (see Fig. 18.3).

The initial approach to development of the information system involved several key steps. First, we created meaningful geographic areas and, for each area, obtained denominator data by age and sex. Second, we developed indicators of socioeconomic risk (note that these are available only at the aggregate level) for these same areas. Third, we developed indicators of health status, and, finally, we developed indicators of use of services. Population-based rates were used to develop all of these indicators. Where possible, they were age- and sex-standardized to permit comparisons across populations. A comparative population-based approach has driven the development of indicators (see Fig. 18.4).

In developing indicators, we developed several additional key concepts. For example, to develop indicators of use of services for relevant data sets, standard approaches to measuring the number of users of services were developed to describe access; and different approaches were used to measure the intensity of ser-

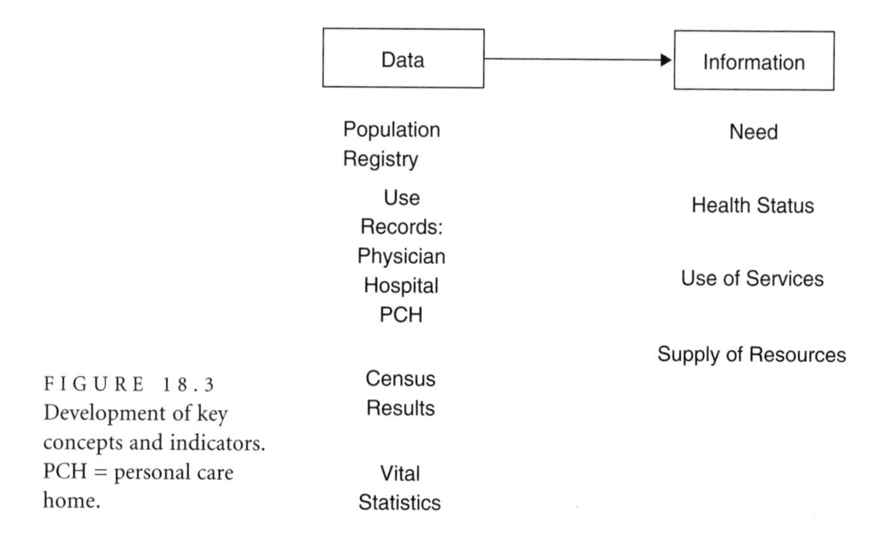

FIGURE 18.3 Development of key concepts and indicators. PCH = personal care home.

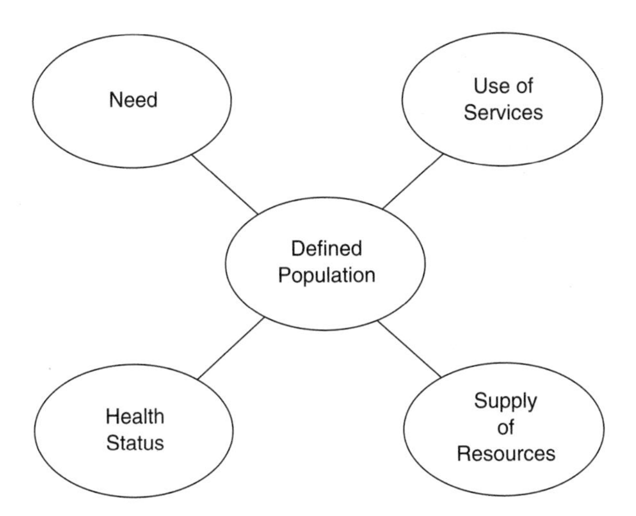

FIGURE 18.4
Transforming data into information: the power of comparative population-based analysis.

vice use, such as frequency, volume, and cost of services. Data on the usual supply parameters of health planning (hospital beds, nursing home beds, and physicians) were also developed, but our system has given equal or more emphasis to measures such as access, focusing on the proportion of individuals resident in a given area who use a service, regardless of where the service is obtained.

Indicators have been developed because of their potential value for health-care system management. The hospital indicators distinguish between medical, surgical, pediatric, psychiatric, and obstetric admissions. Also, use that takes place within the region of residence can be compared with that occurring out of the region. The physician supply indicators distinguish between physicians available to area residents because they live in the area and the physicians effectively available to area residents because patients travel out of the region (Roos et al. 1999).

This information system also permits summing of usage across sectors, using a dollar figure where possible and, in the case of nursing home and hospital use, summing total days of chronic institutional care. Finally, regional profiles showing how each region's health, socioeconomic risk, and health-care use characteristics differ from the provincial norm can be readily created.

Translating Data into Information

Developing these capabilities has been useful for descriptive analyses and for more applied analyses that target the big questions in health and health care, as well as to facilitate more targeted policy-relevant and evaluative research.

Our first steps in developing our health information system focused on conducting population-based analyses in key areas that we felt were critical to underpin such a system. These included focused and comprehensive analyses in key areas where we had data capabilities or needed to develop them—for instance, developing capabilities to measure the health status of the provincial and subprovincial populations. Similar population-based analyses were conducted with key data sets—our hospital discharge data sets, nursing home files, and physician claims files. This involved considerable work to develop and validate measures, understand whether they are all telling us the "same story," and understand which indicators inspire confidence. To consolidate this working knowledge, we have developed the concept dictionary, which focuses on providing a working historical documentation of key developments in a Web-based format (Burchill et al. 2000; Roos et al. 1999).

Our next major steps involved using these data and information tools to develop a general understanding of some of the big issues in health and health care. As a consequence, we have developed this system to help the public understand that more health care is not necessarily better, and to help planners identify the levers for pursuing a policy agenda more oriented to producing health, not health care. The system is organized around issues relevant for policymakers. For example, questions concerning intensity of use can easily be answered: How much do residents of regions vary in their use of high-tech teaching hospitals versus their use of small rural hospitals for acute care? What is the relative use across regions of resource-intensive procedures (e.g., hysterectomy) versus less intensive procedures (such as hysteroscopy)? We can also compare usage patterns across regions in which residents have similar levels of good health, allowing policymakers to approach the question "Which rate is right?" in terms of "What is the least costly rate associated with good health?" Costs incurred by a region's residents will be affected by how often residents access care (e.g., how often they are admitted to a hospital or contact a physician), the average cost of the service incurred (whether the physician was a specialist or whether the hospital day was spent in a teaching hospital or a small rural institution), and the number of services provided per user. Furthermore, POPULIS facilitates an assessment of how each of these factors interacts in contributing to the cost per resident. It has allowed us to develop profiles that juxtapose patterns of health and health-care use for planning (Martens et al. 2003).

The real power of the data and information infrastructure becomes apparent in applying it to more focused policy questions. This became possible once we had developed the basic data and information tools and developed an understanding of some of the big-picture issues from an empirical perspective. Now we are able to identify emerging policy issues and think creatively about applied research that could provide perspective on these issues—and because of the critical and lasting investments in developing data infrastructure, and developing and documenting indicators and approaches—we can now move relatively quickly to conduct analyses that provide a perspective on emerging issues. For instance, once key measures of health status and use were developed, it was possible to study changes in health status over time. We have been able to detect improvements in the health status of some regions and groups, while at the same time detecting significant declines in the health status of other groups. In fact, our work has shown that gradients in health status have increased over time (Mustard et al. 1999), despite the relatively higher use of health care by the less healthy groups in the intervening years.

We have also been able to study how well the system adapted to bed closures, in which 25% of available hospital beds were closed over a 3-year period. Our analyses showed that, in spite of predictions of chaos, the system was able to handle almost the same number of cases with markedly reduced capacity, due largely to a decrease in the length of stay and a shift to outpatient surgery. There was no indication that quality of care, as measured by readmission rates, was affected or that the overall health of the population declined. Moreover, the groups whose health needs were greatest maintained their relatively higher levels of access to hospitals, in comparison to groups whose health need was lower (Brownell et al. 1999). This set of analyses was so critical to policymakers that we were asked to provide two updates to our initial report to determine if the initial findings were sustained.

Another set of projects studied how patterns of flu-like illness contribute to increased hospital use and emergency room crowding in Manitoba hospitals. We demonstrated that annual pressures in hospitals and emergency departments—an issue that has received considerable media attention—are caused by a relatively small number of influenza-related hospital admissions that occur for a fairly circumscribed period during winter months. This study concluded that adding additional hospital beds to the system—the obvious solution, according to many commentators—would not likely solve the problem. It suggested an alternative of finding new strategies for dealing with a fairly predictable annual requirement for more medical admissions (Menec et al. 1999). A subsequent study suggested that with improved tracking methods, a warning system would help predict flu outbreaks and give hospitals time to prepare for an increased number of patients—for example, by discharging patients who no longer required acute care or who could be supported with home-based services (Menec et al. 2001).

A Prototype for the Future

The health information system we have developed in Manitoba has enabled us to use data to develop useful perspectives on health and health care and, from this work, a cohesive set of health statistics that can be used to study health, as well as the impact of factors that influence the health of populations. While the system is still undergoing development, it is fair to say that we have managed to take a data system that is largely based on interactions with the health-care system and develop its capabilities to produce information about health. While its capabilities are still being developed, we believe that it provides some important perspectives for future development of data, statistics, and information systems.

What Aspects Are Critical for Future Development of Health Statistics?

Based on the challenges that supported us in rethinking our approach to health statistics, together with our experience in developing a population-based health information system, several factors emerge as critical to consider in designing systems of the future. Some of these important features are outlined below.

A Focus on Health

The World Health Organization's emphasis on health (denoted by its theme "Health for all") and the emergence of the population health agenda have clearly provided a context in which improving health must be acknowledged as the central goal of health systems. In developing capabilities for the twenty-first century, therefore, the key word is *health.* A system of statistics that will *focus* our attention on health and allow us to make comparisons of health status across individuals, groups, and populations, as well as make it possible to understand how health status changes over time, is needed. Moreover, health statistics must position the improvement of health as the central goal of the health-care system and build capabilities to bring critical analysis to understanding how the set of activities in which society invests can be configured so as to maximize health impacts.

Not Statistics, But an Information System

The term *health statistics* has come to refer to the set of data and aggregate indices that have relevance to health. These statistics often arise from very different perspectives and aim to meet very different needs. In the United States, for instance, they include statistics on births and deaths from the National Vital Statistics System; statistics used for the Healthy People initiatives by the U.S. Department of Health and Human Services; figures released by the National Center for Health Statistics to report on patterns of care (e.g., ambulatory day surgery); manpower data from the Health Resources and Services Administration; disease surveillance systems from the Centers for Disease Control and Prevention; Centers for Medicare and Medicaid Services reports on the Medicare program; and many others.

The population health framework provides a compelling impetus for us to think in a more integrative fashion about health statistics. It provides a big-picture perspective in which all of the existing *stovepipes* of activity can be located. Moreover, it provides a framework that suggests a need for a more interrelated approach to health statistics, one in which all of the activities can be related to the important goal of producing health. Instead of using the all-encompassing term *health statistics*, it is perhaps useful to consider three explicit areas of activity: (*1*) producing data—the raw material that provides the basis of statistics and information systems; (*2*) producing statistics—the indices and measures that are developed to measure specific concepts; and (*3*) producing information—the compilation, comparison, and triangulation of statistics in order to provide a perspective on issues of critical interest. While all of these levels of activity are important, it is this final set of activities—and the development of a health information system—that should receive additional emphasis and be the ultimate goal.

Population-Based

Given the expanding capabilities of computer systems, it is becoming increasingly possible to collect rich and detailed data on the entire population. This, in turn, makes it possible to relate the health characteristics of populations to other factors that influence health—socioeconomic status, health-care use, quality of health care, and supply of health resources. Even small amounts of data on every individual (with appropriate protection of privacy and confidentiality) make it possible to explore and understand the dynamics and distribution of health in a population in a very dynamic manner. In addition, population-based data provide a statistical framework against which more detailed, but less comprehensive data collections (e.g., surveys) can be positioned.

A Focus on the Determinants of Health

Clearly, given the population health framework, a useful health information system must be able to focus attention on understanding the factors that contribute to health. Specifically, it must be able to provide information about medical care and the extent to which investments in medical care contribute to improving health. In addition, a health information system must provide a perspective on factors that influence health but are outside the realm of medical care—for example, the impact of social and living conditions on health. Moreover, information systems must provide capability to track and understand the impact of the large societal investments that are made in domains outside the traditional medical care sector (such as public health, education, support to families with dependent children, food supplementation, and other programs). Finally, this approach requires that we identify and routinely report indicators that can serve as key markers of success or failure in our efforts to influence health.

Mapping Links Across Areas: Determinants of Health, Investments in Improving Health and Health Status

A critical aspect of information systems is the ability to build in capabilities to make links across key areas to examine various types and levels of investment in medical care for different populations. For instance, it must be possible to examine patterns of medical care for populations with the same and with different levels of health status to examine whether they make sense, given our assumptions. It must also be possible to study investments in other areas (as mentioned above) for these same populations. What is critical is the ability to reconfigure information to highlight the distribution of health in relation to the distribution of resources directed toward maintaining or improving health. Only in this way can a health information system provide a critical perspective on the likely effectiveness of societal investments.

A Critical Emphasis on Protecting Privacy and Confidentiality

A centrally important issue for the development of health information systems is the development of standards to protect the privacy and confidentiality of health records. The experience in Manitoba suggests that it is possible to develop systems capable of answering important questions that serve the public interest while at the same time protecting privacy and preserving confidentiality. Without attention to this issue, the ability to develop new knowledge from the study of observational data will likely be sharply curtailed by rising privacy concerns.

SUMMARY

Collectively, we face enormous challenges in developing a system of health statistics for the twenty-first century. Accompanying these challenges is an equally enormous set of opportunities to drastically revamp health statistics: to truly develop a focus on health of the population and to develop an integrative framework that can provide critical intelligence on how to improve health. Experience with the development of a population health information system from Manitoba, Canada, provides some critical lessons for such an undertaking and hints at some of the vastly enhanced capabilities that may be possible in the future.

Given the pluralistic nature of the U.S. system, some may feel that certain features of a health information system would be impossible to implement in the United States. On the other hand, there are examples where significant progress has been made. The United States has been a leader in the development of population-based data sets, most of which fall into three categories: registrations and notifications (such as public health surveillance systems and vital statistics), surveys with ongoing support from federal or state governments, and administrative health data systems (e.g., hospital discharge data sets). Many states have developed useful data collections, and the implementation of the Health Insurance Portability and Accountability Act (HIPAA) of 1996 included a series of *administrative simplification* provisions that required the Department of Health and Human Services to adopt national standards for electronic health care transactions. Theoretically, by ensuring consistency throughout the industry, these national standards will provide more consistent data elements and make it easier to develop more consistent tools across jurisdictions. Moreover, several organizations and jurisdictions have been able to develop more comprehensive approaches to using data for profiling health and health care. In particular, the Dartmouth Atlas project has been able to draw on large health-care claims databases (including Medicare, Blue Cross organizations, and other sources of data) to focus on the accurate description of how medical resources are distributed and used in the United States. The project even provides access to data that makes it possible to answer some very fundamental questions about the U.S. health care system. Examples such as this suggest that, with enough creativity, it will be possible to build more integrated data and information systems in the United States. We believe that the Manitoba model provides a vision for an expanded and more cohesive model as we build health statistics and information systems of the future—systems that can provide critical perspective on what really makes people healthy.

NOTES

1. Recently published research to answer this question has studied the impact of regional variations in Medicare spending across the United States. It has demonstrated that patients in higher-spending regions receive approximately 60% more care, largely explained by a more inpatient-based and specialist-oriented pattern of practice. However, quality of care, access to care, satisfaction with care, and health outcomes *do not* appear to be better for Medicare enrollees who live in higher-spending regions (Fisher et al. 2003a, 2003b).

2. This paragraph provides an oversimplified description of a complex model. Readers who wish to understand its complexities as well as the arguments underpinning the model would be advised to refer to the original publication, as well as further updates and discussions that have been published since.

3. The notable absence of a corresponding population health agenda in the United States during the 1990s was exemplified by John Eisenberg's statement shortly after being appointed Administrator of the U.S. Agency for Health Care and Policy Research (Association for Health Services Research 1997).

> AHCPR is the nation's lead Agency in ensuring that there is a scholarly and scientific foundation for a rapidly changing health care system. . . . Our shared goal is to enhance the way health care services are organized, financed and provided. We want to improve *the care patients receive* . . . [italics added for emphasis]. One of the most critical needs is to ensure that we continue to build capacity for health services research.

Nowhere was there a reference to the health of patients, although no doubt it is assumed that in improving the care patients receive, health would be one of the measuring sticks. More critically, nowhere was there a reference to the health of the population or to understanding the potential contribution that health care does or does not make in determining the health of populations.

REFERENCES

Association for Health Services Research. HSR Reports. Washington, DC: Association for Health Services Research; 1997.

Brownell M, Roos NP, Burchill C. Monitoring the Winnipeg Hospital System: 1990–91 through 1996–97. Winnipeg: Manitoba Centre for Health Policy; 1999 [cited 2004 June 14]. Available at: http://www.umanitoba.ca/centres/mchp/reports/pdfs/bedcloz3.pdf.

Burchill C, Roos LL, Fergusson P, Jebamani L, Turner K, Dueck S. Organizing the present, looking to the future: An online knowledge repository to facilitate collaboration. J Med Internet Res 2000;2(2):e10 [cited 2004 June 14]. Available at: http://www.jmir.org/2000/2/e10/index.htm.

Evans RG, Stoddart GL. Producing health, consuming health care. Soc Sci Med 1990;31(12): 1347–1363.

Fisher ES, Wennberg DE, Stukel TA, Gottlieb DJ, Lucas FL, Pinder EL. The implications of regional variations in Medicare spending. Part 1: The content, quality, and accessibility of care. Ann Intern Med 2003a;138(4):273–287.

Fisher ES, Wennberg DE, Stukel TA, Gottlieb DJ, Lucas FL, Pinder EL. The implications of regional variataions in Medicare spending. Part 2: Health outcomes and satisfaction with care. Ann Intern Med 2003b;138(4):288–299.

Friedman DJ, Hunter EL, Parrish RG, eds. Shaping a Health Statistics Vision for the 21st Century. Final Report, November 2002. Hyattsville, MD: Centers for Disease Control and Prevention, National Center for Health Statistics; Washington, DC: U.S. Department of Health and Human Services Data Council; National Committee on Vital and Health Statistics; 2002 [cited 2004 Mar 17]. Available from: http://www.ncvhs.hhs.gov/reptrecs.htm.

Havens B. Aging in Manitoba: integrating survey and administrative data. In: Warnecke R, ed. Health Survey Research Methods Conference Proceedings. Proceedings of the 6th Annual Conference on Health Survey Research Methods; 1995 Jun 24–26; Breckenridge, CO. Hyattsville, MD: U.S. Department of Health and Human Services; 1996, pp. 197–202 [cited 2004 Jun 14]. Available at: http://www.cdc.gov/nchs/data/misc/proceed.pdf.

Lalonde M. A New Perspective on the Health of Canadians: A Working Document. Ottawa: Health and Welfare Canada; 1974.

Martens P, Fransoo R, The Need to Know Team, Burland E, Jebamani L, Burchill C, et al. The Manitoba RHA Indicators Atlas: Population-Based Comparisons of Health and Health Care Use. Winnipeg: Manitoba Centre for Health Policy; 2003 [cited 2004 Jun 14]. Available at : http://www.umanitoba.ca/centres/mchp/reports/pdfs/rha2pdfs/rha2.pdf.

Menec V, Black C, MacWilliam L, Aoki F, Peterson S, Friesen D. The Impact of Influenza-like Illness on the Winnipeg Health Care System: Is an Early Warning System Possible? Winnipeg: Manitoba Centre for Health Policy; 2001 [cited 2004 Jun 14]. Available at: http://www.umanitoba.ca/centres/mchp/reports/reports_01/flu.htm.

Menec V, Roos N, Nowicki D, MacWilliam L, Finlayson G, Black C. Seasonal Patterns of Winnipeg Hospital Use. Winnipeg: Manitoba Centre for Health Policy; 1999 [cited 2004 Jun 14]. Available at: http://www.umanitoba.ca/centres/mchp/reports/pdfs/seasonal.pdf.

Muhajarine N, Mustard C, Roos LL, Young TK, Gelsky DE. Comparison of survey and physician claims data for detecting hypertension. J Clin Epidemiol 1997;50(6):711–718.

Mustard CA, Derksen S, Black C. Widening inequality in regional mortality trends in Manitoba. Can J Public Health 1999;90:372–376.

Roos NP. From research to policy: What have we learned from designing the Population Health Information System? Med Care 1995;33(12):DS132–DS145.

Roos NP, Black CD, Frohlich N, DeCoster C, Cohen MM, Tataryn DJ, Mustard CA, Toll F, Carriere KC, Burchill CA, MacWilliam L, Bogdanovic B. A population-based health information system. Med Care 1995;33(12):DS13–DS20.

Roos NP, Fransoo R, Bogdanovic B, Carriere KC, Frohlich N, Friesen D, et al. Needs-based planning for generalist physicians. Med Care 1999;37(6 suppl):JS206–JS228.

Roper WL, Winkenwerder W, Hackbarth GM, Krakauer H. Effectiveness in health care. An initiative to evaluate and improve medical practice. N Engl J Med 1988;319:1197–1202.

U.S. Department of Health and Human Services. Briefing On Medical Treatment Effectiveness. Washington, DC: U.S. Department of Health and Human Services; 1990a.

U.S. Department of Health and Human Services. AHCPR. Purpose and Programs. Washington, DC: U.S. Department of Health and Human Services; 1990b.

Watkins W. The Data Liberation Initiative: a new cooperative model. Government Inform Canada 1994;1(5) [cited 2004 Nov 5]. Available at: http://www.usask.ca/library/gic/v1n2/watkins/watkins.html.

CHAPTER 19

Population Health: New Paradigms and Implications for Health Information Systems

Barbara Starfield

Health systems everywhere face three imperatives: to increase the effectiveness of interventions, to increase the efficiency of interventions, and to increase equity in the distribution of health and health services, broadly defined. For the most part, existing health data systems do not facilitate the monitoring of these three objectives. Based largely on a conceptualization of health as the absence of specific diseases, these data systems are primarily oriented to disease as the basic "building block" of ill health, with prevention directed toward eliminating, reducing the likelihood of, or reducing the impact of specific diseases, fostering the assumption that population health can be characterized as the sum of individual health, characterized disease by disease. Thus, there are international, national, and subnational statistics that provide information on causes of death, and health objectives directed at eliminating the incidence, prevalence, or impact of specific diseases or types of diseases. Increasing specialization within the health professions predisposes to such a reductionism, as vested interests compete for resources aimed at their particular area of focus.

Both theoretical and empirical considerations make such approaches increasingly dysfunctional in providing the basis for more effectiveness, efficiency, and equity in the attainment of better health of populations.

Diseases are increasingly less important in understanding the genesis or management of health problems in populations, and in providing a basis for allocating resources (including payment for health services). Because of improved social and economic conditions as well as more effective health services, people with specific illnesses who previously would have died are now surviving, only to become at risk for other diseases. This is leading to increasing burdens of co-morbidity (coexistence of unrelated disease). Most people, particularly as they age, develop more than one health problem, so that co-morbidity becomes a major challenge for health services providers and an important consideration for the quality of health services they provide when they focus primarily on diseases. Although guidelines and standards for care are currently written disease by disease, the extent of their relevance when co-morbidity exists is unknown. Second, there is a wide range of severity within conditions, perhaps even more so than across conditions. Simply characterizing individuals by the presence of a disease provides no information on the impact of that disease or even its likely prognosis. Third, understanding the importance of various risks for disease requires recognition that the presence of some known factors is not associated with subsequent occurrence of disease, that some risk factors predispose to more than one disease, and that some diseases can follow from exposure to any one or a number of types of risk factors (Starfield 1998). Borrowing from terminology used in understanding the risk for genetic diseases, these phenomena are known, respectively, as *incomplete penetrance* (Mayr 1982), *pleiotropism* (Cavalli-Sforza and Bodmer 1971), and *etiologic heterogeneity* (Holtzman 1989). Thus, the characterization of risk factors (as well as diseases) in health information systems must allow for more than is normally provided by disease description and classification.

Moreover, health statistics reflect the existence of a tension between different strategies to achieve better population health. In no society is there such a thing as *average health*, even though statistics make it appear so. Most distributions of health are not normal; health clusters more than would be expected (by chance distributions) in certain subpopulations (van den Akker et al. 1998). Therefore, the goal of improving health might be achieved either by strategies to reduce the occurrence or prevalence of disease overall in the population or by targeting the reduction of disparities between the disadvantaged and advantaged groups, recognizing that the interventions directed at improving overall population health might be most efficiently achieved (at least initially) by focusing on people who are least disadvantaged. That is, the goal of equity might compete with the goals of effectiveness and efficiency (Anand 2002; Wagstaff and Watanabe 2000). (Note that improving the worst-off need not worsen the position of the best-off; if optimal health can be achieved by the most advantaged group with less resources than they now receive, diverting those excess resources could improve the health of the most disadvantaged without compromising the health of the most advantaged.) National and local policies weigh heavily in such decisions; the most common outcome is usually a decision to focus attention on effectiveness and efficiency, because these are perceived to be more conducive to short-term economic growth by increasing the development of ever more sophisticated technology. Systems of health statistics reflect the relative priorities that are placed on average health versus distributions of health as national goals (Kindig 1997).

EXISTING TYPES OF MEASURES OF POPULATION HEALTH

The definition of health is the same whether the focus is on the individual or the population. It is the extent to which an individual or a group is able, on the one hand, to realize its aspirations and satisfy its needs and, on the other hand, to cope with its interpersonal, social, biological, and physical environments. It is a resource for everyday living, not the objective of living; it is a positive concept embracing physical and psychological capacities (Ottawa Charter 1986).

Most existing measures of population health (as represented in health statistics) generally are not consistent with this definition of health (Institute of Medicine 2001; Wolfson 1999). Mortality statistics are based on death rates (the number of deaths per unit of population), sometimes augmented by death rates from selected causes of death, as coded by the International Classification of Diseases, or after stratification by one or more particular demographic characteristics (usually age and/or race and ethnicity).

A somewhat different metric is based on estimates of life expectancy, a method that dates to the seventeenth century and the need for calculation, by actuaries, of annuities. In a given year, given current death rates in different age groups, it provides the expected years of continued life by subtracting from the population those who die in each age range divided by the midyear population. Although it is a synthetic measure (not reflecting the experience of any specific cohort), it has proven useful in comparisons between countries and, within countries, across different population subgroups.

A related measure, years of potential life lost, provides the basis for comparing populations according to the number of years of life "lost" before a particular age (usually age 65, 70, or 75) overall or associated with particular causes of death. The General Accounting Office (GAO), the research arm of the U.S. Congress, considered 17 separate indicators of health (five concerning lifestyle characteristics such as smoking; 4 concerning employment and access to public health and medical care services; 2 concerning occupational health and safety; 3 concerning the specific disease categories of death rates from heart disease, cancer prevalence, and the acquired immunodeficiency syndrome occurrence of (AIDS), tuberculosis, and hepatitis; and 3 concerning mortality: total mortality, infant mortality, and premature mortality) and concluded that premature mortality was the most appropriate indicator for allocating federal funding for core public health functions administered by states (General Accounting Office 1997). This measure of health provides the potential for viewing population health generically (as a composite rather than disease by disease) while also allowing for the possibility of attributing premature deaths to specific diseases.

The International Classification of Primary Care (ICPC) (Lamberts et al. 1993), designed specifically for coding of reasons for visits in primary care, also codes symptoms (such as those associated with undiagnosed disease, inadequately managed diseases, deterioration in disease status, or adverse effects of interventions). Thus, it is theoretically possible to augment population health statistics by the universal coding of both diseases and states of ill health as assessed through symptomatology. To date, this approach has not been implemented.

Health is increasingly measured using reports of individuals in the population. The most common method, which is usually employed in surveys rather than in clinical situations, queries individuals as to whether their health is excellent, very good, good, fair, or poor. These individual assessments can then be aggregated to provide a population measure (the percentage of individuals who report their health in the different categories).

Alternatively, the health of individuals could be calculated as the sum of many separate indicators weighted in an appropriate way. There is no universally agreed-on way to weight the various indicators. In some approaches, such as, health-related quality-of-life assessments, standardized instruments rate the individual on various domains of health (e.g., physical functioning, emotional functioning, social functioning), from which scores are derived and then aggregated to a summary score. Health-related quality-of-life assessments are often weighted based on the values of individuals for either their own health state (patient weights) or the health status of others that are described to them (community weights). Whereas these quality-adjusted health measures (often stated as quality-adjusted life years or QALYs when combined with estimates of survival) (Mushlin et al. 2001) are sometimes used for comparing the effects of various modes of therapy in selected patient populations, they are not used for characterizing population health (Gold et al. 2002).

Disability-adjusted life years (DALYs) measure the gap between a population's health and a hypothetical ideal for health achievement based on life expectancy adjusted for rates of disability associated with individual diseases prevalent in the population. They have been used by global health researchers to quantify the burden of disease in different countries, and they formed the basis for the ranking of countries on health in the World Health Report 2000 (WHO 2000). The standard life expectancy is taken as that from Japan (as it has the longest life expectancy of any country); weights for disability rates were derived from expert judgments and vary with age. Total population disease burden is computed by summing attributable DALYs across diseases. Thus, DALYs are based on the assumption that health is dysfunction associated with individual diseases (Gold et al. 2002).

In 2003, the National Center for Health Statistics reported on the results of a workshop to identify summary measures for monitoring Healthy People 2010 (Molla et al. 2003). It reviewed the advantages and disadvantages of several measures, including healthy life expectancy (HLE), health-adjusted life expectancy (HALE), health-adjusted life years (HALY), and disability-adjusted life years (DALY), as well as newer measures such as years of healthy life (life without disability), years of healthy life (developed for Healthy People 2000), years of life without functioning problems; years of life without specified diseases, years of life in excellent or very good health, and years of life lived with good health behavior. All are constructed with data now available (in the United States) from the National Health Interview Survey, the annual life table for the population, and life tables for the subpopulations of interest. The monograph provided examples of data, by age and sex, for the U.S. population.

A FRAMEWORK FOR HEALTH STATISTICS SYSTEMS

The widespread improvement in individual and population health, consequent to social as well as medical advances, is providing impetus for basing health statistics on a broader conceptualization of health and determinants of health. Figures 19.1 and 19.2 provide one such conceptualization. Figure 19.1 is a parsimonious depiction of types of risks for ill health. Risk factors are not independent of each other; many risk factors predispose to other risk factors. Summing of individual risk factors provides no information on the magnitude of risks in the population, either those for specific diseases or for general states of health. Figure 19.2 provides an equally parsimonious depiction of the web of causation of illness in populations. It differs from Figure 19.1 in two respects: the greater salience of contextual (not individual) influences and the critical features of illness distributions (Diez-Roux 1998; Susser 1998; Susser and Susser 1996). The distinctions between a focus on individuals, aggregated individuals, and populations (or subpopulations) are at the heart of the distinctions among clinical medicine, clinical epidemiology, social medicine, community medicine, and public health. Consider the following questions:

- What disease might this patient have?
- What is the relative likelihood that this patient has or is at risk for this disease?
- Why does this patient have this disease at this particular time?
- Is this disease important? If so, to whom and how important is it?
- What characteristics are most salient in improving overall health and the distribution of health in populations?

The first question is the conventional clinical question; the second is an issue for clinical epidemiology; the third is the subject of social medicine; the fourth is the concern of community medicine; the fifth is the critical concern for public health.

The recognition of the broad range of factors that influence both current health and the potential for future health provides the justification for augmenting conventional health statistics with newer systems that better reflect new imperatives in population health. These include (*1*) increasing disparities across population subgroups; (*2*) increasing recognition of the importance of the social and political contexts in understanding and overcoming their adverse ef-

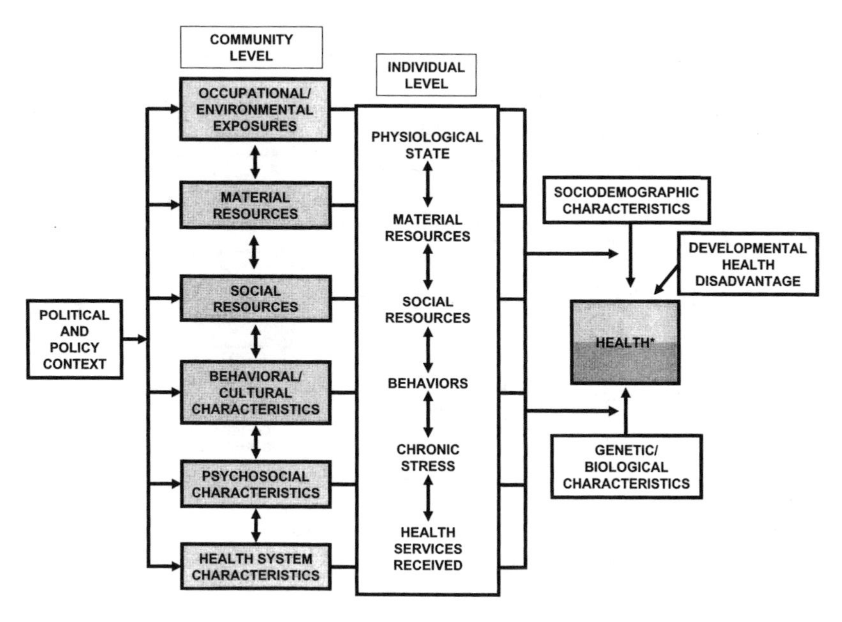

FIGURE 19.1
Influences on health: individual level. Shading represents the degree to which characteristics are measured at the ecological level (lighter color) or at the individual level aggregated to the community level. **Health* has two aspects: occurrence (incidence) and intensity (severity).

fects as well as maximizing their salutary effects; (*3*) a focus on population-attributable risk as well as relative risk; (*4*) increasing co-morbidity in the population; and (*5*) the need for better coordination between public health and clinical medicine in an effort to better protect and promote health and prevent ill health.

DISPARITIES ACROSS POPULATIONS AND POPULATION SUBGROUPS

Disparities across countries and across subpopulations within countries are a worldwide concern (Braveman 1998). Consideration of disparities is an important aspect of the distinction between the population health focus and the individual health focus (Fig. 19.2 vs. Fig. 19.1). No system of national or subnational population health statistics is adequate without attention to characterizing the differences across major population groups. In the past, interpretation of health differences across different areas was made possible by statistically adjusting for differences in the demographic characteristics of populations, thus obscuring the existence of disparities across them. Increasingly, population health statistics will contain mechanisms to stratify populations so that systematic differences across

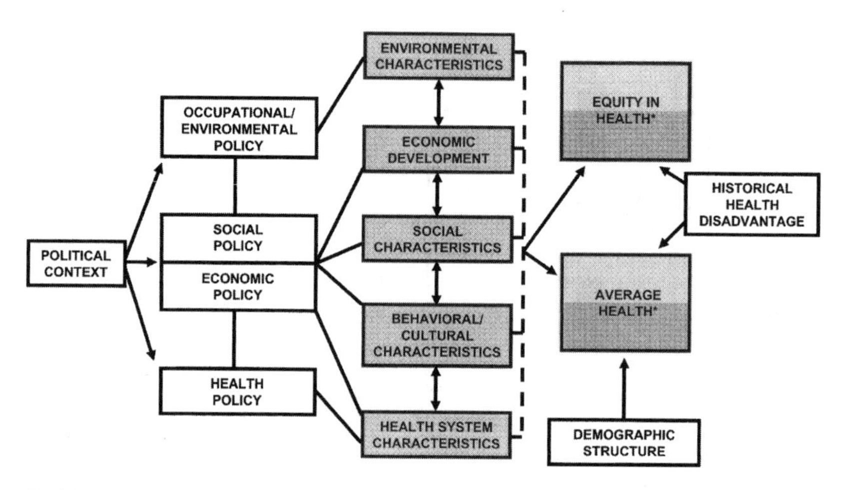

FIGURE 19.2
Influences on health: population level. Dashed lines indicate the existence of pathways through individual-level characteristics that most proximally influence health. Shading represents the degree to which characteristics are measured at the ecological level (lighter color) or at the individual level aggregated to the community level. **Health* has two aspects: occurrence (incidence) and intensity (severity).

them will be sufficiently visible to draw policy attention to them. Although the major subpopulations will differ from country to country and from area to area, each jurisdiction will have to develop a rational plan for analyzing and presenting data according to the most relevant considerations for elucidating existing health disparities.

UNDERSTANDING THE IMPORTANCE OF SOCIAL AND POLITICAL CONTEXT

Although the importance to health of the social context has been recognized for centuries, it is only in the most recent quarter-century that systematic attention has been devoted to clarifying the types and mechanisms of effects of various aspects of the social milieu. The vast literature on the subject has recently been summarized by Berkman and Kawachi (2000). Less well researched is the effect of the political context, although its relevance to policy formulation is self-evident (Fig. 19.2). Szreter (1999) suggested that the state has a role in promoting participatory citizenship, which has direct implications for the design of government and of policies that will determine the relative balance among the various impacts on health. Similarly, Lynch and colleagues (2000) argue for a framework that "embraces structural as well as interpersonal social relationships." Navarro and Shi's (2001) analysis of the impact of the nature of governance on infant mortality is one of the first to consider the relationship between this most distal factor in the web of causality on one aspect of the health of populations. Health statistics will increasingly require expansion to a much wider range of possible influences on the health of populations and subpopulations and a wider variety of measures of health, obtained in ways very different from those used in the past and present. Many of these influences cannot be obtained from individuals, as they are characteristics of environments (Hancock et al. 1999; McKinlay and Marceau 2000; McMichael 1999).

Linkages of different types of statistical data sets will become the imperative in health data systems of the future: individual characteristics linked with characteristics of the areas in which they live and work will provide a much broader base for understanding why some people and some population groups are more ill than others. This will provide the basis for more effective and more efficient interventions to improve overall health as well as to reduce disparities in health.

Policymaking and planning for the deployment of health services require information not only about the types of challenges to health but also about the relative frequency of their distribution in the population. In clinical decision making, relative risks generally dominate: if one risk factor has a higher likelihood of being associated with an adverse outcome, it generally becomes a higher priority for intervention than does a risk factor with a lower relative risk. In planning for population health, the frequency of risks demands consideration; a factor with high relative risk may have little importance as an influence on health if it is very uncommon in the population. Thus, the concepts of *relative risk* and *attributable risk* are of different salience, depending on whether interest is focused on an individual's health or on a population's (or subpopulation's) health.

CO-MORBIDITY

Co-morbidity is the coexistence of two or more unrelated illnesses or types of illness. The clustering of different types of illness within certain individuals and within certain population subgroups has always been a feature of illness, but has only recently been recognized as an important challenge to thinking about the genesis, prevention, and improvement of ill health. An accumulating literature (Starfield 2001a) documents the co-occurrence of otherwise unrelated diseases, and conceptualizations of disease causation provide the theoretical basis for expecting that co-occurrence is of greater magnitude than would be expected by random co-occurrence of two or more unrelated diseases. Figures 19.1 and 19.2 show how risk factors are not independent of one another; many risk factors predispose to other risk factors, and various different risk factors will be represented differently in determining the overall risk for a given health problem (Koopman and Lynch 1999). Summing of individual risk factors provides no information on the magnitude of illness risks in the population; there are many interactions across risk factors and different relative impacts of individual risk factors in different populations and population subgroups. Moreover, simply having a health condition changes the vulnerability to other health problems, usually by increasing it (as a result of debilitated health states with less resistance to new illnesses) but sometimes by decreasing it (through developing biological or psychological coping mechanisms).

As co-morbidity is a major new challenge in characterizing health, it is also a major challenge in characterizing different types of health service interventions. Services received from only one provider or one provider type no longer suffice when people have combinations of different illnesses or types of illnesses; multiple providers are now the rule. This requires the availability of data that are shared across providers and different types of providers. Without shared data, coordination of care becomes impossible. Moreover, a focus on both co-morbidity and co-occurrence of risk factors in populations, as well as on their distribution within populations, calls for an increased role of public health and for coordination of the public health role with the clinical role of health practitioners. The next section discusses the imperative for coordination of these two roles in health services systems using new types of data systems.

DATA REQUIREMENTS FOR COORDINATING PUBLIC HEALTH AND CLINICAL MEDICINE FUNCTIONS

Table 19.1 describes the major types of health activities and their targets. On one axis are the types, divided into three categories: health protection and promotion and primary prevention (improving health and reducing the level of threats to health); secondary prevention (interfering with the progression of ill health at a point where an abnormality can be detected but before manifestations are overt); and tertiary prevention (interfering with progression of ill health after overt manifestations occur and remediation of the overt effects). On the other axis are the targets of activities, divided into those that are addressed at the population level as a whole, those addressed to all individuals within the population (or subpopulations), those addressed uniformly but only for individuals in selected subpopulations, and those directed only at individuals with a particular need for them.

Only in the case of the top row (activities that benefit all individuals in the population) is the locus of responsibility for activities unarguably primarily in the jurisdiction of population medicine (public health). Activities in all other cells in the matrix may be a function of clinical medicine or public health, depending on place and time. A major aspect of policy development, and thus of data systems, concerns decisions on what types of functions are primarily under the aegis of public health or clinical medicine; countries and smaller political

TABLE 19.1
Types of Interventions

Target Group	Primary	Secondary	Tertiary
Population			
As population	Environmental planning	Environmental monitoring and product control	Public advocacy Community mobilization (legal and social remedies)
All individuals	Health education campaigns Immunizations	Phenylketonuria screening Breast cancer screening	Information systems: data standardization, collection, analysis and dissemination
Selective	Genetic engineering	Blood lead screening	Outreach/access (e.g., home visiting)
Indicated	Communicable disease control Prophylactic antibiotics Practice guidelines	Frequent follow-up for disease recurrence	Address problems: quality assessment of clinical services

jurisdictions differ in their decisions. For the most part, activities in the bottom row are in the purview of clinical medicine, although in some countries the activities may be carried out by public health professionals, particularly when the occurrence of disease (such as tuberculosis) in particular individuals carries a threat to other individuals in the population. Differences across jurisdictions and countries are particularly notable in the second and third rows of the matrix, which involve all individuals in the population or individuals in selected target groups in the population.

Although differences among countries or localities in the extent to which the various types of activities are under the jurisdiction of public health or clinical medicine have not been studied or described, some health systems have confronted the issue explicitly. In the United Kingdom, primary care trusts (which are clinical entities) have increasingly been given responsibility for public health functions. This delegation of conventionally public health activity to clinical entities, and hence the responsibility for collecting health statistics, has no strong empirical basis. In fact, there is considerable concern about its likelihood of success, as there are increasing questions about the adequacy of intervention when the populations covered by the clinical entity are too small to support an effective public health function, including health statistics (Gillam et al. 2001).

Clinical medicine rarely covers populations large enough or sufficiently representative for their data systems to show the systematic differences in distribution of risks across population subgroups. Therefore, population health statistics play a critical role in monitoring the existence and degree of disparities across population subgroups. They also can help to provide the basis for deciding which level of services is best suited to carrying out specific activities. Health needs shared by all individuals in the population, such as the need for health protection, are likely to be better served by public health data systems that are derived from intersectoral activities at the population level. The need for preventive activities that are common to all individuals in the population may also be best served by public health data, particularly in countries and areas where health services are not uniformly or equally available to all segments of the population. The new brand of health statistics can greatly inform decisions about the most appropriate locus of action by shedding light on the existence and magnitude of various aspects of health.

POPULATION HEALTH IS MORE THAN THE SUM OF INDIVIDUAL HEALTH

The key to understanding the incidence and prevalence of disease and risk factors lies in characterization of populations, not individuals (Rose 1985; Schwartz et al. 2001).

Is population health the sum of individual health? Although this is commonly assumed, it is not the case, except for very specific aspects of illness and where distributions of health are not of interest.

For each separate manifestation of ill health or health, including predispositions (risks and resiliencies, respectively), the sum of individual health measures, properly adjusted or standardized by sociodemographic characteristics that are inherently related to the occurrence of illness, accurately describes individual aspects of the state of health for a population. Although these sums are accurate, they are increasingly irrelevant for policy and decision making, either because they are not accurate representations of health as now conceptualized or because they assume that the separate components of health and the influences on various aspects of health are randomly distributed in the population. Neither is the case. Morbidity and mortality are not randomly distributed in the population; there is no such characteristic as an *average health* level. Moreover, risk factors are not evenly or randomly distributed in the population; some population groups have more risks factors than are explainable by chance distributions, and some have fewer.

Health statistics are not a heuristic exercise. They are collected for specific purposes. Descriptions of averages, by themselves, provide no useful information. The most basic purpose of health statistics is to provide clues to unmet needs so that resources can be directed appropriately. At the most simple level, needs are manifested as differences in levels of health across populations. This is why the earliest statisticians adjusted their health statistics for differences in major demographic characteristics of populations, so that they could more confidently conclude that any differences were due to health rather than to differences in, for example, the age distribution in the populations that were compared. At their earliest stages, then, health statistics were not simple additions of individual health statistics. However, average health levels, even if age and/or gender adjusted, provide no information on the distribution of health needs in populations; as noted above, consideration of disparities in populations now carries equal weight with poor overall health as a consideration for modern societies. Population health, when characterized as separate disease states, is most certainly not the sum of individual health because of the presence of co-morbidity and the concentration of clusters of types of diseases in particular individuals and population subgroups.

The critical recognition of social and political contexts as determinants of disease is the final reason for considering population health statistics as distinct from a compilation of individual health statistics. If health is determined by factors outside of and separate from the individual, an understanding of the genesis and malleability of population health cannot be obtained by considering population health as a composite of individual health. Many risks and resiliencies derive from factors outside the individual; understanding their impact on population health requires levels of aggregation and analyses that extend to ecological characteristics as well as individual ones.

The recent redefinition of heath statistics as "numerical data that characterize the health of a population and the influences that affect it" provides clear challenges for future health statistics endeavors (see Chapter 1). First, it addresses the issue of *health*, not separate aspects of health. It therefore poses the challenge of developing measures that represent or summarize the state of health of people, many of whom have more than one conventional health condition, as well as maintaining an interest in the individual conditions. Second, it mandates decisions on the nature of these summary measures of health, particularly whether they are to be *morbidity indices* composed of conventional measures of health mortality and morbidity or whether these are to be replaced with alternative constructions of health based on functional disability. Third, the redefinition also speaks to *influences on health*, not only the end results of these influences. Until recently, the concept of health has not included these influences, instead regarding them as of concern for future health and not health per se. Fourth, the worldwide imperative, expressed in many countries as national health goals, not only to improve the overall state of health of the population but also to reduce disparities in health within the population, provides another challenge. Until very recently, health statistics were almost always presented as average values for populations. The fact that these data are often presented separately by age and gender sets the stage for additional stratifications, particularly by social class groupings, ethnicity, and, where relevant, race. Equity is increasingly regarded as equally salient to effectiveness in improving levels of health. Thus, from the viewpoint of health policy, health statistics should not be limited to average levels of health, however measured or specified (Sassi et al. 2001).

Relevance in a world of changing criteria for health provides the imperative for innovation in health statistics. Originally these systems were developed to categorize causes of death. Over time, they were modified to categorize causes of hospitalization and then to categorize diagnoses in visits to physicians. No similar system exists for any other facet of health, although recently, the World Health Organization has developed a new system for classifying functioning. Known as the International Classification of Functioning (ICF) (WHO 2001), it sets out aspects of health that represent the manifestations of activity limitation and disability in the context of people's daily living, including mental and social as well as physical dimensions. As is the case with the International Classification of Diseases, each functional compromise is considered separately.

The World Health Organization has taken the position that health is an attribute of individuals, best measured as deviations from a "threshold level of ability to carry out physical and mental actions and tasks in the current environment" (Chatterji et al. 2002). It recommends that health be understood as a multidimensional phenomenon that can be narrowed to a core set of health domains (such as pain, affect, mobility, cognition, self-care, and usual activities), each characterized by a single cardinal scale of capacity (measured, observed, or self-reported) with the use of currently available personal aids (as distinguished from environmental modifications). A single measure for each individual could be obtained by carrying out health state evaluations for the domains. In this conceptualization of health, inherent capacities (including those modified by personal aids) are distinguished from performance measures, which are dependent on the nature of the environment of the person.

POTENTIALLY PROMISING NEW APPROACHES TO CHARACTERIZATION OF POPULATION HEALTH—A RESEARCH AGENDA

Two main challenges to characterizing population health require attention. The first is a need for a focus on the person rather than on separate diseases or dysfunctions. The second is a need to advance the knowledge of positive health, which includes not only the absence of illness but also the presence of wellness (Singer and Ryff 2001). Two new measures that address these two imperatives are presented next.

Disease Case Mix

The first method, based on clinical data, is the Adjusted Clinical Groupings (ACG) method of characterizing the case mix of diagnoses in individual and populations. The ACG system characterizes people according to the pattern of illnesses they experience in a period of time. Illness is conceptualized as fitting into one of several types: minor illnesses that are generally self-limited if treated appropriately; illnesses that are more major but also are limited in time if treated appropriately; medical illnesses that are generally chronic and not curable by medical therapy; illnesses resulting from anatomic problems (such as hearing, vision, and orthopedic problems); and conditions that are considered psychosocial. The approach involves assigning each of the diagnoses in the International Classification of Diseases—Clinical Modification (ICD-CM) to 1 of 32 categories using the following criteria: likelihood that the condition would persist and the patient would have return visits for it; likelihood of a specialty consultation or referral, currently and in the future; expected need for and cost of diagnostic and therapeutic procedures associated with the condition; likelihood of an associated hospitalization; likelihood of an associated disability; and likelihood of associated decreased life expectancy.

The 32 groupings are collapsed into 12 relatively similar groups (CADGs), which are then aggregated according to their most commonly encountered combinations in clinical practice. Each individual in an enrolled population is characterized by the diagnoses he or she receives in the period of time and placed in the final grouping (the ACG) that represents the constellation of diagnoses for that patient. The case mix of a health facility, or of any practitioner, can be described according to the pattern of ACGs. Practitioners or facilities with greater frequencies of those ACGs that represent sicker patients can be considered to need more resources to care for those patients in their practices.

The important feature of the ACG system is that a single ACG is assigned to an individual based on the pattern of morbidity experienced by that individual over a period of time, generally a year. This assignment of morbidity is not dependent on visit rates per se or on the extent of use or the cost of diagnostic and therapeutic procedures because only diagnoses (including symptoms) coded by the ICD are used for the assignment. An individual may have multiple illnesses of one type, yet be assigned to only one category of illness for the year. Thus, the method is not dependent on the number of illnesses but rather on their type as characterized by the criteria for assignment.

The ACG system has potential utility for describing differences in the patterns of illnesses in different clinical populations; in serving as a method for stratifying populations into clinically meaningful groups for the purpose of profiling the practices of different practitioners or groups of practitioners; and as a method for studying resource use and planning for the resource needs of different populations. It also has applicability in research that seeks to explain the predictiveness of various health system factors on resource use, in that differences in morbidity in different populations can be controlled for when examining the impact of practitioner and system factors on use of services and resources.

For example, a morbidity index based on the ACG case mix system was a far better predictor of premature mortality in a Canadian province than a socioeconomic risk index or use rates in the population (Reid et al. 2002).

Profiles of Health

A second approach, which so far has been developed only for children and youth of ages 6–17, is similar in assuming that population health can be described as the percentage of individuals who fall into each of several mutually exclusive profiles of health. The conceptualization of health that underlies the development of profiles is based on the pattern of scores on the first four of the following domains of health: Symptoms (Discomfort); Satisfaction with Health; Risks; Resilience; Diseases (Disorders); and Achievement of Social Expectations related to health (including Development in Childhood). The profile types were characterized primarily by the number of domains in which health is poor, identifying the unique combinations of problems that characterize different subgroups of children and adolescents. The profiles of health were constructed from the data obtained on the Child Health and Illness Profile–Adolescent Edition (CHIP-AE) and the Child Edition (CHIP-CE), which elicit self-reports of health across these six domains. Several sets of mutually exclusive profile types were defined; 13 profiles can be defined in terms of whether there are zero, one, two, three, to four domains of health need. The actual distributions into these 13 types are significantly different from chance distributions. The best and worst profiles have a much higher proportion of individuals than expected by chance (Riley et al 1998a). Thus this profile method not only describes the health of populations generically but also provides the basis for describing the clustering of good and bad health within and across populations and population subgroups. Tests of its validity confirm that it adequately portrays differences in health by age, gender, and social class groupings (Riley et al 1998b; Starfield et al. 2002a, 2002b).

Many research challenges remain before such alternative or complementary approaches can be converted into useful population health statistics. However, these new alternatives have characteristics that address major challenges for future health statistics. Although the ACG system considers only medically coded diagnoses, it explicitly tackles the issue of characterizing co-morbidity. The profiles-of-health approach addresses the need to go beyond diseases to consider functioning, and to include consideration of the potential for future health as represented by risks and resilience. Its special advantage is its characterization of individuals and populations as patterns of deviation from maximal health in its various categories, thus making it possible to tailor both health policies and clinical services to patterns of needs rather than to needs in separate aspects of health. The eventual utility of any of these innovative methods will be based on wider acceptance of their potential contributions to characterizing population health and more widespread testing of their usefulness in different population subgroups and populations.

SUMMARY

New paradigms for health and changing characteristics of health call for an augmented approach to the design of health statistics. The phenomenon of comorbidity demands a person-oriented rather than a disease focus for depicting the health of people and populations and a new characterization of health services deriving from the increasing need for coordination of care across multiple providers and levels of care, including that between public health and clinical medicine. Increasing and systematic disparities in health across population subgroups and the requirement, in health statistics systems, of a wider variety of political, social, and environmental factors that either predispose to or interfere with the achievement of higher health levels in individuals and populations provide the imperative for a new conceptualization of health data and health statistics systems as the twenty-first century progresses.

REFERENCES

Anand S. The concern for equity in health. J Epidemiol Commun Health 2002;56(7):485–487.

Berkman L, Kawachi I. Social Epidemiology. New York: Oxford University Press; 2000.

Braveman P. Monitoring Equity in Health: A Policy-Oriented Approach in Low- And Middle-Income Countries. (WHO/CHS/HSS/98.1). Geneva: World Health Organization; 1998.

Cavalli-Sforza L, Bodmer W. The Genetics of Human Populations. San Francisco: W.H. Freeman; 1971.

Chatterji S, Ustun B, Sadano R, Salomon J, Mathers C, Murray CJL. The conceptual basis for measuring and reporting on health. Global Programme on Evidence for Health Policy. Discussion Paper No. 45. Geneva: World Health Organization; 2002.

Diez-Roux AV. Bringing context back into epidemiology: variables and fallacies in multilevel analysis. Am J Public Health 1998;88(2):216–222.

General Accounting Office. Public Health: A Health Status Indicator for Targeting Federal Aid to States GAO/HEHS-97-13. Washington, DC; 1997.

Gillam S, Abbott S, Banks-Smith J. Can primary care groups and trusts improve health? BMJ 2001;323(7304):89–92.

Gold MR, Stevenson D, Fryback DG. HALYs and QALYs and DALYs, oh my: similarities and differences in summary measures of population health. Annu Rev Public Health 2002;23:115–134.

Hancock T, Labonte R, Edwards R. Indicators that count! Measuring population health at the community level. Can J Public Health 1999;90(suppl 1):S22–S26.

Holtzman NA. Proceed with Caution: Predicting Genetic Risks in the Recombinant DNA Era. Baltimore: Johns Hopkins University Press; 1989.

Institute of Medicine, Board on Neuroscience and Behavioral Health, Committee on Health and Behavior: Research, Practice, and Policy. Health and Behavior: The Interplay of Biological, Behavioral, and Societal Influences. Washington, DC: National Academy Press; 2001.

Kindig DA. How do you define the health of populations? Physician Exec 1997; 23(7):6–11.
Koopman JS, Lynch JW. Individual causal models and population system models in epidemiology. Am J Public Health 1999; 89(8):1170–1174.
Lamberts H, Wood M, Hofmans-Okkes I. The International Classification of Primary Care in the European Community. Oxford and New York: Oxford University Press; 1993.
Lynch JW, Due P, Muntaner C, Smith GD. Social capital—is it a good investment strategy for public health? J Epidemiol Commun Health 2000; 54(6):404–408.
Mayr E. The Growth of Biological Thought: Diversity, Evolution, and Inheritance. Cambridge, MA: Harvard University Press; 1982.
McKinlay JB, Marceau LD. To boldly go . . . Am J Public Health 2000;90(1):25–33.
McMichael AJ. Prisoners of the proximate: loosening the constraints on epidemiology in an age of change. Am J Epidemiol 1999;149(10):887–897.
Molla MT, Madans JH, Wagener DK, Crimmins EM. Summary Measures of Population Health: Report Of Findings on Methodologic and Data Issues. Hyattsville, MD: National Center for Health Statistics; 2003.
Mushlin AI, Ruchlin HS, Callahan MA. Cost effectiveness of diagnostic tests. Lancet 2001; 358(9290):1353–1355.
Navarro V, Shi L. The political context of social inequalities and health. Soc Sci Med 2001; 52(3):481–491.
Ottawa Charter for Health Promotion. First International Conference on Health Promotion; 1986 Nov 17–21; Ottawa, Canada.
Reid RJ, Roos NP, MacWilliam L, Frohlich N, Black C. Assessing population health care need using a claims-based ACG morbidity measure: a validation analysis in the Province of Manitoba. Health Serv Res 2002;37(5):1345–1364.
Riley AW, Forrest CB, Starfield B, Green B, Kang M, Ensminger M. Reliability and validity of the adolescent health profile-types. Med Care 1998b;36(8):1237–1248.
Riley AW, Green BF, Forrest CB, Starfield B, Kang M, Ensminger ME. A taxonomy of adolescent health: development of the adolescent health profile-types. Med Care 1998a; 36(8):1228–1236.
Rose G. Sick individuals and sick populations. Int J Epidemiol 1985;14(1):32–38. Reprinted in Int J Epidemiol 2001;30(3):427–432; discussion 433–434.
Sassi F, Archard L, Le Grand J. Equity and the economic evaluation of healthcare. Health Technol Assess 2001;5(3):1–138.
Schwartz S, Diez-Roux AV, Diez-Roux R. Commentary: causes of incidence and causes of cases—a Durkheimian perspective on Rose. Int J Epidemiol 2001;30(3):435–439.
Singer BH, Ryff CD, eds. New Horizons in Health: An Integrative Approach. Washington, DC: National Academy Press; 2001.
Starfield B. Primary Care: Balancing Health Needs, Services, and Technology. New York: Oxford University Press; 1998.
Starfield B. New paradigms for quality in primary care. Br J Gen Pract 2001a;51(465):303–309.
Starfield B, Riley AW, Witt WP, Robertson J. Social class gradients in health during adolescence. J Epidemiol Commun Health 2002a;56(5):354–361.
Starfield B, Robertson J, Riley AW. Social class gradients and health in childhood. Ambul Pediatr 2002b;2(4):238–246.
Susser M. Does risk factor epidemiology put epidemiology at risk? Peering into the future. J Epidemiol Commun Health 1998;52(10):608–611.
Susser M, Susser E. Choosing a future for epidemiology: II. From black box to Chinese boxes and eco-epidemiology. Am J Public Health 1996;86(5):674–677.
Szreter S. A new political economy for New Labour—the importance of social capital. Renewal 1999;7:30–44.
van den Akker M, Buntinx F, Metsemakers JF, Roos S, Knottnerus JA. Multimorbidity in

general practice: prevalence, incidence, and determinants of co-occurring chronic and recurrent diseases. J Clin Epidemiol 1998;51(5):367–375.
Wagstaff A, Watanabe N. Socioeconomic Inequalities in Child Malnutrition in the Developing World. Washington, DC: World Bank; 2000 [cited 2004 Mar 10]. Available from: http://econ.worldbank.org/files/1189_wps2434.pdf.
Wolfson M. Measuring health—visions and practicalities. Stat J United Nations 1999;16:1–17.
World Health Organization. The World Health Report 2000. Health Systems: Improving Performance. Geneva: World Health Organization; 2000.
World Health Organization. International Classification of Functioning, Disability, and Health. Geneva: World Health Organization; 2001.

CHAPTER 20

The National Health Information Infrastructure

John R. Lumpkin and Mary Jo Deering

Improving the health of individuals, communities, and nations is the job of more than health-care providers and public health professionals. Successful health improvement efforts must engage policymakers, consumers, patients, and caregivers, all of whom need to make informed decisions based on the best information available.

THE PROBLEM

The people needing specific information often did not collect or analyze it. Health plans and health-care providers need statistical data about such topics as environmental health risks, infant outcomes, communicable diseases, and demographic characteristics of their communities in order to understand, treat, and plan patient care. Public health officials need timely clinical data on emerging health threats to become better prepared and to develop response plans. Health-care services researchers need aggregate data on treatments and outcomes to assess quality and effectiveness. Consumers need information on health-care quality to choose treatments, plans, and providers and information about local environmental health hazards to take action within their homes and communities. Patients need about their own medical histories and information about disease management and treatment options to manage their own health and health care. All need access to synthesized information about individual health and the population's health, accompanied by decision-support tools appropriate to their particular roles.

The data behind the needed information reside in diverse places, reflecting the specific purposes for which those data were collected. Often the data are now kept on paper. When in electronic form, they can be accessed only through dedicated information systems linking the data source to specific categories of end users. All too frequently, because it was presumed that the data were relevant only to a particular group of users, their implications are not translated for other types of users. Consequently, sharing or aggregating data for different types of users and uses is sometimes difficult or impossible. This problem looms increasingly large as health decision making becomes more interconnected and as the vertical and horizontal integration of health-care providers has increased.

If health data and information are to be made more widely available, institutional policies and practices interfering with information exchange must be confronted. Providers, health plans, and researchers who collect and manage health information may view it as proprietary. Concerns about the security and confidentiality of health data may inhibit many stakeholders. Systems for capturing, synthesizing, and presenting data for new uses and users are not widely available. Overcoming these challenges and delivering the right information to the right people at the right time require a comprehensive national health information infrastructure.

WHAT IS THE NATIONAL INFORMATION INFRASTRUCTURE?

The concept of a National Information Infrastructure (NII) emerged from public research and development programs and policies spanning several decades, including developments in networking and computing capability (Shortliffe 2000). The federal NII initiative was announced in September 1993,[1] led by the Information Infrastructure Task Force and the Advisory Council on the National Information Infrastructure, which included industry, labor, universities, public interest groups, and state and local governments (U.S. Department of Commerce 1993). The Information Infrastructure Task Force (IITF) defined the NII as encompassing physical components, the information itself in many different formats, applications and software, network standards and transmission codes, and the people who create information, develop applications and services, construct the facilities, and train others to tap its potential (U.S. Department of Commerce 1993). The IITF looked specifically at opportunities to strengthen manufacturing, electronic commerce, health care, education, environmental monitoring, libraries, and government services through an NII (U.S. Department of Commerce 1994). In 1996, the Next Generation Internet Program was established as a research and development initiative by federal agencies in partnership with academia and industry. The Next Generation Internet Program's goals were to connect at least 100 universities, national laboratories, and research institutions with high-speed networks 100 to 1000 times faster than the current

Internet, invest in research and development to enhance the capabilities of the Internet, and demonstrate new applications supporting important national goals. Also in 1996, a consortium of 200 universities set up the Internet2 initiative to develop advanced network applications and technologies. The Internet2 network is capable of transmitting data at more than 1 billion bits per second, more than 300 times current high-speed broadband connections. Internet2 technology permits the storage and retrieval of vast amounts of information, including images, across multiple sites in ways not previously possible.

THE NATIONAL HEALTH INFORMATION INFRASTRUCTURE

In its 1991 report on computer-based patient records, revised in 1997, the Institute of Medicine envisioned a "national health care information system" to "support the coordination and integration of healthcare services across settings and among providers of care" (Dick et al. 1997). The federal government's 1994 report on *High Performance Computing and Communications: Technology for the National Information Infrastructure* outlined a "national challenge" to improve the quality, effectiveness, and efficiency of health care (National Science and Technology Council 1994). Components of the National Challenge included "testbed networks and collaborative applications to link remote and urban patients and providers to the information they need, database technologies to collect and share patient health records in secure, privacy-assured environments, advanced biomedical devices and sensors, and system architectures to built and maintain the complex health information infrastructure" (National Science and Technology Council 1994). The Information Infrastructure Task Force's Committee on Applications and Technology also addressed the relationship of health care to the NII in its 1994 report, which called for medical information standards for nomenclature, coding, and structure; content of specific data sets; electronic data interchange; unique personal identification; models, requirements, and architecture; federal confidentiality and privacy laws; health data repositories; and computer-based patient record systems (U.S. Department of Commerce 1994). Over the next few years, additional reports added to the idea of a health information infrastructure (Dick et al. 1997; Institute of Medicine 2001; Kohn et al. 2000; Lasker et al. 1995; National Research Council 2000).

Based on a series of national hearings, the National Committee on Vital and Health Statistics (NCVHS), which advises the Secretary of the U.S. Department of Health and Human Services (DHHS) on health information policy, developed a consensus vision of the National Health Information Infrastructure (NHII) in 2000 and 2001. The NCVHS articulated the concept of an infrastructure that emphasizes health-oriented interactions and information sharing among individuals and institutions, rather than just the physical, technical, and data systems that make those interactions possible (National Committee on Vital and Health Statistics 2000, 2001). As set forth by the NCVHS, the NHII includes the values, practices, relationships, laws, standards, systems, applications, and technologies that support all facets of individual health, health care, and population health. The NHII also encompasses tools such as clinical practice guidelines, educational resources for the public and professionals, geographic information systems permitting regional analysis and comparisons, health statistics at all levels of government, and many forms of communication among users (National Committee on Vital and Health Statistics 2001). The NHII would help overcome the problems of inaccessible data and information and enable connectivity and knowledge management (Detmer 2003).

The technical infrastructure of the NHII can be understood as an electronic web of computer and communications technologies enabling each user's computer or communications device to interact with others. The NHII enhances the ability of each individual to control his or her health data and the access by health-care providers to those data. However, the NHII is neither a system of systems nor a centralized government database for storing personal health information. The NHII is envisioned as a way to connect distributed health data and information within the framework of a secure network. Health data and health information will continue to reside in myriad locations in the NHII. Knowledge bases and other intelligent decision-support applications may also be distributed or centralized (National Committee on Vital and Health Statistics 2000, 2001). Information access and exchange will be facilitated by standards for data and technology, by protocols and practices for security and confidentiality, and by supportive public policies.

Delivering health care and protecting the public's health are data and information intensive. The capacity of the NHII will be enhanced by the Next Generation Internet and Internet2 projects. New Internet technologies will enable the transfer of massive amounts of data instantaneously, accurately, and securely. Terms such as *internetworking* and *nomadic computing* illustrate these new developments. For example, current applications in medical care include generating and transmitting a three-dimensional model of a human body, including the skeleton, muscles, and blood vessels; a digital mammogram repository; and off-site medical record storage, including medical images (National Library of Medicine 2002 [hp]). Implicit in this technical foundation is a requirement for the human resources to manage both hardware and software. Experts in computer science, networking, programming, and database management must be available. Staff working in health-care organizations and public health agencies must appreciate the NHII's technical aspects in order to manage and use NHII-enabled activities effectively. Consumers, patients, and health-care providers need to know when and how to use the resources made available by the NHII.

The NHII as a whole is not primarily about data or even about enhancement of information technology; equally important are knowledge exchange and improved communication. Consequently, NHII implementation requires attention to the development, collection, and management of all kinds of content.

Care is needed in identifying the appropriate content (data and nondata) and ensuring that it is accurate, timely, friendly to users, and widely accessible by them. Knowledge management staff with expertise in specific health areas and in cross-cutting information services are essential.

NATIONAL HEALTH INFORMATION INFRASTRUCTURE DIMENSIONS

Just as the NHII can be conceptualized as a circle surrounded by the larger circle of the NII, it can also be conceived as consisting of at least three overlapping circles. Each of the three circles represents a different NHII dimension: the health-care provider dimension, the personal health dimension, and the population health dimension. These three dimensions are equally important in the NHII, and the goal of the NHII is to improve information flows across these dimensions and not just within each dimension.

The health-care provider dimension seeks to enhance the quality and efficiency of clinical health services and is primarily for the use of health-care providers at or near the point of care. It includes information captured during the patient care process, integrated with clinical guidelines, protocols, and other relevant information. The personal health dimension supports the management of wellness and health-care decision making by individuals and their health-care providers. It encompasses information about health status and health care in the form of a personal health record, as well as other information and resources relevant to personal health. The population health dimension encompasses population-based health data, including health statistics, statutorily authorized data in public health and health-care provider systems, and other resources to improve public health. Other dimensions also exist, such as the quality, administrative, and research dimensions, which overlap the three core dimensions (Detmer 2003). Improving information capture, storage, communication, processing, and presentation within each dimension is an important goal of the NHII, but equally or even more important is enhancing the appropriate exchange of information among them. The overlapping information needs of the dimensions are illustrated in Figure 20.1 (National Committee on Vital and Health Statistics 2000, 2001).

While health data constitute the vital foundation of the population health dimension, the broader purposes and users of the population health dimension illustrate why additional content is also important. The population health dimension is intended to promote improvements in public health practice, for example enhanced reporting systems to identify emerging and ongoing health problems; improved population health data to help characterize the whole population and specific subpopulations; mechanisms to identify health needs of subpopulations that are especially at risk because of social or environmental conditions; and expanded potential to identify factors that affect health

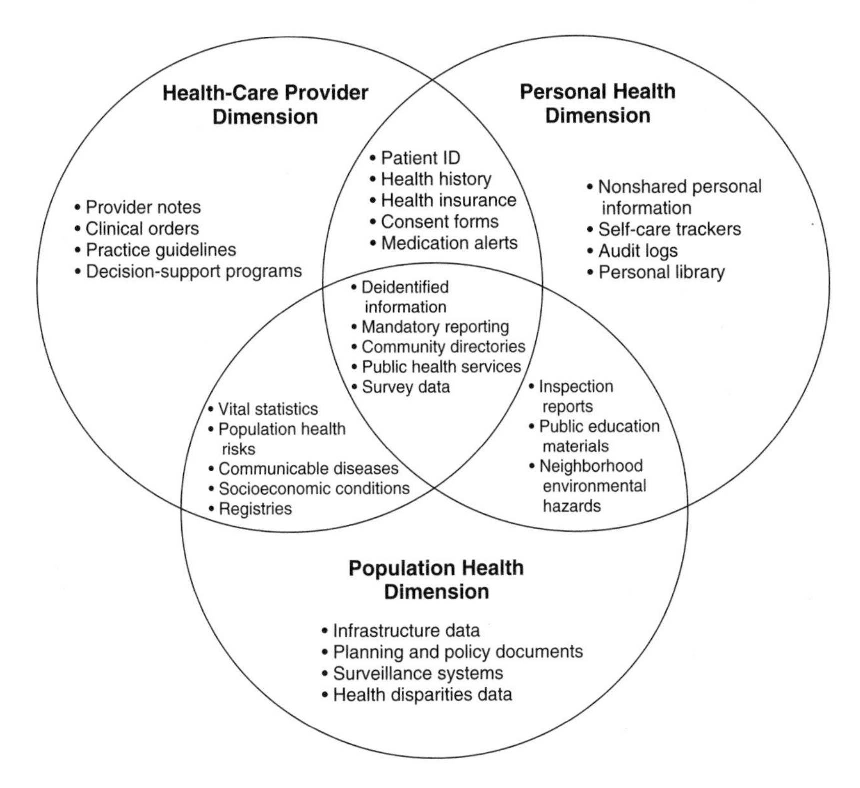

FIGURE 20.1
Dimensions of the National Health Information Infrastructure and examples of content. (Source: National Committee on Vital and Health Statistics 2001.)

throughout life (National Committee on Vital and Health Statistics 2000). Information in the population health dimension focuses on subpopulations and communities defined in many ways: household and family composition, geography, language, race or ethnicity, age, shared risk factors, socioeconomic status, disease status, and so forth. The population health dimension includes information on the health and health care of subpopulations and communities, community attributes affecting health, community health resources, and measures of population health status (see Table 20.1). Regardless of how information in the population health dimension is aggregated, it can be analyzed by looking at individuals, communities, health episodes, or health events. Analyses can be both longitudinal and at a specific point in time (National Committee on Vital and Health Statistics 2000). A robust NHII will facilitate the rapid analysis of population health data and information, facilitating a timely response to health threats and issues.

TABLE 20.1
Core Content of the Population Health Dimension

Public health data and information (most derived from health care encounters)
- Infant mortality, immunization levels, and communicable disease rates
- Environmental, social, and economic conditions
- Measures related to public health infrastructure, individual health-care providers, and health-care institutions
- Other summary measures of population health
- Registries
- Disease surveillance systems
- Survey data
- Data on Healthy People objectives and Leading Health Indicators

Information from health-care providers (with personally identifiable information removed except under legally established public health protocols and strict security)
- Health status and outcomes, health events, health risks, health behaviors, and other individual characteristics
- Health care use and access, health insurance status
- Health care of community members

Other elements
- Directories of community organizations and services
- Planning, evaluation, and policy documents
- Compendia of laws and regulations
- Materials to support public education campaigns
- Practice guidelines and training materials for public health professionals

Source: National Committee on Vital and Health Statistics (2000).

Health Statistics and the National Health Information Infrastructure

Health statistics can be derived from data available through all dimensions of the NHII. An important strength of the NHII will be its capacity to aggregate data from all NHII dimensions into population-based health statistics.

Health Statistics in the Population Health Dimension

Health statistics are a significant portion of the content of the population health dimension. Any data or information that can be aggregated to a geopolitical level could yield useful health statistics, including data on health status, health risks, and community health measures. Public education materials, planning and training documents, knowledge bases, and health-related data that cannot be aggregated or used for statistical purposes also populate the population health dimension.

Health Statistics in the Health-Care Provider Dimension

Aggregated clinical data that are deidentified (except in statutorily mandated circumstances) constitute the most important health statistics generated by the health-care provider dimension. Health-care providers already supply birth, death, cancer incidence, immunization, communicable disease, and other statutorily reportable data to state and local health agencies. Through interoperable electronic health records, much of these data now collected by state and local public health agencies through stand-alone data collection systems will be collected more efficiently and more rapidly in the NHII.

In its 2001 report on *Web-Based Public Health Reporting in California: A Feasibility Study*, the California HealthCare Foundation suggests a strategy for more fully using the World Wide Web as a means of efficiently transporting reportable disease and related public health surveillance data from health-care providers to state and county health departments (Norwell and Warren 2001). The Santa Barbara County Care Data Exchange (SBCCDE) is creating a local infrastructure that includes local public health agencies. When fully operational, the SBCCDE could provide public health agencies with case reporting data from physicians and hospitals and population reporting data from public health plans (Brailer et al. 2003). The Indianapolis Network for Patient Care, based on a citywide electronic health record, is similarly demonstrating how interoperable health records within a health information infrastructure can provide reportable disease data to local public health authorities and ultimately for more rapid development of health statistics (Overhage, Suico, McDonald 2001; Regenstrief Institute for Health Care [hp]). The NHII will enable health-care providers to become more active and frequent users of health statistics. It has been said that health-care providers and public health professionals use the same information, but they just look at it differently. Both use information on patient health risks, conditions, and treatments; however, providers use information to provide the best care for individual patients, and public health professionals use it to provide the best health services to their communities.

Health Statistics in the Personal Health Dimension

The personal health dimension will enable individuals to use, create, and store their own health data for their own uses. Data within the personal health dimension would be only available for aggregation and analysis throughout the NHII based on informed consent and authorization provided by individuals.

The personal health dimension will ultimately include a personal health record that will facilitate authorized sharing and aggregating of individuals' health information. A personal health record could also transform current population-based surveys, perhaps permitting the collection of data for such surveys as the Behavioral Risk Factor Surveillance System and the National Health Interview Survey in a more contemporaneous fashion. The personal health record could also enable individuals to better understand their own health through more ready use of health statistics such as community indicators relevant to their own health or trends regarding a disease or condition that they may be confronting in their own lives.

Health Statistics, The National Information Infrastructure, And The National Health Information Infrastructure

The NII, as the underlying technical infrastructure, and the NHII, as the health sector infrastructure, can expand the scope, timeliness, availability, and utility of health statistics. As the NII develops, it will extend networking and telecommunications across all segments of social, political, and economic life. Homes, schools, government agencies, worksites, industrial plants, commercial stores, and even cars will be electronically linked. Because decisions impacting

Box 20.1

Accelerating Public Health Responses and Outreach

A major city has an Aerometric Information Reporting System that issues emergency alerts when local air quality does not meet National Ambient Air Quality Standards. The alerts trigger a detailed automated air pollution emergency response protocol. Local media, physicians, hospitals, nursing homes, home health agencies, and community information kiosks all receive the emergency notices to alert and protect vulnerable individuals. Some individuals, especially those at risk from poor air quality, have signed up to receive notices electronically. After a few days of poor air quality, automated tracking systems indicate that older persons, infants, and poor, non-English-speaking immigrants close to industrial zones have significantly greater than normal numbers of emergency room (ER) visits. On a short-term basis, the health department intensifies its outreach to these groups with information about how to cope with the situation and immediately sees a decrease in ER visits. On a long-term basis, the health department intensifies its ongoing surveillance of ER visits, creating Web-based graphs and reports that illustrate the over-time relationship between air quality and emergency room visits for specific high-risk groups. Based on simulation modeling that includes surveillance data on ER visits and air quality, predictions are developed of specific temporal periods during which increased ER use can be expected.

health may be made in any of these locations, the NII can facilitate the delivery of essential health information to people in almost any place. As *thing-to-thing* or *ubiquitous* networking links items of daily life, including refrigerators, medicine bottles (and potentially individual pills), and even people themselves, data of interest for public health statistics may be generated directly from these sources (Engels et al. 2001). At the same time, the NII improves the ability of people to obtain information needed for making a particular decision, even if the information is not generated within the health sector. For example, at any Internet-linked workstation with modest computing and communications power, one can access, download, manipulate, and present information from diverse reports, including maps, on waste, water, toxics, air, and land issues from the Environmental Protection Agency Envirofacts Data Warehouse; information on occupational injuries and illnesses or lost work time for a particular occupational population group in a particular industry from the Bureau of Labor Statistics; information on the effectiveness of the Milwaukee lead ordinance or on treatments required by the Maryland lead-based paint risk reduction law from the Department of Housing and Urban Development's Office of Healthy Homes and Lead Hazard Control. The scope of available information seems limitless. The NII creates the platform for making this information available online and supports innovative methods for synthesis and presentation. The NII will stimulate an appreciation for new resources and analytic tools for making health decisions. In short, the NII will open up entirely new areas outside the traditional health sector for health statistics.

The Internet and the World Wide Web have already resulted in an explosion of health data availability. Federal government agencies are making public health information electronically available through gateways such as the DHHS Gateway to Data and Statistics on the Web, which offers easy access to data from DHHS and other federal agencies; the Centers for Diseases Control and Prevention's (CDC's) Wonder, which provides access to CDC reports, guidelines, and numeric public health data; and the Healthy People 2010 Web site, which links to data for the Healthy People 2010 objectives (Centers for Disease Control and Prevention, [db] CDC Wonder; U.S. Department of Health and Human Services, HHS Data Council Gateway; U.S. Department of Health and Human Services [hp]). Increasingly, state and local health departments are using the Internet to disseminate data (Friedman et al. 2001); for example, the Massachusetts Community Health Information Profile (MassCHIP) provides free online access to data from almost 30 major public health, demographic, and related social service data sets, and the Michigan Community Health Information Web site enables citizens to track such topics as infant mortality, nursing facility care, preventable hospitalizations, live births, mortality, population trends, and sexually transmitted diseases in their communities or to compare their own communities to others (Massachusetts Department of Public Health [db]; Michigan Department of Community Health [db]). Voluntary health organizations such as the American Cancer Society publish online data that complement government sources. The North American Association of Central Cancer Registries makes available cancer information by year, geography, sex, race, cancer type, and age and by any combination of these variables through Cina+, a flexible interactive query system providing a choice of custom designed tables, charts, and maps (North American Association of Central Cancer Registries [db]).

The NHII builds on the current capacities of the Internet and the NII's enhanced capacity for sharing information generated by diverse components of the health sector. Through the use of standardized messaging, data and information will be moved easily and rapidly. Interoperability of systems and comparability of data will be maximized. The added computing power of the NHII will enable tailored health statistics to be generated by integrating data and information from disparate sources. Researchers can merge large numbers of Medicare records with U.S. Environmental Protection Agency (EPA) Aerometic Information Retreival System data on particulates, and then display results using Geographic Information Systems to analyze correlations between poor air quality and health-care use by geographic area. In a fully functional NHII, it will be possible (with appropriate legal safeguards for privacy) to merge airline passenger manifests with health-care visits to more rapidly identify groups of people exposed to a communicable disease from a sick traveler. In short, the NHII will facilitate new and better information flows within the health sector.

HEALTH INFORMATION INFRASTRUCTURE DEVELOPMENTS IN OTHER COUNTRIES

Other countries are also developing national information infrastructures and national health information infrastructures. Each of these countries has emphasized different elements in its development efforts, and each country has progressed in different ways and at different speeds. Facilitated by the Internet, substantial international collaboration in the development of essential standards and knowledge transfer has occurred. For example, Australia's development of its National Health Information model has informed the development by the U.S. Centers for Disease Control and Prevention of its Public Health Conceptual Data Model and Logical Data Model. The following sections provide examples of some national health information infrastructure developments in a few example countries. Chapter 17 provides additional information on current developments in health statistics in various countries.

Australia

Australia has made significant strides in developing its public health information infrastructure. In 1999, the Australian Institute for Health and Welfare published a National Public Health Information Development Plan that included recommendations to improve the quality, coverage, and use of public health information across the country (Australian Institute for Health and Welfare 1999). Australia's *National Health Data Dictionary*, now in its tenth version, helps ensure that data are uniform and of high quality; data definitions are organized according to their alignment with entities in the National Health Information Model (Australian Institute for Health and Welfare 2001). Components of the Australian information infrastructure are coordinated in an interactive online resource called the National Health Information Knowledgebase. The Knowledgebase serves as an electronic register and query tool for health metadata, and includes the National Health Information Model and other models, data element definitions (the *National Health Data Dictionary* and the *National Community Services Data Dictionary*), national minimum data sets, indicators and their associated frameworks (including measures of the community at large and the performance health-care services), and tools and feedback functions (Australian Institute for Health and Welfare, The Knowledegebase). Australian progress on the clinical information infrastructure has been regional rather than national; for example, in July 2002, the Northern Territory launched a Primary Care Information System to include medical histories, medication, and health-care coverage (California HealthCare Foundation 2002).

Canada

Canada has established a Roadmap Initiative to modernize health information for assessing the health of Canadians and their health care. Canada budgeted C$95 million in 1999 for this initiative and another C$95 in 2001 for four additional years. The Roadmap Initiative completed numerous projects aimed at improving the quality, timeliness, and comprehensiveness of existing data and developing new data standards and reporting systems by 2004 (Canadian Institute for Health Information, Statistics Canada 2003, [hp]). Progress has been made in developing a health indicators framework and a new array of health indicators, publishing general and special population reports, producing analyses of key and emerging issues, implementing new standards, and establishing the Canadian Population Health Initiative. On a regional basis, the health-care information infrastructure is also developing. In British Columbia, Health Level 7 (HL7) messages and standardized codes are used for all drug prescribing and are under development for linking laboratories (National Committee on Vital and Health Statistics 2001). In Ontario, the Smart Systems for Health will include data and technology standards for services, products, and technologies; a voluntary emergency health record and other secure electronic exchange of personal health information; the Ontario Laboratory Information System; the Integrated Services for Children Information System; and a Health Network System for medications, including a drug interaction checker (Ministry of Health and Long-Term Care 2002).

United Kingdom

The primary focus of infrastructure activity in the United Kingdom is clinical care improvement, including a comprehensive 7-year initiative launched in 1998 to strengthen the National Health Service (NHS). The initiative focuses on building seamless services across whole systems of care in order to create a patient-centered NHS that benefits both health-care providers and also consumers and patients (National Health Service [mg] 1998). NHSnet was created for providing applications and information services to all NHS health-care staff (National Health Service 2001). The United Kingdom is developing an output-based specification (OBS) to support the Integrated Care Records Service (ICRS) program (Department of Health 2004). The OBS is being developed as an iterative process, with input from clinicians, chief information officers, information technology managers, leading clinicians, practitioners, policy advisors, health informaticians, managers, and representatives from the Department of Health, the NHS Information Authority, NHS organizations, general practitioners, academic groups, the Royal Colleges, and other government departments. It includes sections on integration and data and infrastructure services.

BARRIERS, CHALLENGES, AND THE IMPLEMENTATION OF THE NATIONAL HEALTH INFORMATION INFRASTRUCTURE IN THE UNITED STATES

Barriers to the National Health Information Infrastructure

Electronic Health Records

Many barriers stand in the way of achieving the vision of aggregated, anonymous clinical health information, derived from the point of care, available for health statistics use. Chief among these barriers is the lack of widespread adoption of interoperable electronic health records (EHRs) and programs for collecting, deidentifying, and making information derived from them accessible as needed. These barriers will not be overcome without data and technology standards and strict controls to ensure privacy and security. In 2002, 30% of physicians reported using EHRs, compared with only 22% in 2001 (von Knoop et al. 2003). A 2003 survey suggested that the diffusion of EHRs varies by specialty: 42% of internal medicine practices reported using an EHR, 33% of multispecialty practices, and about 30% of family practices (Health Information and Management Systems Society [hp]). A 2004 survey found that 19% of large health-care organizations currently have fully operational EHRs (Health Information and Management Systems Society 2004). However, these systems rarely communicate with each other outside a single health-care organization or voluntary regional initiative. However, Kaiser Permanente is creating a national, self-contained, proprietary EHR system, which will generate health statistics for use within its own provider network. Similarly, the U.S. Departments of Defense and Veterans Affairs are creating interoperable EHR systems that will permit aggregation of clinical information from all beneficiaries of the military health system. Progress toward wider and more rapid diffusion of EHRs will be facilitated by new functional standards that are being developed by the international standards development organization HL7, based on recommendations from the Institute of Medicine (Health Level Seven 2003; National Academy of Sciences 2003). The U.S. Departments of HHS and Veterans Affairs have indicated their support for these efforts.

Connectivity

Recent data on connectivity among users suggest that, while progress is uneven, 89% of U.S. counties had established continuous high-speed Internet connectivity as of December 2002 (Centers for Disease Control and Prevention [hp] Health Alert Network). Ninety-six percent of physicians are online, and 90% of these use the Internet to research clinical information (von Knoop et al. 2003). The public is becoming connected as well, with 51% of households having Internet access in 2001, up from 42% in 2000; this percentage is assumed to be growing steadily (Centers for Disease Control and Prevention [db] CDC Wonder).

Data Standards

The NHII needs data standards to enable sharing of information from multiple sources and aggregating it for health statistics use. Within the public health sector, the CDC has created the National Electronic Disease Surveillance System (NEDSS), which promotes the use of data and information system standards to further the development of efficient, integrated, and interoperable surveillance systems at federal, state, and local levels. The NEDSS is based on a vision of integrated surveillance systems that transfer appropriate public health, laboratory, and clinical data efficiently and securely over the Internet. The NEDSS will make it possible to gather and analyze information more quickly and accurately, and will improve the nation's ability to identify and track emerging infectious diseases and potential bioterrorism attacks, as well as to monitor disease trends (Centers for Disease Control and Prevention [hp] National Electronic Disease Surveillance System). For a fuller discussion of data standards, see Chapter 8.

After the September 11, 2001, terrorist attacks and the subsequent anthrax attacks, substantial federal resources were allocated to enhance the public health infrastructure, including nearly $1 billion in the first year of funding. Grants to states were issued by the CDC and included funding for development of NEDSS-compatible public health surveillance systems (Lumpkin and Richards 2002).

Additionally, the eHealth Initiative created the Public-Private Sector Collaboration for Public Health, which included the CDC, the Centers for Medicare and Medicaid Services (CMS), public health agencies, providers, standards organizations, and health-care information technology suppliers. This Collaboration will develop and implement strategies to transmit electronic data of public health importance (such as laboratory and microbiology results, orders, and chief complaints) using operable standards and NEDSS (eHealth Initiative [hp]). Data standards are also discussed in Chapter 8.

Progress in clinical data standards is uneven. Two efforts—one public, one private—will provide an important basic suite of standards on which to build. The Consolidated Health Informatics (CHI) initiative brings together the U.S. Departments of HHS, Defense, and Veterans Affairs to approve and implement standards that will support exchange of data among their health-care systems. The CHI will provide the basis for a simplified and unified system for sharing and revising medical information among government agencies and their private health-care providers and insurers. The first sets of CHI standards to be approved cover core laboratory and clinical data elements; in March 2003, DHHS Secretary Tommy Thompson announced the adoption of those standards. The Markle Foundation's Connecting for Health initiative brings together leaders from the health-care and health information technology sectors to identify and promote national clinical data standards to facilitate interoperability (Markle Foundation [hp]). The Markle Foundation is coordinating with CHI to ensure mutually reinforcing outcomes and products.

Personal Health Records

Hearings by the NCVHS workgroup on the NHII identified the personal health dimension as the least developed NHII dimension due to limited development of personal health records (PHRs) (National Committee on Vital and Health Statistics 2003a, 2003b). The personal health record enables individuals to store and control pertinent health information and to use decision-support technology to fully participate in their health care. The lack of standards for the PHR is a major obstacle to the development of the PHR. The Markle Foundation's Connecting for Health initiative has made significant strides in identifying the key PHR areas where further work is needed. The Institute of Medicine included the PHR in its report on functional standards for an EHR, and the Health Level Seven EHR standard will support many key functions of the personal health record (Health Level Seven 2003; National Academy of Sciences 2003).

Challenges

While the fundamental purpose of the NHII is to facilitate the flow of information, the need to ensure privacy, security, and confidentiality means that access to information should occur only along a carefully constructed and monitored continuum, depending on the specific use and user of information. At one end of the continuum, authorized public health workers may access individually identifiable data for legally authorized purposes such as contact tracing for highly communicable diseases or identifying high-risk infants in need of intervention. At the other end, the public can access anonymous, aggregated data to identify local public health problems and to set local public health priorities (National Committee on Vital and Health Statistics 2000, 2001). The DHHS issued privacy regulations, which went into effect in April 2003, that fulfill requirements of the Health Insurance Portability and Accountability Act. These regulations establish strong protections for individually identifiable health information held or transmitted by health plans, providers, and health-care clearinghouses, as well as sanctions for its misuse. The regulations also identify how public health programs can obtain timely and complete access to necessary health information. Guidance was issued by the DHHS to clarify the impact of these regulations on public health programs and research (Centers for Disease Control and Prevention 2003; National Institutes of Health [hp]). Experience with the 2003 rules will enable further clarification of the need for additional legal privacy protections or security protocols to ensure that the full potential of the NHII can be achieved.

An important foundation for clinical and public health data standards is being laid by the initiatives mentioned above, but much remains to be done. Many areas of activity crucial to health improvement, including prevention, are not currently encompassed by standards development activities. Standards need to be developed and adopted in these and other areas. Equally important, standards must be widely implemented in the public and private sectors for their value to be realized.

The capital investments needed to build the NHII in both the public and private sectors are sizable. Clinical information systems range from tens of thousands of dollars for individual or small-group medical practices to hundreds of millions for large health-care organizations. For example, Kaiser Permanente announced in 2003 that it was committing $1.8 billion to put all its records online (California HealthCare Foundation 2003). While many leading health-care organizations are making the necessary commitments, funding challenges pose significant barriers for many other health-care organizations and for the public health sector. Future investments by the private sector will depend on the development of a clear business case that identifies the value created and compares it to the capital costs of the systems.

Implementing the National Health Information Infrastructure

Even when privacy, security, standards, and networking infrastructure are in place, it will still be necessary to overcome the reluctance of many key stakeholders to agree to the sharing of information for health statistics use. Concerns about proprietary interests within the health-care sector and concerns about privacy among individuals will require thoughtful solutions with demonstrable benefits. The federal government's leadership through both policy and programs will be crucial. Tying its efforts to vital issues such as patient safety and bioterrorism preparedness may be helpful. The concurrent efforts of the private and public sectors will enable the development and appropriate sharing of health data for decision making at all levels.

NOTE

1. Senator Al Gore was the first to refer to the *national information infrastructure* during the presidential campaign of 1992 (National Coordination Office for Information Technology and Development 1994).

REFERENCES

Australian Institute for Health and Welfare. National Health Data Dictionary, Version 10, 2001 [monograph on the Internet]. Canberra: Australian Institute for Health and Welfare; 2001 [cited 2004 Mar 13]. Available from: http://www.aihw.gov.au/publications/hwi/nhdd10/index.html.

Australian Institute for Health and Welfare [monograph on the Internet]. National Public Health Information Development Plan 1999. Canberra: Australian Institute for Health and Welfare; 1999 [cited 2004 Mar 13]. Available from: http://www.aihw.gov.au/publications/health/nphidp99/index.html#s02.

Australian Institute for Health and Welfare [database on the Internet]. Canberra: Australian Institute for Health and Welfare. The knowledgebase; updated 2002 Jun 20 [cited 2004 Mar 13]. Available from: www.aihw.gov/au/knowledgebase/aboutkb.html.

Brailer DJ, Augustinos N, Evans LM, Karp S [monograph on the Internet]. Moving Toward Electronic Health Information Exchange: Interim Report on the Santa Barbara County Data Exchange. Oakland: California HealthCare Foundation; July 2003 [cited 2004 Mar 13]. Available from: http://www.chcf.org/documents/ihealth/SBCCDEInterimReport.pdf.

California HealthCare Foundation [newsletter on the Internet]. Oakland: California HealthCare Foundation. Australian territory unveils comprehensive health care records system. iHealthBeat; 2002 Jul 26 [cited 2004 Mar 15]. Available from: http://www.ihealthbeat.org.

California HealthCare Foundation [newsletter on the Internet]. Oakland: California HealthCare Foundation. Kaiser Permanente to put patient records online. iHealthBeat; 2003 Feb 4 [cited 2004 Mar 15]. Available from: http://www.ihealthbeat.org.

Canadian Institute for Health Information, Statistics Canada [monograph on the Internet]. Roadmap Initiative, Launching the Process: the Final Year. Ottawa: Canadian Institute for Health Information; 2003 [cited 2004 Mar 15]. Available from: http://secure.cihi.ca/cihiweb/en/downloads/profile_roadmap_e_final_review.pdf.

Canadian Institute for Health Information, Statistics Canada [homepage on the Internet]. Ottawa: Canadian Institute for Health Information. Health information roadmap initiative [cited 2004 Nov 5]. Available from: http://secure.cihi.ca/cihiweb/dispPage.jsp?cw_page=profile_roadmap_e.

Centers for Disease Control and Prevention. HIPAA Privacy Rule and public health: guidance from CDC and the U.S. Department of Health and Human Services. MMWR 2003; 52(suppl):1–20 [cited 2004 Mar 16]. Available from: http://www.cdc.gov/mmwr/pdf/wk/mmsu5201.pdf.

Centers for Disease Control and Prevention [database on the Internet]. Atlanta: Centers for Disease Control and Prevention [updated 2003 Nov 14; cited 2004 Mar 16]. CDC Wonder. Available from: http://wonder.cdc.gov.

Centers for Disease Control and Prevention [database on the Internet]. Atlanta: CDC [updated 2004 Jan 6; cited 2004 Mar 25]. CDC Wonder, Data 2010. The Healthy People 2010 database. Available from: http://wonder.cdc.gov/data2010.

Centers for Disease Control and Prevention [homepage on the Internet]. Atlanta: Centers for Disease Control and Prevention [cited 2004 Mar 15]. National Electronic Disease Surveillance System: surveillance and monitoring component of the Public Health Information Network. Available from: http://www.cdc.gov/nedss.

Centers for Disease Control and Prevention, Public Health Program Office [homepage on the Internet]. Atlanta: Centers for Disease Control and Prevention [cited 2004 Mar 15]. Health Alert Network. http://www.phppo.cdc.gov/HAN/statemap.asp.

Department of Health [monograph on the Internet]. Output Based Specification for the Integrated Care Records Service. London: Department of Health; 2004 Feb 9 [cited 2004 Mar 15]. Available from: http://www.dh.gov.uk/PolicyAndGuidance/InformationTechnology/NationalITProgramme/NationalITProgrammeArticle/fs/en?CONTENT_ID=4071618&chk=FzV2Cm.

Detmer DE [article on the Internet]. Building the National Health Information Infrastructure: personal health, health care services, public health, and research. BMC Med Inform Decis Mak 2003;3(1) [cited 2004 Nov 5]. Available from: http://www.biomedcentral.com/content/pdf/1472-6947-3-1.pdf.

Dick RS, Steen EB, Detmer DE, eds. The Computer-Based Patient Record: An Essential Technology for Health, rev ed. Washington, DC: National Academy Press; 1997.

eHealth Initiative [homepage on the Internet]. Washington, DC: eHealth Initiative; 2002 Feb 12 [cited 2004 Mar 15]. Current state of the health care system: facts at a glance. Available from: http://www.ehealthinitiative.org/events/facts.htm.

Engels DW, Foley J, Waldrop J, Sarma SE, Brock D [article on the Internet]. The networked physical world: an automated identification architecture. Proceedings of the Second IEEE Workshop on Internet Applications (WIAPP '01), 1530–1354/o1. Los Alamitos, CA: IEEE Computer Society; 2001 [cited 2004 Mar 15]. Available from: http://csdl.computer.org/comp/proceedings/wiapp/2001/1137/00/11370076.pdf.

Friedman DJ, Anderka M, Krieger JW, Land G, Solet D 2001. Accessing population health information through interactive systems: lessons learned and future directions. Public Health Rep 2001;116(2):132–147.

Health Information and Management Systems Society [homepage on the Internet]. Chicago: Health Information and Management Systems Society. Fourteenth annual HIMSS leadership survey; 2003 [cited 2004 Mar 15]. Available from: http:// www.himss.org/2003survey.

Health Information and Management Systems Society [homepage on the Internet]. Chicago: Health Information and Management Systems Society. Fifteenth annual HIMSS leadership survey; 2004 [cited 2004 Mar 25]. Available from: http://www.himss.org/2004survey/ASP/healthcarecio_final.asp.

Health Level Seven [monograph on the Internet]. HL7 EHR System Functional Model and Standard: Draft Standard for Trial Use, Release 1.0, August 2003. Ann Arbor, MI: Health Level Seven; 2003 Aug [cited 2004 Mar 15]. Available from: http://www/hl7.org/ehr.

Institute of Medicine, Committee on Quality of Health Care in America. Crossing the Quality Chasm: A New Health System for the 21st Century. Washington, DC: National Academy Press; 2001.

Kohn LT, Corrigan JM, Donaldson MS, eds. To Err Is Human: Building a Safer Health System. Washington, DC: National Academy Press; 2000.

Lasker RD, Humphreys BL, Braithwaite WR. Making a Powerful Connection: The Health of the Public and the National Information Infrastructure, Report of the U.S. Public Health Service Public Health Data Policy Coordinating Committee. Washington, DC: U.S. Public Health Service; 1995 Jul 6.

Lumpkin JR, Richards MS. Transforming the public health iInformation infrastructure. Health Aff 2002;21(6):45–56.

Markle Foundation [homepage on the Internet]. New York: Markle Foundation [cited 2004 Mar 15]. Connecting for health: a public-private collaborative. Available from: www.connectingforhealth.org/aboutus/index.html.

Massachusetts Department of Public Health [database on the Internet]. Boston: Massachusetts Department of Public Health [cited 2004 Mar 16]. Massachusetts Community Health Information Profile (MassCHIP). Available from: http://masschip.state.ma.us.

Michigan Department of Community Health [database on the Internet]. Lansing: Michigan Department of Community Health [cited 2004 Mar 16]. Michigan community health information. Available from: http://www.mdch.state.mi.us/pha/osr/chi/index.asp.

Ministry of Health and Long-Term Care. Notes for Remarks by the Honourable Tony Clement, Minister of Health and Long-Term Care, to the Video Conference with Sweden Event of the Information Technology Association of Canada (ITAC) for Canada. Ontario: Ministry of Health and Long-Term Care; 2002 May 8.

National Academy of Sciences, Institute of Medicine, Committee on Data Standards for Patient Safety, Board of Health Care Services. Key Capabilities of an Electronic Health Record System, Letter Report. Washington, DC: National Academy Press; 2003.

National Committee on Vital and Health Statistics [monograph on the Internet]. Toward a National Health Information Infrastructure, Interim Report, June 2000. Washington, DC: U.S. Department of Health and Human Services; 2000 Jun [cited 2004 Mar 15]. Available from: http://www.ncvhs.hhs.gov/NHII2kReport.htm.

National Committee on Vital and Health Statistics [monograph on the Internet]. Information for Health: A Strategy for Building the National Health Information Infrastructure, Report and Recommendations from the National Committee on Vital and Health Statistics. Washington, DC: U.S. Department of Health and Human Services; 2001 Nov 15 [cited 2004 Mar 15]. Available from: http://aspe.hhs.gov/sp/nhii/Documents/NHIIReport2001/default.htm.

National Committee on Vital and Health Statistics, National Health Information Infrastructure (NHII) Workgroup [hearing minutes on the Internet]. Hearings on Health and the National Information Infrastructure and the NHII, Personal Health Dimension, January 27–28, 2003. Washington, DC: U.S. Department of Health and Human Services; 2003a Jan 27–8 [cited 2004 Mar 15]. Available from: http://ncvhs.hhs.gov/030127mn.htm.

National Committee on Vital and Health Statistics, National Health Information Infrastructure (NHII) Workgroup [meeting minutes on the Internet]. Working Meeting, August 7, 2003. Washington, DC: U.S. Department of Health and Human Services; 2003b [cited 2004 Mar 15]. Available from: http://ncvhs.hhs.gov/030807mn.htm.

National Coordination Office for Information Technology Research and Development, High Performance Computing and Information Technology Subcommittee [monograph on the Internet]. Information Infrastructure Technology and Applications: Report of the IITA Task Group. Arlington, VA: National Coordination Office for Information Technology Research and Development; 1994 Feb [cited 2004 Mar 16]. Available from: http://www.itrd.gov/pubs/iita.

National Health Service [monograph on the Internet]. Information for Health: An Information Strategy for the Modern NHS 1998–2005. Exeter, England: National Health Service; 1998 Sep [cited 2004 Mar 15]. Available from: http://www.nhsia.nhs.uk/def/pages/info4health/contents.asp.

National Health Service Information Authority [monograph on the Internet]. Building the Information Core: Implementing the NHS plan. Exeter, England: National Health Service; 2001 Jan [cited 2004 Mar 13]. Available from: http://www.nhsia.nhs.uk/def/pages/info_core/contents.asp.

National Institutes of Health [homepage on the Internet]. Rockville, MD: National Institutes for Health; updated 2004 Mar 4 [cited 2004 Mar 15. HIPAA privacy rule: information for researchers. Available from: http://privacyruleandresearch.nih.gov.

National Library of Medicine [homepage on the Internet]. Bethesda, MD: National Library of Medicine; 2002 Nov 29 [cited 2004 Mar 15]. National Library of Medicine and Internet2 to demonstrate vast potential of advanced networking for improving delivery of health care. Available from: http://www.nlm.nih.gov/news/press_releases/internet2pr2.html.

National Research Council, Computer Science and Telecommunications Board, Commission on Physical Sciences, Mathematics, and Applications, Committee on Enhancing the Internet for Health Applications: Technical Requirements and Implementation Strategies. Networking Health: Prescriptions for the Internet. Washington, DC: National Academy Press; 2000.

National Science and Technology Council, Committee on Information and Communication [monograph on the Internet]. High Performance Computing and Communications: Technology for the National Information Infrastructure, supplement to the President's Fiscal Year 1995 Budget. Washington, DC: National Science and Technology Council; 1994 [cited 2004 Nov 5]. Available from: http:// www.itrd.gov/pubs/blue95.

North American Association of Central Cancer Registries [database on the Internet]. Springfield, IL: North American Association of Central Cancer Registries [cited 2004 Mar 16]. CiNA+ online. Available from: http://www.naaccr.og/cinap/index.htm.

Norwell DM, Warren FE [monograph on the Internet]. Web-Based Public Health Reporting in California: A Feasibility Study. Oakland: California HealthCare Foundation; 2001 Dec [cited 2004 Mar 13]. Available from: http://www.chcf.org/documents/ihealth/WebbasedPublicHealthReporting.pdf.

Overhage JM, Suico J, McDonald CL. Electronic laboratory reporting: barriers, solutions and findings. J Public Health Manag Pract 2001;7(6):60–66.

Regenstrief Institute for Health Care [homepage on the Internet]. Indianapolis: Regenstrief Institute for Health Care [cited 2004 Mar 15]. Indianapolis Network for Patient Care (INPC)—a community-based electronic medical records. Available from: http://informatics.regenstrief.org/what/?section=inpc.

Shortliffe EH. Networking health: learning from others, taking the lead. Health Aff 2000;19(6):9–22.

U.S. Department of Commerce. The National information infrastructure: Agenda for action. Washington, DC: U.S. Department of Commerce; 1993 [cited 2004 Mar 15]. Available from: http://www.ibiblio.org/nii/toc.html.

U.S. Department of Commerce, National Institute of Standards and Technology. Putting the Information Infrastructure to Work: Report of the Information Infrastructure Task Force Committee on Applications and Technology. NIST Special Publication 857. Gaithersburg, MD: National Institute of Standards and Technology; 1994.

U.S. Department of Health and Human Services, HHS Data Council [database on the Internet]. Washington, DC: U.S. Department of Health and Human Services [cited 2004 Mar 16]. HHS Data Council gateway to data and statistics. Available from: http://hhs-stat.net/index.asp.

U.S. Department of Health and Human Services, Office of Disease Prevention and Health Promotion [homepage on the Internet]. Washington, DC: U.S. Department of Health and Human Services. Healthy People 2010 [cited 2004 Mar 16]. Available from: http://www.healthypeople.gov.

Von Knoop C, Lovich D, Silverstein MB, Tutty M. Vital signs: e-health in the United States [monograph on the Internet]. Boston: Boston Consulting Group; January 2003 [cited 2004 Mar 13]. Available from: www.bcg.com/publications/files/Vital_Signs_Rpt_Jan03/pdf.

CHAPTER 21

Summing Up: Toward a Twenty-First-Century Vision for Health Statistics

Daniel J. Friedman, Edward L. Hunter, and R. Gibson Parrish II

The chapters in this volume define the nature, sources, and uses of health statistics; place efforts to collect and use health statistics in historical and organizational contexts; delineate current and forthcoming issues in health statistics; describe gaps and shortcomings in health statistics, especially as developed and used in the United States; and offer frameworks for conceptualizing and organizing health statistics efforts. These chapters outline an emerging vision that could lead to fundamental improvements in health statistics, which could improve research, health policy, public health practice, and ultimately the population's health. This emerging vision contains

- a more explicit conceptual framework for health statistics;
- suggestions for improving the processes through which health statistics are collected, analyzed, used, and evaluated;
- new approaches to address privacy concerns; and
- ways of seizing opportunities presented by new technologies and methodologies for modeling, linking, and using health statistics.

This chapter will provide a cross-cutting summary of previous chapters and a more explicit vision for health statistics in the twenty-first century.

CURRENT ISSUES IN HEALTH STATISTICS

Conceptual Issues

Political and Social Contexts

Is the generation of health statistics and the data on which health statistics rely essentially a governmental function? Do political considerations ultimately determine the choices that are made about what data are collected, what issues are investigated, and how analyses are conducted by the health statistics enterprise? Do the social assumptions consciously or unconsciously held by developers of health statistics affect their practice? What should be the role of health statistics in the policy process, and what should be the role of the policy process in the health statistics enterprise? Eyler (Chapter 2), Friedman et al. (Chapter 10), and Feder and Levitt (Chapter 11) raise these and other related questions.

Eyler's historical analysis and Feder and Levitt's analysis of the health-care reform debate of the early 1990s indicate that health statistics are both affected by and affect their political and social contexts. Although health statistics are based on scientific methods, those methods often play a subsidiary role in making basic choices about what data are collected and what issues are studied by the health statistics enterprise. Thus, those who develop health statistics must carefully examine their own political and social assumptions, remain aware of the political and social contexts in which they work, and be alert to how those assumptions and contexts affect their work. Such self-awareness and examination should be a realistic goal, whereas isolating the development of health statistics from their political and social contexts may not be a realistic—or even a desirable—goal.

Conceptual Frameworks for Population Health

The U.S. health statistics enterprise has been largely unguided by explicit conceptual frameworks. Numerous chapters in this volume have pointed to this as an ongoing limitation that needs to be addressed. The chapters by Parrish et al. (Chapter 1), Black and Roos (Chapter 9), Stoto (Chapter 13), Wolfson (Chapter 16), Black et al. (Chapter 18), and Starfield (Chapter 19) underscore the importance of guiding national health statistics enterprises with evidence-based conceptual frameworks for population health and the factors that influence it.

Major contributions of a population health framework would be, first, an explicit focus on positive health and well-being as the central variables of interest rather than ill-health or disease; second, concentration on populations rather than on individuals, including recognition of the inherent differences between population and individual health; third, consideration of a full range of influences on population health rather than just the most proximate influences, such as health services; and fourth, awareness of the importance of analyses that include this full range of influences.

Health statistics based on a population health conceptual framework would provide the basis for two types of monitoring. First is the monitoring of population health, including health status, functional status, health outcomes, and influences on population health. Second is the monitoring of what Starfield (Chapter 19) describes as the three imperatives of health systems: increasing the efficiency of interventions, increasing the effectiveness of interventions, and increasing equity.

Traditional health statistics, traditionally presented, perform this role incompletely and fail to provide measures of population health consistent with the World Health Organization's comprehensive definition of health. Driven by disease-oriented data systems, health statistics have been marked largely by a focus on individual illnesses of individual people, rather than by a comprehensive focus on the health of populations and subpopulations.

Health Information Models and National Health Information Infrastructures

In addition to the need for adopting frameworks for understanding population health, various authors emphasize the need for increased adoption of two other types of conceptual frameworks. Zelmer et al. (Chapter 17) point out that health information models, accompanied by data dictionaries and metadata, constitute another important conceptual framework that can be crucial in organizing, rationalizing, and increasing the accessibility of health statistics data holdings. Second, as discussed below, the National Health Information Infrastructure (NHII) in the United States and similar health infostructures in other countries can provide conceptual frameworks to guide advances in national health statistics enterprises.

Little recent attention has been devoted to the structure of the health statistics enterprise in the United States, how that enterprise can be best organized, and how the flow of data that become health statistics can be made more efficient and effective for public health practice, policymaking, and knowledge creation (see Chapter 3). Lumpkin and Deering (Chapter 20) and Detmer and Steen (Chapter 15) indicate that the development of a strong NHII is essential for improving the efficiency and effectiveness of the health statistics enterprise. According to Lumpkin and Deering, the NHII will enable "delivering the right information to the right people at the right time." Through a strong NHII, "we can expect improved depth, breadth, and quality of health data available to generate statistics, reduced costs of gathering and maintaining traditional statistics, and better linkages across data and health statistics systems." Both sets of authors foresee the NHII as the vehicle through which enhanced sharing of deidentified data could occur, including aggregation of clinical data to population levels for use in health statistics. Widespread adoption of interoperable electronic health records—both clinical records and consumer health records maintained by patients themselves—will enable conversion of previously unusable health data into population-level health statistics within the framework of the NHII.

Detmer and Steen envision a health statistics future in which the growth of the NHII in the United States and of similar health information infrastructures in other nations will be dramatically affected by new technologies such as nanotechnology, genomics, and information and communications technology. New technologies will be accompanied by trends, such as the increased automation of traditional health statistics, increased democratization of the use of health statistics, and increased virtual collaboration among developers and users of health statistics through the capabilities of the NHII.

Gaps in Health Statistics

Gaps in the content of the data used to create health statistics exist. Directly or indirectly, many of these gaps result from the absence of a population health framework, especially in the United States, to ensure that data are collected on all major aspects of health and the influences on it. As Starfield (Chapter 19) and Zelmer et al. (Chapter 17) indicate, health statistics focus largely on ill health and disease. As Bailey and colleagues discuss (Chapter 7), inadequate attention is paid to non-health-sector influences on population health. As a consequence, traditional sources of data for health statistics must be supplemented by complementary sources of data that encompass a broader range of the influences on population health; some gaps may be filled by the systematic linkage of data across multiple sources, as described by Black and Roos in Chapter 9.

Gaps in data content also reflect the nature of the health-care delivery system in individual countries, as pointed out by Iezzoni et al. (Chapter 6). In the United States, the health-care delivery system is fragmented and its financing is based on a conglomeration of private and public insurance arrangements. As a result, U.S. administrative health data pertain largely to those who are privately or publicly insured, with minimal administrative health data on the uninsured. Similarly, administrative health data exist for only those specific services that are covered by insurance and that result in paid claims. Content gaps in administrative health data may also exist due to state-to-state differences in Medicaid benefits, again reflecting the fragmented nature of the U.S. health-care system. In contrast, as Black et al. point out (Chapter 18), some of these gaps do not exist in administrative health data produced in some Canadian provinces due to the nature of the Canadian health-care system and the way it is financed.

Finally, in some cases, lack of resources has made it difficult to maintain the collection of health statistics from even traditional data sources (such as those described in Chapters 3, 4, and 5) at levels of completeness and coverage that were once routine.

Methodological and Process Issues

Health statistics should support varied uses and employ appropriate methodologies and measures. Especially important among those uses is community health monitoring, using the population as the patient, as discussed by Stoto (Chapter 13) and Oswald et al. (Chapter 12). To facilitate the dissemination and the understanding of the findings of community health monitoring to and by various communities, the health statistics enterprise should construct "single-number" population-level summary measures (Chapters 13 and 16). The health statistics enterprise should also enable simulation and causal modeling by providing multivariate, multilevel, microdata to appropriate users (Chapter 16).

Many nations are now recognizing the need to build health statistics infrastructures that can support greater integration of different types of micro-level data, especially through the development of electronic health records (Chapter 17). Yet even without the existence of fully developed health statistics infrastructures and electronic health records, steps can be taken to overcome the shortcomings of the current narrowly focused *stovepipe* data systems used for health statistics. As Greenberg and Parrish indicate (Chapter 8), the adoption of standards-based methods can facilitate linkage and sharing of data sets, thus enabling greater integration of microdata. A consistent approach to operationalizing key concepts and indicators, even within the constraints of currently available data, can provide the basis for building integrated research databases and research registries, as has been accomplished by the Manitoba Centre for Health Policy in its POPULIS system (Chapter 18).

Rapidly developing technologies will provide health statistics with new methodological opportunities and new challenges. These technologies will affect the collecting and compiling of health statistics, as well as the uses of health statistics. For example, increasing use of mobile phones, global positioning systems, geographic information systems, and the Internet will impact population survey methods (Chapter 5); increasing use of electronic medical records and electronic consumer health records will affect data derived from administrative health records, registries, and reportable disease systems (Chapter 4). As Black et al. point out in Chapter 18, "given the opportunities, the real challenge before us is to think broadly and boldly enough." A central question confronting health statistics will be "whether it will take advantage of the capabilities offered by technology" (Chapter 15).

New technologies will present significant privacy and confidentiality challenges to the practice of health statistics, as Fanning indicates (Chapter 14). Increased data set linkages, increased use of electronic medical records and consumer health records in health statistics, and increased use of the Internet for data collection and dissemination will test the ability of the health statistics enterprise to protect the privacy of individuals and to maintain the security of individually identifiable data. The success of national health statistics enterprises in adopting new technologies may rest largely on how well they recognize and respond to those privacy and confidentiality challenges.

Health statistics should be employed in monitoring population health, assessing community health, planning programs, targeting interventions, evaluating policies and programs, and informing the public. For health statistics to be successfully used for these purposes, national health statistics enterprises must increase collaboration between data providers and data collectors, among data collectors, between the health statistics enterprise and the public, and among health statistics enterprises across national boundaries (Chapter 3). For the U.S. health statistics enterprise to realize the potential of the emerging NHII, greater collaboration must occur so that the reluctance of data providers to share information for health statistics purposes is overcome (Chapter 20). Additionally, entities responsible for collecting the data used for health statistics must collaborate in overcoming barriers that impede the movement to common standards (Chapter 8). The U.S. health statistics enterprise must also do a better job of collaborating with the public so that the public achieves an appropriate understanding of the value accruing from health statistics, both for society as a whole and for individuals (Chapter 14). Especially important is providing explicit explanations and justifications for any health statistics activities that may be viewed by the public as potentially imposing on privacy or violating confidentiality.

TOWARD A TWENTY-FIRST-CENTURY VISION FOR THE HEALTH STATISTICS ENTERPRISE

National health statistics enterprises reflect the health-care systems in the nations in which they operate. As indicated above and in previous chapters, fragmented health-care delivery systems are reflected in fragmented and poorly coordinated health statistics enterprises. Greater fragmentation and less coordination may be accompanied by less efficiency in data collection, greater burdens on data providers, more overlap among data collection streams, and more one-of-a-kind data systems with fewer linkages among those data systems. Of course, it is not reasonable to expect that individual countries will alter their health-care delivery systems with the sole goal of increasing the efficiency of the health statistics enterprise. But even without reducing fragmentation within health care delivery systems, steps can still be taken to develop more rational, cohesive, and comprehensive national health statistics enterprises. Such enterprises would be better positioned to address the issues and overcome the gaps identified earlier in this chapter and in this volume to support the practice of public health and to foster improvement of the population's health.

In order to develop enhanced national health statistics enterprises, four conditions must be met: first, a clear and explicit mission for the health statistics enterprise; second, use of an overarching conceptual framework; third, consensus on core values; and fourth, agreement on a set of basic principles for further development and reform of the enterprise. The remainder of this chapter presents strategies for meeting these four conditions.[1]

Mission of the Health Statistics Enterprise

The mission of the health statistics enterprise is to provide timely, accurate, and relevant information that can be used to improve the population's health, including information about the status of the population's health, information that can be used to formulate and evaluate the effects of health policy, and information that can be used to manage health interventions and programs. Health statistics must be easily accessible to a wide range of professional and community users.

Overarching Conceptual Framework

An overarching conceptual framework that helps to maintain a focus on needed data must guide the health statistics enterprise. The conceptual framework should delineate major influences on health and place them in an overall context; emphasize the distribution and the level of health in populations; and yield a research agenda relevant to improving the health of populations. The use of an overarching conceptual framework will concentrate the health statistics enterprise on its mission, reduce efforts that are tangential to its mission, and help to accomplish needed changes within the enterprise. Most important, the use of such a framework will focus health policymaking on core influences on the health of populations.

Various alternative conceptual frameworks of the influences on the health of a population have been developed, especially in Canada and by the World Health Organization (Friedman and Starfield 2003). Awareness of the historical and intellectual roots of these frameworks can help participants in the health statistics enterprise to better understand them and why particular frameworks include or omit specific influences (Glouberman 2001; Glouberman and Millar 2003; Szreter 2003). A vigorous debate about the most appropriate conceptual framework and the redirection of focus that it might suggest could enliven the U.S. health statistics enterprise, as it has in Canada, Australia, the United Kingdom, and other European countries (Coburn et al. 2003). Figure 1.3 may help to stimulate such a discussion.

Core Values

The health statistics enterprise rests upon four core values:

1. Maintaining the confidentiality and security of individually identifiable health information;

2. Maximizing the scientific integrity of all aspects of health statistics while acknowledging the specific ways in which the political, cultural, and business contexts may affect data collection, analysis, and interpretation;
3. Optimizing the enterprise's accountability to its users to ensure the availability of the information that is needed for improving the nation's health.
4. Ensuring the enterprise's accountability to its data suppliers to minimize their burden and to provide them with timely feedback.

Guiding Principles

To actualize the four core values, a nation's health statistics enterprise must reinvigorate itself by implementing 10 guiding principles. These will now be discussed.

1. Enterprisewide Planning and Coordination to Ensure Relevance to Local, State, and National Policy and Program Decision Making and to an Overall Conceptual Framework of the Influences on the Health of Populations

Enterprisewide planning and coordination are needed to ensure that the individual components of the nation's health statistics enterprise collectively fulfill the mission of efficiently developing, analyzing, and providing timely, accurate, and relevant information for improving the population's health. Without enterprisewide planning and coordination, the individual components of the health statistics enterprise—those operating at the national, state, and local levels, and in both the public and private sectors—may undertake overlapping and duplicative activities. Enterprisewide planning and coordination can help to concentrate resources on the highest priority policy and programmatic issues, can contribute to efficient use of scarce health statistics resources, and can maximize transfer of new methods and best practices.

Some planning and coordination already occurs within the U.S. health statistics enterprise, most notably at the national level. The Centers for Disease Control and Prevention's (CDC) Public Health Information Network and its component National Electronic Disease Surveillance System activities, the U.S. Department of Health and Human Services' Healthy People goal-setting efforts (U.S. Department of Health and Human Services [hp] Healthy People 2010 implementation), and the implementation of the Health and Insurance Portability and Accountability Act of 1996 have engendered some public and private sector planning and coordination at all geopolitical levels. At the state and local levels, several attempts to foster planning and coordination have occurred, including Louisiana's Turning Point Partnership (2000), Arkansas' Health Improvement Process (Nugent 2000), and the National Association of County and City Health Officials and CDC's Mobilizing for

Action through the Planning and Partnerships process (Upshaw 2000). However, most planning and coordination efforts at all geographic levels are episodic and often confined to compilation of data on individual diseases or groups of diseases.

Enterprisewide planning and coordination will necessarily involve organizations and individuals at all levels of government and in the public and private sectors. Planning and coordination will entail establishing enterprisewide expectations regarding standards for data collection, management, and exchange; for the timeliness, validity, and reliability of data; for access to and use of data; and for the ongoing evaluation of the individual components of the health statistics enterprise. Planning and coordination will also involve joint agenda setting for health statistics organizations throughout the enterprise in such areas as addressing new and emerging health problems, building sampling frames that can produce data generalizable to different units of analysis, expanding and validating the array of survey questions usable by different organizations within the health statistics enterprise, and integrating surveys, registries, surveillance systems, and administrative health data systems.

2. Broad Collaboration Among Data Users, Producers, and Suppliers at Local, State, and National Levels to Ensure the Efficiency of the Enterprise and the Usefulness of the Data that It Produces

The corollary to enterprisewide planning and coordination is broad collaboration and integration to ensure the efficiency of the enterprise's efforts and the usefulness of the data provided by the enterprise. Collaboration must occur in ways, among partners, and on issues that have not typically occurred in the past. Collaboration must occur at all geographic levels among those originally supplying data; among those responsible for compiling, analyzing, and disseminating data; and among those using the data, whether they are in the public or private sector.

Collaboration must rest on mutual recognition of, and respect for, the needs of different organizations and different functions within the enterprise, as well as clear definitions of the roles and responsibilities of organizations within the enterprise. Working toward the shared goal of producing information for improving the population's health, collaboration between those who supply data (e.g., community members and health-care providers) and those who collect and process these data can result in increased awareness among data collectors of the demands and burdens on data suppliers and adjustment of data collection procedures to reduce those burdens. Collaboration among data users and data producers can also result in providing information that more closely meets the needs of data users.

3. *Rigorous Policies and Procedures for Protecting the Privacy of Individuals and the Confidentiality and Security of Data*[2,3]

In protecting data confidentiality, we must distinguish between the confidentiality and security of individual record data and these of aggregate data. The most basic confidentiality and security issues concerning potentially identifiable individual record data include ensuring that the data are collected, released, and used only for specific approved purposes directly related to improving the population's health. The data must be held securely to maximize both the privacy of the data subjects and the integrity of the data themselves. Only the minimum data necessary for specific approved uses must be employed, whether those uses involve the creation of knowledge, the development of health policy, or the practice of public health. The process for determining which uses of potentially identifiable individual record data hold promise for improving the population's health, which uses can be approved, and which data are minimally necessary may vary from data set to data set and from specific use to use. However, clear laws, regulations, or administrative or programmatic rules must delimit all uses of potentially identifiable individual record data.

The most basic confidentiality issues concerning the use of aggregate data include guaranteeing the privacy of individual data subjects by ensuring that their identities cannot be determined from electronic data files, tables, charts, maps, or written documents. This can be accomplished through disclosure limitation techniques, such as algorithms for suppression of cells with potentially high disclosure risk.

The health statistics enterprise confronts new challenges in ensuring the confidentiality and security of individually identifiable health information (e.g., the increasing availability of aggregated health statistics on the World Wide Web and the increasing use of standard formats for data collection, enabling easier linkage of identified and deidentified individual record data). These challenges provide the health statistics enterprise with opportunities for more successfully fulfilling its fundamental mission. But addressing the challenges will require that the health statistics enterprise finds and maintains an appropriate balance between maximizing the confidentiality of data and the privacy of data subjects and collecting and providing information for improving the population's health. Improved security systems can go a long way toward establishing confidence in the integrity of health statistics systems.

The health statistics enterprise must rely on privacy, confidentiality, and security policies and procedures that are clear-cut, easily understandable to the public and to data subjects, and open to external review. Oversight of policies and procedures and their implementation is necessary, and external review of policies and procedures and their implementation should be encouraged or mandated.

4. *Flexibility to Identify and Address Emergent Health Issues and Needs*

The health statistics enterprise must develop the capacity to identify health issues for the population both before and as they emerge. These issues could include the emergence of new at-risk subpopulations; new structures for providing health services; expanded use of certain types of health services, such as alternative medicine; and newly identified health needs. The enterprise should not restrict itself to continually refining retrospective measurements of already identified population health problems. Ongoing data collection efforts must have the flexibility to prospectively identify new influences on the population's health, changing patterns in health, and health issues in new subpopulations. This flexibility should be incorporated into all ongoing data collection efforts, including registries and administrative data sets.

5. *Use of Data Standards to Facilitate Sharing and Comparability of Data*[4]

The U.S. National Committee on Vital and Health Statistics report *Information for Health: A Strategy for Building the National Health Information Infrastructure* (2001) describes standards as "the fundamental building blocks of effective health information systems . . . essential for efficient and effective public health and health care delivery systems." In *Every Manager's Guide to Information Technology*, Peter Keen (1995) offers a more technical definition: "data standards are agreements on formats, procedures, and interfaces that permit designers of hardware, software, databases, and telecommunication facilities to develop products and systems independent of one another with the assurance that they will be compatible with any other product or system that adheres to the same standards."

Standards and consensus approaches can be developed for individual data elements (addressing, for example, definition, nomenclature, taxonomy, vocabulary, and coding); content of specific data sets; the structure of data files (field type and order, file formats, database structures); collection of data (questionnaire design, sampling protocols, laboratory methods, validation of data entry); storage, manipulation, and processing (security and integrity of data, rules for aggregating and analyzing); transmission of data (message format, format and content for each field, format for electronic data interchange security); and the presentation and dissemination of data.

Standards and consensus approaches for the twenty-first century health statistics enterprise must meet five criteria:

First, standards should be applicable to and implemented for multiple purposes on a truly enterprisewide basis. The standards should apply to all geographic levels and to both the public and private sectors. The standards should cut across present disease- and issue-specific data silos, which have historically been fostered by categorical federal funding streams. Standards should be equally appropriate for administrative health data systems, surveillance data systems, survey data, and registries.

Second, standards should extend beyond the health statistics enterprise itself to incorporate multiple purposes. In keeping with the recommendations in *Information for Health: A Strategy for Building the National Health Information Infrastructure,* standards should be equally applicable for population health, personal health, and health-care provider dimensions (National Committee on Vital and Health Statistics 2001).

Third, standards should facilitate data linkage and data sharing while protecting the confidentiality and security of identifiable individual records. Facilitation of data linkage should occur even in the absence of the implementation of the national health identifier initially mandated by the U.S. Health Insurance Portability and Accountability Act; data linkages can be accomplished at the community level even before they are accomplished at the individual level.

Fourth, standards should enhance the comparability of data and results across states, across governmental levels, and between the public and private sectors.

Fifth, standards should be flexible and responsive to the needs of different components of the health statistics enterprise, including local and state health needs.

In short, standards must be intelligently developed and applied for the twenty-first-century health statistics enterprise. The development and application of these standards must constantly return to the touchstones: the purpose of the standards and the five necessary criteria.

6. Sufficient Detail at Different Levels of Aggregation to Support Local, State, and National Policymaking and Programmatic Decision Making

Health policymaking and implementation, as well as the development and management of health programs, occur at the local, state, and national levels. Health statistics must support both policy and program functions at all three governmental levels. Similarly, health statistics must support research employing various units of analysis. Research involving health statistics can employ neighborhood, city or county, state or provincial, or national units of analysis. The specific policy, programmatic, and research uses of each data set must dictate the needed level of detail at different levels of aggregation.

The gold standard for data collection is a data set that can be "rolled up" seamlessly from the neighborhood level, to the city or county level, to the state or provincial level, to the regional level, and to the national level. Such data sets allow the development, implementation, and evaluation of policies and programs at the local, state, and national levels. Some data collection systems of this kind currently exist within the U.S. health statistics enterprise, although they are limited to registries, surveillance systems, and administrative health data systems. Other existing data collection systems, such as population-based surveys, have the potential to be adapted to allow aggregation from local to state to national levels.

In developing data sets with sufficient detail at different levels of aggregation, consideration must be given to both nationally small subpopulations with large local presences and subpopulations with small numbers in local areas but with measurable national presences. Examples of nationally small subpopulations with large local presences include many ethnic groups whose historical migration patterns have resulted in substantial concentrations in small numbers of U.S. cities or counties. Examples of subpopulations with small numbers in local areas but with measurable national presences include groups of individuals with specific chronic conditions or disabilities. Methodological issues inherent in developing data sets with sufficient detail to represent both of these types of subpopulations must be systematically addressed.

The ability to return useful information to data suppliers is an additional consideration in designing data sets at sufficient levels of detail. Through returning information to those who have employed their time, energy, and resources to supply data for statistical purposes, the utility of health statistics generally, as well as of a specific data collection effort, can be shown. Demonstrating such a return on investment is a necessary step in improving the validity, reliability, and completeness of health statistics.

The U.S. health statistics enterprise must devote concentrated and coordinated attention to increasing the number of data sets providing detail at multiple levels of aggregation. This can occur only through the enterprisewide planning, broad collaboration and integration, and compatible standards described in guiding principles 1, 2, and 5 above.

7. Integrated, Streamlined Data Collection for Multiple Purposes

Data collection within the current U.S. health statistics enterprise is distinguished by multiple separate data collection systems. These systems operate at all government levels, cover many diseases, and use various types of data, including administrative health data, surveillance data, survey data, and data from disease or vital event registries. Because most of these systems are not integrated and often not coordinated, an individual data supplier often provides the same data to different data systems within the same health agency. For example, for each birth the obstetric hospital will provide overlapping data on the standard certificate of live birth, the hospital discharge record, claims forms for third-party payment, newborn screening forms, the birth defects registry, and perhaps to condition-specific surveillance systems as well. All of these distinct data collection systems require similar data on the infant's and mother's name, place of birth, date of birth, address, race, ethnicity, and so forth, often including overlapping clinical data. Figure 21.1 uses a workplace injury as the health event to illustrate the wide range of health records that might be generated as an injured

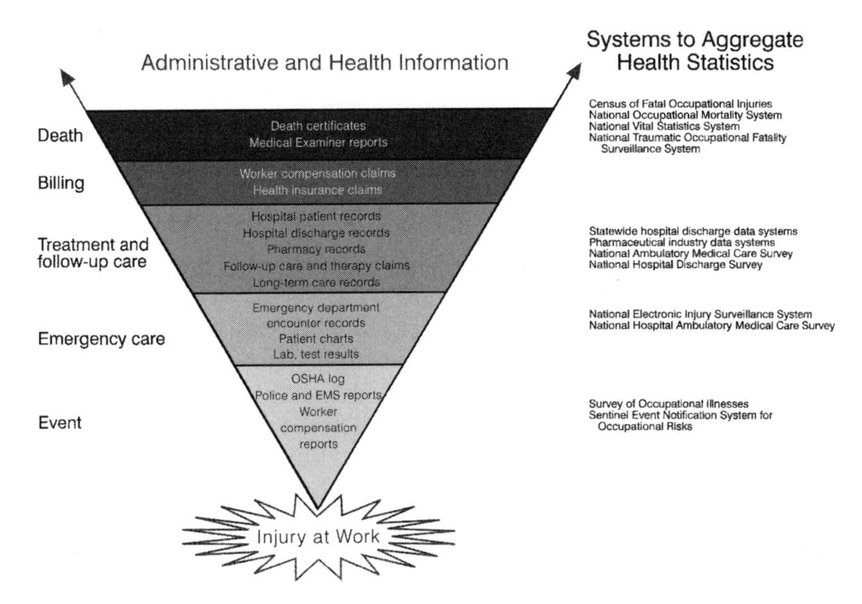

FIGURE 21.1
Multiplicity of data sources and statistical systems. EMS = emergency medical service; OSHA = Occupational Safety and Health Administraion. (Source: Friedman et al. 2002, p. 44.)

worker seeks treatment from an expanding range of health providers, along with administrative records related to the event, to payment for treatment, and to possible death. This demonstrates how multiple systems are used to aggregate health statistics. Few of these efforts to aggregate statistics can currently rely on standardized or integrated systems.

The twenty-first-century health statistics enterprise must rationalize and systematize presently disparate and distinct data collection systems. Multiple purposes or uses for data collection need not necessitate multiple data collection systems. By designing integrated, streamlined data collection for multiple purposes, greater efficiencies at reduced costs will be achieved. The goals of integrated, streamlined data collection systems are three: first, to reduce the burden on data suppliers currently engendered by multiple overlapping data collection systems, by collecting the same data only once and then making them available to other data users; second, to minimize—where appropriate—the technical and administrative barriers between different data collection systems: administrative systems, surveillance systems, surveys, and registries; and third, to enable the use of health data for different purposes by different users, rather than different uses requiring the establishment and maintenance of different data collection systems. Integrated, streamlined data collection for multiple purposes need not imply a loss of confidentiality and security for individually identifiable data. With appropriate laws, policies, procedures, and technologies, the replacement of multiple data collection systems with integrated, streamlined data collection systems can enhance confidentiality and security.

8. Timely Production of Valid and Reliable Health Statistics

Timely production of valid and reliable data is inherent in the mission of the health statistics enterprise. Expectations and standards for the timeliness of health statistics have been changing over the past several years. Although in past years birth data were accepted as timely if published more than 1 year after the conclusion of the data year, individual states and the CDC's National Center for Health Statistics now routinely publish birth data within 12 months of the conclusion of the data year. While previously cancer incidence data were routinely published 2 or even 3 years after the conclusion of the data year, the CDC is now moving states toward publishing these data within 12 months of the conclusion of the data year. The production of more timely health statistics will require careful consideration of whether the considerable investments currently made to achieve small increments in data quality are effective use of resources.

9. Appropriate Access to and Ease of Use of Health Statistics

To fulfill its mission, the health statistics enterprise must provide easy access to health statistics to a broad variety of users. The type and extent of the access must be appropriate for both the particular user and the particular use. Access to the detailed data needed by a health services researcher studying disparities across ethnic groups in the use of different treatment modalities for advanced breast cancer would be inappropriate for community users conducting a local needs assessment. Of course, the extent and the nature of access need to be governed by appropriate statutes, human subjects review committees where appropriate, and the regulations and policies discussed above in principle 3.

The ready availability of data produced by the health statistics enterprise is a significant community resource for improving population health. A wide variety of modes of access to health statistics must be employed, including the Internet, other forms of electronic access, public use data sets where feasible, and print media. Different modes of access must be viewed as complementary rather than as mutually exclusive. The increasing use of the World Wide Web as the backbone for interactive systems for disseminating public health data will provide the health statistics enterprise with new opportunities for customizing access to meet the distinct needs of different communities of users (Friedman et al. 2001). As is already the case in some of the more advanced Web-based interactive systems maintained by state health departments, customization would include providing alternative user interfaces for access to the same data, matched to different levels of user technical skills and goals.

10. Continuous Evaluation of the Scientific Integrity, Accuracy, and Timeliness of Health Statistics and of the Ability of the Health Statistics Enterprise to Fulfill its Mission

Continuous evaluation will aid in ensuring that new and emerging health statistics needs are identified and responded to on an ongoing basis. Evaluation efforts relevant to the health statistics enterprise are now largely limited to peer reviews of articles submitted to professional journals, the review process for competitive applications for federal and foundation grants and cooperative agreements, and legislative review of health statistics programs. Mechanisms must be developed for continually evaluating the extent to which user needs are met, for assessing the scientific integrity, accuracy, and timeliness of health statistics, and for identifying improvements that must be made to meet future user needs. New metrics for evaluating the ability of the health statistics enterprise to meet future needs must be developed. New training is also needed so that those engaged throughout the health statistics enterprise are equipped with the appropriate methods to conduct continuous evaluation. Continuous evaluation must rest on enterprisewide planning and coordination to ensure independence and openness.

As pointed out previously, the health statistics enterprise rests on choices about what to study and how to study it. These choices are based on judgments about what issues merit data collection and analysis. Through aiming for, and exercising self-awareness about, values and choices, through inviting public scrutiny, and through following practices that ensure openness, the health statistics enterprise can maximize its scientific objectivity and its integrity.

NOTES

1. The remainder of this chapter is adapted from Friedman et al. (2002).
2. In this chapter, *privacy* refers to "an individual's desire to limit the disclosure of personal information." *Confidentiality* refers to "a condition in which information is shared or released in a controlled manner. Organizations develop confidentiality policies to codify their rules for controlling the release of personal information in an effort to protect patient privacy." *Security* consists of "a number of measures that organizations implement to protect information and systems. It includes efforts not only to maintain the confidentiality of information, but also to ensure the integrity and availability of that information and the information systems used to access it" (National Research Council 1997).
3. In Chapter 14, Fanning discusses these issues in greater detail.
4. In Chapter 8, Greenberg and Parrish discuss these issues in greater detail.

REFERENCES

Coburn D, Denny K, Mykhalovskiy E, McDonough P, Robertson A, Love R. Population health in Canada: a brief critique. Am J Public Health 2003;93:392–396.

Friedman D, Anderka M, Krieger J, Land G, Solet D. Accessing population health information through interactive systems: lessons learned and future directions. Public Health Rep 2001;116:132–141.

Friedman DJ, Hunter EL, Parrish RG, eds. Shaping a Health Statistics Vision for the 21st Century. Final Report, November 2002. Hyattsville, MD: Centers for Disease Control and Prevention, National Center for Health Statistics; Washington, DC: U.S. Department of Health and Human Services Data Council; National Committee on Vital and Health Statistics; 2002 [cited 2004 Mar 17]. Available from: http://www.ncvhs.hhs.gov/reptrecs.htm.

Friedman D, Starfield B. Models of population health: their value for U.S. public health practice, policy, and research. Am J Public Health 2003;93:366–369.

Glouberman S. Towards a New Perspective on Health Policy. Ottawa: Canadian Policy Research Networks; 2001.

Glouberman S, Millar J. Evolution of the determinants of health, health policy, and health information systems in Canada. Am J Public Health 2003;93:388–392.

Keen P. Every Manager's Guide to Information Technology: A Glossary of Key Terms and Concepts for Today's Business Leader, 2nd ed. Cambridge, MA: Harvard Business School Press; 1995.

Louisiana Turning Point Partnership. Public Health Improvement Plan: A Catalyst for Change. New Orleans: Louisiana Turning Point Partnership; 2000, pp. 38–40 [cited 2004 Jun 9]. Available from: http://www.lphi.org/turning-frameset.html.

National Committee on Vital and Health Statistics. Information for Health: A Strategy for Building the National Health Information Infrastructure. Washington, DC: National Committee on Vital and Health Statistics; 2001 [cited 2002 Sep 24]. Available from: http://ncvhs.hhs.gov/nhiilayo.pdf.

National Research Council. For the Record: Protecting Electronic Health Information. Washington, DC: National Academy Press; 1997, p. 1.

Nugent R. Panel 3: stakeholders for health information. In: National Committee on Vital and Health Statistics, ed. Proceedings of the Joint Hearings of the Workgroups on National Health Information Infrastructure and Health Statistics for the 21st Century; 2000 Jan 11; Washington, DC: [cited 2004 Jun 9]. Available from: http://www.ncvhs.hhs.gov/010111tr.htm.

Szreter S. The population health perspective in historical perspective. Am J Public Health 2003;93:421–431.

Upshaw V. Joint Panel on NHII and health statistics for the 21st century. In: National Committee on Vital and Health Statistics, ed. Proceedings of the Joint Hearings of the Workgroups on National Health Information Infrastructure and Health Statistics for the 21st Century; 2000 Nov 20; Research Triangle Park, NC: [cited 2004 Jun 9]. Available from: http://www.ncvhs.hhs.gov/001120tr.htm.

U.S. Department of Health and Human Services [homepage on the Internet]. Washington, DC: U.S. Department of Health and Human Services [cited 2004 Jun 9]. Healthy People 2010 implementation. Available from: http://www.healthypeople.gov/Implementation.

INDEX

Note: Page numbers followed by b, f, and t refer to boxes, figures, and tables, respectively.